Obstetric Catastrophes

Carlos Montufar • Jorge Hidalgo
Alfredo F. Gei
Editors

Obstetric Catastrophes

A Clinical Guide

Springer

Editors
Carlos Montufar
Critical Care Obstetrics Unit
Hospital Doctor Arnulfo Arias Madrid
Panama City
Panama

Jorge Hidalgo
Division of Critical Care
Karl Heusner Memorial Hospital
Belize City
Belize

Alfredo F. Gei
Houston Center for Maternal-Fetal Medicine
Houston, TX
USA

ISBN 978-3-030-70033-1 ISBN 978-3-030-70034-8 (eBook)
https://doi.org/10.1007/978-3-030-70034-8

This Springer imprint is published by the registered company Springer Nature Switzerland AG
The registered company address is: Gewerbestrasse 11, 6330 Cham, Switzerland

To my parents, my lovely wife Gerhaldine, my daughter Allyson, and my son Benjamin.

—Jorge Hidalgo

To my mentor and late father Orlando Gei Guardia, who guided me through the first steps of this profession. May my efforts always honor his memory.

—Alfredo F. Gei

To Yolanda and Andrea, for putting up with me throughout the book project as I was spending too much time in front of the computer and arriving home late.

—Carlos Montufar

Preface

Obstetric critical care is a relatively new medical field that has grown and gained its critical care space. Every day, the nature of critical illness is better understood at the molecular, cellular, organ, whole patient, and population levels. Diagnostic and monitoring tools, such as point-of-care ultrasound, stroke volume estimating equipment, and biomarkers, have altered the way we examine our critical obstetric patients. New drugs and devices have been devised, tested, and applied. Large clinical trials now inform a broad range of treatments, including respiratory failure, septic shock, and acute kidney injury, and better understanding. The modern intensivist must master a complex science of pathophysiology and be intimately familiar with an increasingly specialized literature. In the twenty-first century, the specialty of critical care has genuinely come of age.

Why have *Obstetric Catastrophes* as textbook at all in the modern era? Whether at home, in the office, or on the road, we can access our patients' vital signs, radiographs, and test results electronically; at the click of a mouse, we can peruse the literature of the world. This is a book that allows us to understand the common mechanisms that transcend all critical illnesses and provides an in-depth, specific discussion of essential procedures and diseases.

Our approach to patient care, teaching, and critical care investigation are energized fundamentally by our clinical practice. In turn, our practice is informed, animated, and balanced by the information and environment arising around learning and research. Clinical excellence is founded in careful history taking, physical examination, and laboratory testing. These data serve to raise questions concerning the patient's disease mechanisms, upon which a complete, prioritized differential diagnosis is formulated and treatment plan initiated. The reality, complexity, and limitations apparent in the ICU drive our search for a better understanding of critical care's pathophysiology and new, effective therapies. We hope that this textbook reflects the interweaving and mutually supporting threads of critical care practice, teaching, and research.

While the field of critical care has changed dramatically, several years ago, Dr. Carlos Montufar and Dr. Alfredo Gei start working together in the pursuit of excellence in the practice, teaching, and study of critical obstetric care. Dr. Jorge Hidalgo has been invited to join them in creating the first edition of this textbook. The chapters reflect the growing scope of critical care obstetrics and the increasing importance and recognition of the hospital structure's field. All intensivists, regardless of primary discipline, must possess a core set of critical care skills to manage critically ill patients. Furthermore, most hospitals today contain intensive care units (ICUs) mixed by intention or by overflow, and multidisciplinary trained intensivists are equipped to recognize and manage the wide range of acute care problems, promoting and keeping the team approach multi-professional nature of critical care delivery.

This textbook, in addition to the practicing critical care physicians and fellows in training, is designed to be a valuable resource for all critical care providers, hospitalists, subspecialty physicians, residents, nurses, physician assistants, nurse practitioners, nutritionists, pharmacists, respiratory therapists, and medical students involved in the care of critically ill obstetric patients.

Panama City, Panama — Carlos Montufar
Belize City, Belize — Jorge Hidalgo
Houston, TX, USA — Alfredo F. Gei

Acknowledgments

We want to take this opportunity to thank the authors, our collaborators, for taking part in this project, who withstood the pressure of a deadline and dedicated their time to answer this call for expertise and help, keeping aside several other tasks and indeed personal time.

We sincerely appreciate the collaboration by the talented staff at Springer and, particularly, Ms. Miranda Finch and Mr. Prakash Jagannathan, who partnered with us all along and took our manuscript and turned it into this book.

Contents

Contributors

Ariatna Arlennys Aguilera Valderrama, MD, ScD Department of Obstetrics and Gynecology, Division of Obstetrics Critical Care, Caja de Seguro Social, Panama City, Panama

Pulmonology Department, Irma de Lourdes Tzanetatos Hospital, Panama City, Panama

Critical Care Obstetrician, Department of Obstetrics and Gynecology, Division of Obstetrics Critical Care, Caja de Seguro Social, Panama City, Panama

Amparo Aguilera Pulmonologist, Pulmonology Department, Irma de Lourdes Tzanetatos Hospital, Panama City, Panama

Ariatna Aguilera Pulmonologist, Pulmonology Department, Irma de Lourdes Tzanetatos Hospital, Panama City, Panama

Rania Magdi Ali Anesthesia, Intensive Care and Pain Management, Faculty of Medicine, Ain Shams University, Cairo, Egypt

Keyra Morales-Allard Department of Obstetrics and Gynecology, Complejo Hospitalario Arnulfo Arias Madrid, Panama City, Panama

Adel Alsisi Prime Healthcare Group LLC, Dubai, UAE

Nares-Torices Miguel Angel Medical Emergencies Specialist, Critical Medicine and Obstetric Critical Medicine Sub-specialist, National Medical Center IMSS "La Raza", México City, Mexico

Hernández-Pacheco José Antonio Internal Medicine Specialist, Critical Medicine and Obstetric Critical Medicine Sub-specialist, National Institute of Perinatology, México City, Mexico

Zulmi Aranda Critical Care Unit, Instituto de Prevision Social, Asunción, Paraguay

Hassan Z. Baig Department of Critical Care Medicine, Mayo Clinic, Jacksonville, FL, USA

Saul Barrera IVI-RMA Global, Panama City, Panama

Juan Carlos Barrientos Rojas Head of the Critical Obstetrics Unit, Gynecology and Obstetrics Department, Hospital General San Juan de Dios, University of San Carlos de Guatemala, Guatemala City, Guatemala

Clinicas Herrera Llerandi, Ala Norte, Guatemala City, Guatemala

Laura Pilar Vélez Batista Hospital Dr. Manuel Amador Guerrero (CSS), Colon City, Panama

Rebecca C. Burnside Department of Critical Care Medicine, Mayo Clinic, Jacksonville, FL, USA

John J. Byrne Department of Obstetrics and Gynecology, University of Texas Southwestern Medical Center, Parkland Health and Hospital Systems, Dallas, TX, USA

Malini Chauhan The University of Arizona College of Medicine – Tucson, Tucson, AZ, USA

Miguel Chung Sang, MD Hospital Gineco Obstétrico y Pediátrico Universitario de Guayaquil, Guayaquil, Ecuador

Universidad Católica de Santiago de Guayaquil, Guayaquil, Ecuador

Leonardo Bonilla Cortés Maternal – Fetal Medicine Division, Hospital Universitario Clínica San Rafael, Bogotá, Colombia

Obstetrics Department at EPS Sanitas, Cali, Colombia

Department of Maternal – Fetal Medicine, Universidad El Bosque, Bogotá, Colombia

F. Gary Cunningham Department of Obstetrics and Gynecology, University of Texas Southwestern Medical Center, Parkland Health and Hospital Systems, Dallas, TX, USA

António Gandra d'Almeida Education and Simulation Coimbra Militar Health Center, Coimbra, Portugal

Head of Education of CSMC, Coimbra, Portugal

The Dr Pure Clinic, Lisbon, Portugal

Sabrina Da Re Gutiérrez Critical and Intensive Care Medicine, Maternal and Child Hospital, Caja Nacional de Salud (CNS), La Paz, Bolivia

Michael Foley The University of Arizona College of Medicine – Phoenix, Phoenix, AZ, USA

Pablo Moreno Franco Department of Critical Care Medicine, Mayo Clinic, Jacksonville, FL, USA

Department of Transplant, Mayo Clinic, Jacksonville, FL, USA

Kendra Gray The University of Arizona College of Medicine – Phoenix, Phoenix, AZ, USA

Bahaa El-Din Ewees Hassan Anesthesia, Intensive Care and Pain Management, Faculty of Medicine, Ain Shams University, Cairo, Egypt

Jorge Hidalgo, MD, MACP, MCCM, FCCP Division of Critical Care, Karl Heusner Memorial Hospital, Belize City, Belize

Flores-Cortés Mildred Ibeth Gynecology and Obstetrics Specialist, Private Medicine, México City, Mexico

Previgliano Ignacio, MD Maimonides University, Buenos Aires, Argentina

Hospital General de Agudos J. A. Fernández, Buenos Aires, Argentina

Jose Miguel Jauregui, MD Gynecological Obstetric and Pediatric University Hospital, Espíritu Santo Specialties University Hospital, Guayaquil, Ecuador

Hospital Gineco Obstétrico y Pediátrico Universitario de Guayaquil, Guayaquil, Ecuador

Universidad de Especialidades Espíritu Santo (UEES), Samborondón, Ecuador

S. Jose Jauregui Hospital Gineco Obstétrico y Pediátrico Universitario de Guayaquil, Universidad de Especialidades Espíritu Santo (UEES), Samborondón, Ecuador

Judy Enamorado National Cardiopulmonary Institute, Tegucigalpa, Honduras

Poliszuk Julieta, MD Hospital General de Agudos J. A. Fernández, Buenos Aires, Argentina

Organ Procurement and Transplantation Section – Hospital General de Agudos J. A. Fernández, Buenos Aires, Argentina

Alex Dagoberto Loarca Chávez Head of the Adult Intensive Care, Quetzaltenango Regional Hospital, Quetzaltenango, Guatemala

President of the Quetzaltenango Chapter, Guatemalan Society of Intensive Care, Guatemala City, Guatemala

Lineth López Department of Hematology, Complejo Hospitalario Dr. Arnulfo Arias Madrid de la Caja de Seguro Social, Panama City, Republic of Panama

Alfredo A. Matos Enteral and Parenteral Nutrition, Head of Surgery Intensive Care Unit, Hospital Social Security Complex, Panama City, Republic of Panama

Maily Velasco Miranda Gynecological Obstetric and Pediatric University Hospital, Guayaquil, Ecuador

Aura Meliza Mejia Monroy General Hospital San Juan de Dios, Ministry of Public Health and Social Assistance of Guatemala, Guatemala, Guatemala

Carlos Montufar Obstetrics Critical Care Unit, Fellowship Program of Critical Care Obstetrics, Complejo Hospitalario, Caja de Seguro Social, Panama City, Panama

José Mora Hospital de SOLCA – Manabí, Portoviejo, Ecuador

Freddy Morales Hospital de SOLCA – Manabí, Portoviejo, Ecuador

Mayka Morgan IVI-RMA Global, Panama City, Panama

David B. Nelson Department of Obstetrics and Gynecology, University of Texas Southwestern Medical Center, Parkland Health and Hospital Systems, Dallas, TX, USA

José Luis Neyro Servicio de Ginecología y Obstetricia, Universidad del País Vasco EHU-UPV, Hospital Universitario Cruces, Bilbao, Spain

Inês Mourato Nunes Hospital das Forças Armadas, Lisboa, Portugal

Hospital de Cascais, Alcabideche, Portugal

Carlos E. Orellana-Jimenez Division of Critical Care, Salvadoran Social Security Institute, San Salvador, El Salvador

Felix Parra Antofagasta University Hospital and Antofagasta University, Antofagasta, Chile

Javier Pérez-Fernández Critical Care Services, Baptist Hospital of Miami, Florida International University, Herbert Wertheim College of Medicine, Miami, FL, USA

Ronald G. Racho Department of Transplant, Mayo Clinic, Jacksonville, FL, USA

Kirenia Petterson Roa Nutritionist and Dietitian, Enteral Therapy and Parenteral Nutrition, Intensive Care Unit, Hospital Social Security Complex, Panama City, Republic of Panama

Bayardo J. Robelo-Pentzke Hospital Dr. Rafael A. Calderon-Guardia, San José, Costa Rica

Maria V. Rodriguez General Verdi Cevallos Hospital, Portoviejo, Ecuador

Gloria Rodríguez-Vega Neurocritical Care Services, HIMA-Caguas, Caguas, Puerto Rico

Angela María Magali Sanchez Department of Intensive Care, Hospital Lagomaggiore, Mendoza, Argentina

Tal E. Sandler University of Nebraska Medical Center, Department of Anesthesiology, Division of Critical Care Medicine, Omaha, NE, USA

Devang K. Sanghavi Department of Critical Care Medicine, Mayo Clinic, Jacksonville, FL, USA

Sofia Santareno, FEBOPRAS Plastic Surgery Department, Burn Unit of University Hospital of Northern, Lisbon, Portugal

The Dr Pure Clinic, Lisbon, Portugal

Juan Ignacio Silesky-Jiménez Critical Care Medicine, Clinical Nutrition, Health Services Administration, Hospital San Juan de Dios and Hospital CIMA, San José, Costa Rica

Costa Rica University, San José, Costa Rica

AMICOR and COCECATI, San José, Costa Rica

Jorge E. Sinclair De Frías Santo Tomas Hospital, Faculty of Medicine University of Panama, Panamá City, Panamá

Jorge Sinclair Ávila Critical Medicine, UCI Hospital Pacifica Salud/Johns Hopkins Medicine, Faculty of Medicine University of Panama, Panama City, Panama

Alberto Sirven Women and Children Department, West Kendall Baptist Hospital, Florida International University, Herbert Wertheim College of Medicine, Miami, FL, USA

Ahmed Reda Taha Cardiac Intensive Care Institute of Critical Care – Cleveland Clinic Abu Dhabi, Abu Dhabi, UAE

Shaun L. Thompson University of Nebraska Medical Center, Department of Anesthesiology, Division of Critical Care Medicine, Omaha, NE, USA

Konstantinos Tserotas Servicio de Ginecología, Complejo Hospitalario "Dr. Arnulfo Arias Madrid", Caja del Seguro Social de Panamá, Ciudad de Panamá, Panamá

Maily Velasco, MD Hospital Gineco Obstétrico y Pediátrico Universitario de Guayaquil, Guayaquil, Ecuador

Fabricio Vera General de Manta Hospital, Manta, Ecuador

Alcibiades E. Villarreal Centro de Neurociencias y Unidad de Investigacion Clínica, Instituto de Investigaciones Científicas y Servicios de Alta Tecnología (INDICASAT AIP), Panama City, Republic of Panama

Ezio Villegas Obstetrics and Gynecological University Hospital Guayaquil, Guayaquil, Ecuador

Hospital Gineco Obstétrico y Pediátrico Universitario de Guayaquil, Guayaquil, Ecuador

Ramoncito Yacab Head of the Oncology Department at Karl Heusner Memorial Hospital, Belize City, Belize

Noura M. Youssri Mahmoud Anesthesia, Intensive Care and Pain Management, Faculty of Medicine, Ain Shams University, Cairo, Egypt

Graciela Raquel Zakalik Department of Intensive Care, Hospital Lagomaggiore, Mendoza, Argentina

Argentine Society of Intensive Therapy (SATI), Buenos Aires, Argentina

Janice Zimmerman Baylor College of Medicine, Houston, TX, USA

Part I
Critical Care

Chapter 1
Critical Care of the Obstetric Patient

Carlos Montufar

The obstetric patient, pregnant or puerperal, is significantly different from the average patient who enters an intensive care unit. These patients have a unique pathophysiology and present specific disorders; in addition, there is the presence of the fetus, an alteration of the pharmacokinetics, diseases that may be aggravated by pregnancy and the scenario of a birth.

The pregnant patient undergoes dramatic physiological changes at the cardiovascular, respiratory, renal, endocrinological, and hematological levels, which make her a different patient [1]. Post-partum hemorrhages, pre-eclampsia, acute fatty liver of pregnancy, and post-partum endometrial infections are unique conditions in an obstetric patient. The management challenge of these patients increases with the presence of the fetus. Publications report that there is a prevalence of critical obstetric patients of 100–900/100,000 gestations (0.1–0.9%) [2, 3], but these statistics are usually from medium- and high-resource countries. Statistical data from low-income countries reach much higher values and often patients do not even manage to be treated in intensive care units. The mortality ratio is also very different between rich and low-income countries, with statistics of 6–24/100,000 live births (LB) in the highest-income countries, and 55–920/100,000 LB in poor countries [4].

It is estimated that 75% of hospitalizations of obstetric patients to intensive care units occur in the puerperium [3], because it is a period susceptible to complications such as pulmonary edema (due to a reduction in oncotic pressure) and a high frequency of hemorrhages, such as uterine atony.

In the ICNARC study in UK 2007, 81.5% of patients were reported as recently pregnant (within 42 days of admission to the ICU) [5], either post-partum or post-abortion.

There are vulnerable populations where the risk of maternal death is multiplied, such as ethnic minorities, extreme maternal ages, and low socioeconomic status [6].

C. Montufar (✉)
Obstetrics Critical Care Unit, Fellowship Program of Critical Care Obstetrics, Complejo Hospitalario, Caja de Seguro Social, Panama City, Panama

C. Montufar et al. (eds.), *Obstetric Catastrophes*,
https://doi.org/10.1007/978-3-030-70034-8_1

These factors usually result in less prenatal care, late hospital admissions, and more serious clinical conditions.

Further, significant pathological conditions can present in the pregnant patient, including hypovolemia, hypotension, hypoxia, and acidosis may result in greatly reduced uteroplacental flow, with subsequent fetal hypoxia and acidosis or even death. Blood product transfusion in the ICU was independently associated with fetal loss in one retrospective series [7].

The causes that lead a pregnant or puerperal patient to a critical state can be direct obstetric disorders (hemorrhagic shock due to uterine atony, puerperal sepsis) in 50–80% of cases and medical disorders (heart disease, diabetes, etc.) between 30% and 60% of patients. Pollock et al. reported that approximately 70% of admissions, in developed and developing countries, were due to obstetrics directly condition [8].

A study in the United Kingdom in 14 intensive care units reported that 1.84% of the admissions was obstetric patients, representing 0.17% of all births, with the most frequent causes being preeclampsia and obstetric hemorrhages [9].

The World Health Organization, in an article published in 2014 [4], for the first time documented hemorrhagic phenomena as the main cause of obstetric death, over and above preeclampsia, both in low-resource countries and in the so-called rich countries.

The evaluation of critical obstetric patients and the analysis of their statistics have led to the knowledge of risk factors that can lead to fetal death. These risk factors are complications in pregnancies far from the term, maternal shock, and the need for blood products in mothers. There are factors inherent to women that increase the risk of death, such as advanced (obstetric) age. Women aged 35–39 years have a 2.6 times higher risk of death and women older than 40 years increase this risk of death to 5.9-fold 95% CI 4.6, 7.7 [1]. Also, black maternal race confers a relative risk of 3.7 (95% CI 3.3, 4.1) for maternal death compared with white women.

There are so dramatic maternal physiological changes that can affect or facilitate conditions that threaten the life of the mother and the fetus. Of these, three are extremely important: decrease in residual functional capacity (transforming it into tidal volume), renal loss of bicarbonate (consequence of respiratory alkalosis), and the prothrombotic state of the pregnant woman. This makes the patient obstetric, intolerant to hypoxia, vulnerable to acidosis, and develops a high risk of thrombosis.

Pregnancy may be associated with an increase in the severity of some medical conditions. The overall risk of ICU admission for pregnant or postpartum women with H1N1 influenza was sevenfold higher than for non-pregnant females [10]. Despite similar rates of bacteriuria in pregnant and non-pregnant women, the rate of pyelonephritis is higher in pregnancy [11]. Further, pregnancy increases the risk of venous embolism [12].

In relation to Public Health and Women's Health Policies, there are factors that can become risk factors for causing maternal deaths: poor or absent prenatal control, and a hospital medical team that does not have the knowledge or skills to care for both patients pregnant and puerperal women, seriously complicated [3, 13].

It is estimated that 80% of pregnant or puerperal patients who develop complications do not have an identified risk factor [13].

Kilpatrick [14] published some interventions that could prevent obstetric complications: use of contraceptives to avoid unwanted pregnancies, providing forms of safe abortions to avoid deaths from complications from abortions, active management of the third stage of labor for the prevention of maternal deaths due to hemorrhage secondary to uterine atony, and the timely interruption of pregnancy in patients with pre-eclampsia.

About 15–20% of pregnancies are complicated, and most of these complications are difficult to predict, and the highest number of maternal deaths occur in patients considered low risk. Therefore, the focus is on preparing effective emergency interventions [15].

The decrease in maternal mortality is based on the correct management of obstetric emergencies and acute medical complications, rather than on identifying risk factors, which requires that the human personnel who take care of pregnant patients must know how to deal with these emergencies and complications. One is considered a qualified provider of obstetric health if one is able to attend a delivery, and also diagnose, treat, and/or refer women who present different obstetric emergencies [15].

In the Green-top Guidelines No 56 of United Kingdom Royal College of Obstetricians and Gynecologists, a systematic review of life-support training showed a significant reduction in maternal morbidity and mortality [15].

In many countries, the reduction in the maternal mortality ratio gave rise to a false perception of an improvement in obstetric care. But it has been found that for every maternal death, there are a considerable number of patients who did not die thanks to timely intervention (near-miss) [3].

The term near-miss or severe maternal morbidity refers to this recent concept of non-fatal maternal morbidity. It is estimated that for each maternal death, there may be a significant number of near-misses, many of which will require care in a general intensive care unit or a specific unit of intensive obstetric care [3]. Hemorrhage and preeclampsia are the most frequent causes that force an obstetric patient to enter a general intensive care unit.

In 2003, the first formal proposals for the structuring of specific intensive care units for pregnant and/or puerperal patients were initiated [16], and by 2009, ACOG had published its first practice bulletin regarding critical care in pregnancy [17].

Subsequently, the first obstetric intensive care units of the United States started coming into existence.

Given the limited specific evidence in the management of obstetric patients in critical condition, many doctors and hospital centers have based their management extrapolation of information on the management of non-obstetric patients.

Critical care in obstetric patients, as a specialty or sub-specialty area, is still underdeveloped [18]. The creation of a program with a multimodal curriculum is considered promising, to have a doctor with an ideal profile to understand an approach an obstetric patient in critical condition, such as: oxygen therapy, mechanical ventilation, transfusion therapy, knowledge of coagulopathy, Adult Respiratory

Distress Syndrome, hemodynamic and respiratory monitoring, septic shock, nutritional support, renal failure and renal replacement therapy, analgesia and sedation, trauma, airway management, and vascular access; in addition, of the knowledge of the different obstetric and medical pathologies that can expose to the death, in the pregnant woman and/or during the puerperium.

The creation of specific intensive care units for obstetric patients can improve the results in terms of management and survival [19] as long as the doctors and all the personnel who work in these units have the physiological knowledge of pregnancy and puerperium, and the knowledge of the pathophysiologies of the different conditions and diseases that occur in these patients. A better understanding of maternal complications will have an impact on maternal mortality statistics.

Critical illness is an uncommon but potentially devastating complication of pregnancy. The priority is to stabilize the mother, with the understanding that what is good for the mother is good for the fetus. Critical-care interventions are like those for non-pregnant patients; however, adjustment of physiologic targets for metabolic, pulmonary, and hemodynamic control may be necessary. The majority of acquired pregnancy-related diseases, such as preeclampsia and acute fatty liver of pregnancy, are abrogated by delivery. However, timing and the state of fetal maturation are crucial to decision-making.

A pregnant patient in critical condition is a challenge. Maternal physiological changes can generate diagnostic errors or prevent the recognition of a pathological condition and overlook a diagnosis. In addition, the fetus imposes obstacles to certain medications or interventions. It is necessary to know the changes of pregnancy and puerperium, as well as the pathophysiology of direct obstetric complications, to improve the clinical results in pregnant patients.

The medical team that takes care of pregnant patients must have the correct training to effectively manage the complications of the pregnant woman are direct obstetric or medical complications.

Similarly, the work team that is responsible for the management of severe obstetric patients must have knowledge about fetal biophysical variables and their pathological states, especially metabolic, gas exchange, and hemodynamic variables. This will be a determinant in obtaining better perinatal results.

References

1. Crozier T. General care of the pregnant patient in the intensive care unit. Semin Respir Crit Care Med. 2017;38:208–17.
2. American College of Obstetricians and Gynecologists. Practice Bulletin No 211: critical are in pregnancy. Obstet Gynecol. 2019;133(5):e303–19.
3. Gaffney A. Critical care in pregnancy- is it different? Semi Perinatol. 2014;38:329–40.
4. Say L, Chou D, Gemmill A, Tunçalp Ö, Moller A, Daniels J, Gülmezoglu A, Temmerman M, Alkema L. Global causes of maternal death: a WHO systematic analysis. www.thelancet.com/lancetgh Vol 2, June 2014.

5. Harrison DA, Penny JA, Yentis SM, Fayek S, Brady AR. Case mix, outcome and activity for obstetric admissions to adult, general critical care units: a secondary analys is of the ICNARC Case Mix Programme Database. Crit Care. 2005;9:S25.
6. Vasquez DN, Estenssoro E, Canales HS, Reina R, Saenz MG, Das Neves AV, Toro MA, Loudet CI. Clinical characteristics and outcomes of obstetric patients requiring ICU admission. Chest. 2007;131(3):718–24.
7. Cartin-Ceba R, Gajic O, Iyer VN, Vlahakis NE. Fetal outcomes of critically ill pregnant women admitted to the intensive care unit for nonobstetric causes. Crit Care Med. 2008;36(10):2746–51.
8. Cartin-Ceba R, Gajic O, Iyer VN. Vlahakis NE- Fetal outcomes of critically ill pregnant women admitted to the intensive care unit for nonobstetric causes. Crit Care Med. 2008;36(10):2746–51.
9. Hazelgrove JF, Price C, Pappachan VJ, Smith GB. Multicentric study of obstetrics admissions to 14 intensive care units in southern England. Crit Care Med. 2001;29(4):770–5.
10. Louie JK, Acosta M, Jamieson DJ, Honein MA. Severe 2009 H1N1 influenza in pregnant and postpartum women in California. N Engl J Med. 2010;362:27–35.
11. Farkash E, Weintraub AY, Sergiento R, Wiznitzer A, Zlotnik A, Sheiner E. Acute ante- partum pyelonephritis in pregnancy: a critical analysis of risk factors and outcomes. Eur J Obstet Gynecol Reprod Biol. 2012;162:24–7.
12. James AH. Venous thromboembolism in pregnancy. Arterioscler Thromb Vasc Biol. 2009;29:326–31.
13. King JC. Strategies to reduce maternal mortality in developed countries. Curr Opin Obstet Gynecol. 2013;25:117–23.
14. Kilpatrick SJ. Next steps to reduce maternal morbidity and mortality in the USA. Womens Health (Lond). 2015 Mar;11(2):193–9.
15. Green–top Guideline No. 56 January 2011 Royal College of Obstetricians and Gynaecologists
16. Zeeman GG, Wendel GD, Cunningham FG. A blueprint for obstetric critical care. Am J Obstet Gynecol. 2003;188(2):532–6.
17. American College of Obstetricians and Gynecologists. ACOG practice bulletin N° 100: critical care in pregnancy. Obstet Gynecol. 2009;113:443–50.
18. Plante L. A curriculum in critical care medicine for maternal-fetal medicine fellows. Crit Care Med. 2006;34:2004–7.
19. Mabie WC, Sibai BM. Treatment in an obstetrical intensive care unit. Am J Obstet Gynecol. 1990;162(1):1–4.

Chapter 2
Hemodynamic Monitoring in Pregnancy and Puerperium

Miguel Chung Sang, Jorge Hidalgo, Jose Miguel Jauregui, and Maily Velasco

Introduction

Maternal mortality is unacceptably high. About 830 women die from pregnancy- or childbirth-related complications around the world every day. It was estimated that in 2015, roughly 303,000 women died during and following pregnancy and childbirth. Almost all of these deaths occurred in low-resource settings, and most could have been prevented. About 73% of all maternal deaths between 2003 and 2009 were due to direct obstetric causes and deaths due to indirect causes accounted for 27.5% of all deaths. Hemorrhage accounted for 27.1%, hypertensive disorders 14%, and sepsis 10.7% of maternal deaths [1].

The overall prevalence of obstetric patients who may require critical care during their pregnancy in our institution ranges from 30 to 40 in 1000 childbirths with a 2.25% of mortality. The main admission causes are hypertensive diseases (eclampsia, preeclampsia, HELLP syndrome) (46%), followed by hemorrhage (uterine atony, lacerations and hematomas, retention of placenta or tissues, abruptio placentae, ectopic gestation) (27%) and then infections (sepsis and septic shock) (16%) (Fig. 2.1).

M. Chung Sang (✉)
Hospital Gineco Obstétrico y Pediátrico Universitario de Guayaquil, Guayaquil, Ecuador

Universidad Católica de Santiago de Guayaquil, Guayaquil, Ecuador

J. Hidalgo
Division of Critical Care, Karl Heusner Memorial Hospital, Belize City, Belize

J. M. Jauregui
Hospital Gineco Obstétrico y Pediátrico Universitario de Guayaquil, Guayaquil, Ecuador

Universidad de Especialidades Espíritu Santo (UEES), Samborondón, Ecuador

M. M. Velasco
Hospital Gineco Obstétrico y Pediátrico Universitario de Guayaquil, Guayaquil, Ecuador

C. Montufar et al. (eds.), *Obstetric Catastrophes*,
https://doi.org/10.1007/978-3-030-70034-8_2

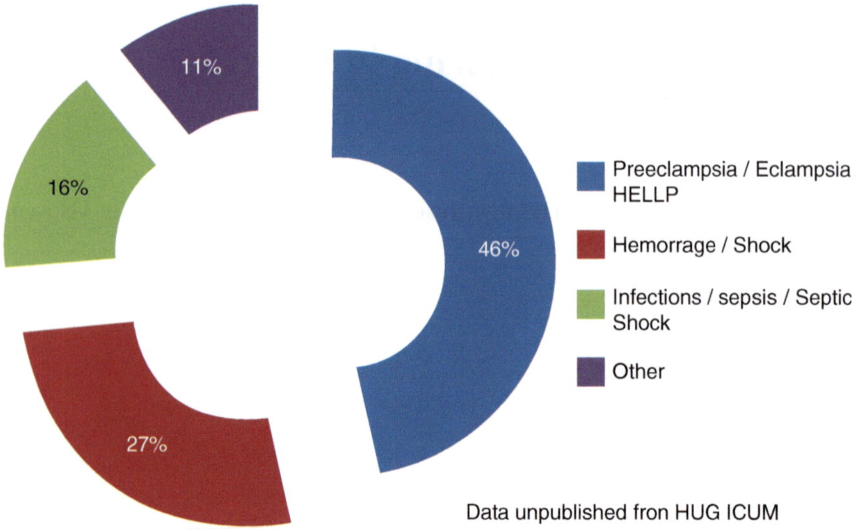

Fig. 2.1 Distribution of admission causes to the Maternal ICU of Hospital Universitario de Guayaquil

In a non-obstetric population, the optimization of cardiac output (CO) had been shown to improve survival and to reduce postoperative complications, organ failure, and the length of stay. So hemodynamic monitoring became a fundamental part of the diagnostic and therapeutic tools of the critical patient, and the obstetric critical patient is not an exception.

In the past decades numerous reports have appeared that show different hemodynamic profiles seen in pregnant patients with a variety of pathologic conditions including pregnancy-induced hypertension, structural cardiac disease, amniotic fluid embolism, and septic shock.

We will review the different modalities of hemodynamic monitoring used, their application to characterize the hemodynamic patterns in normal pregnancy and labor, and their applications in the more common causes of critical illness in the obstetric population, especially in preeclampsia/eclampsia population.

Modalities of Hemodynamic Monitoring in Pregnancy

The different modalities used in hemodynamic monitoring include invasive and noninvasive techniques.

Invasive Techniques

The Pulmonary Artery Catheter (PAC or Swan-Ganz Catheter)

A PAC is placed into the pulmonary artery via a jugular, subclavian, or brachial vascular access. The catheter has several lumens, injection and sampling ports, and a thermistor and balloon at the tip, permitting various pressure (central venous pressure, pulmonary artery pressure, and pulmonary capillary wedge pressure) and output measurements. CO is measured by thermodilution based on the law of conservation of energy. A bolus solution of known volume (5–10 mL) and temperature (either cooled or at room temperature) is injected as an indicator and mixes with blood, thereby cooling it. CO is deducted from curves of temperature difference over time between the injection site and the tip of the PAC using the modified Stewart-Hamilton equation. Intermittent CO values are obtained by averaging 3–5 thermodilution curves or incorporating an electric heating filament into the PAC permitting continuous CO trend measurements of every 30–60 s after initial and regular subsequent calibration with the intermittent bolus technique. The technique is highly invasive with substantial procedure-related risks and limited to ICU settings [7].

In 1980, Benedetti et al. [2] first described the use of PACs in critically ill obstetric patients (10 patients with severe preeclampsia). Since then, it became the standard of care of severe preeclamptic patients and for characterization of hemodynamic profiles of normal pregnant women or preeclamptic/eclamptic patients. A series of publications appeared, but the most relevant were the study of Clark et al., with their pivotal description of hemodynamics in pregnant women, and the study of Cotton et al. [4] in 1988, first describing in detail the changes in a group of 45 preeclamptic patients. A summary of 14 studies about the use of PACs in obstetric patients, published in 1992 by Nolan et al. [5], demonstrated that 64.3% of PACs were used to monitor patients with preeclampsia or eclampsia, specially for control of fluid overload, but none of the studies cited indicate that hemodynamic data would have been helpful in the clinical management of the patients.

In the 2000s Gilbert et al. [6] published a retrospective analysis of 100 medical records of critically ill pregnant women and found that use of PAC in severe preeclampsia complicated with renal failure in 53 cases (53%), pulmonary edema in 30 (30%), and eclampsia in 17 (17%). Subjective evaluation demonstrated that the pulmonary artery catheter was helpful in determining management in 93 cases (93%). The measurements of pulmonary artery wedge pressure and central venous pressure were increased in the cases of pulmonary edema (21.0 ± 2.0 mm Hg and 9.6 ± 1.2 mm Hg, respectively) but were normal in the cases of renal failure and eclampsia. There was a 4.0% complication rate.

Complications of PACs include pneumothorax, ventricular arrhythmias, air embolism, pulmonary infarction, pulmonary artery rupture, sepsis, local vascular thrombosis, intracardiac knotting, and valve damage. Gilbert et al. [6] found in their revision a 0.4% of complications in the obstetric population.

Despite being considered the reference method for CO measurements, it is good to realize that even in optimal conditions the accuracy and precision of the method reflecting the "true actual CO" remains around 10–20% due to inherent technical limitations. It means that PAC, even as a reference technique, can only reliably demonstrate changes in CO of at least 15–30%, being on average 0.75–1.5 L/min for a mean CO of 5 L/min in adults [7–9].

Once popular in intensive care settings and obstetric critical care for hemodynamic monitoring and treatment guidance until the beginning of the twenty-first century, controversy about its risk/benefits ratio and the development of less invasive techniques make the PAC rarely justified, especially in obstetric patients, where most are ambulatory and require a longitudinal follow-up. CO monitoring in pregnant women preferably requires a noninvasive, accessible, and reliable technique that is safe for both the mother and child [7].

Less Invasive Techniques

Pulse Contour Calibrated Devices and Transpulmonary Thermodilution

Pulse contour is based on the analysis of pressure waveforms in a peripheral artery, and assumptions are made to calculate the predicted changes in pulse wave contour to estimate SV and CO. Today, there are numerous commercially available devices, each based on a different algorithm of an arterial pulse pressure waveform analysis. One can differentiate between uncalibrated and calibrated devices, in which the latter need to be externally calibrated once the device is connected with the patient.

The Volume View/EV1000® systems and PiCCO® system use transpulmonary thermodilution similar to thermodilution with PAC. They require a central venous line and femoral or axillary arterial line with thermistor tip, and are only slightly less invasive as compared to PAC, limiting their use to ICU settings. In addition to CO and central venous and intra-arterial pressure, global end diastolic volume (as a measure of preload) and extravascular lung water (as a measure of pulmonary edema) can be obtained. But, there are no studies validating or using the abovementioned technologies in pregnant women, except for a few case reports [7].

The LiDCOplus® device combines pulse contour analysis with lithium indicator dilution for continuous monitoring of CO. It needs the placement of an arterial line, a peripheral or central venous catheter for the lithium bolus, and a lithium sensor. It has the inconvenience that the lithium used for calibration is teratogenic, so in the first trimester of pregnancy, its use must be avoided [7].

Dyer et al. first described a comparison of cardiac output (CO) measurements derived from pulse waveform analysis (LiDCOplus®) with values obtained by thermodilution (TD), in patients with postpartum complications of severe preeclampsia. 18 patients were included at 24–96 h postpartum. Measurements were done at 0, 15, and 30 min after calibration. Bland-Altman Plot was used for comparison between

TD and LiDCOplus; TD exhibited a significant positive bias of 0.58 L/min−1 (95% CI: 0.77–0.39). After peripheral venous calibration, there was no significant bias [0.16 L/min−1 (95% CI: –0.37 to 0.06)] [10].

Noninvasive Techniques

Doppler Echocardiography

Doppler echocardiography is of similar value to PAC, without the complications and invasiveness. Easterling et al. [11, 12] published two studies where they demonstrate the high correlation between Doppler and thermodilution (PAC) with respect to CO. In 1994, Belfort et al. [13, 14] assessed the correlation between Doppler echocardiography and invasive hemodynamic measurements made with the pulmonary artery catheter (PAC) in 11 critically ill obstetric patients. The authors showed a high correlation. There was a good correlation between the two methods for stroke volume ($R^2 = 0.98$), cardiac output ($R^2 = 0.98$), cardiac index ($R^2 = 0.96$), left ventricular filling pressure ($R^2 = 0.79$), pulmonary artery systolic pressure ($R^2 = 0.85$), and right atrial pressure ($R^2 = 0.86$). The same authors demonstrate the clinical utilization of Doppler echocardiography to guide therapeutics and to avoid unnecessary placement of PAC in 10 out of 12 critically ill obstetric patients.

Bioimpedance and Bioreactance

Bioimpedance techniques are another noninvasive tool of central hemodynamic assessment, but in contrast to Doppler, they do not require specific training. In 1989, Masaki et al. [15] did a comparison between thoracic electrical bioimpedance (TEB) and PAC in 11 pregnant women. 9 patients completed the study, and there was an agreement (within ±20%) between the two methods. Bivariate linear regression showed excellent correlation ($r = 0.91$, p less than 0.001) with a slope of 1.04, which indicated a one-to-one relationship between thoracic electrical bioimpedance and thermodilution. However, a study conducted by Clark et al. [16] assessing cardiac index in normal term pregnancy with thoracic electrical bioimpedance and oxygen extraction techniques showed that the results of thoracic electrical bioimpedance were influenced by maternal position.

Doherty et al. [17] compared bioreactance (BRT) with Doppler and found in 35 healthy pregnant women at 21–29 weeks of gestation that there was good agreement between measured stroke volume (SV) [mean bias 6 ml (limits of agreement −18 to 29); ICC 0.8 (95% confidence interval 0.6–0.9), $p < 0.001$] and CO [mean bias 0.2 L (limits of agreement −1.3–1.7); ICC 0.8 (95% confidence interval 0.7–0.9), $p < 0.001$.

Changes in Normal Cardiovascular Physiology Induced by Pregnancy

Hemodynamic Changes Observed in Pregnancy Compared with Non-pregnancy

30 years ago in a pivotal study conducted by Clark et al. [3], 10 carefully screened normal pregnant patients between 36 and 38 weeks (in left lateral decubitus position) of gestation were studied using current clinical techniques. Each patient served as their own control during the postpartum period (between 11 and 13 weeks of puerperium). They place a pulmonary and radial artery catheters and central hemodynamics described; finding a significant ($p < 0.05$ compared with the non-pregnant state) fall in systemic vascular resistance (21%), pulmonary vascular resistance (34%), and colloid oncotic pressure (14%) and a significant rise in cardiac output (43%) and heart rate (17%) in all patients. But there was no significant change in pulmonary capillary wedge pressure, central venous pressure, left ventricular stroke work index, or mean arterial pressure. See (Fig. 2.2).

Robson et al. [18] published a study where longitudinal maternal hemodynamics measurements were done, using echocardiography and Doppler; 13 healthy women complete the study. They were measured 2 times before conception, every month during pregnancy and after partum. Cardiac output had increased by 5 weeks of pregnancy, and the increase continued to 24 weeks when it was 47% above the non-pregnant level, but no further changes were noted in the rest of pregnancy, and it was

Hemodynamic parameter	Non Pregnant	Pregnant	Change
Cardiac Output (L/minute)	4.3 ± 0.9	6.2 ± 10	43%
Hear rate (bpm)	71 ± 10	83 ± 10	17%
Sytemic Vascular Resistance (dines.cm.sec^{-5})	1530 ± 520	1210 ± 266	–21%
Mean arterial pressure (mmHg)	86.4 ± 7.5	90.3 ± 5.8	NS
Pulmonary artery occlussion pressure	6.3 ± 2.1	7.5 ± 1.8	NS
Central venous pressure (mmHg)	3.7 ± 2.6	3.6 ± 2.5	NS
Adapted from Clark SL et al: Central hemodynamic assessment of normal term pregnancy. Am J Obstet Gynecol 1989; 161: 1439–1442			

Fig. 2.2 Central hemodynamic changes in pregnant vs. non-pregnant women

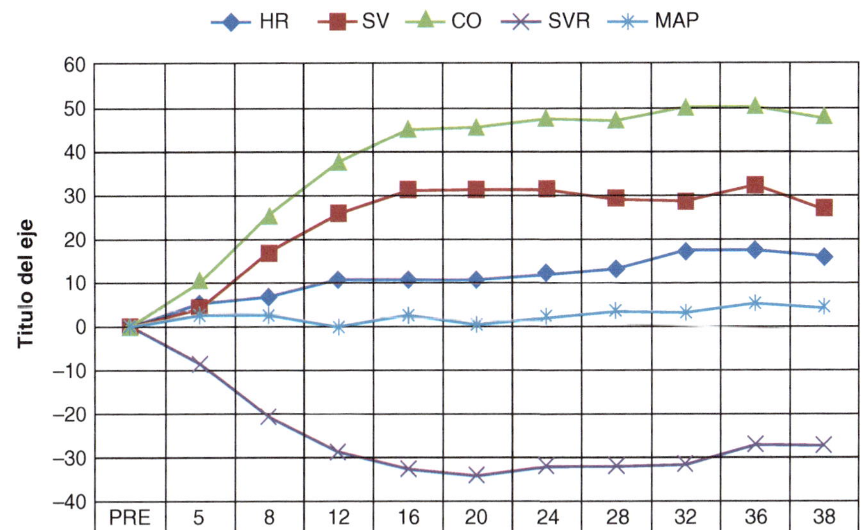

	PRE	5	8	12	16	20	24	28	32	36	38
HR	0	5.33	6.67	10.67	10.67	10.67	12.00	13.33	17.33	17.33	16.00
SV	0	4.26	17.02	25.84	31.16	31.46	31.46	29.33	28.72	32.22	27.05
CO	0	10.66	25.41	37.70	45.29	45.70	47.75	47.13	50.20	50.41	47.95
SVR	0	–8.60	–20.66	–28.88	–32.65	–34.01	–31.98	–31.83	–31.52	–27.15	–27.15
MAP	0	2.64	2.64	0.01	2.64	0.53	2.11	3.69	3.16	5.27	4.22

Fig. 2.3 Hemodynamic changes induced by pregnancy

stated that these changes are the result of heart rate and stroke volume elevations. The heart rate increase was seen by 5 weeks' gestation and continued till 32 weeks. The stroke volume increase occurred a little later at 8 weeks and reached its maximum at about 20 weeks. There was a slight fall in stroke volume after 38 weeks but this was not significant. See (Fig. 2.3).

Vårtun et al. [19], using thoracic impedance cardiotocography, conducted a prospective longitudinal study on 98 healthy pregnant women who were examined 3–5 times during 20–40 weeks of gestation (a total of 441 observations) and found that the SV increased from 83.0 ± 15.83 ml during 20–24 weeks to a maximum of 84.6 ± 16.74 ml at 28–32 weeks and then decreased to 81.7 ± 16.62 ml during 36–40 weeks. The CO was 6.58 ± 1.34 L/min at 20–24 weeks, increased to 7.14 ± 1.46 L/min (8.5%) at 28–32 weeks, and then decreased to 7.03 ± 1.57 L/min at 32–36 weeks and 7.11 L/min at 36–40 weeks. The HR and TFC increased steadily from 82/min to 90/min and from 28.63/kOhm to 30.16/kOhm, respectively, during 20–40 weeks. The blood pressure was lowest at 24–28 weeks, and then there was a steady increase toward term. The SVR was lowest (899 dyne s/cm5) at 28–32 weeks; thereafter it increased slightly to 971 dyne s/cm5 at term (Fig. 2.4).

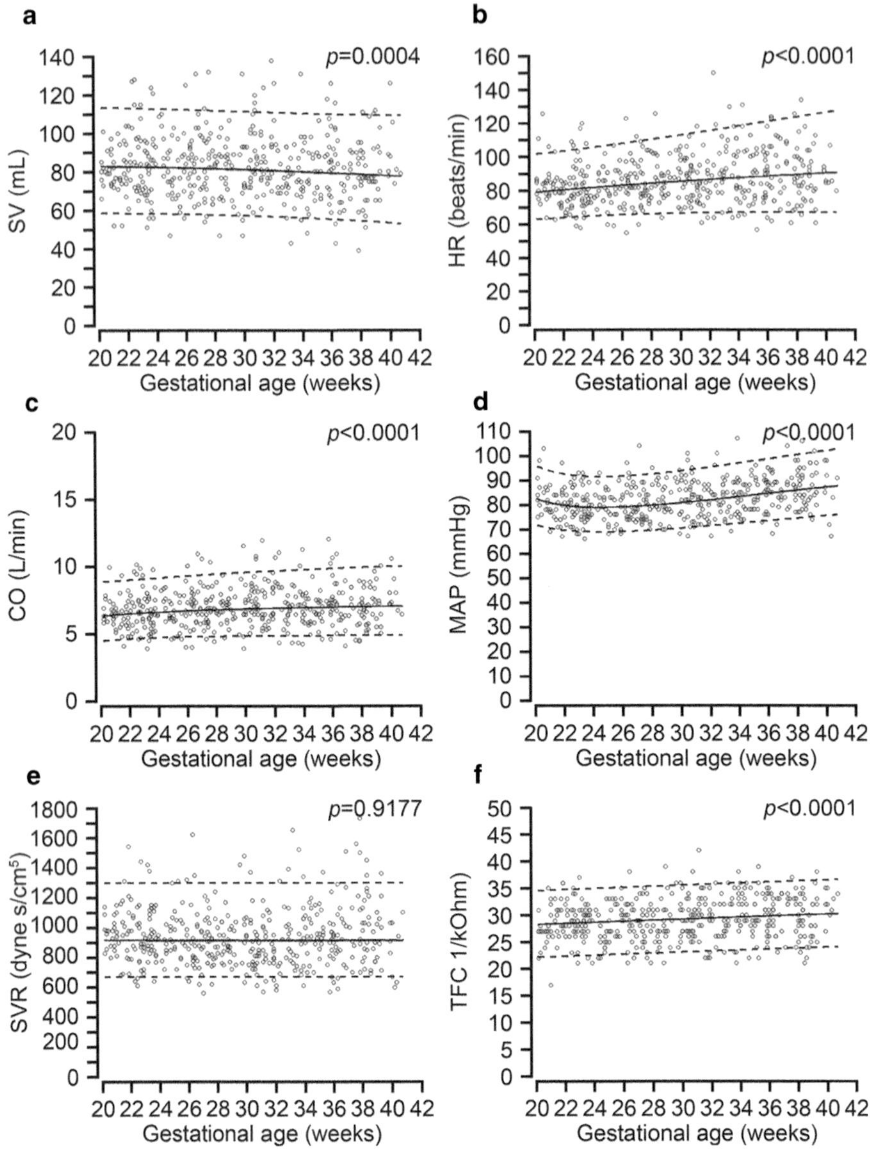

Fig. 2.4 Maternal functional hemodynamics in the second half of pregnancy. A. SV, stroke volume; B. HR, heart rate; C. CO, cardiac output; D. MAP, mean arterial pressure; E. SVR, systemic vascular resistance and F. TFC, thoracic fluid content Adapted from Vårtun Å, Flo K, Wilsgaard T, Acharya G (2015) Maternal Functional Hemodynamics in the Second Half of Pregnancy: A Longitudinal Study. PLoS ONE 10(8): e0135300. https://doi.org/10.1371/journal.pone.0135300

Hemodynamic Changes Observed During Labor and Early Postpartum

Robson et al. [20] conducted a study in 15 women during the first stage of labor and at 24 h after delivery. They measure CO by Doppler and cross-sectional echocardiography. They found basal cardiac output (between uterine contractions) increased from a prelabor mean of 6.99 L/min to 7.88 L/min. During uterine contractions, there was a further increase in cardiac output (7.88 L/min to 10.57 L/min). Mean arterial pressure also increased during the labor. One hour after delivery the heart rate and cardiac output had returned to prelabor values except arterial pressure, and 24 h after delivery all hemodynamic variables had returned to prelabor values.

Ashwal et al. [21] described the hemodynamic patterns (using impedance cardiography) seen in 37 healthy pregnant women pre- (latent phase), intra- (active phases), and post labor. They found that in the prelabor after the administration of epidural analgesia, a decrease in mean cardiac index (CI), cardiac output (CO), stroke volume (SV), and heart rate (HR) and an increase in total peripheral resistance (TPR) were observed; during the labor phase, an increase in CI, CO, SV, and HR and a decrease in TPV in comparison to the prelabor and no significant changes during the rest of the labor and after 1 h postpartum; but within 1–48 h after

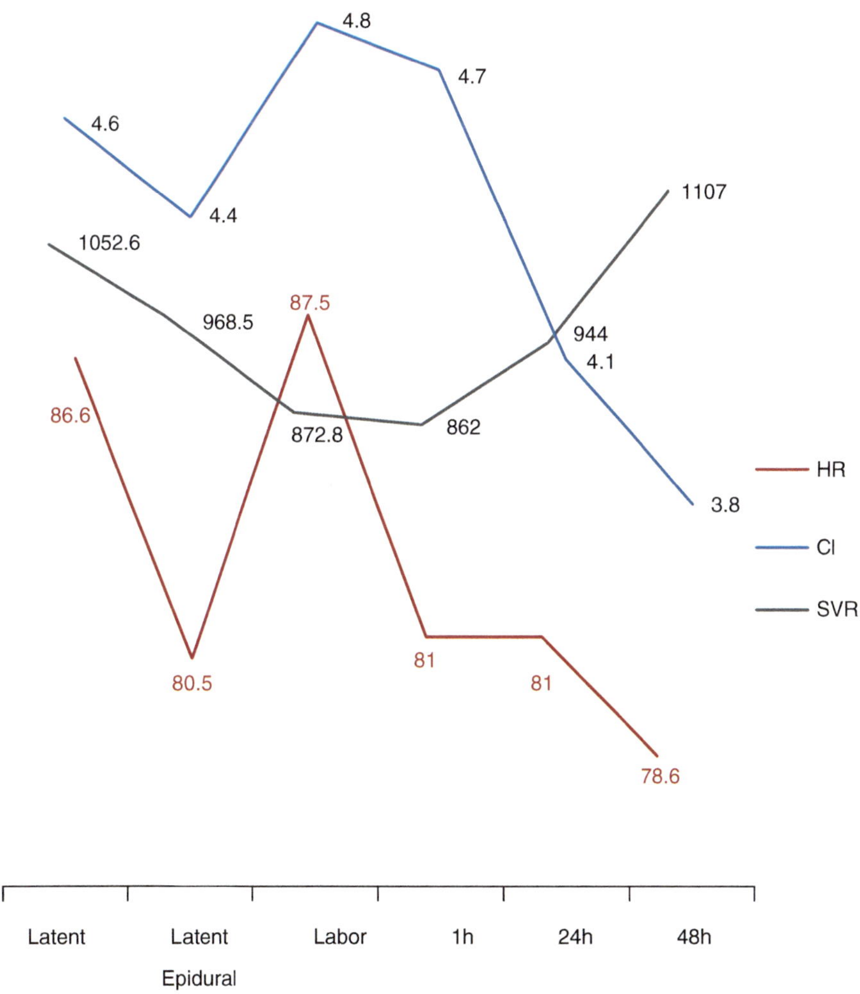

Fig. 2.5 Hemodynamics in labor and postpartum

delivery, CI, CO, SV, and HR decrease to lower values and TPR increases to higher values in comparison to the latent phase (Fig. 2.5).

When do cardiovascular parameters return to their preconception values? This is the question that Capeless et al. tried to answer in a study where 35 healthy women were recruited before they became pregnant and studied their hemodynamic parameters at that time and 6 and 12 weeks after partum. The technique used was echocardiography. What do they found? Stroke volume and end diastolic volume remained consistently elevated over preconception values at 6 and 12 weeks. Systemic vascular resistance remained decreased, compared with baseline, at 12 weeks [22].

In conclusion, using noninvasive and invasive techniques, the general consensus is that CO rises in the first trimester and peaks by the end of the second trimester at approximately 30–50% of non-pregnant values (3.5–6.0 L/min), and SV and HR augment during pregnancy while SVR (TPR) diminishes. But there is still debate with CO and SV in the last trimester: some studies found a decline; others show no change or an increase. These differences may be related to the techniques or methodology or the population participating. During labor CO, SV, and HR increase due to the injection of 400–500 mL of blood from the uterus, every time it contracts. Finally, it is unknown how long CO, SV, and SVR remain elevated [23].

Indications of Hemodynamic Monitoring in Pregnancy [7]

Cardiac indications

- Severe valvular heart disease (aortic stenosis or mitral stenosis associated with pulmonary hypertension)
- Cardiomyopathy with ejection fraction 15–20%
- Sudden cardiovascular collapse (suspected amniotic fluid embolism or pulmonary embolism)

Pulmonary indications

- Adult respiratory distress syndrome with positive end-expiratory pressure 15 mm Hg
- Severe pulmonary disease with secondary pulmonary hypertension
- Pulmonary edema associated with severe preeclampsia

Renal indications

- Persistent oliguria despite fluid resuscitation (e.g., severe preeclampsia)

Miscellaneous

- Septic shock refractory to fluid resuscitation and vasopressor therapy

Hemodynamic Monitoring in Preeclampsia/Eclampsia

Characterization of Hemodynamic Profiles of Preeclamptic/ Eclamptic Women

Cotton et al. [4] studied 45 women with severe preeclampsia/eclampsia with the placement of a PAC to describe their hemodynamic profile. They found that these women could not be easily categorized into one specific hemodynamic pattern. The mean heart rate was 95 ± 2 beats/min. The mean arterial blood pressure was 138 ± 3 mm Hg. The mean arterial blood pressure from the women with severe preeclampsia (145 ± 2 mm Hg) was significantly higher than that of patients with eclampsia (122 ± 2 mm Hg) ($p < 0.001$). Stroke volume and cardiac output varied markedly in this population; when these parameters were normalized for body surface area, they were not appreciably different from the values reported for normal pregnancy. Mean SVI was 44 ± 1 ml.beat.m^2 and CI 4.14 ± 0.13 L/min/m^2 but in 9 patients the CI was >5 L/min/m^2. The mean central venous pressure was 4 ± I mm Hg. The mean pulmonary artery and pulmonary capillary wedge pressures were 17 ± 1 and 10 ± 1 mm Hg, respectively. The percentage distribution of this patient population to the "normal" pregnancy parameters were as follows: 69% had normal cardiac indices, and 20% had elevated cardiac indices compared with 11% with low values; 71% were noted to have elevated systemic vascular resistance indices, with the majority of the remaining patients having high normal values; 53% demonstrated pulmonary capillary wedge pressures in the normal range. 31% had pulmonary capillary wedge pressure measurements >12 mm Hg while only seven patients 16% were observed to have low values. A graphic analysis of left ventricular function (pulmonary capillary wedge pressure versus left ventricular stroke work index) revealed that 80% had hyperdynamic left ventricular function characterized by a Starling curve shifted upward and to the left (Fig. 2.6).

Ohashi et al. [24] in Brazil conducted a study where they compared hemodynamic profiles of healthy and mildly preeclamptic pregnant women at term, as well as those of non-pregnant controls, using a new noninvasive cardiac output monitor (NICOM) based on bioreactance. The preeclamptic group showed higher HR, CO, and SVR (85.4 ± 8.4 beats.min^{-1}; 6.6 ± 0.7 L.min^{-1}; 1369.9 ± 173.5 dyne.sec.cm^{-5}, 221.6 ± 22.4 ms) compared to the non-pregnant group (67.9 ± 9.5 beats.min^{-1}; 5.6 ± 0.7 L.min^{-1}; 1136.9 ± 149.8 dyne.sec.cm^{-5}, 265.0 ± 28.8 ms), but there were no statically significant differences in these parameters between preeclamptic and pregnant women.

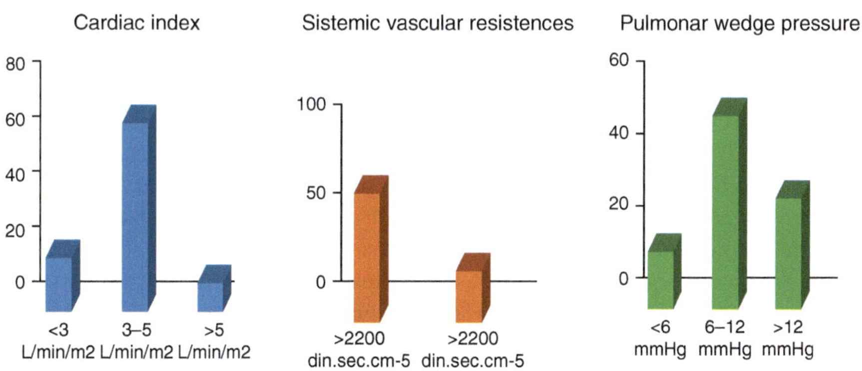

Fig. 2.6 Hemodynamic profile of severe pregnancy-induced hypertension

Hemodynamic Monitoring as a Tool to Identify Different Phenotypes of Preeclampsia

Recent investigations have identified striking differences in the maternal hemodynamic profiles of early-onset and late-onset preeclampsia, leading to the hypothesis that these hypertensive disorders of pregnancy most likely arise from different pathoetiologies. Early-onset preeclampsia seems to be mediated predominantly by placental dysfunction, whereas late-onset preeclampsia more likely relates to maternal constitutional factors associated with the metabolic syndrome and abnormalities in vascular function.

Valensise et al. [25] compared maternal hemodynamics (calculated using echocardiography) at 24 weeks gestation in a group of normotensive asymptomatic patients with subsequent development of early (<34 weeks gestation) and late (≥34 weeks gestation) preeclampsia. Women who develop early-onset preeclampsia demonstrate significantly higher blood pressure and systemic vascular resistance with lower heart rate, stroke volume, and cardiac output and exhibit significantly higher levels of placental-derived antiangiogenic proteins and significantly lower levels of proangiogenic proteins, when compared with healthy pregnant women. By contrast, pregnant women who subsequently develop late-onset preeclampsia manifest higher stoke volume, cardiac output, and heart rate with significantly lower vascular resistance compared with normotensive pregnant women; is less frequently associated with placental pathology and more normal levels of placental-derived angiogenic proteins compared with early-onset preeclampsia; and is associated with more favorable maternal and infant outcomes, with a normal or even large for gestational age birth weight. Total vascular resistance was 1605 ± 248 versus 739 ± 244 dyn·s·cm^{-5}, and cardiac output was 4.49 ± 1.09 versus 8.96 ± 1.83 L in early versus late PE ($p < 0.001$). Prepregnancy body mass index was higher in late versus early preeclampsia (28 ± 6 versus 24 ± 2 kg/m^2; $p < 0.001$).

McLaughlin et al. [26] conducted a study where 26 normotensive pregnant women at high risk to develop hypertension and 20 normotensive healthy women (controls) were recruited between 22 and 26 weeks of gestation. Transthoracic bioreactance was used to estimate stroke volume continuously for 15 min. They identify three groups of patients: (1) ("low risk" of hypertension) was characterized by a high volume, low resistance hemodynamic profile with normal levels of circulating angiogenic proteins and maternal blood pressure, along with normal birth weight and 4% incidence of hypertensive disorders of pregnancy; (2) ("moderate risk" of hypertension) was characterized by a lower volume, higher resistance hemodynamic profile compared with group 1, with higher sFlt-1 (an angiogenic protein) and blood pressure levels, along with lower birth weight and a 27% incidence of hypertension during pregnancy; and (3) ("high risk" of hypertension) exhibited a low volume, high resistance hemodynamic profile with an elevated antiangiogenic protein profile and higher blood pressure levels. They also report that total peripheral resistance was the most significant distinguishing parameter between these groups ($p < 0.0001$), followed by placental growth factor, endoglin, and cardiac output ($p < 0.0001$). Using these four parameters, a receiver operating curve was constructed with an area under the curve of 0.975 (95% confidence interval 0.93–1) for the prediction of developing hypertension in pregnancy.

Miranda et al. [27] conducted a prospective observational study in an obstetric-referral center in Cartagena, Colombia. 30 pregnant women presenting with PE were recruited, and hemodynamics were obtained through bioreactance. Preeclampsia with high SVR had worse hemodynamic parameters than those with normal SVR, and significantly lower cardiac output, stroke volume, and oxygen delivery index compared to controls (all p values <0.05). Furthermore, preeclampsia with high SVR had a trend toward higher brain natriuretic peptide and longer length of hospital stay, but also their newborns have significantly lower birth weight.

Hemodynamic-Guided Antihypertensive Therapy in Preeclampsia

The management of preeclampsia is primarily focused on the therapy of maternal hypertension to reduce the risk of severe hypertensive episodes and to safely prolong gestation. In general, the current standard of care follows the principle that optimum timing and effectiveness of antihypertensive therapy have favorable influence on maternal and fetal outcomes.

Current recommendations for antihypertensive therapy during pregnancy do not differentiate therapy based on an assessment of maternal hemodynamics and is based mereley in empirical recommendations when blood pressure is above a certain threshold. Furthermore, the choice of antihypertensive medications for the management of hypertensive disorders of pregnancy is recommended to be primarily based on the physician's familiarity and experience, adverse effects and contraindications to the prescribed drug, local availability, and cost.

Although the theory of guiding antihypertensive treatment in pregnancy through hemodynamic assessment is not novel, only a small number of trials have evaluated maternal hemodynamics in pregnant women receiving antihypertensive therapies [28].

Cornette et al. [29] studied the hemodynamic effects of intravenous nicardipine in 10 severely preeclamptic pregnant women and found a significantly reduced mean arterial blood pressure (median difference, 26 mmHg; $p = 0.002$) and total vascular resistance (median difference, 791 dynes × s/cm^5; $p = 0.002$) in all patients. This induced a reflex tachycardia with consequent increase in cardiac output of 1.55 L/min ($p = 0.004$), without affecting uteroplacental or fetal perfusion.

Scardo et al. [30] evaluated the hemodynamic effects of oral nifedipine in 10 severely preeclamptic women. Patients were hemodynamically monitored in the lateral recumbent position by thoracic electrical bioimpedance before, during, and after oral nifedipine dosing. A steady decrease in mean arterial pressure was noted, and cardiac index increased over time ($p = 0.0011$). There was no significant effect on maternal heart rate or stroke index. No periodic fetal heart rate changes were noted.

Easterling et al. [31], in a randomized, placebo-controlled trial, found that atenolol decreased the incidence of late-onset preeclampsia in nulliparous women with a high cardiac output hyperdynamic state (>7.4 L/m at 24 week of gestation), compared with placebo treatment (18 vs. 3.8% $p < 0.04$).

Stott et al. [32] conducted a study where 134 pregnant women presenting with hypertension at a UK hospital were treated with labetalol and monitored hemodynamically (bioreactance) at presentation and at 1 h and 24 h after commencement of treatment. They found that who were unresponsive to labetalol were characterized as being more likely to be of black ethnicity and to have higher blood pressure and total peripheral resistance and lower heart rate and cardiac output at the time of clinical presentation, as assessed through thoracic bioreactance; and these unresponsive women also delivered significantly earlier in pregnancy with lower fetal birth weight, were twice as likely to develop preeclampsia, and over 10× as likely to develop severe hypertension. In another study [33] found that antihypertensive therapy for pregnant women presenting with any type of hypertension being referred for antihypertensive therapy that was guided by hemodynamic monitoring significantly reduced the rates of severe maternal hypertension from 18% to 3.8%.

Hemodynamic Monitoring in Septic Shock

There is a paucity of studies of hemodynamic monitoring specifically in septic pregnant or postpartum patients. An old study conducted by Lee et al. [34] using PACs for monitoring 10 pregnant women complicated with septic shock showed the classical hemodynamic picture of reduced systemic vascular resistance with depressed myocardial function. The mean initial systemic vascular resistance index in eight surviving women was 885 +/− 253 dyne.sec/cm^5.m^2, mean cardiac index of 4.20 +/− 2.01 L/min/m^2, and in 50% of the patients, there were evidence of myocardial depression based on analysis of their left ventricular function curves. A hemodynamic algorithm based on volume therapy, vasopressors, and inotropes was administered, producing an improvement in the hemodynamic parameters.

More recently, Guinn et al. [35] in an essay recommended the Early Goal Directed Therapy for Sepsis (EGDT) during pregnancy, the same way that was stated by Rivers et al. [36] and the Surviving Sepsis Campaign. But as stated by Joseph et al. [37] there is no evidence-based goal-directed recommendations for this group, and noted that normal pregnancy-induced physiological changes confound the application of EGDT during pregnancy because the CVP may be increased to 10 mmHg, the MAP is decreased, and the Scv02 may be as high as 80%. CO monitoring may be useful to guide fluid resuscitation but has not been studied formally in this setting.

References

1. Alkema L, Chou D, Hogan D, Zhang S, Moller AB, Gemmill A, Fat DM, Boerma T, Temmerman M, Mathers C, Say L, United Nations Maternal Mortality Estimation Inter-Agency Group collaborators and technical advisory group. Global, regional, and national lev-

els and trends in maternal mortality between 1990 and 2015, with scenario-based projections to 2030: a systematic analysis by the UN Maternal Mortality Estimation Inter-Agency Group. Lancet. 2016;387(10017):462–74.
2. Benedetti TJ, Cotton DB, Read JC, Miller FC. Hemodynamic observations in severe pre-eclampsia with a flow-directed pulmonary artery catheter. Am J Obstet Gynecol. 1980;136:465–708.
3. Clark SL, Cotton DB, Lee W, et al. Central hemodynamic assessment of normal term pregnancy. Am J Obstet Gynecol. 1989;161:1439–42.
4. Cotton DB, Lee W, Huhta JC, Dorman KF. Hemodynamic profile of severe pregnancy-induced hypertension. Am J Obstet Gynecol. 1988;158(3 Pt 1):523–9.
5. Nolan TE, Wakefield ML, Devoe LD. Invasive hemodynamic monitoring in obstetrics. A critical review of its indications, benefits, complications, and alternatives. Chest. 1992;101(5):1429–33.
6. Gilbert WM, Towner DR, Field NT, Anthony J. The safety and utility of pulmonary artery catheterization in severe preeclampsia and eclampsia. Am J Obstet Gynecol. 2000;182(6):1397–403.
7. Bijl RC, Valensise H, Novelli GP, Vasapollo B, Wilkinson I, Thilaganathan B, Stöhr EJ, Lees C, van der Marel CD, Cornette JMJ, International Working Group on Maternal Hemodynamics. Methods and considerations concerning cardiac output measurement in pregnant women: recommendations of the International Working Group on Maternal Hemodynamics. Ultrasound Obstet Gynecol. 2019;54(1):35–50.
8. Cecconi M, Rhodes A, Poloniecki J, Della Rocca G, Grounds RM. Bench-to bedside review: the importance of the precision of the reference technique in method comparison studies–with specific reference to the measurement of cardiac output. Crit Care. 2009;13:201.
9. Hapfelmeier A, Cecconi M, Saugel B. Cardiac output method comparison studies: the relation of the precision of agreement and the precision of method. J Clin Monit Comput. 2016;30:149–55.
10. Dyer RA, Piercy JL, Reed AR, Strathie GW, Lombard CJ, Anthony JA, James MF. Comparison between pulse waveform analysis and thermodilution cardiac output determination in patients with severe pre-eclampsia. Br J Anaesth. 2011;106(1):77–81.
11. Easterling TR, Watts DH, Schmucker BC, Benedetti TJ. Measurement of cardiac output during pregnancy: validation of Doppler technique and clinical observations in preeclampsia. Obstet Gynecol. 1987;69:845.
12. Easterling TR, Carlson KL, Schmucker BC, Brateng DA, Benedetti TJ. Measurement of cardiac output in pregnancy by Doppler technique. Am J Perinatol. 1990;7(3):220–2.
13. Belfort MA, Rokey R, Saade GR, Moise KJ Jr. Rapid echocardiographic assessment of left and right heart hemodynamics in critically ill obstetric patients. Am J Obstet Gynecol. 1994;171(4):884–92.
14. Belfort MA, Mares A, Saade G, et al. Two dimensional echocardiography and Doppler ultrasound in managing obstetric patients. Obstet Gynecol. 1997;90:326–30.
15. Masaki DI, Greenspoon JS, Ouzounian JG. Measurement of cardiac output in pregnancy by thoracic electrical bioimpedance and thermodilution. A preliminary report. Am J Obstet Gynecol. 1989;161(3):680–4.
16. Clark SL, Southwick J, Pivarnik JM, Cotton DB, Hankins GD, Phelan JP. A comparison of cardiac index in normal term pregnancy using thoracic electrical bio-impedance and oxygen extraction (Fick) techniques. Obstet Gynecol. 1994;83(5 Pt 1):669–72.
17. Doherty A, El-Khuffash A, Monteith C, McSweeney L, Breatnach C, Kent E, Tully E, Malone F, Thornton P. Comparison of bioreactance and echocardiographic non-invasive cardiac output monitoring and myocardial function assessment in primagravida women. Br J Anaesth. 2017;118(4):527–32.
18. Robson SC, Hunter S, Boys RJ, Dunlop W. Serial study of factors influencing changes in cardiac output during human pregnancy. Am J Phys. 1989;256(4 Pt 2):H1060–5.
19. Vårtun Å, Flo K, Wilsgaard T, Acharya G. Maternal functional hemodynamics in the second half of pregnancy: a longitudinal study. PLoS One. 2015;10(8):e0135300.
20. Robson SC, Hunter S, Moore M, Dunlop W. Haemodynamic changes during the puerperium: a Doppler and M-mode echocardiographic study. Br J Obstet Gynaecol. 1987;94(11):1028–39.
21. Ashwal E, et al. Cardiac hemodynamics in labor and postpartum. A new look into physiology. Am J Obstet Gynecol. 2015;212(1):S167–8.

22. Capeless EL, Clapp JF. When do cardiovascular parameters return to their preconception values? Am J Obstet Gynecol. 1991;165(4 Pt 1):883–6.
23. Carlin A, Alfirevic Z. Physiological changes of pregnancy and monitoring. Best Pract Res Clin Obstet Gynaecol. 2008;22(5):801–23.
24. Ohashi Y, Ibrahim H, Furtado L, Kingdom J, Carvalho JC. Non-invasive hemodynamic assessment of non-pregnant, healthy pregnant and preeclamptic women using bioreactance. Rev Bras Anestesiol. 2010;60(6):603–13. https://doi.org/10.1016/S0034-7094(10)70075-1.
25. Valensise H, Vasapollo B, Gagliardi G, Novelli GP. Early and late preeclampsia: two different maternal hemodynamic states in the latent phase of the disease. Hypertension. 2008;52:873–80.
26. McLaughlin K, Zhang J, Lye SJ, Parker JD, Kingdom JC. Phenotypes of pregnant women who subsequently develop hypertension in pregnancy. J Am Heart Assoc. 2018;7(14):e009595.
27. Miranda J, et al. Maternal cardiovascular hemodynamics in preeclampsia allows identification of patients with a more severe clinical phenotype. Am J Obstet Gynecol. 2019;220(1):S299–300.
28. American College of Obstetricians and Gynecologists; Task Force on Hypertension in Pregnancy. Hypertension in pregnancy. Report of the American College of Obstetricians and Gynecologists' Task Force on Hypertension in Pregnancy. Obstet Gynecol. 2013;122:1122–31.
29. Cornette J, Buijs EA, Duvekot JJ, Herzog E, Roos-Hesselink JW, Rizopoulos D, Meima M, Steegers EA. Hemodynamic effects of intravenous nicardipine in severely pre-eclamptic women with a hypertensive crisis. Ultrasound Obstet Gynecol. 2016;47:89–95.
30. Scardo JA, Vermillion ST, Hogg BB, Newman RB. Hemodynamic effects of oral nifedipine in preeclamptic hypertensive emergencies. Am J Obstet Gynecol. 1996;175:336–8.
31. Easterling TR, Brateng D, Schmucker B, Brown Z, Millard SP. Prevention of preeclampsia: a randomized trial of atenolol in hyperdynamic patients before onset of hypertension. Obstet Gynecol. 1999;93(5 pt 1):725–33.
32. Stott D, Bolten M, Paraschiv D, Papastefanou I, Chambers JB, Kametas NA. Longitudinal hemodynamics in acute phase of treatment with labetalol in hypertensive pregnant women to predict need for vasodilatory therapy. Ultrasound Obstet Gynecol. 2017;49:85–94.
33. Stott D, Papastefanou I, Paraschiv D, Clark K, Kametas NA. Serial hemodynamic monitoring to guide treatment of maternal hypertension leads to reduction in severe hypertension. Ultrasound Obstet Gynecol. 2017;49:95–103. https://doi.org/10.1002/uog.17341.
34. Lee W, Clark SL, Cotton DB, Gonik B, Phelan J, Faro S, Giebel R. Septic shock during pregnancy. Am J Obstet Gynecol. 1988;159(2):410–6.
35. Guinn DA, Abel DE, Tomlinson MW. Early goal directed therapy for sepsis during pregnancy. Obstet Gynecol Clin N Am. 2007;34(3):459–79.
36. Rivers E, Nguyen B, Havstad S, Ressler J, Muzzin A, Knoblich B, Peterson E, Tomlanovich M, Early Goal-Directed Therapy Collaborative Group. Early goal-directed therapy in the treatment of severe sepsis and septic shock. N Engl J Med. 2001;345(19):1368–77.
37. Joseph J, Sinha A, Paech M, Walters BN. Sepsis in pregnancy and early goal-directed therapy. Obstet Med. 2009;2(3):93–9.

Part II
Critical Care, Special Consideration

Chapter 3
Eclampsia

Keyra Morales-Allard

Introduction

Eclampsia represents an obstetric catastrophe resulting from the umbrella of hypertensive disorders, which complicates about 10% of pregnancies [1]; these disorders are one of the leading causes of maternal death worldwide, only surpassed by obstetric hemorrhage, and most of these deaths occur in developing countries [2]. Around the world 76,000 women and 500,000 babies die from these disorders each year [3].

Preeclampsia is a multisystem disorder; even though the brain is just one of several organs affected, cerebrovascular events in the context of hypertensive disorders during pregnancy represent a direct cause of death in about 40% of cases [4]. In a published study of 53 pregnant women who were complicated with eclampsia, only 13% had been diagnosed with severe preeclampsia prior to the convulsive episode [5].

The incidence of eclampsia and its complications is significantly low in developed countries. In the United States, it has declined from 8 per 10,000 births in 2001 to 5.6 cases per 10,000 births in 2007. On the other hand, in underdeveloped countries the incidence of eclampsia is very high [6]. In the Western world a range of incidence is reported from 1 in 2000 to 1 in 3448 pregnancies [7].

It's crucial to develop capacities for the suspicion and recognition of complications of preeclampsia and its management. Eclampsia, although, it's probably the most florid and easiest to diagnose, the same can't be said about its management, especially if progression occurs to other complications resulting from the convulsive episode such as bleeding, brain herniation, and convulsive status. This chapter

K. Morales-Allard (✉)
Department of Obstetrics and Gynecology, Complejo Hospitalario Arnulfo Arias Madrid, Panama City, Panama

C. Montufar et al. (eds.), *Obstetric Catastrophes*,
https://doi.org/10.1007/978-3-030-70034-8_3

will develop key points for the diagnosis and management of eclampsia and its main complications.

Definitions

Preeclampsia is a multisystem disorder that can define as high blood pressure (systolic blood pressure ≥140 and/or diastolic blood pressure ≥90 mmHg) after 20 weeks of gestation and postpartum, associated with proteinuria and/or target organ damage.

Any hypertensive disorder during pregnancy can result in preeclampsia. This way, 35% of patients diagnosed with gestational hypertension will develop preeclampsia and the same goes for 25% of patients with chronic hypertension, which is called superimposed preeclampsia [1].

Understanding that preeclampsia originates from a reduction in placental perfusion and hypoxia, which ultimately triggers pathophysiological mechanisms that result in systemic vascular endothelial dysfunction [8], the disease therefore resolves with the interruption of pregnancy. Its natural history implies that it's progressive; therefore once the diagnosis is made, it's time to decide optimal time for delivery, and this decision takes into account the development of maternal and fetal complications, and the latter concept is mainly related to the gestational age at which the diagnosis is made and the fetal condition.

One of the maternal complications we face is the development of eclampsia; although rare, important maternal and fetal morbidity occurs because of it. Eclampsia is defined as the occurrence of one or more new convulsive episodes superimposed on a preeclamptic syndrome [9] during pregnancy or postpartum, up to a period of 10 days [10].

Eclampsia is directly related to neurological events that are a potential cause of death. Acute seizures can result in severe complications such as stroke, bleeding, edema, and brain herniation [11]. Despite of the usually self-limiting nature of eclamptic seizures, catastrophic events can occur and progression to a convulsive status is possible. This status is characterized by both clinical and electroencephalography epileptic activity that persists beyond 5 min, or if there is no recovery between the seizure events in this period of time [12].

Pathophysiology

The pathophysiological mechanisms of eclamptic episode have been the subject of research over the years. In order to understand the concept, we must take into account the non-expansive nature of the human skull as a continent.

Preeclampsia can produce severe and acute elevation of systemic blood pressure, and this causes a loss of cerebral compensatory mechanisms. Cerebral blood flow is regulated mainly by changes in the vascular caliber to maintain cerebral perfusion pressure [4]. Increased blood pressure causes an increase in hydrostatic pressure and a state of cerebral hyperperfusion that is initially regulated by increasing cerebrovascular resistances through vasoconstriction; finally these compensatory mechanisms are depleted causing loss of the vascular resistances, resulting in the abrupt increase in the permeability of the blood-brain barrier generating a vasogenic cerebral edema and increasing intracranial pressure [4, 11]. The expansion of extracellular space during vasogenic edema occurs in the closed space of the skull causing progressive cerebral compression, which causes classic symptoms like headache, nausea, vomiting, visual disturbances, and seizure [11, 13]. The global endothelial injury and the oxidative stress typical of preeclampsia also causes alterations in the permeability of the blood-brain barrier allowing access to pro-inflammatory cytokines exacerbating cerebral injury and edema [14]. This final concept explains cases of eclampsia that are not accompanied by hypertensive crisis.

The primary explanation of edema pathogenesis and the neurological symptoms of eclampsia is that they represent a form of posterior reversible encephalopathy syndrome (PRES) [4]. This syndrome is characterized by clinical symptoms such as headache, visual disturbances, and seizures, associated with white matter abnormalities suggestive of cerebral edema observed in neuroimaging studies, which is precipitated in this case by endothelial dysfunction and hypertension [6, 15]. The syndrome is called this way to allude to the propensity of the posterior brain developing the pathology, which is not yet clearly explained. Some theories have been exposed including decreased vascular sympathetic innervation and the increased capillary density of the posterior brain region [11]. The truth is that in neuroimaging studies such as MRI, injuries are not only confined to the posterior brain, they have been described in the parietal brain, cerebellum, middle brain, and basal ganglia [6]. On the other hand, follow-up studies of patients using neuroimaging have been published, where it's observed that the lesions don't disappear or do so partially [2].

Diagnosis

As we mentioned, the diagnosis of eclampsia is made when we are faced with a new convulsive episode during pregnancy, or in the postpartum period, this patient may not been known with the diagnosis of preeclampsia. If the patient hadn't been diagnosed with hypertension, in our first contact we should suspect that the cause of convulsions is eclampsia, and in this emergency scenario it's reasonable to begin management even before having a thorough clinical analysis and anamnesis.

The eclamptic seizure is usually a generalized tonic-clonic type and self-limiting, and typically doesn't last more than 3 or 4 min. In some some patients when the origin is occipital, the episode may be preceded by auras and visual hallucinations [6].

One of the aspects associated with seizure is hypertension that can be severe (systolic pressure ≥160 mmHg and/or diastolic pressure ≥110 mmHg) in which case it must be treated immediately, or mild hypertension (systolic pressure between 140 and 159 mmHg and/or diastolic pressure between 90 and 109) [16]. However, there's a significant percentage of patients in which hypertension can be absent, the same with proteinuria, suggesting that the diagnosis of preeclampsia isn't necessarily a prerequisite for eclampsia [7, 11, 16].

In relation to symptomatology in the context of preeclampsia, in 2013 the American College of Obstetrics and Gynecology published the Task Force for Hypertension in Pregnancy describing the new onset of cerebral and visual disturbances as one of the six diagnostic criteria for severity of preeclampsia and superimposed preeclampsia [17]. They mentioned that some symptoms such as persistent occipital or frontal headache, blurred vision, photophobia, severe persistent right upper quadrant or epigastric pain, and altered mental status have potential utility in predicting an eclamptic seizure [7].

It has been established that headache in a preeclamptic patient is characterized for being severe, persistent, progressive, and unresponsive to medication, in a very imprecise way [17–19]. And this represents a premonitory symptom of an eclamptic seizure.

It's described in some publications that more than half of patients reported severe headache prior the eclamptic seizure [19, 20]. However, it's important that it's unknown how many patients with preeclampsia and severe headache will develop eclampsia [20]. In fact, headache may be a benign symptom in 60% of women in their reproductive lives. On the other the other hand, a severe headache may be the initial symptom in more than half of patients with intracranial hemorrhage, limiting its utility in the diagnosis of preeclampsia [20, 21]. In 2011 a systematic review was published showing that the sensitivity and specificity of headache as a predictor of maternal adverse outcome were 54% and 59%, respectively, and the area under the curve for prediction of maternal complications was 0.58 [22]. This study suggests that using headache as a diagnostic criteria for severe preeclampsia or as an indication of immediate delivery is unreliable, is imprecise, and is unable to predict maternal and perinatal adverse outcomes [20].

Visual disturbances are described in about 32% of patients who experience an eclamptic seizure and ranges from scotomas to bright flashes [7, 19].

Sensorium alteration is sudden, is acute, and usually follows the seizure, and a prolonged decrease of mental status must be assessed for possible complications, which should be treated, such as convulsive status or severe metabolic alteration like uremia [23].

Maternal and Fetal Adverse Outcomes of the Seizure Episode

As we have mentioned, eclampsia is associated with a high risk of maternal and perinatal death, mainly in developing countries. Seizures during pregnancy can result in both maternal and fetal acute complications, also long-term adverse outcomes. Pregnancies complicated with eclampsia have an increased maternal risk of abruptio placentae, disseminated intravascular coagulation, pulmonary edema, acute kidney failure, aspiration pneumonia, and cardiac arrest [7, 16].

Prolonged tonic-clonic seizures can cause maternal acidosis, hypoxia, head trauma, and bleeding. It's necessary to perform an appropriate physical examination after the convulsive episode looking for focal neurologic signs that are suggestive of complications.

The fetus has an important risk of perinatal death that has been reported from 5.6% to 11.8%, which is related to prematurity, abruptio placentae, and severe growth restriction [7, 10]. A prolonged eclamptic seizure can lead to such a state of hypoxia that there may be a fetal bradycardia, late decelerations, minimal variability, and a transient tachycardia for more than 20 min in fetal monitoring, especially if we haven't started resuscitation maneuvers [11]. It isn't right to perform an emergency c-section, particularly if the mother is unstable. An increase in uterine dynamics and tone may occur, which can be resolved spontaneously in the next 3–10 min. If bradycardia and late decelerations persist for more than 10–15 min despite proper resuscitation, we should suspect abruptio placentae and nonreassuring fetal status [7].

Differential Diagnosis

The main cause of seizures during pregnancy is eclampsia. Discarding other diagnoses becomes important when we witness an atypical eclamptic seizure, focal neurologic signs, or prolonged coma [7].

Seizures without neurological deficit may be associated with metabolic disorders (hydroelectrolytic imbalance and hypoglycemia), toxic drugs (abuse drugs and medication such as oxytocin), and infections (encephalitis, meningitis, sepsis) [24]. However, not finding focal neurological deficit doesn't rule out anatomical abnormalities, such as, stroke, tumors, and bleeding. In order to optimize the diagnosis, an adequate medical history is necessary if it's possible and a rigorous physical examination.

Neuroimaging studies such as computed tomography and MRI are not routinely performed, but they can be used to show complications secondary to vasogenic cerebral edema, like brain herniation, and to rule out other diagnostic alternatives [11] especially in those patients who are refractory to initial treatment.

Management

The initial approach of the eclamptic patient is based on the following:

1. Prevent traumatic injuries. It's necessary to prevent a patient injury with objects around her during the convulsive episode. In-hospital, we must adapt the patient's bed to prevent falls or wounds with sharp objects.
2. Ensure airway permeability and oxygen intake. Despite the self-limiting condition of the eclamptic seizure, its prolongation results in a state of maternal hypoxia, which we can correct by administering supplemental oxygen through a face mask to 8–10 Lpm, only if it's necessary.
3. Preventive bronchoaspiration measures. Place the patient in lateral decubitus position, and suction secretions to prevent fluid aspiration.
4. Managing the hypertensive crisis if present. There is no controversy that blood pressure should be treated until it's less than 160/110, which is considered severe hypertension. In case of eclampsia, which is considered a "target organ damage," a rapid reduction in blood pressure is recommended. However, there isn't enough evidence on the blood pressure targets to be achieved in women with preeclampsia and cerebrovascular complications. We should take into account that a failure in the treatment of severe hypertension is associated with maternal death by intracranial hemorrhage and aortic dissection [25] and a blood pressure level below 110/80 compromises the blood perfusion to vital organs, so abrupt reduction in mean arterial pressure should be avoided.

   In order to control severe hypertension, it's recommended the use of three antihypertensives [1]:

   - Labetalol intravenous: 10–20 mg, then 20–80 mg every 15 min. Maximum 300 mg. Infusion 1–2 mg/min
   - Hydralazine intravenous: 5 mg, then 5–10 mg every 20 min. Maximum 20 mg. Infusion at 0.5–10 mg/h
   - Nifedipine oral immediate release 10–20 mg every 2–6 h. Maximum 180 mg/d

5. Preventing seizure recurrence: magnesium sulfate is the treatment of choice. Magnesium sulfate is credited with advantages over decreased cerebral edema and blood-brain barrier disruption, in addition to its anticonvulsive effect [26]. The Magpie study showed that MgSO4 is able to improve maternal mortality and reduce the risk of eclampsia by 58% of women with preeclampsia [9]. Systematic reviews show their superiority over diazepam, phenytoin, nimodipine, and placebo. In a publication by the Eclampsia Trial Collaborative Group, $MgSO_4$ was able to reduce the risk of seizure recurrence in eclamptic women by 52% when it was compared with diazepam and by 67% when it was compared with phenytoin [27]. The serum concentration of MgSO4 to be achieved for the treatment of eclamptic seizures should be 3.5–7 mEq/L (4.2–8.4 mg/dL), which can be achieved with intravenous administration of 4–6 g in bolus, followed by a maintenance dose of 1–2 g/h for 24 h after birth or the last convulsive episode [17]. Approximately 10% of patients will repeat another seizure after starting treat-

ment; it's advisable to administer an additional bolus of 2 g of magnesium sulfate [7]. It's of utmost importance to be alert of the development of a convulsive status and start its management quickly.
6. Pregnancy interruption. Once the patient is stable, if there is fetal viability we should start fetal heart rate monitoring and start pregnancy termination regardless of gestational age. This goal should be achieved as soon as possible. Eclampsia isn't an indication for cesarean delivery. The decision on the route of pregnancy termination should be based on obstetric indications and whether we have the favorable conditions to benefit a timely vaginal birth.

Once the initial measures have been established, if the patient has regained her mental status, we should perform a rigorous physical examination aimed at detecting possible complications secondary to the convulsive episode, such as maternal traumatic injuries. Non-invasive monitoring of maternal vital signs, including fetal heart rate and pulse oximetry, will provide evidence of other complications such as bronchoaspiration and abruptio placentae, especially when clinical expression isn't as florid.

If the hypertensive crisis has been overcomed (blood pressure ≤160/110), subsequent blood pressure measurements should be recorded every 10 min for an hour, then every 15 min for an hour, then every 30 min for an hour, and then every hour [28]. The same as measuring diuresis should be every hour.

We must obtain laboratory tests of the patient, to analyze their liver, kidney, and hematological function, glycemia, and electrolytes, to rule out other disorders that need to be treated immediately.

Magnesium sulfate intoxication is always a concern. Diuresis, patellar reflexes, and respiratory pattern should be monitored. Plasma levels of 8–10 mEq/L are enough to abolish the patellar reflex, and respiratory arrest occurs when reaching 13 mEq/L. We must have calcium gluconate and endotracheal intubation equipment available to respond to clinical suspicion of intoxication. The dose of 10% calcium gluconate is 1 g administered in bolus intravenously [12].

Considerations in the Management of the Convulsive Status

Convulsive status is an obstetric emergency that carries high maternal and fetal mortality [29]. Quick and proper management should be performed in the obstetric intensive care unit and aims to reduce the occurrence of possible maternal and fetal neurological sequelae. Initially, it's necessary to focus on maternal resuscitation. Once the mother is stable, if fetus is viable its indicated to start fetal monitoring.

In those patients who are refractory to initial treatment and who persist in convulsion, despite maintaining therapeutic doses of magnesium sulfate, endotracheal intubation and sedation is required. First thing we need to ensure is oxygen input by administering oxygen therapy enough to maintain adequate O2 saturation. If the patient is still pregnant, an O2 saturation >95% is necessary to ensure the correct fetal oxygenation [12]. Sedation can be achieved with midazolam administration (0.02–0.1 mg/kg/h), propofol (5–50 μg/kg/min, starts at 5 g/kg/min for 5 min and then increases at a dose of 5–10 g/kg/min every 5–10 min until the desired effect), or pentobarbital/thiopental (maintenance dose 1 mg/kg/h) [12, 30]. The patient's epileptic activity should be monitored by electroencephalography, and if it's necessary, antiepileptic medications such as phenytoin and levetiracetam should be administered.

It's necessary to keep in mind the physiological changes that involve convulsive status, which result mainly from the release of catecholamines into the systemic circulation, as well as from possible adverse effects of medication used. Close maternal hemodynamic monitoring is crucial. Termination of pregnancy in this scenario should be a cesarean delivery and it should be performed once we achieve maternal stability.

Neuroimaging studies performed to an eclamptic patient who has progressed to a convulsive status are indicated to rule out differential diagnoses that need to be treated, such as hemorrhage and brain herniation. While brain MRI gives us a better anatomical detail, the time and complexity of the study puts it at a disadvantage compared to computed tomography, which meets the needs of immediate urgency.

Long-Term Consequences of Eclampsia

According to the pathophysiology of eclampsia, a delay in the recognition and management of the disease could result in irreversible changes in maternal brain. The development of vasogenic brain edema with progressive pattern can eventually lead to cerebral ischemia and cytotoxic edema. This has been evident in neuroimaging studies conducted as a follow-up to these patients, where lesions have been observed in the white matter of the frontal, parietal, insular, and temporal lobe, mainly [31]. Neurological sequelae have been reported, such as permanent vision loss and long-term cognitive deficit [6].

The increased risk of cardiovascular disease has been known for several years in patients who have had preeclampsia/eclampsia. This is probably related to the hemodynamic changes these patients undergo that don't revert in the postpartum and are maintained after this period, such as increased peripheral vascular resistances and cardiac contractility dysfunction [32, 33].

Follow-up of complicated patients with preeclampsia/eclampsia is mandatory. Blood pressure monitoring is necessary until normalization, and some authors recommend cardiac function studies such as an echocardiogram at 6 and 12 months after pregnancy, where we can evaluate the ventricular function [32]. Little is known about the prevention of the hemodynamic impact of preeclampsia/eclampsia, so timely diagnosis and proper management are the best methods for decreasing cardiovascular risk.

Eclampsia is a complication of preeclampsia that has important immediate and long-term clinical implications. Timely diagnosis recognition and administration of anticonvulsant prophylaxis with magnesium sulfate is crucial. When the convulsive episode is associated with severe hypertension, it should be managed immediately to prevent exacerbation of brain injury. Knowing the pathophysiology of the disease, preeclampsia/eclampsia is a systemic and progressive disorder, and once the target organ damage is stablished, termination of pregnancy is necessary regardless of gestational age. Such interruption should be made in a timely manner as provided for maternal and fetal conditions. We must be prepared for the management of acute complications secondary to the grand mal seizure and for proper follow-up of the patient, in order to reduce the risk of long-term complications.

References

1. Braunthal S, Brateanu A. Hypertension in pregnancy: pathophysiology and treatment. SAGE Open Med. 2019;7:1–15.
2. Say L, Chou D, Tuncalp GA. Global causes of maternal death: a WHO systematic analysis. Lancet Glob Health. 2014;2:e323–33.
3. Poon LC, Hyett JA. The International Federation of Gynecology and Obstetrics (FIGO) initiative on pre-eclampsia: a pragmatic guide for first trimester screening and prevention. Int J Gynecol Obstet. 2019;145:1–33.
4. Cipolla MJ. Cerebrovascular function in pregnancy and eclampsia. Hypertension. 2007;50(1):14–24.
5. Sibai BM. Eclampsia. Am J Obstet Gynecol. 1990;163(3):1049–54.
6. Garg RK, Kumar N, Malhotra HS. Posterior reversible encephalopathy syndrome in eclampsia. Neurology. 2018;66:1316–23.
7. Sibai BM. Diagnosis, prevention and management of eclampsia. Obstet Gynecol. 2005;105(2):297–302.
8. Granger JP, Alexander BT, Bennet WA, et al. Pathophysiology of pregnancy induced hypertension. Am J Hypertens. 2001;14:178S–85S.
9. The Magpie Trial Collaborative Group. Do women with preeclampsia, and their babies, benefit from magnesium sulphate? The Magpie Trial: a randomised placebo controlled trial. Lancet. 2002;359:1877–90.
10. Douglas KA, Redman CW. Eclampsia in the United Kingdom. BMJ. 1994;309(6966):1395–400.
11. Cipolla MJ, Kraig RP. Seizure in women with preeclampsia: mechanisms and management. Fetal Mater Med. 2011;22(02):91–108.
12. Phelan JP, Pacheco LD, Foley MR. Critical care obstetrics. 6th ed. Hoboken: Wiley Blackwell; 2019.
13. Barnett Henry JM, Mohr JP, Bennet M, Stein Bennet M, Yatsu FM. Hypertensive encephalopathy. 3rd ed. New York: Stroke. Pathophysiology, Diagnosis and Management; 2019.
14. Matthiesen L, Berg G, Ernerudh J, Ekerfelt C, Jonsson Y, Sharma S. Immunology of preeclampsia. Chem Immunol Allergy. 2005;89:49–61.
15. Zambrano MD, Miller EC. Maternal stroke: an update. Curr Atheroscler Rep. 2019;21(9):33.
16. Mattar F, Sibai B. Eclampsia VIII Risk factors for maternal morbidity. Am J Obstet Gynecol. 2000;182(2):307–12.
17. American College of Obstetricians and Gynecologists. Task Force on Hypertension in pregnancy. Obstet Gynecol. 2013;122:1122–31.
18. American College of Obstetricians and Gynecologists. Practice bulletin No 202: gestational hypertension and preeclampsia. Obstet Gynecol. 2019;133:e1–e25.
19. Katz VL, Farmer R, Kuller JA. Preeclampsia into eclampsia: toward a new paradigm. Am J Obstet Gynecol. 2000;182(6):1389–96.

20. Sperling JD, Dahlke JD, Huber WJ, Sibai BM. The tole of headache in the classification and management of Hypertensive Disorder in Pregnancy. Obstet Gynecol. 2015;126(2):297–302.
21. MacGregor EA. Headache in pregnancy. Neurol Clin. 2012;30:835–66.
22. Thangaratinam S, Gallos I, Meah N, Usman S, Ismail K, Khan KS. TIPPS (Tests in prediction of preeclampsia's severity. Review Group). How accurate are maternal symptoms in predicting impending complications in women with preeclampsia? A systematic review and meta-analysis. Acta Obstet Gynecol Scand. 2011;90:564–73.
23. Wright WL. Neurologic complications in critically ill pregnant patients. Handb Clin Neurol. 2017;141:657–74.
24. Peracoli JC, VTM B, JGL R. Preeclampsia/Eclampsia. Rev Bras Ginecol Obstet. 2019;41(5):318–32.
25. Cantwell R, Clutton-Brock T, Cooper G, et al. Saving mothers' lives: reviewing maternal deaths to make motherhood safer: 2006–2008. The eighth report of the confidential enquiries into maternal deaths in the United Kingdom. BJOG. 2011;118(Suppl 1):1–203.
26. Euser AG, Cipolla MJ. Magnesium sulfate for the treatment of eclampsia: a brief review. Stroke. 2009;40:1169–75.
27. The Eclampsia Trial Collaborative Group. Which anticonvulsant for women with eclampsia? Evidence from the collaborative eclampsia trial. Lancet. 1995;345:1455–63.
28. American College of Obstetricians and Gynecologists. Committee Opinion No. 623. Emergent therapy for acute onset, severe hypertension during pregnancy and postpartum period. Obstet Gynecol. 2015;125:521–5.
29. RJ DL, HauserWA TAR, Boggs JG, Pellock JM, Penberthy L, et al. A prospective, population based epidemiology study of status epilepticus in Richmond, Virginia. Neurology. 1996;46:1029–35.
30. Shorvon S, Ferlisi M. The outcome of therapies in refractory and super-refractory convulsive status epilepticus and recommendations for therapy. Brain. 2012;135(8):2314–28.
31. Postma IR, Slager S, Kremer HPH, de Groot JC, Zeeman GG. Long-term consequences of the posterior reversible encephalopathy syndrome in eclampsia and preeclampsia: a review of the obstetric and nonobstetric literature. Obstet Gynecol Surv. 2014;69:287–300.
32. Timokhina E, Kuzmina T, Strizhakov A, Pitskhelauri E. Maternal cardiac function after normal delivery, preeclampsia and eclampsia: a prospective study. J Pregnancy. 2019;2019:1–8.
33. Bellamy L, Casas JP, Hingorani AD, Williams DJ. Pre-eclampsia and risk of cardiovascular disease and cancer in later life: systematic review and meta-analysis. Br Med J. 2007;335:974–86.

Chapter 4
HELLP Syndrome

Carlos Montufar

Introduction

In 1982, Weinstein described a "sub-group" of preeclamptic patients who collected a triad composed of hemolysis, elevated liver enzymes (hepatic dysfunction), and thrombocytopenia [1].

The interest of separating these patients from the rest of the preeclampsias was based on the higher rate of maternal and perinatal mortality and morbidity. There is a clear overlap between preeclampsia and HELLP syndrome, and it is unclear whether the latter is a primary or secondary disease process.

But the hematologic and hepatic abnormalities of three cases were described previously by Pritchard et al. in 1954 [2].

Chesley described the long-standing recognition that preeclampsia was associated with microthrombi and platelet consumption and that the overt development of a coagulopathy carried a poor prognosis [3].

Kitzmiller et al. identified significant thrombocytopenia in a group of patients with severe preeclampsia [4]. Weinstein began, with the description of his original 29 patients with HELLP, the process that has led him and others to provide a better understanding of the entity he named [1, 5].

Hemolysis

The decrease in the number of erythrocytes is secondary to the fragmentation of red cells, which is the result of (1) the weakening of the cell membrane by lipid

C. Montufar (✉)
Obstetrics Critical Care Unit, Fellowship Program of Critical Care Obstetrics, Complejo Hospitalario, Caja de Seguro Social, Panama City, Panama

C. Montufar et al. (eds.), *Obstetric Catastrophes*,
https://doi.org/10.1007/978-3-030-70034-8_4

peroxidation carried out by free radicals and (2) the presence of fibrin deposits that develop in the microvasculature, which facilitate the rupture of the erythrocyte [6, 7].

Liver Enzymes Elevation

Fibrin deposits at the vascular level can lead to an obstruction of the hepatic sinusoids, with consequent congestion and elevation of intrahepatic pressure, resulting in periportal necrosis and elevation of liver enzymes [8, 9].

Low Platelet Count

Platelets are activated as a result of endothelial damage. The presence of thromboxane A2 and serotonin lead to platelet agglutination in order to repair the sites of endothelial rupture of the entire microvasculature, with the consequent consumption.

Due to the platelet activation, the homeostatic mechanisms result in an increased number of released megakaryocytes circulating in the vessels, resulting in circulation of platelets with a shorter mean lifespan, since the "newly created" cells are adhered to the exposed collagen of the traumatized endothelium.

High Mortality and Complications

This group of patients, with HELLP syndrome, is associated with an increased risk of adverse maternal events, with serious complications such as cerebral hemorrhage and hepatic hematoma (liver rupture). There are other various life-threatening complications, such as placental abruption, pulmonary edema followed by acute respiratory distress, disseminated intravascular coagulation (DIC), cerebral hemorrhage, acute renal failure, and hepatic hemorrhage due to hepatic rupture [10].

Women with preeclampsia complicated by HELLP syndrome have an increased risk of adverse maternal events compared to women with preeclampsia alone. Risks of perinatal morbidity and mortality are also increased [11].

In a multicentric study, Haddad et al. [12] described 183 patients with HELLP syndrome. Adverse outcomes occurred in almost 40% of cases, and two women died.

In pregnancies complicated by HELLP syndrome, multiorgan system derangement can ensue, which can lead to produce acute renal impairment and third spacing of intravascular volume resulting in ascites and pleural effusion [13].

Also, postpartum hemorrhage, disseminated intravascular hemolysis (DIC), and transfusion of blood products are also more common in pregnancies complicated by

HELLP. Maternal death has traditionally been reported in up to 24% of cases of HELLP syndrome [13]. More recently, due to timely management, case-fatality rates have decreased.

HELLP syndrome complicates 0.2–0.8% of pregnancies and 12–20% of preeclampsia [14].

Despite this recent literature, the diagnosis, management, and pregnancy outcome of HELLP syndrome remain controversial.

Within the differential diagnosis of HELLP syndrome, we have thrombotic thrombocytopenic purpura, hemolytic uremic syndrome, and acute fatty liver of pregnancy. All are similar in the increase of liver enzymes, the presence of proteinuria, and the possibility of developing a kidney injury. The main differences are based on the severity of hypertension, fibrinogen levels, and the platelet count.

It is likely that the patient with HELLP syndrome will have a more severe liver dysfunction, potentially complicated by hepatic infarction or subcapsular hematoma [10].

The Sibai criteria [13] is the most widely accepted diagnostic criteria for HELLP syndrome; it is defined by all three of thrombocytopenia, hemolysis, and liver function derangement and is best at predicting those women at risk of serious morbidity and mortality.

Thrombocytopenia is defined as a platelet count less than 100,000/μL. Hemolysis is characterized by blood film changes (schistocytes, burr cells, or falling hemoglobin) or other markers of intravascular erythrocyte destruction including high reticulocyte count, elevated indirect bilirubin (>1.2 mg/dL), or low haptoglobin, coupled with an elevated lactate dehydrogenase (LDH) >600 IU/L [15].

Elevated transaminases may accompany other liver function derangement, but aspartate aminotransferase (AST) and/or alanine aminotransferase (ALT) derangement ≥70 U/L is diagnostic [15].

The diagnostic requires the presence of (1) microangiopathic hemolytic anemia with abnormal blood smear, low serum haptoglobin, and elevated LDH levels, (2) elevation of AST above 70 IU/L and LDH above 600 IU/L (both enzyme levels more than twice the upper limit of normal values) or bilirubin more than 1.2 mg/dL, and (3) a platelet count below 100, 000 mm^3 [15].

Clotting parameters, such as the prothrombin time, partial thromboplastin time, fibrinogen, and bleeding time, in the patient with HELLP syndrome are generally normal in the absence of abruptio placenta or fetal demise [16].

Clinical Features

The typical clinical characteristics are the development of the described triad of the syndrome, associated with a clinical scenario with findings of arterial hypertension as a criterion of preeclampsia.

A group of patients with HELLP syndrome do not meet the parameters of classical hypertension of preeclampsia. In one series of 112 women with severe preeclampsia–eclampsia complicated by HELLP syndrome, diastolic BP was less than 110 mmHg in 31% of cases and less than 90 mmHg in 15% at admission [17].

The majority of patients present with signs or symptoms of liver compromise. Patients may present with nonspecific symptoms, mostly nausea, vomiting, malaise/fatigue, and viral-like symptoms, as well as more specific ones, as mid-epigastric/right upper quadrant discomfort, blurred vision, altered consciousness, clonus, bleeding diathesis, and pulmonary edema, abdominal distension, and hypertension or hypovolemic shock [18]. In most series, hepatic or right upper quadrant tenderness to palpation is seen consistently in HELLP syndrome patients [5, 19].

The incidence of recurrent HELLP syndrome was 19–27%, and the recurrence of any form of preeclampsia–eclampsia was 42–43% [20].

Treatment

The management of patients with preeclampsia and HELLP syndrome is controversial. Most therapeutic modalities are similar to those applied for severe preeclampsia. What is certain is the decision to terminate the pregnancy by the most expeditious route. The mode of delivery should depend on the state of the cervix and other obstetric indications for cesarean birth. HELLP syndrome, by itself, is not an indication for cesarean delivery. At least half of patients with HELLP syndrome, however, will undergo operative delivery.

When the HELLP syndrome is diagnosed, clinically and by laboratory testing, the main priority is to assess and stabilize the woman's condition, especially coagulation dysfunction. Thereafter, fetal wellbeing should be evaluated by ultrasound biophysical profile, umbilical artery Doppler, and/or cardiotocography. Third, a decision needs to be made as to whether immediate delivery is indicated.

In severe cases, control of hypertension and immediate delivery, usually by caesarean section, is the treatment of choice. A woman with HELLP at a gestational age greater than 34 weeks should also be delivered immediately. Before 34 weeks, the woman should be delivered if her condition cannot be controlled rapidly.

Several clinical trials have been performed since 1994 because it was expected that corticosteroid therapy, primarily with dexamethasone, accelerates recovery after delivery.

However, the effect of dexamethasone therapy in cases of HELLP syndrome with less than 50,000mm^3 platelets is unclear [21, 22], although the evidence seems to indicate that it has no utility because it fails to reduce maternal mortality.

The Cochrane Database Systematic Review in 2010 also concluded that there was insufficient evidence to support the routine use of corticosteroids [23].

The patient must be transferred to a tertiary level center for their care, and if possible, be treated in an Intensive Care Unit either a Surgical Intensive Care Unit or a specific Unit of Critical Care Obstetric.

The patient with HELLP syndrome should receive her infusion of MgSO4 as prophylaxis for seizures, to avoid a neurological catastrophe (cerebral hemorrhage), as a result of the combination of eclampsia and thrombocytopenia [24].

Eclampsia associated with HELLP syndrome is a dangerous complication in a pregnant woman. Low platelet count (100,000 mm^3) secondary to HELLP syndrome and severe systolic hypertension can be associated with maternal mortality from eclampsia [24].

Similarly, in the presence of high blood pressure levels, antihypertensive drugs should be used for the management of hypertensive crises. The approved antihypertensive for this purpose are labetalol, nifedipine, and/or hydralazine as first-line drugs [25].

The administration of magnesium sulfate intravenously as a measure of prophylaxis against seizures is considered to be essential and should be administered at the same dose used in preeclampsia [26]. The patient should receive the proper medication of antihypertensive drugs, such as hydralazine, nifedipine, or labetalol, in order to stabilize blood pressure and prevent further cardiovascular and renal complications, which may lead to systematic dysfunction [25].

Platelet transfusion is indicated if there is significant maternal bleeding (spontaneous or from surgical incisions), or if the platelet count is less than 10,000 cells/μl. If caesarean delivery is planned, then some experts recommend platelet transfusion, as necessary, to achieve a preoperative platelet count greater than 40,000–50,000 cells/μl [27]. If it is necessary to perform a regional anesthetic block, it is necessary to reach a platelet level of 70,000–80,000 cells/μl [27].

The major life-threatening complications of HELLP syndrome are hepatic hemorrhage, subcapsular hematoma, liver rupture, and multiorgan failure. Liver hemorrhage is managed conservatively where possible with aggressive blood product resuscitation to reverse the coagulopathy and ensure adequate oxygen-carrying capacity. The development of a subcapsular hematoma may lead to hepatic rupture, which is potentially life-threatening for the mother and fetus.

Most authors and experts agree that the HELLP syndrome is not the appropriate scenario for expectant management in a pregnant patient, and the termination of pregnancy is suggested in the most expeditious manner.

The early identification of a patient with preeclampsia complicated with HELLP syndrome is crucial to carry out supportive and timely management, as well as the decision to terminate the pregnancy.

References

1. Weinstein L. Syndrome of hemolysis, elevated liver enzymes, and low platelet count: a severe consequence of hypertension in pregnancy. Am J Obstet Gynecol. 1982;142:159–67.
2. Pritchard JA, Weisman R, Ratnoff OD, Vosburgh GJ. Intravascular hemolysis, thrombocytopenia, and other hematologic abnormalities associated with severe toxemia of pregnancy. N Engl J Med. 1954;150:89–98.

3. Chesley L. Hypertensive disorders in pregnancy. 1st ed. New York: Appleton-Century-Crofts; 1978.
4. Kitzmiller JL, LangJE YPF, et al. Hematologic assays in pre-eclampsia. Am J Obstet Gynecol. 1974;118:362–7.
5. Weinstein L. Preeclampsia/eclampsia with hemolysis, elevated liver enzymes, and thrombocytopenia. Obstet Gynecol. 1985;66:657–60.
6. Doshi S, Zucker SD. Liver emergencies during pregnancy. Gastroenterol Clin N Am. 2003;32:1213–27.
7. Moake J. Thrombotic thrombocytopenia purpura (TTP) and other thrombotic microangiopathies. Best Practice and Research. Clin Hematol. 2009;22:567–76.
8. Baxter JK, Weinstein L. HELLP syndrome: the state of the art. Obstet Gynecol Surv. 2004;59:838–45.
9. Tsokos M, Longauer F, et al. Maternal death in pregnancy from HELLP syndrome. A report of three medico-legal autopsy cases with special reference to distinctive histopathological alterations. Int J Legal Med. 2002;116:50–3.
10. Barton JR, Sibai BM. Gastrointestinal complications of pre-eclampsia. Semin Perinatol. 2009;33:179–88.
11. Dötsch J, Hohmann M, Kühl P. Neonatal morbidity and mortality associated with maternal haemolysis elevated liver enzymes and low platelets syndrome. Eur J Pediatr. 1997;156(5):389–91.
12. Haddad B, Barton JR, Livingston JC, et al. Risk factors for adverse maternal outcomes among women with HELLP (hemolysis, elevated liver enzymes, and low platelet count) Syndrome. Am J Obstet Gynecol. 2000;183:444–8.
13. Sibai B. The HELLP syndrome (hemolysis, elevated liver enzymes, and low platelets): much ado about nothing? Am J Obstet Gynecol. 1990;162(2):311–6.
14. Sibai BM, Ramadan MK, Usta I, Salama M, Mercer BM, Friedman SA. Maternal morbidity and mortality in 442 pregnancies with hemolysis, elevated liver enzymes, and low platelets (HELLP syndrome). Am J Obstet Gynecol. 1993;169:1000–6.
15. Sibai B. Diagnosis, controversies, and management of the syndrome of hemolysis, elevated liver enzymes, and low platelet count. Obstet Gynecol. 2004;103(5 Part 1):981–91.
16. Sibai BM, Taslimi MM, et al. Maternal – perinatal outcome associated with the syndrome of hemolysis, elevated liver enzymes, and low platelets in severe preeclampsia – eclampsia. Am J Obstet Gynecol. 1986;155:501–9.
17. Sibai BM, Mercer B, Sarinoglu C. Severe preeclampsia in the second trimester: recurrence risk and long - term prognosis. Am J Obstet Gynecol. 1991;165:1408–12.
18. Thangaratinam S, Gallos ID, Meah N, Usman S, Ismail KM, Khan KS. How accurate are maternal symptoms in predicting impending complications in women with preeclampsia? A systematic review and meta-analysis. Acta Obstet Gynecol Scand. 2011;90:564–73.
19. MacKenna J, Dover NL, Brame RG. Preeclampsia associated with hemolysis, elevated liver enzymes, and low platelets: an obstetric emergency? Obstet Gynecol. 1983;62:751–4.
20. Sullivan CA, Magann EF, Perry KG, et al. The recurrence risk of the syndrome of hemolysis, elevated liver enzymes, and low platelets (HELLP) in subsequent gestations. Am J Obstet Gynecol. 1994;171:940–3.
21. Magann EF, Perry KG, Meydrech EF, Harris RL, Chauhan SP, Martin JN. Postpartum corticosteroids: accelerated recovery from the syndrome of hemolysis, elevated liver enzymes, and low platelets (HELLP). Am J Obstet Gynecol. 1994;171:1154–8.
22. Fonseca JE, Mendez F, Cataño C, Arias F. Dexamethasone treatment does not improve the outcome of women with HELLP syndrome: a double-blind, placebo-controlled, randomized clinical trial. Am J Obstet Gynecol. 2005;193:1591–8.
23. Woudstra DM, Chandra S, Hofmeyr GJ, Dowswell T. Corticosteroids for HELLP (hemolysis, elevated liver enzymes, low platelets) syndrome in pregnancy. Cochrane Database Syst Rev. 2010;9:CD008148.
24. Lucas MJ, Leveno KJ, Cunningham FG. A comparison of magnesium sulfate with phenytoin for the prevention of eclampsia. N Engl J Med. 1995;333(4):201–5.

25. ACOG Committee Opinion No. 767 summary: emergent therapy for acute-onset, severe hypertension during pregnancy and the postpartum period. Obstet Gynecol. 2019;133(2):409–12.
26. Altman D, Carroli G, Duley L, Farrell B, Moodley J, Neilson J, Smith D, Magpie Trial Collaboration Group. Do women with pre-eclampsia, and their babies, benefit from magnesium sulphate? The Magpie Trial: a randomized placebo-controlled trial. Lancet. 2002;359(9321):1877–90.
27. British Committee for Standards in Haematology, Blood Transfusion Task Force. Guidelines for the use of platelet transfusion. Br J Haematol. 2003;122:10–23.

Chapter 5
Acute Fatty Liver of Pregnancy

David B. Nelson, John J. Byrne, and F. Gary Cunningham

Introduction

Acute liver failure was first described in pregnancy by Tarnier in 1857 as microvesicular fatty infiltration of the liver [1]. Evidence regarding this link was further described by Lomer in 1884, at which time he described 30 cases of fatty liver during pregnancy at time of autopsy [2]. J. Whitridge Williams termed this *acute yellow atrophy* in the first edition of his textbook and stated that pregnancy appeared to be a predisposing factor [3]. Over the next few decades, there were sporadic case reports of women who died near term from acute liver failure with fatty infiltration; however, elucidation of its etiopathogenesis remained obscure [4].

Major progress in understanding the cause of acute liver failure in pregnancy was reported by Sheehan in 1940 [5]. At that time, he concluded that the majority of maternal deaths secondary to fatty liver were related to the common use of chloroform anesthesia which was popular from the mid-1800s through 1940. After excluding cases attributed to hepatotoxins, such as chloroform, and from infectious etiologies, he termed the remaining cases as *obstetric acute yellow atrophy*. During the late 1940s, however there were still case reports reviewing the difficulty of differentiation between end-stage hepatitis and acute fatty liver of pregnancy [6, 7]. But while fulminant viral hepatitis does have clinical similarities with acute fatty liver of pregnancy, the two appear to be distinctly different histologically [8].

In 1982, Burroughs and colleagues [9] described the clinicopathological findings of idiopathic fatty liver of pregnancy, more contemporaneously known as acute fatty liver of pregnancy (AFLP). They described 12 women who were admitted to the Liver Unit at the Royal Free Hospital in London. Importantly, none of these women

D. B. Nelson (✉) · J. J. Byrne · F. G. Cunningham
Department of Obstetrics and Gynecology, University of Texas Southwestern Medical Center, Parkland Health and Hospital Systems, Dallas, TX, USA
e-mail: DavidB.Nelson@utsouthwestern.edu; John.Byrne@utsouthwestern.edu; Gary.Cunningham@utsouthwestern.edu

C. Montufar et al. (eds.), *Obstetric Catastrophes*,
https://doi.org/10.1007/978-3-030-70034-8_5

had been exposed to chloroform, tetracycline, or other hepatotoxic agents. Indeed, the diagnosis in all but one case was biopsy proven. These investigators carefully characterized symptomatology, laboratory findings, light- and electron-microscopic histopathology, pregnancy outcomes, and complications. They reported that these women had characteristic clinical findings of acute liver failure to include encephalopathy and severe metabolic acidosis. The biopsy findings disclosed widespread microvesicular fat infiltration with swollen hepatocytes, minimal necrosis, and cholestasis. They also reported that acute kidney injury was common, and three women required dialysis. Another recognized manifestation was coagulopathy; however, it was reported as seldom clinically significant and infrequent. Common hematological findings included thrombocytopenia and hemolysis.

Epidemiology

The incidence of acute fatty liver of pregnancy varies depending on diagnostic criteria and population studied and ranges from 1 in 7000 to 1 in 20,000 pregnancies [10–13]. There does not appear to be geographic or ethnic differences in the severity or incidence of the disease; however there are limited population-specific data [14]. Although there are a few cases reported in the second trimester, most develop in the late third trimester [12, 15].

AFLP has a number of associated risk factors. Fetal acid oxidation disorders, multifetal gestation, and male fetuses all have been reported to predispose a woman to develop AFLP [12, 16, 17]. Lesser reported risk factors include metabolic disorders, obesity, and hepatic disorders such as intrahepatic cholestasis of pregnancy [12, 14, 18]. Preeclampsia syndrome is also a well-known association; however, cause-and-effect with AFLP are uncertain.

Pathophysiology

An important finding regarding the pathogenesis of fatty liver disease of pregnancy was provided by Reye and colleagues [19], who described a similar syndrome in children. Subsequent research suggested that microvesicular fatty hepatocyte infiltration was caused by deficiency of one or more of the mitochondrial fatty-acid oxidative enzymes or fetal fatty acid oxidation defects [20]. In this scheme, the fetal-placental unit metabolizes free fatty acids for growth and development during pregnancy, and the placenta contains enzymes involved in the fatty acid metabolism pathway. Placental enzymes metabolize triglycerides into free fatty acids which enter the fetal compartment. Because the products of this metabolism are transferred to the fetus, defects in the fatty acid oxidation pathway of the fetal-placental unit result in accumulation of intermediate products of fatty acids in the maternal circulation. These metabolites are taken up by the maternal liver along with reactive oxygen species that activate inflammatory processes and cause cellular hepatic necrosis [20, 21].

To date, there have been a number of mutations reported for genes that encode for enzymes in this pathway [21]. Of all of these oxidation disorders, maternal deficiency of long-chain 3-hydroxyacyl-CoA dehydrogenase (LCHAD) has been most strongly linked with pregnancy-associated fatty liver disease [22, 23]. Other, less common, fatty acid oxidation defects have been associated with AFLP, such as medium-chain acyl CoA dehydrogenase (MCAD) deficiency, very long-chain acyl-CoA dehydrogenase (VLCAD) deficiency, and carnitine palmitoyltransferase 1 (CPT1) deficiency [24, 25].

LCHAD deficiency is caused by a defect in the mitochondrial trifunctional protein along the inner mitochondrial membrane, specifically on the C-terminal protein of the alpha subunit. The most common defect seen in LCHAD deficiency is a 1528 G-to-C nucleotide change in exon 15 of the alpha subunit, which causes a change of glutamate-to-glutamine [26]. Because the third step in the oxidation of long-chain fatty acids is catalyzed by LCHAD, a buildup of intermediate products of metabolism is seen in individuals with LCHAD deficiency.

There are two proposed scenarios wherein accumulation of fatty acids and metabolites can accrue within the maternal compartment. In the first, a homozygous enzymatic defect is shared by the fetus and placenta. In the second, a heterozygous mother has decreased ability to perform fatty acid oxidation in late pregnancy. As seen in Fig. 5.1, homozygous enzymatic defects in the fetal-placental fatty acid oxidation pathway lead to an accumulation of fatty acid metabolites that are transferred to a heterozygous mother.

Clinical Presentation

The woman with acute fatty liver will typically present in late pregnancy with a variety of nonspecific symptoms, such as persistent anorexia, nausea, vomiting, and abdominal pain. Some will have findings of encephalopathy or polydipsia and polyuria [10, 12, 27]. Nelson and colleagues [10] described 51 women with AFLP who presented to Parkland Hospital at a mean gestational age of 37 weeks. Most of these had a variety of the symptoms mentioned above; however, approximately 10% were asymptomatic. Almost half of the women had associated hypertension, with or without proteinuria. In some of these women, these clinical findings progressed to liver failure with associated renal failure, coagulopathy, and hypoglycemia. Figure 5.2 demonstrates the spectrum of clinical consequence to this disorder.

Classically, the initial laboratory findings in AFLP depend on the degree of hepatic dysfunction. Some of these abnormalities include elevated levels of hepatic transaminases, creatinine, bilirubin, ammonia, and uric acid, along with hypoglycemia. There can also be associated coagulopathy [28]. This dysfunction can be profound and typically manifests as a prolonged prothrombin time and international normalized ratio (INR) with varying degrees of hypofibrinogenemia and elevated

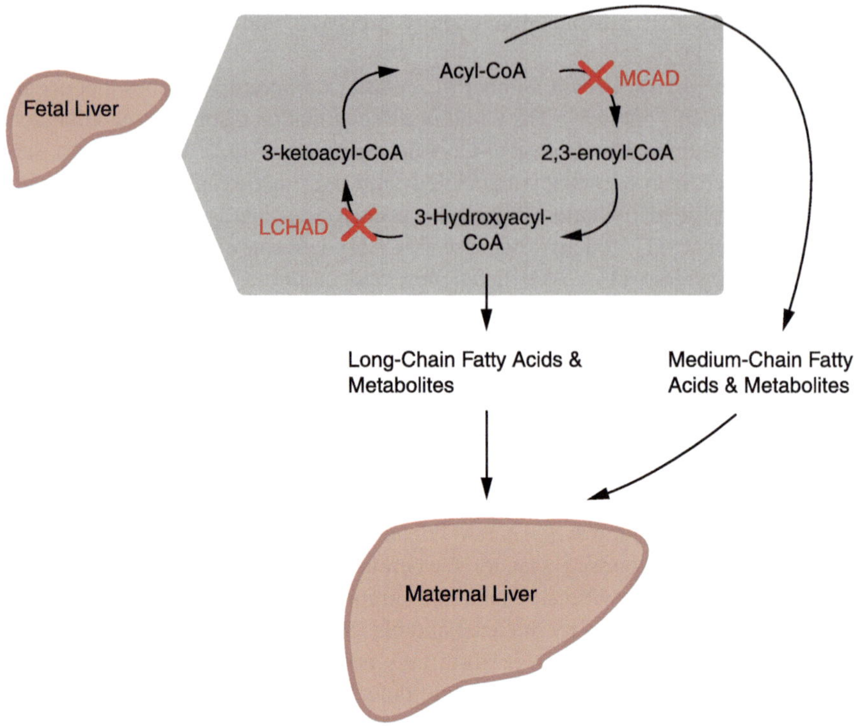

Fig. 5.1 Organ-specific effects of acute fatty liver of pregnancy. (Adapted from Nelson et al. [63])

D-dimer levels [10, 27–30]. There is also usually some degree of hypocholesterolemia concordant with hepatic dysfunction, and antithrombin III levels are also decreased [10, 31]. The peripheral smear shows echinocytosis caused by hypocholesterolemia [32], and there is typically a modest leukocytosis. Hemolysis with reticulocytosis and nucleated erythrocytes are also frequently seen [10].

Hemoconcentration is caused by endothelial cell activation with capillary leakage. There may be polycythemia, but with concomitant hemolysis, the hematocrit may be normal or even low. This "endotheliopathy" ultimately results in prerenal azotemia, compounding acute kidney injury. Intravascular volume depletion can be further intensified by associated ascites [33]. Hypovolemia combined with metabolic acidosis from liver injury can cause a reduction in uteroplacental perfusion that can have profound adverse fetal affects to include death.

Diagnosis

For clinical diagnosis, some recommend application of the Swansea criteria, as described by Ch'ng and colleagues (Table 5.1) [29]. These diagnostic criteria have since been validated by Knight and colleagues [12], and when six of these criteria are

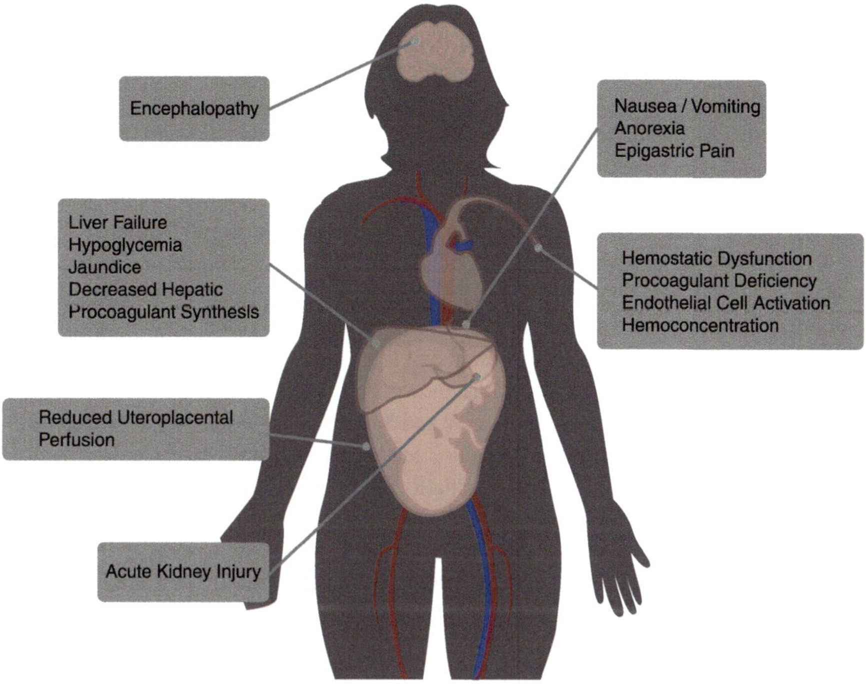

Fig. 5.2 Pathophysiology of acute fatty liver of pregnancy. The oxidation of long-chain fatty acids is catalyzed by long-chain 3-hydroxyacyl-CoA dehydrogenase (LCHAD) and medium-chain acyl CoA dehydrogenase (MCAD). When a homozygous enzymatic defect occurs in the fetal/placental fatty acid oxidation pathway, this leads to an accumulation of intermediate products of metabolism that are transferred to a heterozygous mother

Table 5.1 Diagnostic criteria using the Swansea criteria – six of these criteria satisfy the diagnosis of AFLP

Swansea criteria	Vomiting Encephalopathy Abdominal pain Ascites Polydipsia/polyuria Bilirubin >0.8 mg/dL Hypoglycemia <72 mg/dL White blood cell count >11 × 10^9/l Elevated urea >340 μmol/L ALT >42 U/L AKI or Cr >1.7 mg/dl Ammonia >47 μmol/L Coagulopathy or PT >14s Echogenic liver on ultrasound Microvesicular steatosis on liver biopsy

identified, the diagnosis of AFLP is suggested. These criteria are helpful because diagnosis may not be readily apparent, because of the previously described vague symptomatology. For the woman who presents with persistent nausea and vomiting, abdominal pain and jaundice and encephalopathy, the diagnosis is seemingly more straightforward. But for most women the differential diagnosis is wide. Specifically, AFLP is frequently confused with the more commonly associated obstetric conditions [34]. One of the most difficult conditions to distinguish is hemolysis, elevated liver enzymes, low platelets (HELLP) syndrome, which is considered an "imitator" [34].

To establish the diagnosis of AFLP, both clinical findings and laboratory evaluation are essential. Shown in Fig. 5.3 is a suggested testing algorithm. Initially, serum creatinine and hepatic transaminase levels are measured along with a hemogram with platelet quantification. With evidence of liver failure and laboratory abnormalities, these women should undergo further workup to differentiate between related disorders such as acetaminophen toxicity and hepatitis – as discussed in Differential Diagnosis. If abnormal laboratory values are identified, then targeted studies are performed including evaluation for hepatic function and disordered coagulation. Serum cholesterol and plasma fibrinogen levels can be a good measure of liver function. It is important to consider that both of these analytes are markedly influenced by the physiologic changes of normal pregnancy and increase substantially above nonpregnant values. Thus, these analytes can be dramatically abnormal when

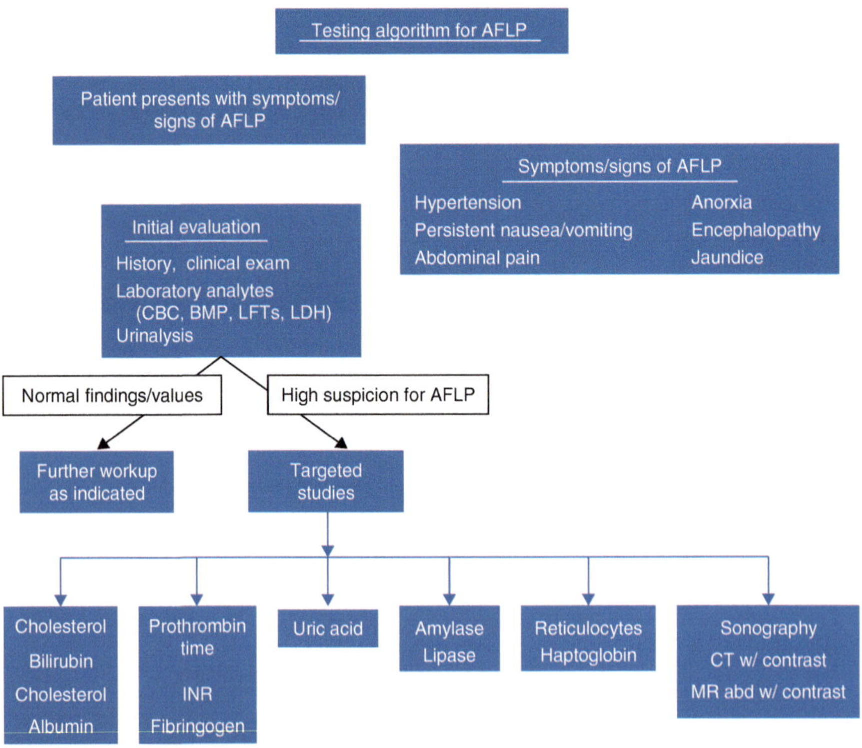

Fig. 5.3 Algorithm to identify acute fatty liver of pregnancy. (Adapted from Nelson et al. [63])

considered in the context of the third trimester of pregnancy. For example, plasma fibrinogen levels in nonpregnant women range from 233 to 496 mg/dL; however, in the third trimester these range between 373 and 619 mg/dL [35].

Although imaging studies are recommended by some [14], in our experience, these are of limited value in the diagnosis of AFLP [10]. For example, although sonographic findings are one element of the Swansea criteria, only a fourth of women had the classic ultrasound findings in a prospective evaluation [12]. Using computed tomography, sonography, and magnetic resonance imaging, Castro and colleagues [11] attempted to confirm the diagnosis; however, they were only able to do so in 30% of patients. The highest yield was 50% with computed tomography [11].

In the past, liver biopsy was considered necessary to confirm the diagnosis of AFLP; however, it is now accepted that it is not the case if characteristic clinical and laboratory findings are present. In women in whom the diagnosis is uncertain, liver biopsy may still be beneficial. As described by Sheehan, pathognomonic histopathologic findings include swollen hepatocytes with central nuclei along with microvesicular fatty infiltration of hepatocytes [5]. In some cases, fat droplets may not be easily identified on hematoxylin and eosin staining; thus a special *oil-red-O stain* must be performed on specimens [36].

Differential Diagnosis

A number of general as well as pregnancy-related disorders may initially be confused with AFLP. In addition to the HELLP syndrome already mentioned, consideration is given to viral hepatitis, acetaminophen toxicity, thrombotic microangiopathies, preeclampsia, and exacerbation of systemic lupus erythematosus [34]. HELLP syndrome is by far the most common disorder that may be mistaken for AFLP and vice versa. The two disorders are characterized by a constellation of similar symptoms and laboratory values; however, there are a number of significant – albeit sometimes subtle – differences. As initially reported by Vigil-de Gracia et al. [37], hepatic, renal, and hemostatic dysfunction is more severe in AFLP. Recent observations by Byrne and colleagues [38, 39] showed that women with AFLP were more likely than those with HELLP syndrome to have hypofibrinogemia, acute kidney injury, hyperbilirubinemia, hypoglycemia, and hypocholesterolemia at the time of admission (Table 5.2). Although initial management is similar and both conditions warrant delivery, the recovery and associated morbidity can be substantially different.

Management

Clinical management may vary because AFLP manifests as a spectrum from mild metabolic and coagulopathic disturbances to overt liver failure and hepatic encephalopathy. The cornerstone of management of AFLP includes (1) prompt recognition

Table 5.2 Most abnormal laboratory findings among women from Parkland Hospital with AFLP and HELLP syndrome

Analyte	AFLP $N = 67$	HELLP $N = 67$
Fibrinogen (mg/dL)	158 [87, 245]	422 [342, 482]
AST (U/L)	278 [146, 564]	135 [77, 250]
Creatinine (mg/dL)	2 [1, 2]	1 [1,1]
Cholesterol (mg/dL)	88 [70, 122]	168 [137, 227]
Total bilirubin (mg/dL)	5 [2, 8]	1 [1,2]
Platelets (/μL)	106,000 [57, 137]	44,000 [33, 63]
LDH (U/L)	512 [398, 865]	678 [530, 850]
Glucose (mg/dL)	88 [70, 122]	98 [137, 227]
White blood cell count ($\times 10^3/mm^3$)	23 [18, 28]	16 [13, 20]

Data are presented as median [Q_1, Q_3]
Data from Byrne et al. [37, 38]

and evaluation of mother and fetus; (2) plan for supportive care such as reversal of coagulopathy; (3) preparation for delivery as soon as feasible; (4) and postpartum supportive care. Until the fetus is delivered, it is thought that the ongoing liver failure will continue with its attendant constellation of abnormalities. After delivery, there is a slow return to metabolic normalcy that frequently requires considerable supportive care for days and even weeks.

Thus, the clinical course of women with AFLP may be characterized by subacute or acute changes in either the maternal or fetal condition. Therefore, women who present with symptoms concerning for AFLP should be admitted to the labor and delivery unit of a hospital with the ability to transition care to an intensive care unit [40]. While evaluating the maternal status, the fetus should undergo fetal heart rate monitoring. Given the proclivity for maternal lactic acidosis with diminished uteroplacental blood flow in the setting AFLP, fetal condition may be nonreassuring. Indeed, fetal jeopardy accounts for the high rate of cesarean delivery. Although the definitive treatment is delivery, AFLP, per se, is not an indication for cesarean delivery, and vaginal delivery is preferable considering the sometimes profound coagulopathy that accompanies the syndrome. In the setting of a vaginal delivery, care is taken to prevent vaginal trauma and lacerations – including episiotomy – given these bleeding risks.

A number of preparations are carried out quickly and as simultaneously as possible. Among these is consultation with anesthesiology colleagues. If the woman is obtunded, airway protection is paramount. Because of vomiting, consideration is given to a nasogastric tube with antacids to neutralize gastric contents. And for the woman with obvious hepatic encephalopathy, tracheal intubation should be considered. Two large-bore intravenous catheters are placed in anticipation of severe hemorrhage. As indicated above, continuous fetal monitoring is performed. Magnesium sulfate infusion is begun for neuroprophylaxis for those women who have evidence for preeclampsia which is seen in up to 70%. Finally, antihypertensive agents are given to treat dangerously high blood pressure levels [41].

Delivery

Although vaginal delivery is preferred, the majority of these women will undergo cesarean delivery because of the high incidence of nonreassuring fetal status associated with maternal acidosis and decreased blood volume due to the endotheliopathy. We prefer a midline skin incision because there is less subcutaneous bleeding than with a Pfannenstiel incision. Some prefer to use a drain such as a Blake or Jackson-Pratt device given the possibility of ascitic fluid and bleeding. At Parkland Hospital, routine draine placement is not our practice.

Given the high risk of coagulopathy at time of delivery, preparations need to be made regarding the potential for massive hemorrhage [42, 43]. Restoration of procoagulants and improvement of hypovolemia are integral especially if cesarean delivery is indicated. Because whole blood is not available in most institutions, resuscitation is done with packed red cells and fresh frozen plasma. Again, especially with operative delivery, maintenance of plasma fibrinogen levels >150 mg/dL is important [42]. Finally, platelet transfusions may be necessary if there is severe thrombocytopenia [43].

Analgesia and Anesthesia

The choice of analgesia depends on the degree of hepatic dysfunction and coagulopathy, especially with consideration for cerebral edema and intracranial hypertension [30]. Cited again is the high incidence of cesarean delivery. For the majority of women who have a limited coagulopathy and only moderate thrombocytopenia, it is reasonable to place neuraxial analgesia with the proviso that the nadir of some of the analytes, vis-à-vis platelets, may not recover until several days postpartum. In other cases, the use of general anesthesia may be necessitated by profound coagulopathy with severe thrombocytopenia, serious hemorrhage, or fetal compromise mandating emergency cesarean delivery.

Postpartum Course

After delivery, even though the AFLP pathophysiology begins to reverse, there will be continuation of the changes for periods up to 7–10 days. Because these women have a high incidence of postpartum hemorrhage, disseminated intravascular coagulopathy, acute renal failure, and gastrointestinal bleeding, continued care is necessary in an acute care unit [40]. Serial measurements of hematologic, hepatic, and renal function is performed every 6 h within the first 1–2 days [10]. Anemia is common from brisk hemolysis, and multiple transfusions are usually required. If there is a recent surgical incision, then clotting function is monitored and transfusion with fresh-frozen plasma, cryoprecipitate, or platelets may be indicated. Given the risk of hypoglycemia, serial blood glucose levels are monitored every 2–3 h, and if these are less than 60 mg/dL, then an infusion with 10% glucose is begun.

In most women, evidence of liver failure will begin to improve 2–3 days after delivery. Typically, hepatic transaminase values decline in a linear fashion to values at or below 100 IU/L after which values plateau for several weeks [10]. Other markers of liver failure, specifically total bilirubin and cholesterol levels, will start to improve after 3–4 days [44]. Acute kidney injury results from both prerenal and intrinsic pathology. The prerenal component can be seen in the swift decline in serum creatinine values after delivery, recovering to within a normal range within 7–10 days; however, the intrinsic kidney injury component is evidenced by the persistence of elevated serum creatinine for several weeks.

There are also two associated conditions that may be identified in the postpartum period – transient diabetes insipidus and acute pancreatitis. As many as a fourth of women develop diabetes insipidus, which is thought to be from elevated vasopressinase concentrations stemming from diminished hepatic production of its inactivating enzyme. Also, acute pancreatitis develops in up to 20% of the women [45].

More recently, postpartum artificial liver support therapy (ALST) has been described [46]. This includes plasma exchange which removes toxic metabolites, improves electrolyte management and acid-base balance, and supports coagulation factors [47, 48]. While plasmapheresis may result in an improvement of oxidative stress markers and hasten hepatic function recovery, there has not been an improvement in mortality [48, 49]. And although the data are limited, continuous renal replacement therapy (CRRT) along with plasma exchange has been shown to improve clinical symptoms and laboratory analyte recovery [50].

For the woman with persistent profound hepatic failure with hypotension and acidosis, liver transplantation must be considered [51]. Usually, the need for transplantation is typically later in the recovery period remote from delivery. Of the 51 women whom we previously described at Parkland Hospital, only two were considered candidates for transplantation. One woman died from intractable liver failure, and the other survived after a long hospital course with application of CRRT.

Experimental Treatment

One proposed treatment with possible benefits in AFLP is molecular absorbent recirculating system therapy [52, 53]. This system functionally replaces the liver in removing albumin-bound toxic metabolites from the blood via albumin dialysis, which results in stabilization of liver function and improvement in the hyperbilirubinemia. However, there has been no clear mortality benefit. This modality can be considered in patients with acute liver failure who are awaiting liver transplantation.

Maternal and Perinatal Outcomes

Since there has been broad acceptance for relatively uniform criteria for diagnosis, there are at least 10 reports that are listed in Table 5.3 and that include 18 or more pregnancies complicated by acute fatty liver [11, 27, 54–59]. The largest was a multicenter cohort study that identified 133 cases from four tertiary hospitals in China from January 2009 to April 2014 [59]. The single-center studies from Taiwan and California hospitals each reported an incidence of about 1:7000 deliveries in contrast to that of 1:20,000 from the UK nationwide audit [11, 12, 54]. It seems likely that these higher reported incidences result from regional referrals. Uniform to all 12 reports are three major causes of maternal morbidity and mortality, including various combinations and severities of liver failure, renal failure, and hemorrhage. These reports stress that delivery is necessary to reverse ongoing organ dysfunction, but also recognize that cesarean delivery is more likely performed because of associated fetal compromise and that operative delivery has more hemorrhagic complications.

These reports also cite maternal and perinatal survival rates that are much improved compared with earlier reports. In fact, maternal mortality rates in women with AFLP have improved dramatically over the last several decades. In the 1980s, the maternal mortality rate was as high as 80–90%, but this is now below 10% in the most recent literature [12, 59–61]. Many of these cases will trigger as a severe maternal morbidity ("SMM") event, given their increased risk of acute kidney injury, ICU admission, and need for blood and component transfusions. Early diagnosis, prompt delivery, and improved supportive care have led to this improvement in severe morbidity and mortality over time. Although maternal mortality rates have improved over the last several decades, perinatal mortality rates continue to remain substantively increased. As seen in Table 5.3, perinatal mortality over a 20-year period was about 20%. Furthermore, there is still substantive maternal morbidity.

Subsequent Pregnancy

Reports of AFLP recurrence in subsequent pregnancies are unusual [62]. In the setting of women who are heterozygous or carriers of the long chain 3-hydroxyacyconezyme A dehydrogenase mutation, the risk of recurrence is increased. This is contingent upon the fetus being affected during that subsequent pregnancy. If a woman has developed AFLP in a previous pregnancy, it is prudent to screen the fetus for fatty acid oxidation disorder, specifically LCHAD deficiency. At this time, there have only been case reports of recurrent AFLP outside of this proposed pathogenesis [16].

Disclosure Statement The authors report no conflict of interest.

Table 5.3 Selected maternal and perinatal outcomes in women with acute fatty liver of pregnancy

		Diagnosis		Liver failure	Renal failure[a]	Coagulopathy	CD rate	Maternal	Perinatal
Investigator	N	AP	PP	(encephalopathy)				deaths	deaths[b]
Castro (1999) Los Angeles	28	10	18	21%	NS	100%	50%	0	2/30
Knight (2008) UK	57	42	15	9%	14%	52%	74%	1	7/67
Lau (2010) Taipei, Taiwan	18	6	12	11%	83%	61%	72%	2	3/22
Vigil-De Gracia (2011) Panama	35	NS	NS	40%	94%	77%	89%	4	4/39
Mellouli (2012) Tunisia	19	19	0	11%	63%	58%	79%	2	4/22
Nelson (2013) Dallas	51	NS	NS	16%	4%	80%	49%	2	7/58
Cheng (2014) China	32	NS	NS	53%	81%	16%	69%	14	8/41
Zhang (2016) China	56	NS	NS	20%	39%	54%	80%	4	10/61
Gao (2018) China	133	120	13	33%	10%	86%	85%	22	36/161
Ilham (2019) Indonesia	18	16	2	61%	83%	72%	50%	12	11/19
Estimated average	*447*						*298/447 (67%)*	*63/447 (14%)*	*92/520 (18%)*[c]

AP antepartum, *NS* not stated, *PP* postpartum
Adapted from Nelson et al. [63]
[a]Renal failure is variably defined
[b]Fetal demise or neonatal death <28 days
[c]Total 520 includes 92 multifetal pregnancies

References

1. Tarnier. Note sur l'etat graisseux du foie dans la fievre peurperale. C R Soc Biol. 1857;3:209–14.
2. Lomer O. Ueber die Bedeutung des Icterus gravidarum, etc. Zeitschr f Geb u Gyn. 1886;xiii:169–85.
3. Williams JW. Obstetrics: a textbook for students and practitioners. London: D Appelton and Company; 1903. p. 444.
4. Stander H, Cadden B. Acute yellow atrophy of the liver in pregnancy. Am J Obstet Gynecol. 1934;28:61–9.
5. Sheehan HL. The pathology of acute yellow atrophy and delayed chloroform poisoning. J Obstet Gynecol. 1940;47:49–62.
6. Lucke B. the pathology of fatal epidemic hepatitis. Am J Pathol. 1944;20:471–593.
7. Zondek B, Bromberg YM. Infectious hepatitis in pregnancy. J Mt Sinai Hosp N Y. 1947;14:222–43.
8. Sherlock S. Acute fatty liver of pregnancy and the microvesicular fat diseases. Gut. 1983;24:265–9.
9. Burroughs AK, Seong NH, Dojcinov DM, et al. Idiopathic acute fatty liver of pregnancy in 12 patients. Q J Med. 1982;51:481–97.
10. Nelson DB, Yost NP, Cunningham FG. Acute fatty liver of pregnancy: clinical outcomes and expected duration of recovery. Am J Obstet Gynecol. 2013;209:456, e1–7.
11. Castro MA, Fassett MJ, Reynolds TB, et al. Reversible peripartum liver failure: a new perspective on the diagnosis, treatment, and cause of acute fatty liver of pregnancy, based on 28 consecutive cases. Am J Obstet Gynecol. 1999;18:389–95.
12. Knight M, Nelson-Piercy C, Kurinczuk JJ, et al. A prospective national study of acute fatty liver of pregnancy in the UK. Gut. 2008;57:951–6.
13. Reyes H, Sandoval L, Wainstein A, et al. Acute fatty liver of pregnancy: a clinical study of 12 episodes in 11 patients. Gut. 1994;35:101–6.
14. Lui J, Ghaziani TT, Wolf JL. Acute fatty liver disease of pregnancy: updates in pathogenesis, diagnosis, and management. Am J Gastroenterol. 2017;112:838–46.
15. Monga M, Katz AR. Acute fatty liver in the second trimester. Obstet Gynecol. 1999;93:811–3.
16. Bacq Y. Liver disease unique to pregnancy: a 2010 update. Clin Res Hepatol Gastroenterol. 2011;35:182–93.
17. Davidson KM, Simpson LL, Knox TA, et al. Acute fatty liver of pregnancy in triplet gestation. Obstet Gynecol. 1998;91:806–8.
18. Chen H, Yuan L, Tan J, et al. Severe liver disease in pregnancy. Int J Gynaecol Obstet. 2008;101:277–80.
19. Reye RD, Morgan G, Baral J. Encephalopathy and fatty degeneration of the viscera. A disease entity in childhood. Lancet. 1963;2:749–52.
20. Strauss AW, Bennett MJ, Rinaldo P, et al. Inherited long –chain 3-hydroxyacyl-CoA dehydrogenase deficiency and a fetal-maternal interaction cause maternal liver disease and other pregnancy complications. Semin Perinatol. 1999;23:100–12.
21. Browning MF, Levy HL, Wilkins-Haug LE, et al. Fetal fatty acid oxidation defects and maternal liver disease in pregnancy. Obstet Gynecol. 2006;107:115–20.
22. Ibdah JA, Bennett MJ, Rinaldo P, et al. A fetal fatty-acid oxidation disorder as a cause of liver disease in pregnant women. N Engl J Med. 1999;340:1723–31.
23. Tyni T, Ekholm E, Pihko H. Pregnancy complications are frequent in long-chain 3-hydroxyacyl-coenzyme A dehydrogenase deficiency. Am J Obstet Gynecol. 1998;178:603–8.
24. Santos L, Patterson A, Moreea SM, et al. Acute liver failure in pregnancy associated with maternal MCAD deficiency. J Inhert Metab Dis. 2007;30:103.
25. Ylitalo K, Vanttinen T, Halmesmaki E, et al. Serious pregnancy complications in a patient with previously undiagnosed carnitine palmitoyltransferase 1 deficiency. Am J Obstet Gynecol. 2005;193:2060–2.

26. Sims HF, Brackett JC, Powell CK, et al. The molecular basis of pediatric long chain 3-hydroxyacyl-Co-A dehydrogenase deficiency associated with maternal acute fatty liver of pregnancy. Proc Natl Acad Sci U S A. 1995;92:841–5.
27. Vigil-de Gracia P, Montufar-Rueda C. Acute fatty liver of pregnancy: diagnosis, treatment, and outcome based on 35 consecutive cases. J Matern Fetal Neonatal Med. 2011;24:1143–6.
28. Nelson DB, Yost NP, Cunningham FG. Hemostatic dysfunction with acute fatty liver of pregnancy. Obstet Gynecol. 2014;124:40–6.
29. Ch'ng CL, Morgan M, Hainsworth I, et al. Prospective study of liver dysfunction in pregnancy in Southwester Wales. Gut. 2002;51:876–80.
30. Naoum EE, Leffert LR, Chitilian HV, et al. Acute fatty liver of pregnancy. Anesthesiology. 2019;130:446–61.
31. Kerr R, Newsome P, Germain L, et al. Effects of acute liver injury on blood coagulation. J Thromb Haemost. 2003;1:754–9.
32. Cunningham FG, Lowe T, Guss S, et al. Erythrocyte morphology in women with severe preeclampsia and eclampsia. Preliminary observations with scanning electron microscopy. Am J Obstet Gynecol. 1985;153:358–63.
33. Bernal W, Wendon J. Acute liver failure. N Engl J Med. 2013;369:2525–34.
34. Sibai BM. Imitators of severe preeclampsia. Obstet Gyncol. 2007;109:956–66.
35. Abbassi-Ghanavati M, Greer LG, Cunningham FG. Pregnancy and laboratory studies: a reference table for clinicians. Obstet Gynecol. 2009;114:1326–31.
36. Mabie WC. Acute fatty liver of pregnancy. Crit Care Clin. 1991;7:799–808.
37. Vigil-De Gracia P. Acute fatty liver and HELLP syndrome: two distinct pregnancy disorders. Int J Gynecol Obstet. 2001;73:215–20.
38. Byrne JJ, Seasely A, McIntire DD, Nelson DB, Cunningham FG. Pragmatic acute fatty liver of pregnancy and HELLP syndrome on admission. Am J Obstet Gynecol. 2019;220:863.
39. Byrne JJ, Seasely A, McIntire DD, Nelson DB, Cunningham FG. AFLP versus HELLP syndrome: pregnancy outcomes and recovery. Am J Obstet Gynecol. 2019;220:563.
40. ACOG Practice Bulletin No. 211: Critical care in Pregnancy. Obstet Gynecol. 2019;133:e303–19.
41. American College of Obstetricians and Gynecologists: Hypertension in pregnancy. Report of the American college of obstetricians and gynecologists' task force on hypertension in pregnancy. Obstet Gynecol. 2013;122:1122–31.
42. Alexander JM, Sarode R, McIntire DD, et al. Use of whole blood in the management of hypovolemia due to obstetric hemorrhage. Obstet Gynecol. 2009;113:1320–6.
43. Kenny L, McCrae K, Cunningham FG. Platelets, coagulation, and the liver. In: Taylor R, Roberts JM, Cunningham FG, editors. Chesley's hypertension in pregnancy. 4th ed. Amsterdam: Academic Press; 2015.
44. Rolfes DB, Ishak KG. Acute fatty liver of pregnancy: a clinicopathologic study of 35 cases. Hepatology. 1985;5:1149–58.
45. Moldenhauer JS, O'brien JM, Barton JR, et al. Acute fatty liver of pregnancy with pancreatitis: a life-threatening complication. Am J Obstet Gynecol. 2004;190:502–5.
46. Wu Z, Huang P, Gong Y, et al. Treating acute fatty liver of pregnancy with artificial liver support therapy: systematic review. Medicine (Baltimore). 2018;97:e12473. https://doi.org/10.1097/MD.0000000000012473.
47. Martin JN, Briery NM, Rose CH, et al. Postpartum plasma exchange as adjunctive therapy for severe acute fatty liver of pregnancy. J Clin Apher. 2008;47:113–5.
48. Yu CB, Chen JJ, Du WB, et al. Effects of plasma exchange combined with continuous renal replacement therapy on acute fatty liver of pregnancy. Hepatobiliary Pancreat Dis Int. 2014;13:179–83.
49. Tang W, Huang Z, Wang Y, et al. Effect of plasma exchange on hepatocyte oxidative stress, mitochondria function, and apoptosis in patients with acute fatty liver of pregnancy. Artif Organs. 2012;36:E39–47.

50. Ding J, Han LP, Lou XP, et al. Effectiveness of combining plasma exchange with plasma perfusion in acute fatty liver of pregnancy: a retrospective analysis. Gynecol Obstet Investig. 2015;79:97–100.
51. Kushner T, Tholey D, Dodge J, et al. Outcomes of liver transplantation for acute fatty liver disease of pregnancy. Am J Transplant. 2019;19:2101–7.
52. de Naeyer S, Ysebaert D, van Utterbeeck M, et al. Acute fatty liver of pregnancy and molecular absorbent recirculating system (MARS)- therapy: a case report. J Matern Fetal Neonatal Med. 2008;21:587–9.
53. Saliba F. The molecular absorbent recirculating system (MARS) in the intensive care unit: a rescue therapy for patients with hepatic failure. Crit Care. 2006;10:118.
54. Lau HH, Chen YY, Huang JP, et al. Acute fatty liver of pregnancy in a Taiwanese tertiary care center: a retrospective review. Taiwan J Obstet Gynecol. 2010;49:156–9.
55. Mellouli MM, Amara FB, Maghrebi H, et al. Acute fatty liver of pregnancy over a 10-year period at a Tunisian tertiary care center. Int J Gynaecol Obstet. 2012;117:88–9.
56. Cheng N, Xiang T, Wu X, et al. Acute fatty liver of pregnancy: a retrospective study of 32 cases in South China. J Matern Fetal Neonatal Med. 2014;27:1693–7.
57. Zhang YP, Kong WQ, Zhou SP, et al. Acute fatty liver of pregnancy: a retrospective analysis of 56 cases. Chin Med J. 2016;129:1208–14.
58. Aldika Akbar MI, Mayang Sari I, Aditiawarman DEG, Dekker G. Clinical characteristics of acute fatty liver of pregnancy in a tertiary Indonesian hospital. J Matern Fetal Neonatal Med. 2019;32:826–32.
59. Gao Q, Qu X, Chen X, et al. Outcomes and risk factors of patients with acute fatty liver of pregnancy: a multicenter retrospective study. Singap Med J. 2018;59:425–30.
60. Varner M, Rinderknecht NK. Acute fatty metamorphosis of pregnancy. A maternal mortality and literature review. J Reprod Med. 1980;24:177–80.
61. den Boer ME, Wanders RJ, Morris AA, et al. Long-chain 3-hydroxyacyl-CoA dehydrogenase deficiency: clinical presentation and follow-up of 50 patients. Pediatrics. 2002;109:99–104.
62. Usta IM, Barton JR, Amon EA, et al. Acute fatty liver of pregnancy: an experience in diagnosis and management of fourteen cases. Am J Obstet Gynecol. 1994;171:1342–7.
63. Nelson DB, Byrne JJ, Cunningham FG. Acute fatty liver of pregnancy. Clin Obstet Gynecol. 2020;63(1):152–64.

Chapter 6
Liver Failure and Hepatic Encephalopathy in Pregnancy

Devang K. Sanghavi, Rebecca C. Burnside, Ronald G. Racho, Hassan Z. Baig, and Pablo Moreno Franco

Introduction

Liver disease in pregnancy presents a challenging proposition as effects of liver dysfunction impact both maternal and fetal mortality and morbidity. The causes of liver disease in pregnancy can be classified into two types: the first type is conditions which are unique to pregnancy such as HELLP (hemolysis, elevated liver enzymes, low platelets) syndrome, preeclampsia, acute fatty liver of the pregnancy, etc. The second type of liver disease in pregnancy is coincidental liver disorders and is not unique to pregnancy. The occurrences of this match the epidemiology of the general population. Pregnancy-related liver disease usually occurs around the third trimester of pregnancy. In this chapter we will discuss hepatic encephalopathy, acute liver failure in pregnancy, and extracorporeal liver support during acute liver failure.

D. K. Sanghavi · R. C. Burnside · H. Z. Baig
Department of Critical Care Medicine, Mayo Clinic, Jacksonville, FL, USA
e-mail: Sanghavi.Devang@mayo.edu; Burnside.Rebecca@mayo.edu; Baig.Hassan@mayo.edu

R. G. Racho
Department of Transplant, Mayo Clinic, Jacksonville, FL, USA
e-mail: Racho.Ronald@mayo.edu

P. M. Franco (✉)
Department of Critical Care Medicine, Mayo Clinic, Jacksonville, FL, USA

Department of Transplant, Mayo Clinic, Jacksonville, FL, USA
e-mail: MorenoFranco.Pablo@mayo.edu

C. Montufar et al. (eds.), *Obstetric Catastrophes*,
https://doi.org/10.1007/978-3-030-70034-8_6

Normal Liver Function in Pregnancy

The normal blood flow to the liver is around 25–33% of the cardiac output. This is essentially unchanged during pregnancy. Pregnancy does not induce hepatomegaly, and any hepatomegaly seen in pregnancy should be promptly evaluated. One potential confounder is that during pregnancy the gravid uterus increases in size and the liver is pushed upward toward the diaphragm. Liver enzymes are usually normal if there is a slight decline seen in their levels. Alkaline phosphatase increases with the advancing gestation.

Hepatic Encephalopathy

Alteration in cognitive function is a hallmark feature of liver failure. This entity has traditionally been referred to as hepatic encephalopathy (HE). Precisely defining this condition has proven to be difficult due to variability in its presentation and course. Potential symptoms range from mild cognitive impairment, unrecognizable by standard physical exam, to cerebral edema, coma, and even death. The acuity of symptoms and prognosis differs depending on whether HE is a product of acute liver failure (ALF) or chronic liver disease (CLD). For patients with liver disease in pregnancy, HE is more likely to be an acute process. Not only do pregnant patients carry the same risk for developing acute liver failure as the general population, but they also are at risk for pregnancy-specific causes of ALF. HE as a complication of CLD is less likely in pregnancy as CLD leads to a reduced ability to conceive [1].

The identification of HE is of utmost importance due to the associated prognostic implications. In patients with ALF, intracranial hypertension and brain herniation are the leading causes of mortality [2]. In patients with CLD, onset of HE marks a predicted mortality of more than 50% within the following 12 months [3].

Evaluation of HE should be focused on rapid identification of associated end organ damage along with an exhaustive search for precipitating factors. Appropriate triage to specialized centers and higher level of care is often necessary.

Epidemiology

A. Acute Liver Failure

Very limited information exists regarding the epidemiology of ALF. One study looking at the burden of hepatic encephalopathy in the United States (US) between 2010 and 2014 showed that approximately 4% of treated cases of HE could be attributed to ALF [4].

B. Chronic Liver Disease

Cirrhosis is scarring in the liver that over time replaces healthy tissue. Cirrhosis is a CLD that eventually leads to liver failure. At the time of diagnosis of cirrhosis, approximately 10–14% of individuals are found to have obvious symptoms of HE. In patients who undergo transjugular intrahepatic portosystemic shunt (TIPS), HE can be identified in as many as 50% of patients. Following an episode of HE, a patient's risk for recurrent episodes increases and the time to a next episode decreases. HE related to CLD accounted for approximately 110,000 hospitalizations between 2005 and 2009 in the United States [5].

Pathogenesis

Pathogenesis of HE remains only partially understood. There have been multiple coexisting mechanisms that have been described, and there is variability depending on underlying etiology of liver dysfunction. The proposed mechanisms leading to HE are summarized in Table 6.1.

A. Toxins

In most cases, the accumulation of toxins has been implicated in the central nervous system dysfunction and injury related to HE. Specifically, ammonia has been the topic of much discussion and research as well as the target of most accepted

Table 6.1 Implicated processes of CNS injury in liver failure

Category		Proposed mechanism
Toxins	Ammonia	Decreased clearance by the liver Increased portosystemic shunting Astrocyte alteration – see below
	Glutamine	Increased synthesis through combination of ammonia and glutamate Osmolyte leading to cerebral edema
	Lactate	Increased intracranial hypertension and cellular swelling Increase activation of microglia – see below
Cellular alterations	Astrocyte	Cellular swelling secondary to ammonia and lactate accumulation Impaired gene coding for structural proteins, neurotransmitter transporters, and receptors
	Microglia	Activation by increased levels of lactate leads to release of pro-inflammatory cytokines – see below
Pro-inflammatory state	Bacteria	Dysregulation of the blood-brain barrier leading to vasogenic edema Increased production in endogenous benzodiazepines leading to GABA receptor activation and neuro-inhibition
	Cytokines (IL-1b, IL-6)	Increased permeability of the blood-brain barrier Increased diffusion of ammonia into astrocytes

therapies for HE. During digestion, protein is broken down by colonic bacteria and gut enzymes. This process produces ammonia, which is transported through the portal circulation to the liver for participation in the urea cycle. In the setting of liver failure, less detoxification by the liver leads to ammonia accumulation and shunting of ammonia directly into the systemic circulation.

In normal physiology, ammonia is removed from the central nervous system (CNS) through the function of astrocytes. Astrocytes are the sole location of glutamine synthetase, which is able to synthetize glutamine from a combination of glutamate and ammonia. In liver failure, the increased ammonia crosses the blood-brain barrier, which in turn leads to a larger amount of glutamine synthesis within the CNS. One proposed mechanism for the development of cerebral edema is that the increased CNS glutamine acts as an osmolyte and increases cerebral volume. In the setting of ALF and infection, there has been evidence that the blood-brain barrier can be altered leading to an acceleration of edema through vasogenic injury as well [2].

In addition to hyperammonemia and elevation in glutamine, there is also evidence that increased lactate accumulation in the CNS has downstream negative effects. Increases in lactate concentration have been correlated with worsening neurological status, intracranial hypertension, and astrocyte swelling in animal models [2].

B. Cellular Alterations

There have been multiple other actions of ammonia in the CNS that have been identified: excitatory and inhibitory neurotransmission, stimulation of glycolysis, inhibition of pyruvate oxidation, and altered mitochondrial function [2]. Overall, these effects have been referred to as brain energy failure.

When weighing the impact of ammonia and glutamine accumulation, it has been proposed that the more injurious is ammonia. Glutamine accumulates within the cytoplasm but is transported into the mitochondria and converted back to glutamate and ammonia by glutaminase. The proposition that accumulation of glutamine is a benign intermediate has led to description of this process as the "Trojan Horse Hypothesis."

Hyperammonemia has also been linked to alterations in gene expression for astrocytic proteins. Identified genes code for structural proteins of astrocytes (glial fibrillary acidic protein or GFAP), key amino acid neurotransmitter transporters (EAAT-2, GLYT-1, SNAT-3, and SNAT-5), and receptors (translocator protein or TLP.) [6].

In CLD, exposure to chronically elevated levels of ammonia in the CNS has been linked to downregulation of glutamate receptors and development of Alzheimer type II astrocytosis [7].

C. Pro-inflammatory State

In ALF, increased lactate in the CNS has been linked to microglia activation and release of various cytokines, such as TNFα, IL-1b, and IL-6, which also suggests a pro-inflammatory response [2].

It seems that in CLD, states of increased inflammation, such as GI bleeding or infections, contribute to an increased likelihood of HE. This systemic inflammation triggers the previously described pro-inflammatory response. Increased levels of CRP, IL-6, and white blood cells have been correlated with the development of HE [7]. Steroids synthesized within the CNS have been discovered and termed "neurosteroids." These neurosteroids have been shown to act as neurotransmitters and have been implicated in development of HE through their action on GABA receptors. GABA receptors are inhibitory receptors and have been shown to be upregulated in the setting of HE. Both exogenous benzodiazepines and endogenous benzodiazepines have action on GABA receptors. Increased endogenous benzodiazepines are produced by certain bacteria and can lead to activation of GABA receptors and contribute to HE [7].

Diagnosis, Methods of Classification, and Grading Severity

There is no single exam finding, laboratory test, or imaging study that can unilaterally lead to diagnosis of HE. The diagnosis remains one that requires an appropriate clinical context and is a diagnosis of exclusion.

A. Ammonia Level

A major focus of laboratory investigations has been measurement of ammonia levels within the blood. There has not been consistent correlation demonstrated between ammonia level and severity or likelihood of HE. One study by *Ong* et al. published in *The American Journal of Medicine* in 2003 showed a strong overall correlation ($r = 0.61$, $p < 0.001$) between ammonia levels and severity of HE. However, results also demonstrated a large degree of overlap between different grades of HE and absolute values of ammonia levels. Based on these results ammonia levels can suggest the presence of HE in the correct clinical context and can be a useful marker to guide treatment response. However, a dichotomous grading system for HE based on the level of serum ammonia alone has not been established [8]. While the level of ammonia in isolation cannot definitively diagnose HE, there have been studies showing correlation between the level of ammonia and prognosis in HE, which are outlined later in the chapter.

B. Methods of Classification

There are multiple grading classification systems currently used to describe HE. Approaches include descriptors for (1) underlying disease, (2) time course, (3) symptoms at presentation, and (4) precipitating factors.

(a) Based on criteria from the 11th World Congress of Gastroenterology [9], HE should be defined based on the underlying disease state:

  (i) Type A hepatic encephalopathy: acute liver failure
  (ii) Type B hepatic encephalopathy: portosystemic shunt without intrinsic liver disease

(iii) Type C hepatic encephalopathy: cirrhosis with portosystemic shunt or portal hypertension, which can be further subclassified based on time course: [5]

1. Episodic
   (a) First occurrence or recurrence
   (b) Spontaneous or related to precipitating factors
2. Persistent

(b) West Haven Criteria (WHC)
The WHC is the most recognized form of symptom classification of HE in cirrhotic patients. This system classifies HE into discrete grades 0–IV based on symptoms [10].

(c) International Society for Hepatic Encephalopathy and Nitrogen Metabolism (ISHEN)
The most recent consensus established by the ISHEN focused on classifying the degree of impairment as a continuum rather than categorically. This classification system defines the presentation of HE as a continuum ranging from very mild changes in cognition to coma and potentially even death from herniation in the most severe cases [7, 11] (Fig. 6.1). This is described as covert hepatic encephalopathy (CHE) or overt hepatic encephalopathy (OHE). The ISHEN has defined CHE as the presence of neuropsychometric/neurophysiological abnormalities in the absence of disorientation and asterixis [11]. In cases of CHE, there are various proposed tools to identify deficits that may not be readily apparent by tradition history and physical exam [12]. Some of the available tools are listed in Table 6.2. It is recommended that CHE is confirmed with at least two different neuropsychometric or neurophysiologic assessments [7]. CHE is a topic under much investigation in the setting of CLD, but is poorly understood as a feature of ALF at the present time.

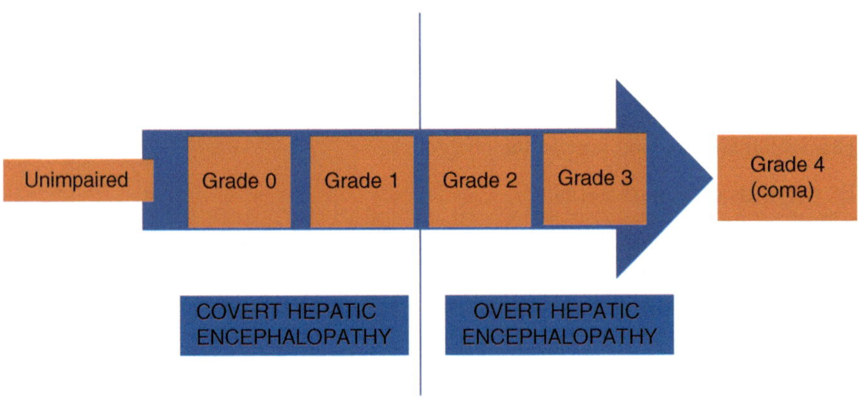

Fig. 6.1 ISHEN classification of hepatic encephalopathy (covert and overt) and West Haven Criteria (Grades 0–4)

Table 6.2 Tools for assessment of CHE

Psychometric tests
Psychometric hepatic encephalopathy score (PHES)
Repeatable battery for the assessment of neuropsychological status (RBANS)
Choice tests and Sternberg paradigm
Inhibitory control test (ICT)
Cognitive drug research computerized assessment system (CDR)
Immediate postconcussion assessment and cognitive testing (ImPACT)
Central nervous system vital signs (CNSVS)
Neurophysiological tests
Electroencephalogram (EEG)
Critical flicker frequency (CFF)

(d) Full Outline of UnResponsive (FOUR) Score

In patients with altered consciousness, the WHC does not give a precise stratification of acuity. For this subset of patients, the use of the FOUR score has been proposed [13, 14]. This scoring system has been validated for use in the setting of coma. It has been studied in patients with OHE in the setting of cirrhosis. It was shown to accurately predict severe stages of OHE, as well as discriminate between grades III and IV OHE, which traditionally have had a greater degree of interobserver variability. This scoring system uses an aggregate of scores 0–4 for four separate components: eye response, motor response, brainstem reflexes, and respiration. A lower score indicates a greater degree of impairment [15]

Prognosis

In acute liver failure, ammonia levels have been shown to have prognostic significance. An ammonia level ≥211 μg/dL (124 μmol/l) has been associated with a higher probability of cerebral edema, seizures, higher grade of encephalopathy, and death [16]. In addition, one study showed a combination of a MELD of 32 or greater and ammonia level greater than 170 μg/dL (100 μmol/l) predicted the onset of advanced HE alone or with even more specificity in combination. In the same study, there was a positive correlation between rise in ammonia level and probability of intracerebral hemorrhage (ICH) [17].

While the presence of CHE is not routinely screened for in the clinical setting, there have been identified downstream consequences. These include reduced health-related quality of life scores, sleep derangements, more frequent falls, decreased ability to perform complex tasks, and a higher probability of developing overt hepatic encephalopathy [7, 11].

In CLD, the onset of HE has been associated with a poor prognosis with a 12-month and 36-month mortality of 58% and 77%, respectively [18].

Acute Liver Failure in Pregnancy

Acute liver failure (ALF) in pregnancy is rare and can occur at any time during the pregnancy. Acute fatty liver of pregnancy (AFLP) and HELLP (hemolysis, elevated liver enzymes, low platelets) syndrome are unique to pregnancy and typically occur in the late second trimester and third trimester. Management of these pregnancy-related liver diseases is focused on supportive care and prompt delivery of the fetus. AFLP and HELLP syndrome are discussed in detail elsewhere in this book. In this section, we will focus on the epidemiology, clinical characteristics, diagnosis, and management of the critically ill pregnant patient with ALF and hepatic encephalopathy. Liver diseases that are not unique to pregnancy such as acute viral hepatitis and drug-induced liver injury can precipitate ALF in any trimester. In cases of ALF related to viral hepatitis and drug-induced liver injury, pregnant patients should be managed similarly as non-pregnant patients.

HELLP Syndrome

HELLP syndrome is unique to pregnancy and presents in the late second trimester to third trimester with hemolysis, elevated liver enzymes, and low platelet count. HELLP syndrome occurs in less than 1% of pregnancies and up to 20% of cases of severe preeclampsia [26, 27]. The exact pathogenesis of preeclampsia and HELLP syndrome remains unclear, but the abnormal development of the placenta, endothelial dysfunction, systemic inflammation, and defects in beta-oxidation of fatty acids have been described [28–30].

Patients may present with right upper quadrant pain, nausea, or vomiting. Features of preeclampsia include hypertension, proteinuria, and edema. Other end-organ damage may be present and manifest with acute renal failure, pulmonary edema, retinal detachment, disseminated intravascular hemolysis (DIC), and placental abruption. Hepatic rupture and acute liver failure are rare occurrences and have been managed with liver transplantation [31].

Lactate dehydrogenase, haptoglobin, complete blood count, and serum uric acid should be obtained as part of the workup when HELLP syndrome is suspected. The diagnosis of HELLP syndrome according to the Tennessee Classification is defined by having a platelet count $\leq 100 \times 10^9$/L, AST ≥ 70 units/L, and LDH ≥ 600 units/L [26]. Imaging to detect intrahepatic hematoma and/or hepatic infarction should be obtained to evaluate for complications of preeclampsia and HELLP syndrome.

Management includes treatment of hypertension, coagulopathy, and prevention of seizures. Definitive therapy is delivery of the fetus.

Acute Hepatic Hematoma and Rupture

Hepatic hematoma and rupture can occur in the setting of severe preeclampsia and HELLP syndrome [32, 33]. Imaging studies such as CT and MRI can detect complications of hepatic infarct, hematoma, and rupture [34]. Ultrasonography is recommended as a first line test due to its non-invasive nature. Non-specific imaging findings may show perihepatic free fluid, hepatic steatosis, hepatomegaly, and periportal edema. Doppler US may detect decreased arterial and portal venous blood flow in patients with severe preeclampsia and HELLP syndrome. Only if ultrasonography shows abnormal findings should cross-sectional imaging with CT or MRI be obtained to confirm hematoma or infarction [35].

A contained hematoma can be managed with supportive care along with blood transfusions. For enlarging hematomas with active bleeding, management may require surgery, hepatic artery embolization, and liver transplantation [36–38].

Acute Fatty Liver of Pregnancy

Acute fatty liver of pregnancy (AFLP) is rare (5 cases per 100,000 maternities) and occurs in the third trimester with signs and symptoms of ALF including jaundice, ascites, encephalopathy, and coagulopathy [39]. The pathogenesis involves defects in fatty acid metabolism with about 20% of AFLP attributed to fetal long-chain 3-hydroxyacyl-CoA dehydrogenase deficiency (LCHAD) [30, 40]. Maternal heterozygosity for LCHAD deficiency leads to the inability of the mother to oxidize long-chain fatty acids from the liver and placenta which subjects the mother to increasing circulating hepatotoxic metabolites.

Patients may present with headache, fatigue, nausea, vomiting, right upper quadrant pain, and jaundice. Hepatic encephalopathy and coagulopathy are late complications and hallmarks of the development of ALF which can be further complicated by multi-system organ failure.

Histology typically shows microvesicular fatty infiltration of the liver [41, 42].

Maternal and fetal mortality rate is high. Management is supportive care and prompt delivery of the fetus.

Acute Viral Hepatitis

Acute hepatitis A virus (HAV), hepatitis B virus (HBV), and hepatitis E virus (HEV) can cause ALF. Non-hepatotrophic viral infections such as herpes simplex virus (HSV), varicella-zoster virus (VZV), Epstein-Barr virus (EBV), adenovirus, and cytomegalovirus (CMV) have also been associated with ALF. Of all the viral infections listed above, only acute hepatitis related to HEV and HSV are known to have an increased risk of ALF in pregnant patients compared to non-pregnant patients [43].

Pregnant patients presenting with any combination of jaundice, right upper quadrant pain, elevated transaminases, or thrombocytopenia should have serological testing to evaluate for pre-existing or acutely acquired viral hepatitis. All pregnant patients should be screened for hepatitis B with HBsAg. Pregnant patients with chronic hepatitis B may have hepatitis flares within the first months after delivery. Cases of acute liver failure can occur in the peripartum period.

Hepatitis A

HAV and HEV are transmitted through the fecal-oral route and do not progress to chronic infections with the exception of chronic HEV in immunocompromised patients [44]. While HAV infection is the most common cause of acute viral hepatitis in the general population, there is no evidence that pregnant women are at increased risk of severe liver injury or ALF from HAV infection [45, 46]. Complications such as premature contractions, placental separation, premature rupture of membranes, and vaginal bleeding have been reported in acute HAV infection in pregnancy and may lead to preterm labor [45].

Hepatitis E

In parts of the world where HEV is endemic, such as India, Southeast Asia, the Middle East, and Africa, it is a major cause of maternal and fetal mortality [14, 47–50]. In a study from India, ALF was more common in the third trimester [51]. In the United States, HEV is an uncommon cause of acute liver failure; however it appears to be more likely in pregnant patients as well as in patients that are malnourished or have underlying chronic liver disease [43]. Supporting the idea that pregnancy is a risk for viral replication, HEV viral loads were found to be significantly higher in pregnant versus non-pregnant patients [52]. Additionally, diminished cellular immunity and increased level of steroid hormones may also impact viral replication during pregnancy [51]. Ribavirin is a teratogen and therefore should not be used in pregnant patients.

Hepatitis B

HBV can cause ALF by de novo infection, delta superinfection, or reactivation in the setting of previous HBV infection [53]. Among patients with acute HBV, about 1% will develop ALF. The risk of ALF is increased in patients with hepatitis D virus (HDV) coinfection, chronic hepatitis C virus (HCV) infection, and older age patients [54–56]. The clinical course of acute HBV in pregnant patients is similar to non-pregnant patients, but the risk of HBV transmission to the neonate increases in later part of gestation [57]. After delivery, women with chronic HBV may develop reactivation and even ALF [58]. Antiviral therapies may be considered in patients with acute HBV.

Herpes Simplex Virus

ALF due to herpes virus infection is exceedingly rare. While immunocompromised individuals are at risk, herpes virus ALF has occurred in immunocompetent individuals. Women in the third trimester of pregnancy are at increased risk of herpes virus ALF. HSV1 and HSV2 in pregnancy can cause disseminated infection as well as acute liver failure, particularly in the third trimester [59]. HSV hepatitis characteristically presents without jaundice and is characterized as an anicteric hepatitis, where transaminases can be quite high and the bilirubin normal [60]. The typical lesions of herpes virus are only present in half of cases. Treatment includes supportive care and prompt initiation of acyclovir (5–10 mg/kg every 8 h for at least 7 days) [50, 59, 61–67].

Drug-Induced Acute Liver Failure

While certain medications such as acetaminophen (APAP) have predictable dose-dependent hepatotoxicity, DILI and ALF can be the result of an idiosyncratic reaction from a variety of drug classes including antimicrobials, herbals, and dietary supplements [68]. Anti-hypertensives such as methyldopa and labetalol, antimicrobials, antiretroviral agents, and propylthiouracil have been reported to cause DILI and ALF in pregnant patients [68, 69]. Drug-induced liver injury (DILI) and resultant ALF is not unique to pregnant patients; however gender and pregnancy may impact the risk for both DILI and ALF [70]. Compared to men, women appear to be more prone to DILI from minocycline, methyldopa, diclofenac, isoniazid, and nitrofurantoin [70, 71]. Along the same lines, tetracycline-induced hepatic microvesicular steatosis occurs most often in pregnant patients when given in high doses intravenously [70].

Acetaminophen (APAP) is the most common cause of drug-induced ALF in developed countries and accounts for almost 50% of cases of ALF in adults [72, 73]. Acetaminophen is commonly used for analgesia with a typical therapeutic dose of 1–4 grams daily. Hepatotoxicity can occur through intentional ingestion of high doses often in the setting of a suicidal gesture, but can also occur as a consequence of chronic use or a therapeutic misadventure. Toxic doses are generally greater than 7–10 grams daily. In the liver, APAP is converted to glucuronide or sulfate metabolites, then excreted in the urine [74]. Toxic doses of APAP saturate these pathways, and the remaining APAP is metabolized by hepatic cytochrome P450 oxidase pathways creating the toxic metabolite N-acetyl-p-benzoquinoneimine (NAPQI). Glutathione (GSH) forms a nontoxic APAP-GSH conjugate. However, when GSH is depleted, NAPQI forms irreversible NAPQI-protein adducts leading to oxidative hepatocyte injury and hepatocellular necrosis [75–77]. Chronic alcohol use can make patients more susceptible to APAP hepatotoxicity by increasing CYP2E1 activity and decreasing glutathione (GSH) synthesis and storage. Pregnancy can increase activity of glucuronidation and increase oxidative pathways. Based on experimental data from mice, it appears that pregnant mice are at risk of acetaminophen-induced DILI from decreased GSH levels as a consequence of fetal and placental demand [78]. As is the case in non-pregnant patients, early therapy with IV N-acetylcysteine is likely beneficial and can reduce risk of miscarriage and fetal death.

Management of Acute Liver Failure

ALF can be a rapidly progressive process with a high degree of morbidity and mortality.

A. Diagnosis requires identification of the constellation of:

   (a) Elevated transaminases (twofold increase from upper limits of normal)
   (b) Altered coagulation (INR >1.5)
   (c) Hepatic encephalopathy

B. ALF is subcategorized based on duration of illness:

   (a) Hyperacute (<7 days)
   (b) Acute (7–21 days)
   (c) Subacute (>21 days and <26 weeks)

It is imperative that patients with ALF are hospitalized for further monitoring.

A. Initial Assessment

Laboratory investigation should include lab markers for severity of disease and identification of potential precipitating factors. It is important to note that an elevation in alkaline phosphatase, especially in later trimesters, is a normal finding in pregnancy as it is produced by both the placenta and fetal bone development [19]. Close attention should be made to home medications, and investigation into additional over-the-counter supplements is necessary to rule out drug or toxin-induced injury.

B. Imaging

Abdominal imaging is necessary in patients with pregnancy related liver dysfunction to rule out the presence of hepatic infarction, rupture, or hematoma. Hepatic rupture and hematoma are life threatening and associated with mortality of up to 50% [19]. Ultrasound imaging is the preferred initial modality given its lack of radiation. However, in scenarios where further characterization of the parenchyma is necessary, non-contrasted MRI or CT can be performed in the second and third trimester. When utilizing CT, it is recommended that protocols utilizing the lowest possible radiation (2–5 rads) should be employed. [21]

C. Critical Care and Specialty Center Consultation

Patients with progressive coagulopathy, hemodynamic instability, or high grades (III-IV) of HE should be monitored in the intensive care unit (ICU). Consultation with a transplant center should take place early in the process of supportive care, and consideration for transfer should be made [20]. In the case of pregnancy specific ALF, such as AFLP or HELLP syndrome, prompt delivery is crucial to recovery. If the gestational age is greater than 34 weeks, induction should occur immediately. If the gestational age is between 24 and 34 weeks, corticosteroids should be given and delivery should be delayed for 48 h if possible [22]. Common regimens of antenatal steroids include:

(a) Betamethasone 12 mg intramuscular given 24 h apart for two doses
(b) Dexamethasone 6 mg intramuscular given 12 h apart for four doses

If recovery is not rapid following delivery, consideration for transplantation should not be delayed [20]. However, transplant will likely be unnecessary in up to half of cases. The most recent US data suggests superior outcomes in pregnancy-related ALF, acetaminophen toxicity, hepatitis A, or shock liver when compared to all other causes. These etiologies demonstrate a greater than 50% transplant-free survival compared to less than 25% in all other causes.

Organ System Specific Considerations

A. Central Nervous System

a. Cerebral Edema and Intracranial Hypertension

Central nervous dysfunction in the form of HE is a hallmark feature of ALF. While any degree of HE or rate of onset of liver disease has been associated with downstream morbidity, the acuity of consequences increases in both the setting of ALF and with increasing grades of HE. Patients with grades III–IV HE are at risk for increased intracranial pressure (ICP). The American Association for the Study of Liver Diseases (AASLD) recommends hourly neurologic checks in all patients with grades III–IV HE to detect signs of elevated ICP at the earliest point. In centers with expertise, invasive ICP monitoring should be considered. In the absence of quantitative ICP monitoring, clinical signs of elevated ICP include Cushing's triad (systemic hypertension, bradycardia, and irregular respirations), pupillary dilation, or decerebrate posturing. However, these are not consistently present and may only appear late in the course.

The goal of therapy is to reduce ICP (less than 20 mmHg) but maintain mean arterial pressure (MAP) as to preserve cerebral perfusion pressure (CPP), ideally greater than 60 mmHg. Strategies to reduce ICP include osmotic diuresis with mannitol and the use of hypertonic saline with a goal sodium level of 145–155 mmol/L. Hyperventilation with a goal $PaCO_2$ of 25–30 mmHg effectively produces cerebral vasoconstriction resulting in ICP reduction. However, this is very short-lived and only recommended as a bridge to additional therapies when there is impending herniation. In experimental models, hypothermia (core temperature of 33–34 °C) has been shown to prevent development of brain edema [20].

b. Hepatic Encephalopathy

As HE is considered a diagnosis of exclusion, it is important to confirm there is no coexisting abnormality that could explain an acute change in mental status or sensorium. Once HE is confirmed, a search for precipitating factors should ensue. Initial management should focus on directed therapy at the underlying precipitating factors as well as targeted therapy for HE. Gold standard therapy for acute HE includes agents that enhance the removal of ammonia in the gastrointestinal tract or reduce its production altogether. Several oral antibiotics including metronidazole, neomycin, and rifaximin have been studied, which all are effective at reducing the urease-producing bacteria in the gut. However, rifaximin has been proven superior to the others due to its minimal absorption, which leads to a higher long-term safety profile and reduction in side effects. Lactulose can be given in oral or rectal forms, and when compared to non-absorbable antibiotics, it has been shown to be inferior in reducing symptoms of HE with long-term use in patients with chronic liver disease. Neither non-absorbable antibiotics nor synthetic disaccharides, such as lactulose, have shown a mortality benefit in ALF. In addition, caution should be taken when dosing lactulose in the critically ill as it can produce significant gastrointestinal side effects such as gaseous distention and even ileus [23]. These side effects may make transplantation more difficult.

Other supplements have been used to promote ammonia clearance including zinc, L-ornithine L-aspartate, sodium benzoate, sodium phenylacetate, and L-carnitine. These have been studied in the setting of chronic liver disease with variable outcomes.

B. Cardiovascular

Hypotension is a common feature of ALF due to low systemic vascular resistance. Maintaining an adequate mean arterial pressure is imperative to maintain adequate cerebral and renal perfusion. Given the likelihood of altered mental status and lack of oral intake prior to admission along with transudative extravascular fluid shifts, there is a typically a component of intravascular volume depletion as well. Fluid resuscitation with an isotonic solution is recommended as the initial therapy of hypotension.

In patients who are not fluid responsive, vasopressors are necessary. The recommended initial vasopressor for shock in ALF is norepinephrine (NE). NE has greater $\alpha 1$ activity than cardiac $\beta 1$ activity leading to increased SVR with less pronounced tachycardia when compared to other agents such as epinephrine. Vasopressin and its analogs have also been shown to help reduce the dose of NE and associated ischemia in peripheral tissues. Caution should be taken in patients with evidence of elevated ICP as there has been some evidence that it may increase cerebral vasodilation and ICP [20].

Adrenal insufficiency has been associated with both acute and chronic liver failure. This is thought to be related to reduced synthesis of cortisol binding globulin by the liver [24]. Hypotension despite vasopressor use and volume resuscitation should prompt consideration of adrenal insufficiency and a trial of hydrocortisone.

C. Coagulopathy

In the absence of liver failure, pregnancy is characterized by a procoagulant state. There are increases in clotting factors I, II, V, VII, X, XII, and fibrinogen. In ALF, there is typically an increase in INR, consumption of clotting factors, and onset of thrombocytopenia, which might suggest a predilection toward abnormal bleeding. However, when measuring hemostasis using thromboelastography (TEG) results are typically normal. Prophylactic transfusion or blood products should not be performed unless invasive testing or a planned procedure is performed, unless platelet count is $<10{,}000/\text{mm}^3$. In preparation for invasive procedures or during a bleeding event, platelet transfusion with a goal of $>50{,}000/\text{mm}^3$ is recommended. However, in centers where TEG is available and rapid, this can be a useful tool for guiding correction of coagulation deficits. Prophylaxis for gastrointestinal bleeding is recommended, and use of H_2 blocking agents, such as ranitidine, or sucralfate is considered safe in pregnancy.

D. Renal

The presence of coexisting renal failure in ALF ranges from 40% to 85% depending on the etiology of ALF. Typically, the cause of acute renal failure (ARF) can be linked to the relative pre-renal state that is induced by decreased SVR. The kidneys lose their ability to autoregulate and are dependent on systemic blood pressure to receive adequate flow. Other factors that may limit renal blood flow include the development of tense ascites or hepatorenal syndrome (HRS). Depending on the underlying etiology of ALF, there may also be direct injury to the kidneys causing acute tubular necrosis. This is common with paracetamol overdose or viral hepatitis [25].

The combination of ALF and ARF should prompt admission to the ICU. This combination makes acute life-threatening derangements in acid/base status, electrolytes, volume status, and coagulation more likely. Early initiation of hemodialysis should be considered, especially in patients with cerebral edema or elevated ICP. The method of choice to reduce rapid shifts in systemic and intracranial hemodynamics is continuous renal replacement therapy [20].

E. Liver Transplantation

The available literature concerning timing and indication for orthotopic liver transplantation (OLT) in the pregnant patient with liver failure is sparse. There have been case reports of prepartum OLT performed pre-viable delivery and post-viable delivery with variable outcomes for the neonate [22].

While those with prepartum cirrhosis have a reduction in fertility, it has been shown that fertility is restored shortly following OLT. However, subsequent pregnancy is not without increased risk. Acute cellular rejection occurs in 10–17% of patients with a subsequent pregnancy, but can be reduced by delaying pregnancy for greater than 1 year following OLT. Infections occur in 27% of these pregnancies. There is also a 30% increased risk of prematurity and low birth weight. Immunosuppression is typically safe for the fetus, with most common regimens including azathioprine, tacrolimus, cyclosporine, and steroids. Mycophenolate has been associated with congenital facial abnormalities such as external ear malformation, cleft lip, and cleft palate. A 6-month gap between cessation of mycophenolate and pregnancy is recommended [19].

Molecular Adsorbent Recirculating System (MARS®) Indications, Considerations, and Contraindications

Extracorporeal liver support system (ELS) using Molecular Adsorbent Recirculating System (MARS®) is an infrequent but very useful rescue strategy used in our institution to be used in certain severe cases with acute liver failure (ALF), acute-on-chronic liver failure (AOCLF), or certain intoxications. In this section we describe in more detail our decision-making process to initiate MARS®. Figure 6.2 depicts a sketch of a typical MARS® setup which includes albumin circuit and MARS® dialyzer.

a. ELS indications:

   1. Portosystemic encephalopathy (PSE) is the main indication for which MARS® received FDA approval. We consider it for patients with ALF or AOCLF once the PSE has reached grade 3–4 and is refractory to maximum medical therapy with the rationale to maintain/improve cerebral perfusion pressure (CPP).

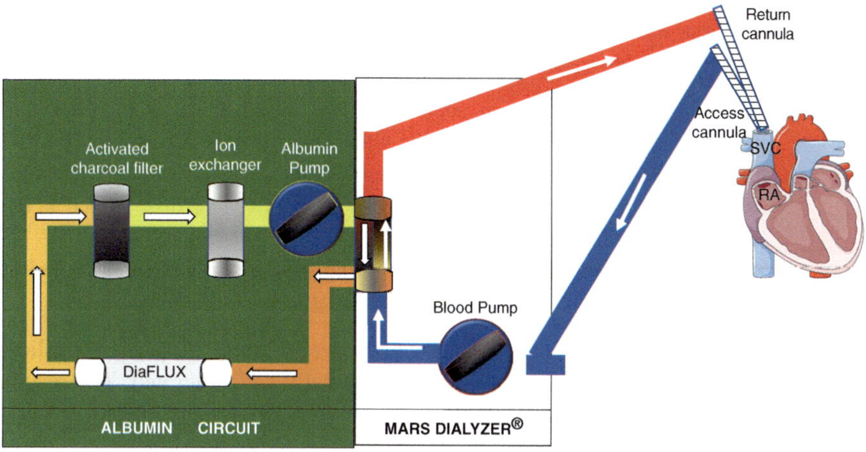

Fig. 6.2 Typical MARS® setup. Nothing in this manuscript implies Mayo Clinic's endorsement of MARS or DiaFLUX

Table 6.3 ELS may be considered for some poisonings related and unrelated to liver failure

ELS indication for poisoning with albumin bound substances in patients presenting with other toxin-related organ dysfunctions not associated with liver failure
1. Phenytoin [80]
2. Lamotrigine [81]
3. Theophylline [82]
4. Calcium channel blocker – diltiazem [83, 84]
ELS indication for poisoning associated with liver failure due to the following substances:
1. Chromium [85]
2. Copper [85, 86]
3. Paracetamol [87–91]
4. Amanita phalloides [92–97]
5. Diazepam [98]
6. Midazolam [99]
7. Fentanyl [99]
8. Cocaine [100]
9. Amphetamines [101]
10. Thiocyanate [102]
11. Allopurinol [103]

MARS® is used until PSE improves or as a bridge to transplant in patients who are liver transplant candidates. We typically include the following patient categories: Those who are listed or those who are undergoing liver transplant evaluation and do not have contraindications for transplantation [79].

2. Intoxications and poisoning. As a general rule ELS use is more widely accepted in poisonings associated with liver failure. But ELS can also be considered in the setting of selected poisonings without liver failure that are

due to albumin bound substances and causing other organ dysfunction/s related to that substance. ELS may be considered for selected cases of poisoning without liver failure with other organ dysfunction/s related to substances described on Table 6.3.

a. Acute hepatic failure from acetaminophen overdose. This includes two possible groups: early on, meaning when there is still acetaminophen circulating blood/plasma levels and such levels are high enough to cause severe hepatic injury. Later on (i.e., >24 h post overdose) once acute hepatic failure has become evident.
b. Acute severe alcoholic hepatitis. Including Maddrey discrimination factor value >32 and/or spontaneous encephalopathy.

3. Patients with cholestatic liver disease that have pruritus refractory to medical therapy. The procedure is low risk and typically well tolerated. The results tend to be only transient.

b. ELS may be considered under the following circumstances:

1. ELS will be considered in selected cases of AOCLF with hepatorenal syndrome as a combined decision between transplant (Tx) nephrology, Tx hepatology, and Tx critical care.
2. ELS may also be considered in patients with ALF as part of management to determine if the liver failure is reversible (e.g., acute liver failure due to hepatitis or shock liver). These patients should not have any of the contraindications listed (see below) and ideally would be considered liver transplant patients if the liver does not recover.
3. We also consider ELS initiation and other forms of intracranial pressure (ICP) control therapies in ALF or AOLF patients with an acute and significant increase in ammonia level or with signs of increased ICP.

c. ELS contraindications:

The decision to initiate MARS® treatment at our institution is made with input from Tx critical care, Tx nephrology, Tx hepatology, and Tx surgery. The following is a partial list of absolute and relative contraindications for MARS® per the manufacturers' recommendations, based on research and clinical data that was provided to the FDA for its approval:

Relative contraindications:

1. International normalized ratio (INR) >2.3
2. Platelet count <50K
3. Disseminated intravascular coagulation
4. Severe sepsis or septic shock unresponsive to antibiotics
5. Acute hemorrhage unresponsive to standard treatment
6. Unstable hemodynamics

Absolute contraindications:

This is a partial list of absolute contraindications:

1. Portal vein thrombosis in patients with HCC and malignant vascular invasion

Conflict of Interest None.

References

1. Aggarwal R. Hepatic encephalopathy in pregnancy. Indian J Gastroenterol. 2003;22(Suppl 2):S78–80.
2. Butterworth RF. Pathogenesis of hepatic encephalopathy and brain edema in acute liver failure. J Clin Exp Hepatol. 2015;5(Suppl 1):S96–S103.
3. Wijdicks EF. Hepatic encephalopathy. N Engl J Med. 2016;375(17):1660–70.
4. Hirode G, Vittinghoff E, Wong RJ. Increasing burden of hepatic encephalopathy among hospitalized adults: an analysis of the 2010–2014 national inpatient sample. Dig Dis Sci. 2019;64(6):1448–57.
5. Vilstrup H, Amodio P, Bajaj J, Cordoba J, Ferenci P, Mullen KD, et al. Hepatic encephalopathy in chronic liver disease: 2014 Practice Guideline by the American Association for the Study of Liver Diseases and the European Association for the Study of the Liver. Hepatology. 2014;60(2):715–35.
6. Albrecht J, Norenberg MD. Glutamine: a Trojan horse in ammonia neurotoxicity. Hepatology. 2006;44(4):788–94.
7. Kappus MR, Bajaj JS. Covert hepatic encephalopathy: not as minimal as you might think. Clin Gastroenterol Hepatol. 2012;10(11):1208–19.
8. Ong JP, Aggarwal A, Krieger D, Easley KA, Karafa MT, Van Lente F, et al. Correlation between ammonia levels and the severity of hepatic encephalopathy. Am J Med. 2003;114(3):188–93.
9. Ferenci P, Lockwood A, Mullen K, Tarter R, Weissenborn K, Blei AT. Hepatic encephalopathy–definition, nomenclature, diagnosis, and quantification: final report of the working party at the 11th World Congresses of Gastroenterology, Vienna, 1998. Hepatology. 2002;35(3):716–21.
10. Conn HO, Leevy CM, Vlahcevic ZR, Rodgers JB, Maddrey WC, Seeff L, et al. Comparison of lactulose and neomycin in the treatment of chronic portal-systemic encephalopathy. A double blind controlled trial. Gastroenterology. 1977;72(4 Pt 1):573–83.
11. Bajaj JS, Cordoba J, Mullen KD, Amodio P, Shawcross DL, Butterworth RF, et al. Review article: the design of clinical trials in hepatic encephalopathy–an International Society for Hepatic Encephalopathy and Nitrogen Metabolism (ISHEN) consensus statement. Aliment Pharmacol Ther. 2011;33(7):739–47.
12. Ge PS, Runyon BA. Serum ammonia level for the evaluation of hepatic encephalopathy. JAMA. 2014;312(6):643–4.
13. Iyer VN, Mandrekar JN, Danielson RD, Zubkov AY, Elmer JL, Wijdicks EF. Validity of the FOUR score coma scale in the medical intensive care unit. Mayo Clin Proc. 2009;84(8):694–701.
14. Perumpail RB, Ahmed A, Higgins JP, et al. Fatal accelerated cirrhosis after imported HEV genotype 4 infection. Emerg Infect Dis. 2015;21(9):1679–81.
15. Mouri S, Tripon S, Rudler M, Mallet M, Mayaux J, Thabut D, et al. FOUR score, a reliable score for assessing overt hepatic encephalopathy in cirrhotic patients. Neurocrit Care. 2015;22(2):251–7.
16. Bhatia V, Singh R, Acharya SK. Predictive value of arterial ammonia for complications and outcome in acute liver failure. Gut. 2006;55(1):98–104.
17. Bernal W, Hall C, Karvellas CJ, Auzinger G, Sizer E, Wendon J. Arterial ammonia and clinical risk factors for encephalopathy and intracranial hypertension in acute liver failure. Hepatology. 2007;46(6):1844–52.
18. Saad WE. Portosystemic shunt syndrome and endovascular management of hepatic encephalopathy. Semin Intervent Radiol. 2014;31(3):262–5.
19. Westbrook RH, Dusheiko G, Williamson C. Pregnancy and liver disease. J Hepatol. 2016;64(4):933–45.

20. Lee WM. AASLD position paper: the management of acute liver failure: update 2011. American association for the study of liver diseases, 2011, p. 1–88.
21. Tran TT, Ahn J, Reau NS. ACG clinical guideline: liver disease and pregnancy. Am J Gastroenterol. 2016;111(2):176–94. quiz 96
22. Pandey CK, Karna ST, Pandey VK, Tandon M. Acute liver failure in pregnancy: challenges and management. Indian J Anaesth. 2015;59(3):144–9.
23. Bass NM. Review article: the current pharmacological therapies for hepatic encephalopathy. Aliment Pharmacol Ther. 2007;25(Suppl 1):23–31.
24. Kharb S, Garg MK, Puri P, Nandi B, Brar KS, Gundgurthi A, et al. Assessment of adrenal function in liver diseases. Indian J Endocrinol Metab. 2013;17(3):465–71.
25. Betrosian AP, Agarwal B, Douzinas EE. Acute renal dysfunction in liver diseases. World J Gastroenterol. 2007;13(42):5552–9.
26. Sibai BM, Ramadan MK, Usta I, Salama M, Mercer BM, Friedman SA. Maternal morbidity and mortality in 442 pregnancies with hemolysis, elevated liver enzymes, and low platelets (HELLP syndrome). Am J Obstet Gynecol. 1993;169(4):1000–6.
27. Magann EF, Perry KG Jr, Chauhan SP, Graves GR, Blake PG, Martin JN Jr. Neonatal salvage by week's gestation in pregnancies complicated by HELLP syndrome. J Soc Gynecol Investig. 1994;1(3):206–9.
28. Rahman TM, Wendon J. Severe hepatic dysfunction in pregnancy. QJM. 2002;95(6):343–57.
29. Salmon JE, Heuser C, Triebwasser M, et al. Mutations in complement regulatory proteins predispose to preeclampsia: a genetic analysis of the PROMISSE cohort. PLoS Med. 2011;8(3):e1001013.
30. Ibdah JA, Bennett MJ, Rinaldo P, et al. A fetal fatty-acid oxidation disorder as a cause of liver disease in pregnant women. N Engl J Med. 1999;340(22):1723–31.
31. Shames BD, Fernandez LA, Sollinger HW, et al. Liver transplantation for HELLP syndrome. Liver Transpl. 2005;11(2):224–8.
32. Kozic JR, Benton SJ, Hutcheon JA, Payne BA, Magee LA, von Dadelszen P. Abnormal liver function tests as predictors of adverse maternal outcomes in women with preeclampsia. J Obstet Gynaecol Can. 2011;33(10):995–1004.
33. Vigil-De Gracia P, Ortega-Paz L. Pre-eclampsia/eclampsia and hepatic rupture. Int J Gynaecol Obstet. 2012;118(3):186–9.
34. Schwartz ML, Lien JM. Spontaneous liver hematoma in pregnancy not clearly associated with preeclampsia: a case presentation and literature review. Am J Obstet Gynecol. 1997;176(6):1328–32; discussion 1332–1323.
35. Perronne L, Dohan A, Bazeries P, et al. Hepatic involvement in HELLP syndrome: an update with emphasis on imaging features. Abdom Imaging. 2015;40(7):2839–49.
36. Zarrinpar A, Farmer DG, Ghobrial RM, et al. Liver transplantation for HELLP syndrome. Am Surg. 2007;73(10):1013–6.
37. Grand'Maison S, Sauve N, Weber F, Dagenais M, Durand M, Mahone M. Hepatic rupture in hemolysis, elevated liver enzymes, low platelets syndrome. Obstet Gynecol. 2012;119(3):617–25.
38. Zissin R, Yaffe D, Fejgin M, Olsfanger D, Shapiro-Feinberg M. Hepatic infarction in preeclampsia as part of the HELLP syndrome: CT appearance. Abdom Imaging. 1999;24(6):594–6.
39. Knight M, Nelson-Piercy C, Kurinczuk JJ, Spark P, Brocklehurst P. A prospective national study of acute fatty liver of pregnancy in the UK. Gut. 2008;57(7):951–6.
40. Yang Z, Yamada J, Zhao Y, Strauss AW, Ibdah JA. Prospective screening for pediatric mitochondrial trifunctional protein defects in pregnancies complicated by liver disease. JAMA. 2002;288(17):2163–6.
41. Bacq Y. Acute fatty liver of pregnancy. Semin Perinatol. 1998;22(2):134–40.
42. Rolfes DB, Ishak KG. Acute fatty liver of pregnancy: a clinicopathologic study of 35 cases. Hepatology. 1985;5(6):1149–58.
43. Fontana RJ, Engle RE, Scaglione S, et al. The role of hepatitis E virus infection in adult Americans with acute liver failure. Hepatology. 2016;64(6):1870–80.

44. Behrendt P, Steinmann E, Manns MP, Wedemeyer H. The impact of hepatitis E in the liver transplant setting. J Hepatol. 2014;61(6):1418–29.
45. Elinav E, Ben-Dov IZ, Shapira Y, et al. Acute hepatitis A infection in pregnancy is associated with high rates of gestational complications and preterm labor. Gastroenterology. 2006;130(4):1129–34.
46. Willner IR, Uhl MD, Howard SC, Williams EQ, Riely CA, Waters B. Serious hepatitis A: an analysis of patients hospitalized during an urban epidemic in the United States. Ann Intern Med. 1998;128(2):111–4.
47. Khuroo MS, Kamili S. Aetiology and prognostic factors in acute liver failure in India. J Viral Hepat. 2003;10(3):224–31.
48. Kumar A, Beniwal M, Kar P, Sharma JB, Murthy NS. Hepatitis E in pregnancy. Int J Gynaecol Obstet. 2004;85(3):240–4.
49. Kourtis AP, Read JS, Jamieson DJ. Pregnancy and infection. N Engl J Med. 2014;370(23):2211–8.
50. Patra S, Kumar A, Trivedi SS, Puri M, Sarin SK. Maternal and fetal outcomes in pregnant women with acute hepatitis E virus infection. Ann Intern Med. 2007;147(1):28–33.
51. Jilani N, Das BC, Husain SA, et al. Hepatitis E virus infection and fulminant hepatic failure during pregnancy. J Gastroenterol Hepatol. 2007;22(5):676–82.
52. Kar P, Jilani N, Husain SA, et al. Does hepatitis E viral load and genotypes influence the final outcome of acute liver failure during pregnancy? Am J Gastroenterol. 2008;103(10):2495–501.
53. Chang ML, Liaw YF. Hepatitis B flares in chronic hepatitis B: pathogenesis, natural course, and management. J Hepatol. 2014;61(6):1407–17.
54. Shukla NB, Poles MA. Hepatitis B virus infection: co-infection with hepatitis C virus, hepatitis D virus, and human immunodeficiency virus. Clin Liver Dis. 2004;8(2):445–60, viii.
55. Wai CT, Fontana RJ, Polson J, et al. Clinical outcome and virological characteristics of hepatitis B-related acute liver failure in the United States. J Viral Hepat. 2005;12(2):192–8.
56. Sagnelli E, Coppola N, Pisaturo M, et al. HBV superinfection in HCV chronic carriers: a disease that is frequently severe but associated with the eradication of HCV. Hepatology. 2009;49(4):1090–7.
57. Jonas MM. Hepatitis B and pregnancy: an underestimated issue. Liver Int. 2009;29(Suppl 1):133–9.
58. Lin HH, Chen PJ, Chen DS, et al. Postpartum subsidence of hepatitis B viral replication in HBeAg-positive carrier mothers. J Med Virol. 1989;29(1):1–6.
59. Kang AH, Graves CR. Herpes simplex hepatitis in pregnancy: a case report and review of the literature. Obstet Gynecol Surv. 1999;54(7):463–8.
60. Goyert GL, Bottoms SF, Sokol RJ. Anicteric presentation of fatal herpetic hepatitis in pregnancy. Obstet Gynecol. 1985;65(4):585–8.
61. Bernal W, Auzinger G, Dhawan A, Wendon J. Acute liver failure. Lancet. 2010;376(9736):190–201.
62. Lee WM. Etiologies of acute liver failure. Semin Liver Dis. 2008;28(2):142–52.
63. Lee WM, Squires RH Jr, Nyberg SL, Doo E, Hoofnagle JH. Acute liver failure: summary of a workshop. Hepatology. 2008;47(4):1401–15.
64. Levitsky J, Duddempudi AT, Lakeman FD, et al. Detection and diagnosis of herpes simplex virus infection in adults with acute liver failure. Liver Transpl. 2008;14(10):1498–504.
65. Ostapowicz G, Fontana RJ, Schiodt FV, et al. Results of a prospective study of acute liver failure at 17 tertiary care centers in the United States. Ann Intern Med. 2002;137(12):947–54.
66. Peters DJ, Greene WH, Ruggiero F, McGarrity TJ. Herpes simplex-induced fulminant hepatitis in adults: a call for empiric therapy. Dig Dis Sci. 2000;45(12):2399–404.
67. Schiodt FV, Davern TJ, Shakil AO, McGuire B, Samuel G, Lee WM. Viral hepatitis-related acute liver failure. Am J Gastroenterol. 2003;98(2):448–53.
68. Chalasani NP, Hayashi PH, Bonkovsky HL, Navarro VJ, Lee WM, Fontana RJ. ACG Clinical Guideline: the diagnosis and management of idiosyncratic drug-induced liver injury. Am J Gastroenterol. 2014;109(7):950–66; quiz 967.

69. Bartnik CM, Maheshwari RN, Subramanian RM. Beating the odds: a full-term delivery after liver transplantation of a pregnant hyperthyroid patient at 19 weeks' gestation for propylthiouracil-induced acute liver failure. Transplant Proc. 2018;50(10):3995–9.
70. Larrey D. Epidemiology and individual susceptibility to adverse drug reactions affecting the liver. Semin Liver Dis. 2002;22(2):145–55.
71. Yu YC, Mao YM, Chen CW, et al. CSH guidelines for the diagnosis and treatment of drug-induced liver injury. Hepatol Int. 2017;11(3):221–41.
72. Gill RQ, Sterling RK. Acute liver failure. J Clin Gastroenterol. 2001;33(3):191–8.
73. Nourjah P, Ahmad SR, Karwoski C, Willy M. Estimates of acetaminophen (Paracetomal)-associated overdoses in the United States. Pharmacoepidemiol Drug Saf. 2006;15(6):398–405.
74. Manyike PT, Kharasch ED, Kalhorn TF, Slattery JT. Contribution of CYP2E1 and CYP3A to acetaminophen reactive metabolite formation. Clin Pharmacol Ther. 2000;67(3):275–82.
75. Thummel KE, Lee CA, Kunze KL, Nelson SD, Slattery JT. Oxidation of acetaminophen to N-acetyl-p-aminobenzoquinone imine by human CYP3A4. Biochem Pharmacol. 1993;45(8):1563–9.
76. James LP, Mayeux PR, Hinson JA. Acetaminophen-induced hepatotoxicity. Drug Metab Dispos. 2003;31(12):1499–506.
77. Roberts DW, Pumford NR, Potter DW, Benson RW, Hinson JA. A sensitive immunochemical assay for acetaminophen-protein adducts. J Pharmacol Exp Ther. 1987;241(2):527–33.
78. Larrey D, Letteron P, Foliot A, et al. Effects of pregnancy on the toxicity and metabolism of acetaminophen in mice. J Pharmacol Exp Ther. 1986;237(1):283–91.
79. Hassanein T, et al. Hepatology. 2007;46:1853–62.
80. Mecarelli O, Pulitano P, Mingoia M, Ferretti G, Rossi M, Berloco PB, Muda AO. Acute hepatitis associated with lamotrigin and managed with the molecular adsorbent recirculating system (MARS®). Epilepsia. 2005;46:1687–9.
81. Stange J, Ramlow W, Mitzner S, Schmidt R, Klinkmann H. Dialysis against a recycled albumin solution enables the removal of albumin bound toxins. Artif Organs. 1993;17:809–81.
82. Korsheed S, Selby NM, Fluck RJ. Treatment of severe theophylline poisoning with the molecular adsorbent recirculating system (MARS®). Nephrol Dial Transplant. 2007;22:969–70.
83. Pichon N, François B, Clavel M, Vignon P, Chevreuil C, Michel Gaulier J. Albumin dialysis: a new therapeutic alternative for severe diltiazem intoxication. Clin Toxicol. 2006;44:195–6.
84. Belleflamme M, et al. Survival despite extremely high plasma diltiazem level in a case of acute poisoning treated by the molecular-adsorbent recirculating system. Eur J Emerg Med. 2012;19:59–61.
85. Prokurat S, Grenda R, Lipowski D, Kalicinski P, Migdal M. MARS® procedure as a bridge to combined kidney-liver transplantation in severe chromium-copper acute intoxication: a paediatric case report. Liver. 2002;22:76–7.
86. Kreymann B, Seyge M, Schweigart U, Kopp KF, Classen M. Albumin dialysis: effective removal of copper in a patient with fulminant Wilson disease and successful bridging to liver transplantation: a new possibility for the elimination of protein-bound toxins. J Hepatol. 1999;31:1080–5.
87. de Geus H, Mathôt R, van der Hoven B, Tjoa M, Bakker J. Enhanced paracetamol clearance with molecular adsorbents recirculating system (MARS®) in severe autointoxication. Blood Purif. 2010;30:118–9.
88. McIntyre CW, Fluck RJ, Freeman JG, Lambie SH. Use of albumin dialysis in the treatment of hepatic and renal dysfunction due to paracetamol intoxication. Nephrol Dial Transplant. 2002;17:316–7.
89. Felldin M, Friman S, Backman L, Siewert-Delle A, Henriksson BA, Larsson B, Olausson M. Treatment with the molecular adsorbent recirculating system in patients with acute liver failure. Transplant Proc. 2003;35:822–3.
90. Koivusalo AM, Yldirim Y, Vakkuri A, Lindgren L, Höckerstedt K, Isoniemi H. Experience with albumin dialysis in five patients with severe overdoses of paracetamol. Acta Anaesthesiol Scand. 2003;47:1145–50.

91. Hydzik P, Drozdz M, Sulowicz W, Groszek B. Liver albumin dialysis – application in acetaminophen poisoning. Przegl Lek. 2004;61:377–82.
92. Hydzik P, Gawlikowski T, Ciszowski K, Kwella N, Sein Anand J, Wojcicki M, et al. Liver albumin dialysis (MARS®) – treatment of choice in Amanita phalloides poisoning? Przegl Lek. 2005;62:475–9.
93. Lionte C, Sorodoc L, Simionescu V. Successful treatment of an adult with Amanita phalloides – induced fulminant liver failure with Molecular Adsorbent Recirculating System. Rom J Gastroenterol. 2005;14:267–71.
94. Sein Anand J, Chodorowski Z, Hydzik P. Molecular Adsorbent Recirculating System – MARS® as a bridge to liver transplantation in Amanita phalloides intoxication. Przegl Lek. 2005;62:480–1.
95. Sein Anand J, Chodorowski Z, Wisniewski M, Waldman W. The assessment of albumin liver dialysis—MARS® efficacy in the treatment of Amanita phalloides poisoning. Przegl Lek. 2007;64:255–7.
96. Wisniewski M, Lukasik-Glebocka M, Chodorowski Z, Sein AJ. Albumin dialysis (MARS®) vs standard therapy in management of Amanita phalloides poisoning (Abstract). Clin Toxicol. 2008;46:402–3.
97. Kantola T, Kantola T, Koivusalo AM, Höckerstedt K, Isoniemi H. Early molecular adsorbents recirculating system treatment in Amanita mushroom poisoning. Ther Apher Dial. 2009;13:399–403.
98. Peszynski P, Stange J, Mitzner S, Klammt S, Majcher-Peszynska J, Wacke R, Drewelow B, Schmidt R. Removal of benzodiazepine-like substances as a cause of improvement of hepatic encephalopathy during albumin dialysis. Z Gastroenterol. 2001;39:53.
99. Sen S, Ytrebo LM, Rose C, Fuskevaag OM, Davies NA, Nedredal GI, et al. Albumin dialysis: a new therapeutic strategy for intoxication from protein-bound drugs. Intensive Care Med. 2004;30:496–501.
100. Kramer L, Bauer E, Schenk P, Steininger R, Vigl M, Mallek R. Successful treatment of refractory cerebral edema in ecstasy/cocaine-induced fulminant hepatic failure using a new high-efficacy liver detoxifi cation device (FPSA-Prometheus). Wien Klin Wochenschr. 2003;115:599–603.
101. Sein Anand J, Chodorowski Z, Wisniewski M. Molecular Adsorbent Recirculating System (MARS®) a helpful procedure in acute liver failure caused by synthetic amphetamines intoxication. Przegl Lek. 2006;63:514–5.
102. Braun RC, Birck R, Singer MV, Schnuelle P, van der Woude FJ, Löhr M. Life-threatening intoxication with methylenebis(thiocyanate): clinical picture and pitfalls. A case report. BMC Emerg Med. 2006;6:5.
103. Fagugli RM, Gentile G, Ferrara G, Brugnano R. Acute renal and hepatic failure associated with allopurinol treatment. Clin Nephrol. 2008;70:523–36.

Chapter 7
Liver Hematoma and Hepatic Rupture

Carlos Montufar

Introduction

Preeclampsia is a syndrome with multisystem expression and involvement, due to its pathophysiology, which has an endothelial component. In this way, preeclampsia has the ability to damage almost any organ or system, leading to serious complications such as cerebral hemorrhage, acute pulmonary edema, and hepatic rupture [1].

Another important complication of preeclampsia is the development of the triad consisting of hemolysis, elevated liver enzymes, and thrombocytopenia (HELLP syndrome), which increases maternal and perinatal mortality and morbidity [1]. This complication (HELLP syndrome), in turn, facilitates the formation of hepatic hematomas.

In 1844, Abercrombie published in the London Medic Gazette the "first case" of a liver rupture in a pregnant woman who, after 26 hours of labor and normal delivery, presented a circulatory collapse and death. The necropsy revealed a hemoperitoneum of approximately two liters and two sites of rupture of the hepatic parenchyma [2].

Hepatic rupture is a rare complication, but lethal. It is associated with preeclampsia, and more specifically HELLP syndrome, with very few cases presented with preeclampsia without HELLP syndrome [3, 4]. Reported maternal mortality is 16% to 100% [5], depending on the capacity of the hospital center to solve these cases, according to its resources and medical technology, as well as the training of its medical personnel.

The actual frequency of hepatic hematomas in pregnant patients is unknown, since not all liver hematomas rupture. A considerable number of liver hematomas can remain intact, and are not diagnosed. The incidence is estimated to be at one per

---

C. Montufar (✉)
Obstetrics Critical Care Unit, Fellowship Program of Critical Care Obstetrics, Complejo Hospitalario, Caja de Seguro Social, Panama City, Panama

C. Montufar et al. (eds.), *Obstetric Catastrophes*,
https://doi.org/10.1007/978-3-030-70034-8_7

67,000 births or one per 2000 patients with preeclampsia, eclampsia, or HELLP syndrome [6]. It is probable that only cases of liver rupture with successful outcomes will be published, and the literature will not expose the cases with poor results.

The rupture of a hepatic hematoma in patients with HELLP syndrome usually occurs during pregnancy and a third occurs within the first 48 hours of puerperium [7], although hepatic ruptures have been described up to six weeks post-partum [8]. Regardless of when it occurs, hepatic hematoma is a serious condition, especially with the rupture thereof, which becomes an obstetric catastrophe.

Pathophysiology

Its pathophysiology includes hemorrhage and periportal congestion, and fibrin deposits, which leads to sinusoidal obstruction and intrahepatic vascular congestion, producing ischemia of the liver and necrosis [9, 10].

Sensitization of the reticuloendothelial system of the liver by preeclampsia may render it unable to clear the fibrin thrombi from the circulation, resulting in infarction with vascular disruption, leading to intrahepatic hemorrhage and parenchyma destruction [11]. The initial phase leads to the formation of "microhematomas."

This liver damage leads to intrahepatic hemorrhage and the possible development of a hepatic hematoma, which can cause a rupture within the peritoneal space, resulting in profound hemorrhagic shock and death [11].

Clinical Presentation

Some patients present with a "mild" clinical presentation with the formation of a hematoma that is asymptomatic and without hemodynamic impact, while others may reach the catastrophic scenario of ruptured liver, severe coagulopathy, and deep circulatory collapse. Among its clinical manifestations is pain in the upper right quadrant or epigastric pain in 90% of cases, shoulder pain, vomiting, and sudden circulatory collapse [4].

Henny et al. described a biphasic sequence of events in which the patient initiates the described symptoms, with worsening of the epigastric pain and/or upper right quadrant of the abdomen, nausea, and vomiting; and a second phase where deep vascular collapse, shock and death, both maternal and fetal, develop [12].

Spontaneous hepatic hemorrhage/rupture has been reported to occur most commonly in the right lobe of the liver [13], with a group of patients that presents hematomas in both hepatic lobes, and a smaller percentage of patients who present hematomas specifically in the left lobe of the liver. Thus, in almost 98% of cases, patients with preeclampsia/HELLP syndrome, who have a hepatic hematoma, have the right lobe of the liver involved [13].

Diagnosis

The diagnosis of liver rupture secondary to a hepatic hematoma in patients with preeclampsia/HELLP syndrome is based on clinical suspicion. The presence of a circulatory collapse and confirmation, either by imaging studies (ultrasonography, computed tomography, and magnetic resonance imaging) or from the finding of hemoperitoneum during a cesarean, make the diagnosis of liver hematoma. Both the ultrasound and the computed tomography are useful for the diagnosis by images of the hepatic hematoma. But sonography is more easily available and it is feasible to perform at the bedside of the patient wherever it is. In cases of having diagnostic doubts after performing a liver ultrasound, you can support by performing a Computed Tomography [14]. Magnetic resonance is more expensive and more difficult to dispose of this technological resource.

Given the lack of specificity regarding these symptoms, the variable clinical presentation, and the low incidence of this complication, diagnosis is often delayed until the rupture has already occurred and the patient is in hypovolemic shock.

The prevalence of liver hematomas in pregnant women with HELLP syndrome laboratory criteria and severe right upper quadrant pain was 39% in a series of 34 cases [15].

Treatment

There has been much disagreement about what would be the correct approach to liver hematoma, especially when it causes the rupture of the liver. The majority considers that a hematoma without a hepatic rupture can have a conservation approach, with clinical surveillance and through image studies.

In cases with bleeding without rupture of the capsule, conservative treatment with volume replacement and transfusion of blood products is the treatment of choice. Surgery is the treatment of choice in patients with hemodynamic instability despite adequate resuscitation and when the hematoma ruptures into the peritoneal cavity.

When the diagnosis of hepatic hematoma (not broken) is suspected or confirmed during the antepartum period, an exploratory laparotomy and fetal extraction via cesarean section should be performed to avoid rupture of the liver due to increased intra-abdominal pressure during labor, or some other event such as vomiting or an eclamptic convulsions [12].

If the hepatic hematoma is diagnosed during the puerperium, conservative management is possible, following up with imaging studies, and in case of coagulation alteration, blood products will be transfused [4].

Even in the presence of a non-ruptured hepatic hematoma, laboratory alteration can occur with elevated aminotransferases and alterations in the parameters of coagulation. In case of alterations of the coagulation, this should be corrected with the transfusion of blood products: plasma, platelets, and cryoprecipitate. In cases where the hematoma is large and causes anemia, stored red blood cell should be transfused.

To avoid massive bleeding with a subsequent circulatory collapse due to a hepatic rupture secondary to a parenchyma hematoma, hepatic artery ligation [4, 16], embolization of the hepatic artery [17, 18], suture of the hepatic parenchyma [7, 8], packing [4, 7, 8, 19], placement of absorbable hemostatic material [8], laser argon [6], until liver transplantation [7, 20] have been described.

The surgical approach by liver packing is the intervention with the lowest mortality rate (20–30%) for patients with a hepatic rupture described in the literature [8, 21]. Other approaches such as hepatic lobectomy, hepatic artery ligation, and hepatic embolization have mortality rates of 75 [8], 40 and 35% [21], respectively.

The literature has shown that the performance of a hepatic lobectomy leads to higher maternal mortality when compared to the packing approach (82% vs 24% survival, respectively) [22].

The management of patients with hemodynamic and/or coagulopathic compromise consists in a complex approach of different surgical options and correction of coagulation in an intensive care unit. In patients where rupture of the liver occurs, with a circulatory collapse due to hypovolemia, resuscitation with crystalloids, such as Ringer's Lactate, is necessary. To the extent that massive bleeding stops, the use of crystalloids will be less necessary, and therefore, we will have less-known negative effects of the use of fluids. In many cases, due to the multisystemic impact of a massive hemorrhage, the use of vasopressors, such as norepinephrine, will be necessary.

Because cases of hepatic rupture secondary to HELLP syndrome are infrequent, there are no agreements regarding the best management of these patients. The most commonly used techniques are liver packing, hepatic artery ligation, and embolization of the hepatic artery by specialists in interventional radiology [23].

Surgical options (hepatic artery ligation, embolization of the hepatic artery, hepatic parenchyma suture, liver packing, placement of absorbable mesh, laser argon, and liver transplant) will depend on the experience of the surgeon, as well as the availability of equipment and materials for the realization of the chosen procedure.

Another important factor is whether the patient responds to support management and stability is achieved. Only in this way it will be possible to perform procedures, such as embolization of the hepatic artery, by interventional radiology.

Liver transplantation is necessary in the presence of liver necrosis data, data of fulminant hepatic failure, or inability to stop liver bleeding.

Few cases of pregnancy following a liver rupture due to HELLP syndrome have been reported [24]. In most of these cases, a recurrence of hepatic rupture has not been published, except in one case [25].

There is still much to investigate and know about the pathophysiology of hepatic rupture in HELLP syndrome, as per the findings described by Greenstein [26], who, through a liver arteriogram, showed numerous pseudoaneurysms in the area of bleeding, suggesting that vasculopathy plays a primary role in the pathogenesis of the intrahepatic hemorrhage associated with pregnancy.

Despite all the diagnostic, preventive, predictive, and therapeutic efforts, preeclampsia remains one of the main causes of maternal death in the world. This syndrome has the capacity to generate complications with high lethality, such as the development of a hepatic hematoma with its consequent rupture and maternal death.

The early identification or suspicion of a hepatic hematoma or hepatic rupture, together with the transfusion of blood products for the correction of coagulopathy, and the choice of a surgical intervention to stop the bleeding, will be key to achieving the survival of patients with diagnoses of preeclampsia/HELLP syndrome.

References

1. Magee LA, Pels A, Helewa M, Rey E, Dadelszen P, On behalf of the Canadian Hypertensive Disorders of Pregnancy (HDP) Working Group. Diagnosis, evaluation, and management of the hypertensive disorders of pregnancy. Pregnancy Hypertens. 2014;4(2):105–45.
2. Abercrombie J. Hemorrhage of the liver. Lon Med Gaz. 1844;34:792–4.
3. Martin JN Jr, Rinehart BK, May WL, Magann EF, Terrone DA, Blake PG. The spectrum of severe preeclampsia: comparative analysis by HELLP (hemolysis, elevated liver enzyme level, and low platelet count) syndrome classification. Am J Obstet Gynecol. 1999;180:1373–84.
4. Araujo AC, Leao MD, Nobrega MH, Bezerra PF, Pereira FV, Dantas EM, et al. Characteristics and treatment of hepatic rupture caused by HELLP syndrome. Am J Obstet Gynecol. 2006;195:129–33.
5. Barton JR, Sibai BM. Care of the pregnancy complicated by HELLP syndrome. Obstet Gynecol Clin N Am. 1991;18(2):165–79.
6. Pavlis T, Aloizos S, Aravosita P, Mystakelli C, Petrochilou D, Dimopoulos N, Gourgiotis S. Diagnosis and surgical management of spontaneous hepatic rupture associated with HELLP syndrome. J Surg Educ. 2009;66(3):163–7.
7. Reck T, Bussenius-Kammerer M, Ott R, et al. Surgical treatment of HELLP syndrome-associated liver rupture—an update. Eur J Obstet Gynecol Reprod Biol. 2001;99(1):57–65.
8. Marsh FA, Kaufmann SJ, Bhabra K. Surviving hepatic rupture in pregnancy—a literature review with an illustrative case report. J Obstet Gynaecol. 2003;23(2):109–13.
9. Agatisa PK, Ness RB, Roberts JM, et al. Impairment of endothelial function in women with a history of preeclampsia: an indicator of cardiovascular risk. Am J Physiol Heart Circ Physiol. 2004;286:1389–93.
10. Levine RJ, Maynard SE, Qian C, et al. Circulating angiogenic factors and the risk of preeclampsia. N Engl J Med. 2004;350:672–83.
11. Arias F, Mancilla-Jimenez R. Hepatic fibrinogen deposits in preeclampsia: immunofluorescent evidence. N Engl J Med. 1976;295(11):578–82.
12. Henny CP, Lim AE, Brummelkamp WH, et al. A review of the importance of acute multidisciplinary treatment following spontaneous rupture of the liver capsule during pregnancy. Surg Gynecol Obstet. 1983;156:593–8.
13. Poo JL, Góngora J. Hepatic hematoma and hepatic rupture in pregnancy. Ann Hepatol. 2006;5(3):224–6.
14. Rinehart BK, Terrone DA, Magann EF, Martin RW, May WL, Martin JN Jr. Preeclampsia-associated hepatic hemorrhage and rupture: mode of management related to maternal and perinatal outcome. Obstet Gynecol Surv. 1999;54(3):196–202.
15. Barton JR, Sibai BM. Hepatic imaging in HELLP syndrome (hemolysis, elevated liver enzymes, and low platelet count). Am J Obstet Gynecol. 1996;174(6):1820–5.
16. El Youssoufi S, Nsiri A, Salmi S, Miguil M. Liver rupture in peripartum: about 8 cases. J Gynecol Obstet Biol Reprod (Paris). 2007;36(1):57–61.

17. Pilco P, McCormack L, Perez D, Clavien PA. Ruptured subcapsular hepatic hematoma associated with HELLP syndrome. Rev Gastroenterol Peru. 2006;26(2):207–10.
18. Harris BM, Kuczkowski KM. Diagnostic dilemma: hepatic rupture due to HELLP syndrome vs. trauma. Arch Gynecol Obstet. 2005;272(2):176–8.
19. Miguelote RF, Costa V, Vivas J, Gonzaga L, Menezes CA. Postpartum spontaneous rupture of a liver hematoma associated with preeclampsia and HELLP syndrome. Arch Gynecol Obstet. 2009;279(6):923–6.
20. Shames BD, Fernandez LA, Sollinger HW, Chin LT, D'Alessandro AM, Knechtle SJ, et al. Liver transplantation for HELLP syndrome. Liver Transpl. 2005;11(2):224–8.
21. Dildy GA, Belfort M. Complications of pre-eclampsia. In: Lyall F, Belfort M, editors. Pre-eclampsia etiology and clinical practice. London: Cambridge University Press; 2007. p. 406–24.
22. Smith LG, Moise KJ, Dildy GA, Carpenter RJ. Spontaneous rupture of the liver during pregnancy: current therapy. Obstet Gynecol. 1991;77:171–5.
23. Singh Y, Kochar S, Biswas M, et al. Hepatic rupture complicating HELLP syndrome in pregnancy. Med J Armed Forces India. 2009;65(1):89–90.
24. Sakala EP, Moore WD. Successful term delivery after previous pregnancy with ruptured liver. Obstet Gynecol. 1986;68:124–6.
25. Greenstein D, Henderson JM, Boyer TD. Liver hemorrhage: recurrent episodes during pregnancy complicated by preeclampsia. Gastroenterology. 1994;106:1668–71.
26. Greenstein D, Henderson JM, Boyer TD. Liver hemorrhage: recurrent episodes during pregnancy complicated by preeclampsia. Gastroenterology. 1994;106(6):1668–71.

Chapter 8
Pregnancy-Associated Thrombotic Thrombocytopenic Purpura and Hemolytic-Uremic Syndrome

Rania Magdi Ali, Bahaa El-Din Ewees Hassan, and Noura M. Youssri Mahmoud

Introduction

Thrombotic thrombocytopenic purpura (TTP) and hemolytic-uremic syndrome (HUS) are part of thrombotic microangiopathy (TMA) syndromes, which represent a spectrum of disorders characterized by endothelial damage resulting in microvascular thrombosis that leads to the mechanical shearing of erythrocytes and the consumption of platelets. The microvascular thrombi also lead to end-organ damage, such as renal abnormalities and neurological symptoms. Accordingly, TMA typically presents with microangiopathic hemolytic anemia (MAHA), thrombocytopenia, and organ failure of variable severity [1]. Both TTP and HUS are not pregnancy-specific pathologic conditions but occur with higher incidence in pregnancy [2].

TMA during pregnancy represents a heterogeneous group that also includes hemolysis, elevated liver enzymes, low platelets (HELLP) syndrome, acute fatty liver of pregnancy (AFLP), antiphospholipid syndrome (APS), and systemic lupus erythematosus (SLE) besides TTP and HUS. It is important to note other pregnancy-related complications, like sepsis, placental abruption, and postpartum hemorrhage; they can present as TMA since they can cause MAHA, thrombocytopenia in addition to acute kidney injury [3].

Efficient differentiation of the causes of TMA diagnosed during pregnancy is sometimes difficult due to overlapping clinical and laboratory features. A high index of suspicion and collaboration of multi-dispensary approach of different specialties that include nephrologists, hematologists, obstetricians, and intensivists are essential to a timely diagnosis and treatment.

R. M. Ali (✉) · B. E.-D. E. Hassan · N. M. Y. Mahmoud
Anesthesia, Intensive Care and Pain Management, Faculty of Medicine, Ain Shams University, Cairo, Egypt

C. Montufar et al. (eds.), *Obstetric Catastrophes*,
https://doi.org/10.1007/978-3-030-70034-8_8

Hemostatic Changes of Normal Pregnancy

Normal gestation is associated with marked hemostatic changes, which lead to a hypercoagulable state and provide a protective effect against hemorrhage at delivery. There is an increase in procoagulant activity, together with a decrease in fibrinolytic activity [4].

ADAMTS13, a disintegrin and metalloprotease with thrombospondin type 1 motif, member 13, is an enzyme required to break down ultra-large von Willebrand factor multimers (VWF), which increase platelet adhesion with subsequent thrombotic occlusion of the microvasculature and platelet consumption [5]. VWF increase in pregnancy and return to normal levels over the puerperium period. In normal pregnant women, ADAMTS13 activity normally decreases in the second and third trimesters of pregnancy and return to pre-gestational levels over the puerperium period. In women with hereditary TTP, the increase in VWF may consume an already severely reduced ADAMTS13 level. Therefore, late-onset hereditary TTP can be revealed by pregnancy. Therefore, hereditary TTP can be revealed by pregnancy and complications is usually noted in untreated cases from the second trimester whereas the requirements for plasma increase to maintain a normal platelet count in cases under treatment [6].

During pregnancy, there is a reduction in the platelet count to 10% less than the pre-pregnancy level, particularly during the last trimester. The mechanisms are a combination of dilutional effects and acceleration of platelet destruction across the placenta. Most women still have platelet counts within the normal range at term. Nevertheless, if the starting count is at the lower end of the normal range, or there is a more severe reduction, thrombocytopenia occurs [7]. Hence, thrombocytopenia is often an incidental feature, but it might also provide a biomarker of a coexisting systemic or gestational disorder.

Pathologic Feature

The central pathologic feature of TMA is the formation of platelet thrombi in the microvasculature which may produce tissue ischemia and infarction. In TTP, the platelet thrombi contain large amounts of von Willebrand factor (VWF). These thrombi cause shearing stress on the red blood cells passing through the Plasma antithrombin III causing fragmentation and thrombotic microangiopathic hemolytic anemia [1].

In HUS, hyperactivation of complement results in diffuse endothelial injury, with subsequent formation of fibrin and platelet microthrombi in the vasculature, leading to hemolysis, thrombocytopenia, and acute kidney injury [8]. In atypical HUS associated with pregnancy, the primary pathology is in the renal arterioles and interlobular arteries. Widespread endothelial cell swelling leading to exposure of the underlying basement membrane is the main manifestation. Hence, the vessel lumens are occluded by red cells and platelet fibrin thrombi [6]. In atypical HUS associated with pregnancy, the primary pathology is in the renal arterioles and interlobular arteries, with widespread endothelial cell swelling, leading to exposure of the underlying basement membrane. The vessel lumens are occluded by red cells and platelet fibrin thrombi [6].

Although TTP and HUS have pathologic features similar to those of TMA and similar clinical features, they are distinct entities with distinct etiologies and pathogenesis.

Etiologies of TTP and HUS

TTP

TTP is more common in women and at least half of all cases of TTP occur in women of childbearing age [6]. Pregnancy can be the trigger event for approximately 5–25% of TTP cases [2]. TTP usually occurs in the second part of pregnancy and sometimes in postpartum, but it is not ruled out during the first trimester of gestation [9].

TTP is characterized by a severe deficiency of ADAMTS13 [5]. There are two types of TTP: the acquired type caused by anti-ADAMTS13 immunoglobulin G and the hereditary type caused by the mutation of genes resulting in persisting ultra-large von Willebrand factor multimers. The acquired type is much more common than the hereditary type [7].

A deficiency in ADAMTS 13 activity, less than 40% but greater than 10%, can be seen in disseminated intravascular coagulopathy (DIC), HUS, preeclampsia, and the HELLP syndrome, but a severe deficiency of less than 5–10% of the normal activity and the presence of IgG antibodies are specific to TTP [10]. Altered ADAMTS13 activity and presence of antibody can be found in secondary causes of TTP such as human immunodeficiency virus infection (HIV), hepatitis B and C virus, or iatrogenic by some drugs [11].

Although hereditary TTP is much less common than acquired TTP, the relative frequency of hereditary TTP is higher among women presenting during their first pregnancy. Approximately 10% of women with acquired TTP and up to half of those with hereditary TTP present for the first-time during pregnancy or postpartum, often the first pregnancy [12].

HUS

There are two forms of HUS: typical and atypical forms. Typical HUS is more common in children than in adults; the most common cause is infection with Shiga-toxin producing Escherichia coli. It can also be associated with HIV, oral contraceptive pills, autoimmune diseases like systemic lupus erythematosus, bone marrow transplantation, cancer, and cyclosporin and other medications [2].

Pregnancy usually triggers atypical HUS—20% of all women present with atypical HUS for the first-time during pregnancy [12]. HUS is estimated to occur in 1 in 25,000 pregnancies and up to 20% of them present with atypical HUS during the initial pregnancy, while the others have had previous unaffected gestations [12]. Further, 80% of affected women develop HUS postpartum, with the remainder distributed throughout all trimesters [8].

Atypical HUS associated with pregnancy is caused by dysregulation of the alternative complement pathway. It is most commonly hereditary with mutations of genes encoding complement regulatory proteins and pregnancy acts as a trigger in those with an underlying genetic predisposition. Also, it may also be acquired with antibodies to complement factor H, the major regulatory protein of the alternative complement pathway [3]. Several factors such as inflammation, drugs, cancer, preeclampsia, maternal–fetal hemorrhage, and infections may act as a trigger for complement activation in an already genetically susceptible individual [8]. In atypical HUS, ADAMTS13 activity may be normal or moderately reduced more than 10% but with no antibodies to ADAMTS13 [13].

Diagnostic Criteria for TTP and HUS

Presentation of a TMA requires careful review of clinical features and laboratory parameters to aid in differential diagnosis.

Clinical Features

The diagnostic criteria for TTP and HUS consist of a classic pentad of MAHA, thrombocytopenia, central nervous system abnormalities, fever, and renal impairment [14]. The differentiation between TTP and HUS depends on the severity of thrombocytopenia, neurologic abnormalities, and kidney injury.

Patients with TTP typically have severe thrombocytopenia ranging between 10 and 30,000/μL and may have overt neurologic abnormalities but rarely have severe kidney injury. Thrombocytopenia presents as petechiae, nose bleeding and, more rarely, hematuria and gastrointestinal bleeding. It is unusual to have any clinical signs or symptoms when the platelet count is greater than 50,000/μL, unless platelet function is also defective [7]. Neurological presentation could include loads of signs as headache, altered personality, reduced cognition, and transient ischemic attacks up to coma [15]. In HUS, generally the platelet count does not drop severely, overt neurological abnormalities are rare, and the most distinctive feature is the more severe kidney impairment that requires dialysis. In HUS, severe hypertension, congestive heart failure, and neurologic symptoms develop secondary to uncontrolled renal failure [8].

The classic pentad occurs in less than half of the patients of TTP and HUS. The triad of anemia, thrombocytopenia, and fluctuating neurologic abnormalities can be observed in up to 75% of the patients of TTP and the triad of anemia, thrombocytopenia, and renal impairment is the typical presentation in atypical HUS [6]. Hence, the diagnosis of TTP and HUS is often made by a dyad of thrombocytopenia and MAHA because of the discrepancy of non-hematological findings, whether fever, neurologic abnormalities, or renal impairment [14].

The gestation at presentation is a factor that promotes distinguishing diagnosis. Although pregnancy-associated TTP most commonly presents in the third trimester or postpartum period, TTP remains the most likely diagnosis of a TMA presenting in the first trimester. Also, most cases of HUS occur postpartum [6]. Diagnosis is clear when a previously healthy woman presents in the first trimester with severe MAHA, thrombocytopenia, and neurologic dysfunction, which may be accompanied by renal insufficiency and fever. On the contrary, as term approaches, the overlap with the features of severe pre-eclampsia (PE) progressively increases [12].

The diagnosis of atypical HUS becomes clear when a pregnant woman presents with progressive renal failure, thrombocytopenia with platelet counts above 50,000/μL, MAHA, and, occasionally, evidence of ischemic tissue injury elsewhere in the absence of meeting the criteria for PE and HELLP. Meanwhile, in women, rapidly progressive postpartum acute kidney injury without an apparent cause for acute tubular necrosis implies atypical HUS. Before renal failure becomes the predominant feature, it is hard to reach a definitive diagnosis, especially when thrombocytopenia is severe or when extrarenal manifestations occur [12]. Extrarenal manifestations incorporate neurological involvement including seizures and altered consciousness, pancreatitis, cardiac involvement and myocardial infarction, cerebral artery thrombosis, digital gangrene, ocular involvement, and pulmonary involvement. It is not known whether they are a consequence of the TMA, a direct effect of complement activation, or complications of AKI, such as severe hypertension and uremia [16].

Differential Diagnosis

The diagnosis of TTP or HUS should be considered in the appropriate clinical context after exclusion of other causes of TMA and thrombocytopenia.

Pregnancy-Specific TMA

In pregnancy, the differentiation of TTP or HUS from other TMAs may be very difficult. The primary diagnostic challenge is the differentiation from acute fatty liver of pregnancy (AFLP), PE, and HELLP syndrome.

1. *PE and HELLP syndrome*

When a pregnant or postpartum woman develops severe MAHA and thrombocytopenia, three syndromes must be considered: preeclampsia with severe features and HELLP syndrome, TTP, and HUS in spite of the fact that other conditions can cause them.

PE is a multisystem disorder resulting from endothelial damage. PE is the most common cause of thrombocytopenia associated with TMA presenting after 20 weeks of gestation and uncommonly postpartum. Most women with PE develop thrombocytopenia, with platelet counts generally above 100,000/μL and not below 50,000/μL unless there are superimposed complications [12].

Although MAHA is not among the criteria defining PE with severe features, it commonly occurs with the HELLP syndrome. HELLP syndrome is a variant of PE. TMA-like presentation occurs more profoundly in HELLP syndrome and is characterized by more severely elevated liver function tests than in PE. Biochemical changes consistent with DIC may be present in up to 10% of women and can be a marker of disease progression [12].

Features of PE and HELLP syndrome may be the initial presentation prior to the subsequent diagnosis of TTP or HUS [5]. Due to overlapping clinical and laboratory features, TTP and HUS are often mistaken for PE or HELLP. Unfortunately, delays in appropriate diagnosis and treatment may be life-threatening.

Development of seizures in woman with TMA proposes the differential diagnosis of eclampsia in addition to TTP. In such conditions, PE and HELLP syndrome could exclude the diagnosis of TTP by providing an alternative etiology for MAHA and thrombocytopenia, particularly that TTP is much less common than PE and HELLP syndrome [3].

TTP confers an increased risk of PE and HELLP syndrome particularly among women who have recovered from an acute episode of acquired TTP and who are at risk of recurrent acute episodes [10]. Therefore, the diagnosis of TTP must be considered in women with severe preeclampsia who have severe MAHA and thrombocytopenia. Moreover, the presence of transient focal abnormalities, such as weakness, numbness, and aphasia, in women with PE and HELLP syndrome suggests the diagnosis of TTP [17]. Instantly, renal involvement may be seen with PE, whereas in HUS, it is so aggressive that two-thirds of cases eventually develop end-stage renal failure [6].

In PE and HELLP syndrome, delivery of the baby is the definitive treatment and the clinical course after delivery may alter the diagnosis. In women with PE and HELLP syndrome, the average time for platelet recovery above 100,000/μL is 3 days postdelivery [18]. LDH recovery may be slower than thrombocytopenia. Increasing platelet counts, in addition to decreasing LDH and creatinine, can be considered hallmark to exclude TTP or HUS. Whereas in women with PE and HELLP syndrome who do not show clinical and laboratory improvement within 48–72 hours postdelivery, TTP should be considered as an alternative diagnosis [12]. Likewise, if women develop severe and progressive renal insufficiency postdelivery, it suggests the diagnosis of HUS [3].

2. *Acute fatty liver of pregnancy*

Acute fatty liver of pregnancy (AFLP) may result from mitochondrial dysfunction and typically presents in the third trimester, although it rarely presents in the first and second trimesters. Most women presentation is non-specific, it usually presents with nausea or vomiting and pain in right upper quadrant or epigastric or else presents with signs and symptoms consistent with PE. AFLP is characterized by impaired hepatic function reflected as encephalopathy, marked elevations in transaminases and bilirubin together with hypoglycemia. Hypoglycemia is a key diagnostic feature not seen in related conditions. Reduction in plasma antithrombin III may be an early marker of AFLP, and coagulopathy up to DIC picture can develop. Thrombocytopenia is not uncommon, and usually mild to moderate. Renal impairment with elevated creatinine associated with blood pressures in the normal range can help the diagnosis of AFLP [13].

Diagnosis is made by combination of clinical and biochemical features and can be supported by using Swansea criteria [19] which require 6 or more of 14 features in the absence of another explanation. The 14 features include vomiting, abdominal pain, polydipsia/ polyuria, encephalopathy, hyperbilirubinemia, elevated transaminases, hypoglycemia, coagulopathy, hyperuricemia, hyperammonemia, renal impairment, leukocytosis, ascites or bright liver on ultrasound scan, micro vesicular steatosis on liver biopsy. However, it is usually impossible to undertake liver biopsy because of the coagulopathy [6].

Pregnancy Non-specific TMA

TMA can develop in patients with APS, SLE, and DIC in addition to other forms of vasculitis or scleroderma, allogeneic bone marrow transplantation, allograft rejection, and graft-versus-host disease. They present as MAHA in association with thrombocytopenia. There is insufficient information to determine whether pregnancy poses an increased risk of TMA in these settings or not [12]. The clinical picture of TMA, SLE, and APS may overlap and, if any of them coexist in the same patient, the diagnosis may be difficult at the time of initial presentation.

1. *Systemic lupus erythematosus*

SLE can mimic all clinical features of TTP. SLE may present with hemolytic anemia, thrombocytopenia, neurologic deficits, fever, renal insufficiency and even can present with low levels of ADAMTS-13. TTP can present in approximately 2% of the patients with SLE, commonly in patients with active SLE disease. Patients present with antiphospholipid and/or lupus anticoagulant have an increased risk of thromboembolism compared with those who lack these antibodies. TTP occurring in pregnant patients with SLE has potentially higher mortality than either disease alone [20].

2. *Antiphospholipid syndromes*

APL may be associated with PE in addition to thrombosis and recurrent fetal loss, and have been described in patients with HELLP, HUS, or TTP [20].

3. *Disseminated intravascular coagulation*

DIC is characterized by the activation of the coagulation system, microvascular thrombus formation in different organs, and multiple organ failure. In pregnancy, DIC is caused by several causes, the most important being placental abruption, amniotic embolus, and uterine rupture. It is defined by an increase in the prothrombin time (PT), aPTT, thrombocytopenia, decreased fibrinogen, fibrin degradation product accumulation, and the presence of D-dimers. Notably, the degree of hemolysis and thrombocytopenia is less profound [12].

It can be very difficult to differentiate DIC from HUS and TTP. The very low platelet count with normal international normalized ratio (INR), partial thromboplastin time (PTT), and D-dimer in a patient with marked thrombocytopenia makes DIC less likely. Notably, some patients initially diagnosed with TTP were later confirmed to have DIC [2].

Sepsis, disseminated malignancy, and systemic vasculitis may all be associated with microangiopathy, primarily due to associated DIC. Sepsis with DIC must be excluded in acutely ill patients with fever, thrombocytopenia, and multiorgan dysfunction. High spiking fevers and rigors are not characteristic of TTP and suggest sepsis [2].

Pregnancy-Related Thrombocytopenia

Thrombocytopenia develops in 5–10% of women during pregnancy or in the immediate postpartum period. A low platelet count is often an incidental feature of pregnancy, but it might also provide a biomarker of a coexisting systemic or gestational disorder.

1. *Pseudo thrombocytopenia*

They induce platelet aggregation, resulting in false low platelet count. Pseudo thrombocytopenia is often seen when anticoagulants such as EDTA are used when collecting blood. A peripheral blood smear is important for establishing the diagnosis; the platelets are seen arranged in stacks [2].

2. *Immune thrombocytopenia (ITP)*

ITP is the most common cause of a decrease in platelet count below 50,000/μL in the first and second trimesters [12]. There is no laboratory test to distinguish ITP from other causes of maternal thrombocytopenia. Patients could be completely asymptomatic or present ecchymosis, petechiae, purpura, gum bleeding, or menorrhagia. The diagnosis is clinical and based on a personal history of bleeding, a low platelet count prior to pregnancy or may present with other immune mediated diseases. The therapeutic response to steroids or intravenous immunoglobulins can contribute to the diagnosis of ITP. A peripheral blood smear reflects only thrombocytopenia without unusually small or giant platelets [2].

3. *Von Willebrand disease type IIb*

It is a rare cause of thrombocytopenia in pregnancy. Thrombocytopenia is justified by increased platelet aggregation as a result to von Willebrand factor elevated affinity to the platelet receptor of glycoprotein 1b. Women with this condition may present with thrombocytopenia for the first time in pregnancy and platelets can drop to values below 20-30 000/μL [2].

4. *Drug-induced thrombocytopenia*

Thrombocytopenia is a frequent adverse effect of commonly used drugs. Heparin-induced thrombocytopenia (HIT) can rarely occur with the administration of unfractionated heparin but not with the use of low-molecular-weight heparin in pregnancy [7]. In HIT, thrombosis is the cause of thrombocytopenia and ischemic manifestations. HIT can be distinguished from TTP and HUS by the absence of hemolysis and red blood cell fragmentation.

5. *Viral infection*

Almost any virus, particularly HIV and cytomegalovirus infections, can cause a reduction in platelet count. This is usually transient but may extend for several weeks [7].

Laboratory Parameters

Laboratory investigations are useful in establishing the diagnosis of TTP and HUS.

Laboratory Investigations to Identify TMA

Thrombotic microangiopathy should be suspected in any patient presenting with unexplained MAHA and thrombocytopenia. Corresponding blood film changes include anemia, polychromasia (abnormally large number of immature red blood cells in the bloodstream), reticulocytosis, thrombocytopenia, and fragmented red blood cells. Schistocytes usually form more than 1% of red cells in the blood smear [1]. However, in the appropriate clinical context, the mere presence of schistocytes is adequate. TMA may present without schistocytosis, just at initial presentation and in the setting of early relapse. The coagulation screen, prothrombin time, activated partial thromboplastin time, fibrinogen, and D-dimers are often normal [21].

Thrombocytopenia is defined as a platelet count of less than 150,000/μL and only a platelet count less than 100,000/μL is clinically significant [22]. The severity of thrombocytopenia is an important biomarker of a coexisting systemic or gestational disorder. Although thrombocytopenia always occurs in PE and HELLP syndrome, it is typically not severe. In contrast, thrombocytopenia among TTP patients is always severe. The platelet count typically ranges from 10,000/μL to 30,000/μL [23], while in HUS, the platelet count is usually above 50,000/μL [24].

Classic biochemical evidence of nonimmune hemolysis includes high lactate dehydrogenase (LDH) and indirect bilirubin and low haptoglobin levels in addition to a negative direct antiglobulin test [21]. Serum lactate dehydrogenase (LDH) levels may be very high in TTP and HUS, as well as PE and HELLP syndrome. LDH is often increased out of proportion to the degree of hemolysis due to associated tissue ischemia. Nevertheless, it has a diagnostic and prognostic value. Notably, the LDH reference range changes with pregnancy and is more than twice the non-pregnant level in the third trimester [3].

Laboratory Investigations to Determine the Cause of TMA

The cause of TMA may not be obvious initially, but the differential diagnosis can be narrowed down quickly by performing multiple laboratory investigations.

TTP is characterized by a severe ADAMTS13 deficiency of less than 5–10%, and its activity should be measured in all patients in whom the diagnosis of TTP is suspected. However, because the results of ADAMTS13 activity measurements may not be available for several days and because it is not always available, the initial diagnosis of TTP and the decision to begin plasma exchange treatment are based on clinical judgment [25].

The diagnosis of atypical HUS is suspected when a woman presents with TMA and progressive renal impairment. Shiga-toxin-induced HUS is excluded by performing a stool culture and a molecular detection of Shiga toxin using polymerase chain reaction assay [1]. Renal impairment can be identified by raised serum creatinine levels above 2.2 mg/dl. Urinalysis may reveal only mild proteinuria, microscopic hematuria, and few casts. A progressive rise in serum creatinine or the need for dialysis on initial presentation of women with PE and HELLP syndrome suggests the diagnosis of HUS regardless of the fact that the criteria for acute kidney injury at diagnosis can be part of PE and HELLP syndrome [24].

The role of genetic testing during the initial evaluation of atypical HUS remains limited as patients with a confident clinical diagnosis of HUS do not have an identified complement mutation. The greatest value of genetic testing is to provide information about the risk of recurrence and for planning long-term management. Consumption of plasma C3 and C4 and generation of soluble C5b-9 complexes are seen in some forms of HUS but are not diagnostic [26].

A marked increase in liver function tests suggests PE and HELLP syndrome or AFL. Antiphospholipid antibodies and lupus anticoagulant, and serologies for systemic lupus erythematosus are done if laboratory data, history, and physical examination suspect the diagnosis. Viral screening for HIV, hepatitis C virus, and hepatitis

B virus, and *Helicobacter pylori* testing are also recommended [1]. Plasma antithrombin III level is helpful in differentiating among the various causes of TMA, being reduced in PE and normal in TTP [12].

Management of TTP and HUS

The cause of TMA is usually established after a complete evaluation. However, the results of the investigations are not available immediately, while immediate management decisions are required. Acute decision-making is time-critical. The priority should be the consideration of TTP, because maternal mortality can be reduced by 80–90% in women who are promptly treated [12]. Therefore, plasma exchange should be instituted, after obtaining a sample for ADAMTS13 activity testing if available, on the presumption that it is TTP until proved otherwise. If the ADAMTS13 result excludes TTP, then complement-mediated atypical HUS is assumed and treatment with eculizumab is recommended if it is yet again available [16].

The goal of treatment in TTP or HUS is to continue the pregnancy until an appropriate time for delivery. There is no evidence to suggest that either anticomplement treatment or plasma exchange is harmful for the fetus. There is no evidence to suggest that delivery is beneficial for either TTP or HUS. The postpartum period appears to have as much risk as during gestation for TTP and particularly for HUS [3].

Although the clinical features of both TTP and HUS appear to be alike, they get different treatment modalities.

Plasma Therapy

TTP

The efficacy of plasma therapy depends on the supplement of large amounts of ADAMTS13 in addition to removal of the inhibitory antibodies such as in case of plasma exchange. In the hereditary cases, infusion of fresh frozen plasma is enough since they do not have antibodies [7].

Plasma infusion of 10–15 mL/kg IV is recommended with attention to avoid volume overload. If the volume of plasma to be infused cannot be tolerated, then plasma exchange is recommended [1]. The half-life of ADAMTS13 is 2–3 days, nevertheless the optimal frequency of plasma replacement during pregnancy is variable. Every 1–2 week initially may be enough while maintenance infusions is individually guided by the platelet counts and serum LDH concentrations [5].

The plasma exchange treatment course consists of daily 1–1.5 plasma volume exchanges using plasma as the replacement fluid. Various types of plasma are treated to reduce the viral transmission or manipulated to reduce the level of vWF multimers like the cryosupernatant plasma, which is plasma that remains after the cryoprecipitate is prepared. Nevertheless, none of these products has shown superiority over regular plasma as plasma exchange replacement fluid [27].

Similarly, the frequency of exchange is based on platelet count and LDH concentrations, and is repeated until the normal levels are reached [5]. Noting that absence of schistocytes is not necessary before discontinuation of plasma exchange. Once platelet counts have normalized, plasma exchange can either be stopped abruptly or weaned, with increasing time between procedures. It is important to note that there is no evidence demonstrating the superiority of weaning compared with abruptly stopping therapy [1].

Afterward and up until the postpartum period, platelet count and LDH concentrations are monitored and subsequently plasma infusion can be administered. However, if there is poor response plasma exchange can be restarted according to the platelet count [6].

HUS

Plasma exchange should be started in the acute setting with identification of the dyad of thrombocytopenia and MAHA. However, once endorsement of ADAMTS13 levels, if available, complement inhibition with eculizumab is the therapy of choice [16].

In atypical HUS, the mainstay of plasma exchange is replacing the mutant dysfunctional forms of proteins with normal regular proteins. Although plasma therapy may improve the hematologic parameters, especially if associated with acquired anti-complement factor H antibodies, but unfortunately with lesser renal improvement [28]. It is recommended to start plasma exchange before hemodialysis if the latter is also necessary [1].

Eculizumab is not always available. In many parts of the world, the cost of eculizumab precludes its use, and plasma exchange remains the only treatment for atypical HUS [29]. The installation of both plasma therapy and eculizumab concurrently requires the need for additional eculizumab doses and therefore increases the cost of treatment significantly [3].

PE and HELLP Syndrome

Plasma exchange is applicable for severe preeclampsia and HELLP syndrome when spontaneous recovery following delivery is doubtful and clinical worsening or mortality is expected [14].

Anticomplement Eculizumab

Eculizumab is a monoclonal anti-C5 inhibitor and has been used in pregnancy in women with paroxysmal nocturnal hematuria. Eculizumab is safe in pregnancy and in lactating mothers. The main concerns are the high costs and the risk of Neisseria infection, thus vaccination prior to treatment is required and long-term antibiotic prophylaxis is recommended for up to three months after withdrawal [6, 12].

Eculizumab increases platelet counts, improves renal function, reduces the need for renal replacement therapy, and improves the overall quality of life for patients with HUS [2]. Pregnancy may require an increase in the dosage and/or frequency of eculizumab infusions due to the increase in the distribution volume or C5 synthesis. Thus, a careful monitoring of complement blockade is mandatory [30].

It is worth mentioning that there is subjective experience with the use of eculizumab in some patients with HELLP as some abnormalities in complement regulatory pathways have been described in HELLP [16]. However, preeclampsia has occurred in women taking eculizumab for paroxysmal nocturnal hemoglobinuria [31] and aHUS [30].

Platelet Transfusions

TMA is a disorder of microcirculatory thrombosis and severe hemorrhage is rare. In HELLP syndrome and AFL, platelet transfusions may be useful in severely affected mothers. Conversely, administration of platelets to a patient with TTP or HUS may deteriorate the clinical picture by increasing thrombosis. Therefore, platelet transfusion should be avoided and reserved to cases with life-threatening bleeding or when an invasive procedure is required. Nevertheless, platelets should not be withheld in a bleeding patient due to this concern [32].

Glucocorticoids

In the era of plasma therapy, assessing the additional benefit of secondary therapies is difficult. Steroids can reduce the production of the ADAMTS13 inhibitor in patients with hereditary TTP [33]. Although evidence from randomized clinical trial is lacking, either prednisone 1 mg per kg daily orally or methylprednisolone 125 mg IV 2–4 times daily has been recommended at the same time as plasma exchange, then gradually tapered off once remission is achieved [1].

Others

Rituximab, anti-CD20 therapy, is reserved for the refractory situations. Rituximab has been used in pregnancy for a variety of other autoimmune conditions [34]. The evidence on the use of azathioprine, or other modalities in women with TTP who do not respond to plasmapheresis, is limited. Factor VIII preparation containing ADAMTS13 has been used; data on the use of recombinant ADAMTS13 are needed [12].

Antiplatelet and Anti-coagulant Agents

Low-dose aspirin and low-molecular-weight heparin augment the potential for hemorrhagic complications without proven benefit. They can only be advocated once the platelet count is greater than 500,000/μL during pregnancy to avoid the effect of microthrombi formation on placenta [5]. Women with a previous pregnancy loss due to TTP or with low ADAMTS13 activity at the onset of pregnancy can be assumed to be at increased risk of further placental disorder in subsequent pregnancies. However, recommendations for the use of anticoagulants in these patients have low evidence [6].

Supportive Care

These often critically ill patients require appropriately intensive supportive care. Red blood cell transfusions are usually indicated based on the initial hemoglobin level and degree of hemolysis. Hypertension may necessitate medical intervention. Hemodialysis may be indicated for severe renal insufficiency. Seizures may develop during illness, and anti-convulsant therapy is indicated in such patients.

Mode of Delivery

If delivery is required urgently, for instance, because of progressive clinical symptoms or fetal distress, cesarean section is usually performed. Intensive plasma exchange pre-cesarean should be considered if time permits. Pulsed methylprednisolone 500–1000 mg IV daily for 2–4 consecutive days in those with acquired TTP could be given post-plasma exchange [6].

It is advisable to consider delivery at a maximum of 37-week gestation [6]. Induction of labor and vaginal delivery is encouraged. Vaginal delivery is safe when the platelet count is higher than 30,000/μL. For operative vaginal or cesarean deliveries, the safe platelet count should be at least 50,000/μL. The exact platelet number needed to achieve a safe epidural anesthesia is not established but 75,000–85,000/μL is considered appropriate as there is a theoretical concern over the risk of epidural hematoma with lower platelet counts. Spontaneous bleeding may occur with less than 20,000/μL and the risk of internal bleeding is increased if the platelet count falls below 10,000/μL [2].

Fetal Outcomes

When TTP occurs in the first and second trimesters, the stillbirth rate in TTP is frequent, mainly due to intrauterine fetal death, spontaneous abortions, and prematurity caused by widespread placental ischemia. Conversely, when TTP develops closer to term and when maternal treatment has been effective, the incidence of healthy live births approaches 75–90% [10]. It is worth noting that no cases of fetal thrombocytopenia or hemolytic anemia have been described, although the anti-ADAMTS13 antibodies cross the placental barrier [12]. On the other hand, in women with atypical HUS, the risk of fetal loss is lower, ranging from 10% to 20%, which may reflect the capture of microthrombi by the maternal renal microvasculature [9].

Long-Term Outcomes

Women who have recovered from TTP or HUS have significant long-term morbidities. Concerning TTP, they have increased frequency of abnormal kidney function [35], minor cognitive impairment, severe depression, and systemic lupus erythematosus [36]. Then again, regarding atypical HUS greater than 75% of cases develop ESRD despite plasma exchange [24] whereas in the era of eculizumab, this high prevalence of ESRD is diminishing [3].

Considerations for Subsequent Pregnancies

TTP and HUS are not contraindications to pregnancy in women who have had a history of either acute TTP or HUS unrelated to pregnancy. Accordingly, there should be a multidisciplinary supervision with hematologists and obstetricians, and patients should have regular fetal growth scans and uterine artery Doppler studies during pregnancy [6]. Women who have recovered from TTP or atypical HUS may also have an increased risk of PE during subsequent pregnancies [6, 12].

TTP

In TTP, close monitoring of ADAMTS13 activity and antibody is an absolute requirement prior to or early in the first trimester of pregnancy to identify women at highest risk who require close surveillance.

In women with a history of acquired TTP who subsequently become pregnant, it is not as easy to predict who may relapse. The risk of recurrence and the negative impact on the pregnancy itself are not clear as supporting data are limited. ADAMTS13 activity at the onset of pregnancy is a useful prognostic marker. Platelet counts should be followed monthly in case of normal levels of ADAMTS13 at the onset of pregnancy. If ADAMTS13 activity is lower than 10% at the onset of pregnancy, regular plasma exchange throughout pregnancy is recommended [6].

In women with a history of hereditary ADAMTS13 deficiency, the risk of relapse in the subsequent pregnancies is absolute. Prophylaxis with serial plasma infusions should be strongly considered throughout subsequent gestations. Plasma exchange may be required, particularly later in pregnancy [37].

Atypical HUS

In patients with a known history of atypical HUS, there is 10–30% risk of recurrence in subsequent pregnancies [24]. As soon as pregnancy is confirmed in women on anti-hypertensive therapy, antihypertensive drugs should be revised to ensure that they are appropriate during pregnancy particularly if the patient is on angiotensin-converting-enzyme inhibitors. Whereas in women not on anti-hypertensive therapy, strict monitoring of the blood pressure is mandatory. It is common for renal protein leak to increase during pregnancy associated HUS. Hence, monitoring of protein-creatinine ratios in conjunction with creatinine levels is vital in such cases of pregnancy associated HUS [6].

In women on anticomplement therapy prior to pregnancy, eculizumab should continue to the postpartum period, which is the greatest period of relapse. Conversely, in women who are not already on eculizumab, it is difficult to predict a relapse using routine laboratory parameters. Like in hereditary TTP, starting eculizumab at least by the second trimester and until the end of the postpartum period is appropriate [6].

References

1. Go RS, Winters JL, Leung N, Murray DL, Willrich MA, Abraham RS, Amer H, Hogan WJ, Marshall AL, Sethi S, Tran CL, Chen D, Pruthi RK, Ashrani AA, Fervenza FC, Cramer CH 2nd, Rodriguez V, Wolanskyj AP, Thomé SD, Hook CC. Thrombotic microangiopathy care pathway: a consensus statement for the Mayo clinic complement alternative pathway-thrombotic microangiopathy (CAP-TMA) dsease-oriented group. Mayo Clin Proc. 2016;91(9):1189–211.

2. Ciobanu AM, Colibaba S, Cimpoca B, Peltecu G, Panaitescu AM. Thrombocytopenia in pregnancy. Maedica (Buchar). 2016;11(1):55–60.
3. George JN, Nester CM, McIntosh JJ. Syndromes of thrombotic microangiopathy associated with pregnancy. Hematology Am Soc Hematol Educ Program. 2015;2015:644–8.
4. Laganà AS, Sofo V, Salmeri F, Chiofalo B, Ciancimino L, Triolo O. Post-partum management in a patient affected by Thrombotic thrombocytopenic purpura: case report and review of literature. Clin Exp Obstet Gynecol. 2015;42:90–4.
5. Scully M, Thomas M, Underwood M, Watson H, Langley K, Camilleri RS, Clark A, Creagh D, Rayment R, McDonald V, Roy A, Evans G, McGuckin S, Ni Ainle F, Maclean R, Lester W, Nash M, Scott R, O'Brien P, Collaborators of the UK TTP Registry. Thrombotic thrombocytopenic purpura and pregnancy: presentation, management, and subsequent pregnancy outcomes. Blood. 2014;124:211–9.
6. Thomas MR, Robinson S, Scully MA. How we manage thrombotic microangiopathies in pregnancy. Br J Haematol. 2016;173(6):821–30.
7. Myers B. Thrombocytopenia in pregnancy. Obstet Gynaecol. 2009;11:177–83.
8. Saad AF, Roman J, Wyble A, Pacheco LD. Pregnancy-associated atypical hemolytic-uremic syndrome. AJP Rep. 2016;6(1):e125–8.
9. Scully M. Thrombotic thrombocytopenic purpura and atypical hemolytic uremic syndrome microangiopathy in pregnancy. Semin Thromb Hemost. 2016;42(7):774–9.
10. Jiang Y, McIntosh JJ, Reese JA, Deford CC, Kremer Hovinga JA, Lämmle B, Terrell DR, Vesely SK, Knudtson EJ, George JN. Pregnancy outcomes following recovery from acquired thrombotic thrombocytopenic purpura. Blood. 2014;123(11):1674–80.
11. Birkhoelzer S, Belcher A, Peet H. Diagnostic dilemma: severe thrombotic microangiopathy in pregnancy. J Intensive Care Soc. 2017;18(4):348–51.
12. Cines DB, Levine LD. Thrombocytopenia in pregnancy. Blood. 2017;130(21):2271–7.
13. Hassan S, Westwood JP, Ellis D, Laing C, Mc Guckin S, Benjamin S, Scully M. The utility of ADAMTS13 in differentiating TTP from other acute thrombotic microangiopathies: results from the UK TTP Registry. Br J Haematol. 2015;171:830–5.
14. Mwita JC, Vento S, Benti T. Thrombotic thrombocytopenic purpura-haemolytic uremic syndrome and pregnancy. Pan Afr Med J. 2014;17:255.
15. Scully M, Hunt BJ, Benjamin S, Liesner R, Rose P, Peyvandi F, Cheung B, Machin SJ, British Committee for Standards in Haematology. Guidelines on the diagnosis and management of thrombotic thrombocytopenic purpura and other thrombotic microangiopathies. Br J Haematol. 2012;158:323–35.
16. Brocklebank V, Wood KM, Kavanagh D. Thrombotic microangiopathy and the kidney. Clin J Am Soc Nephrol. 2018;13(2):300–17.
17. Kremer Hovinga JA, Vesely SK, Terrell DR, Lämmle B, George JN. Survival and relapse in patients with thrombotic thrombocytopenic purpura. Blood. 2010;115(8):1500–11.
18. Martin JN, Blake PG, Perry KG, McCaul JF, Hess LW, Martin RW. The natural history of HELLP syndrome: patterns of disease progression and regression. Am J Obstet Gynecol. 1991;164(6):1500–13.
19. Kingham JG. Swansea criteria for diagnosis of acute fatty liver of pregnancy. Gut. 2011;60:139–40.
20. McCrae KR. Thrombocytopenia in pregnancy: differential diagnosis, pathogenesis, and management. Blood Rev. 2003;17:7–14.
21. Nester CM, Thomas CP. Atypical hemolytic uremic syndrome: what is it, how is it diagnosed, and how is it treated? Hematology Am Soc Hematol Educ Program. 2012;2012:617–25.
22. Pranas M, Shiner E, Shoham-Vardi I, Burstein E, Yeridah T, Levi I, Hochberg G, Yerushalmi R. Moderate to severe thrombocytopenia during pregnancy. Eur J Obstet Gynecol Reprod Biol. 2006;128:163–8.
23. Kremer Hovinga JA, Vesely SK, Terrell DR, Lämmle B, George JN. Survival and relapse in patients with thrombotic thrombocytopenic purpura. Blood. 2010;115(8):1500–11.
24. Fakhouri F, Roumenina L, Provot F, Sallée M, Caillard S, Couzi L, Essig M, Ribes D, Dragon-Durey MA, Bridoux F, Rondeau E, Frémeaux-Bacchi V. Pregnancy-associated hemolytic

uremic syndrome revisited in the era of complement gene mutations. J Am Soc Nephrol. 2010;21(5):859–67.
25. George JN. Measuring ADAMTS13 activity in patients with suspected thrombotic thrombocytopenic purpura: when, how, why. Transfusion. 2015;55(1):11–3.
26. Legendre CM, Licht C, Muus P, Greenbaum LA, Babu S, Bedrosian C, Bingham C, Cohen DJ, Delmas Y, Douglas K, Eitner F, Feldkamp T, Fouque D, Furman RR, Gaber O, Herthelius M, Hourmant M, Karpman D, Lebranchu Y, Mariat C, Menne J, Moulin B, Nürnberger J, Ogawa M, Remuzzi G, Richard T, Sberro-Soussan R, Severino B, Sheerin NS, Trivelli A, Zimmerhackl LB, Goodship T, Loirat C. Terminal complement inhibitor eculizumab in atypical hemolytic-uremic syndrome. New Engl J Med. 2013;368(23):2169–81.
27. Rock G, Anderson D, Clark W, Leblond P, Palmer D, Sternbach M, Sutton D, Wells G, Canadian Apheresis Group. Does cryosupernatant plasma improve outcome in thrombotic thrombocytopenic purpura? No answer yet. Br J Haematol. 2005;129(1):79–86.
28. McClain RS, Terrell DR, Vesely SK, George JN. Plasma exchange complications in patients treated for thrombotic thrombocytopenic purpura-hemolytic uremic syndrome: 2011–2014. Transfusion. 2014;52(12):3257–9.
29. Hofer J, Giner T, Safouh H. Diagnosis and treatment of the hemolytic uremic syndrome disease spectrum in developing regions. Semin Thromb Hemost. 2014;40:478–86.
30. Servais A, Devillard N, Frémeaux-Bacchi V, Hummel A, Salomon L, Contin-Bordes C, Gomer H, Legendre C, Delmas Y. Atypical haemolytic uraemic syndrome and pregnancy: outcome with ongoing eculizumab. Nephrol Dial Transplant. 2016;31:2122–30.
31. Kelly RJ, Höchsmann B, Szer J, Kulasekararaj A, de Guibert S, Röth A, Weitz IC, Armstrong E, Risitano AM, Patriquin CJ, Terriou L, Muus P, Hill A, Turner MP, Schrezenmeier H, Peffault de Latour R. Eculizumab in pregnant patients with paroxysmal nocturnal hemoglobinuria. N Engl J Med. 2015;373:1032–9.
32. Patnaik MM, Deshpande AK, Nagar V, Algotar K. Thrombotic microangiopathies presenting as an obstetric emergency. J Assoc Physicians India. 2004;52:152–3.
33. Basta M. Thrombotic thrombocytopenic purpura during pregnancy and its overlap with the HELLP syndrome, a clinical dilemma: a case report and review of the literature. J Obstet Anaesth Crit Care. 2019;9:50–2.
34. Page EE, Kremer Hovinga JA, Terrell DR, Vesely SK, George JN. Rituximab reduces risk for relapse in patients with thrombotic thrombocytopenic purpura. Blood. 2016;127:3092–4.
35. Little DJ, Reese JA, Vesely SK, George JN. Increased urinary albumin excretion following recovery from acquired thrombotic thrombocytopenic purpura. Am J Kidney Dis. 2014;64(2):317–8.
36. Deford CC, Reese JA, Schwartz LH, Perdue JJ, Kremer Hovinga JA, Lämmle B, Terrell DR, Vesely SK, George JN. Multiple major morbidities and increased mortality during long-term follow-up after recovery from thrombotic thrombocytopenic purpura. Blood. 2013;122(12):2023–9.
37. Battinelli EM. TTP and pregnancy. Blood. 2014;123(11):1624–5.

Chapter 9
Hyperemesis Gravidarum

V. Ariatna Aguilera

Introduction

Antoine Dubois, a consultant surgeon and a head obstetrician to Napoleon Bonaparte and his second wife Empress Marie Louise, as a physician who first identified the condition in 1852. Dubois is thought to have first described the syndrome during his address before the French Academy of Medicine when he spoke about the finding of "pernicious vomiting of pregnancy" [1].

The prevalence of hyperemesis gravidarum is approximately 0.3–3% of pregnancies and varies on account of different diagnostic criteria and ethnic variation in study populations. Notwithstanding, most studies agree that hyperemesis gravidarum is more common among young, primiparous mothers who are non-Caucasian and nonsmokers [2].

The etiology of hyperemesis gravidarum is likely multifactorial. With typical onset at 4–8 weeks of pregnancy and continuing through weeks 14–16 of pregnancy [3].

Clinical Diagnosis

According to the latest American College of Obstetricians and Gynecologists (ACOG) guidelines on Nausea and Vomiting during pregnancy (2015), there still is no single accepted definition of hyperemesis gravidarum (HG).

V. A. Aguilera (✉)
Critical Care Obstetrician, Department of Gynecology and Obstetrics, Division of Obstetrics Critical Care, Caja de Seguro Social, Panamá, Panama

C. Montufar et al. (eds.), *Obstetric Catastrophes*,
https://doi.org/10.1007/978-3-030-70034-8_9

The most commonly cited criteria for diagnosis of hyperemesis gravidarum include the following:

- Persistent vomiting not related to other causes
- An objective measure of acute starvation (usually large ketonuria on urine analysis)
- Electrolyte abnormalities and acid-base disturbances, as well as weight loss Weight loss is often cited as at least 5% loss of pre-pregnancy weight [3].

Recently, a classification system was created to categorize hyperemesis gravidarum called the pregnancy-unique quantification of emesis and nausea (PUQE) scoring index. This index accounts for the daily number of vomiting episodes, the length of nausea per day in hours, and the number of retching episodes per day [4].

Of note, the ACOG 2015 guidelines recommend that serum thyroid function studies should be obtained only in the presence of other signs of hyperthyroidism such as a palpable goiter. Several studies also recommend testing for *Helicobacter pylori* infection, as gastric ulcers can be a contributing factor to persistent, refractory hyperemesis gravidarum [3].

Etiology

No discrete mechanism of pathogenesis has yet been established, but the number of proposed associations continues to suggest that the etiology of hyperemesis gravidarum (HG) is likely multifactorial [5]. Mechanism such as:

- Psychiatric Background: Current studies regarding this topic are targeted at evaluating the development of depression, anxiety, posttraumatic stress disorder, and other psychiatric disorders as an effect of hyperemesis gravidarum, rather than a cause.
- There exists a number of hypotheses regarding hormonal causes of hyperemesis gravidarum like levels of serum human chorionic gonadotropin (hCG), estrogen, and progesterone.
- Genetics: One of the more prevailing theories on the etiology of hyperemesis gravidarum is the importance of genetic factors in its pathogenesis [5].
- Thyroid hormone: In early pregnancy, physiological stimulation of the thyroid gland occasionally leads to gestational transient thyrotoxicosis (GTT). GTT has been observed in up to two-thirds of women suffering from hyperemesis [5].

Therapeutic Options

A wide range of interventions have been studied in randomized control trials (RCTs) for management of hyperemesis gravidarum, starting from supportive measures, such as hydration, to preconception supplementation with prenatal vitamins for

3 months prior to conception. Various outpatient and inpatient pharmacological methods and alternative medicine methods such as acupuncture [3] have also been described [5].

Some drugs described in the management of hyperemesis are [5] as follows:

- Diclegis is an antihistamine (H1 blocker) with vitamin B6 (cofactor in enzymatic reactions), with a clinical benefit mainly in nausea/vomiting of pregnancy. May aid in pretreatment of HG. Pregnancy category A.
- Ondansetron is a selective 5-HT3 receptor antagonist. It is consider first-line treatment in HG. Pregnancy category B.
- Metoclopramide is an anti-HT3 with antidopaminergic properties. Prokinetic agent first-line treatment in HG. Pregnancy category B.
- Clonidine is a centrally acting alpha-agonist. Pilot studies show benefit in refractory HG. Pregnancy category C.
- Promethazine is a weak antidopaminergic and antiserotonin receptor activity in CNS, antimuscarinic, long-lasting antihistamine action. Small-scale studies for refractory HG show benefit of addition of promethazine to first-line treatment. Pregnancy category C.
- Prednisone with multifactorial mechanism of action. Small-scale studies show addition of prednisone decreases daily episodes of emesis. Pregnancy category C.
- Mirtazapine with multifactorial mechanism of action: adrenergic alpha2 antagonist, serotonin 5-HT2, and 5-HT3 antagonism with histaminergic and muscarinic effects. It shows benefit in symptomatic relief in small-scale studies of refractory HG. Pregnancy category C; Strong association of prednisone exposure and fetal oral cleft defects [5].

Maternal Complications

A. Wernicke's Encephalopathy

Introduction

Wernicke's encephalopathy (WE) is an acute neurological condition caused by vitamin B1 or thiamine deficiency, which is potentially fatal that can lead to *Korsakoff syndrome*, coma, and death [6]. It was first described in 1881, by the polish neurologist Carl Wernicke, as a clinical triad characterized by ophthalmoplegia, ataxia, and mental confusion [7].

In the United States, the majority of cases appear in alcoholics, patients with malnutrition secondary to hyperemesis gravidarum (HG), starvation, diabetic ketosis, cancer, acquired immunodeficiency syndrome (AIDS), or administration of parenteral glucose in a state of low thiamine reserve [8].

Wernicke's encephalopathy complicates 0.1–0.5% of pregnancies and has a 10–20% of mortality [10].

Thiamine deficiency causes significant decrease on utilization of cerebral glucose utilization and causes mitochondrial damage [11].

The diagnosis should be suspected in patients with a history of neurological symptoms (apathy and mental confusion). Magnetic resonance imaging (MRI) is the gold standard method, and it demarcates hyperdense, bilateral, and symmetric lesions around the fourth ventricle. However, the best diagnostic method is measuring the level of neurological response to the administration of thiamine [12–15].

Symptoms usually reverse in the first hours or days after the administration of thiamine. In 53% of cases, symptoms reverse during the first three months [16]. In an English literature review of Di Gangi and his group [15] that included 62 publications of Wernicke's encephalopathy (WE), it was observed that the average gestational age at which the disease was presented was 14.6 ± 3.9 weeks. The vomiting clinic was 7.3 ± 3.2 weeks prior to encephalopathy. Of these patients, 26% required parenteral treatment.

It can be developed in patients with hyperemesis gravidarum (HG), since thiamine deposits are altered by the needs of the growing fetus, and the presence of incoercible vomiting leads to a decrease in food intake, malnutrition, and malabsorption [18].

It has been suggested that almost 70% of WE cases are not diagnosed before severe complications occur [17]. As of June 2008, only 45 cases of pregnant patients had been reported in the world literature [19].

Risk Factors

Main causes of thiamine deficiency [20, 21]

Chronic alcoholism
Hyperemesis gravidarum (HG)
Malnutrition
Fast
Vomiting
Anorexia nervosa
Dialysis and kidney diseases
Infections
Intoxications
Thyroid diseases
Cancer
Acquired immunodeficiency syndrome
Gastrointestinal surgery/digestive tract pathology

The most common cause of thiamine deficiency is malnutrition secondary to alcoholism. Other causes may be due to dietary deficiency (beriberi, anorexia nervosa), systemic diseases (disseminated tuberculosis), treatment with diuretics, iatrogenic (chronic hemodialysis), and hyperemesis gravidarum, although this remains a diagnosis little recognized by its low frequency [22].

For its part, hyperemesis gravidarum is a syndrome that occurs in the first half of pregnancy, affecting pregnant women in 0.3–2%, is characterized by incoercible nausea and vomiting causing weight loss, dehydration, ketoneuria, and hydroelectrolytic disorders attributed to the hormonal peak of hCG and estradiol [23, 24].

Some predisposing risk factors for HG are the history of multiple gestation, previous caesarean section, previous HG, conception by assisted reproduction techniques, molar pregnancy, gestational diabetes, depressive disorders, hyperthyroid disorders, peptic ulcer, and asthma [25, 26].

HG occurs in young, primiparous, low social strata women, and with female products 55.6% compared to male products 44.4%.

Pathogenesis

Thiamine was the first vitamin B identified, so it was called B12. It is a water-soluble vitamin, which is actively reabsorbed in the duodenum [28, 29] and is deposited in the muscle, heart, liver, kidneys and brain, although its most important place of storage is muscle [29, 30]. Thiamine pyrophosphate is the biological active form, an essential coenzyme in many brain biochemical processes [31]. Thiamine is a cofactor of several enzymes such as transketolase, pyruvate dehydrogenase, and alpha-ketoglutarate dehydrogenase.

The Sources of Thiamine

The primary sources of this vitamin are yeasts, pork, legumes, beef, whole grains and nuts, and the average intake from food is 2 mg/day. Tea, coffee, raw fish, and shellfish contain thiamines that destroy vitamins, so that the consumption of these foods decreases the reserve of this vitamin [27].

Body reserves are 25–30 mg (approximately 18 days of storage), so they can be depleted in 2 weeks if not replenished [31].

Thiamine Deficiency

There is a decrease in the activity of transketolase, which involves focal lactic acidosis, cerebral energetic alteration, and depolarization of neurons by *n*-methyl-D-aspartate. This causes alterations of the blood-brain barrier, generation of free radicals, and cell death due to apoptosis and necrosis [19].

Nearly 46.9% of patients have the classic triad of ophthalmoplegia, ataxia, and mental confusion. It is possible that at first, only one or two nonspecific symptoms appear such as apathy, decreased attention, disorientation, tachycardia, hypotension, hypothermia, and seizures [6].

It is important to take into account that in these pregnant patients the picture may be precipitated if glucose serums are administered repeatedly or in situations of hyperthyroidism or thyrotoxicosis.

Di Gangi and his collaborators [15] observed that ocular alterations appear in 95.2% of patients and of them horizontal nystagmus is the most frequent.

Brain alterations appear in 82.5%, ataxia in 74.6% and confusion and hypotonia in 60.3% of cases. Mild memory impairments arise in 52.3% of cases and severe disorders of consciousness in 30.1%.

Chiosii and his group2 carried out a review in 49 patients with hyperemesis gravidarum, in which only 47% had the classic triad.

The ocular symptoms appeared in 96% of the cases, and manifested as: nystagmus, weakness, or paralysis of the straight muscles producing diplopia, ptosis, arreactive myotic pupils, small retinal hemorrhages, and papillae edema. The ataxia appeared in 96%, and manifested itself as alterations of gait and posture, with slow and staggered gait.

Among the cognitive alterations, amnestic syndrome-confabulation, restlessness, stupor and, in severe cases, coma stand out. It has been reported that 80% of patients who survive have *Korsakoff syndrome*, characterized by behavioral abnormalities, confabulations, and memory impairment (anterograde and retrograde amnesia) [20, 31].

Diagnosis

Suspicion before any pregnant patient with hyperemesis gravidarum and neurological alteration. The diagnosis can be made by ataxia, mental confusion, and visual disturbances that are present in almost all cases. Horizontal nystagmus is the most frequent. 10% of patients with WE do not have alterations in mental status, but alterations in memory and cognitive deficits are detected [33].

Magnetic resonance imaging (MRI) is the gold standard for diagnosis. This has a sensitivity of 53% and specificity of 93%. It is important for the initial diagnosis and the exclusion of other causes. The characteristic lesions are hyperintense, bilateral, and symmetrical and involve the mammillary bodies, hypothalamic nuclei, periaqueductal gray matter, superior cerebellar vermis, midline, third, and fourth ventricles [21, 32]. There is often endothelial proliferation, demyelination, and some neuronal loss. The amnestic defect is related to the presence of lesions in the internal dorsal nuclei of the thalamus [11].

Serum determinations of thiamine and transketolase activity in erythrocytes are difficult to interpret and are not performed routinely.

The best diagnostic test is the response to the administration of thiamine.

Treatment and Prognosis

Wernicke's encephalopathy is a medical emergency and requires the immediate administration of thiamine [9].

At present there is no consensus about the optimal daily dose. The half-life of thiamine is 96 minutes, so administration in several doses can achieve better brain penetration than with only one dose [34].

When a pregnant woman presents with characteristic symptoms, a dose of 0.5–2 grams of intravenous thiamine should be received prior to providing oral or parenteral carbohydrates, since in a state of poor vitamin B1 reserve the administration of dextrose exacerbates the process of cerebral apoptosis by providing more substrate for biochemical pathways without the necessary coenzymes.

Guidelines of the European Federation of Neurological Societies (EFNS) recommend a dose of 200 mg three times a day, intravenously, before any carbohydrate, until symptoms and signs diminish [21].

The Royal College of Physicians of London developed a protocol through a high-potency complex of vitamin B, with a minimum of 500 mg of thiamine intravenously, three times a day for 3 days, in case of good response should continue with 500 mg daily for 5 days or until clinical improvement occurs [30]. In patients with risk factors for WE, prophylactic thiamine treatment should be initiated at a dose of 250 mg daily for 3 or 5 days, and in case of requiring glucose serums, they should always be supplemented with thiamine. They recommend continuing a dose of 30 mg of thiamine twice daily for a minimum of 3 months [21].

Symptoms may reverse within the first hours or days after the administration of thiamine. In 53.9% of the cases, the symptoms revert during the first 3 months [15], leaving the nystagmus, ataxia, memory disorders, difficulty in coordination, vertigo, and paresthesia as a residual clinic.

Magnesium sulfate should be administered concomitantly, as it is known that these patients are involved with hypomagnesemia and, as this functions as a cofactor in neuronal transmission; therefore, it must be corrected so that the treatment with parenteral thiamine is effective [33–37].

A joint treatment with intensive physical, occupational, and swallowing rehabilitation should be performed.

Di Gangi and his group observed that 34.5% of the patients had spontaneous abortions, 9% legal interruptions of pregnancy, and 3.6% fetal deaths.

B. Mallory–Weiss Syndrome

Esophageal laceration associated with hematemesis, known as Mallory–Weiss syndrome (WMS), may result from the repetitive wrenching associated with hyperemesis. The American scientists Mallory and Weiss, in 1929 and 1932, respectively, revealed the cause of upper gastrointestinal bleedings: mucosal tears at the junction of the stomach and esophagus. This syndrome was associated with recurrent vomiting after drinking and a heavy meal [38]. It is estimated that WMS is the cause of 8–15% of nonvariceal upper gastrointestinal bleeding [38].

When this barotrauma causes rupture of the esophagus (Boerhaave syndrome), pneumomediastinum may result (Hamman's syndrome). While some patients with this complication may tolerate conservative management, others may require surgical intervention. This complication may be suspected in patients presenting with subcutaneous emphysema on physical exam or imaging [39].

Pathogenesis

The pathogenesis of Mallory–Weiss syndrome has not been fully studied by now. The authors have presented its mechanism as follows: in retching, the pylorus is closed, and the cardiac part of the stomach and the esophagus are dilated. The gastric contents, due to antiperistalsis and a sudden increase in intra-abdominal pressure, impetuously move forward to the gastroesophageal hole. The result is that intra-gastric pressure is rapidly increased, the cardiac part of the stomach is hyperextended, and its mucosa is lacerated [38]. The presence of a hiatal hernia has been documented as a predisposing factor because it is present in 40–80% of these patients. During vomiting, the transmural pressure gradient is thought to be greater in the hiatal hernia than that in rest of the stomach, causing the lacerations [39].

Symptoms and Diagnosis

An acute onset of hematemesis, that is, either frank red blood or coffee ground in appearance, is present in the majority of patients. This upper gastrointestinal bleeding is often preceded by an episode of vomiting, retching, straining, or coughing. Additional symptoms include back or epigastric pain, melena, or hematochezia. Signs of shock such as hypotension and tachycardia may be present depending on the blood loss volume [40, 41].

Obtaining a medical history to identify the presence of risk factors, medication use, and comorbid conditions assists in differentiating potential bleeding causes. Baseline laboratory tests include a complete blood count, serum electrolytes, blood urea nitrogen, creatinine liver function, and coagulation tests to assess the patient's current status [41]. Use of a risk stratification scale such as the Rockall scoring system aids the physician in identifying those patients at risk for adverse outcomes of rebleeding or death [42].

Treatment

The initial management of any patient with upper gastrointestinal bleeding includes assessing for hemodynamic instability, subsequent patient stabilization with intravenous (IV) fluid resuscitation, and, if indicated, blood product transfusions. The patient is kept nothing by mouth (NPO) until bleeding is controlled, and the endoscopic evaluation is done [41].

Therapeutic endoscopy may appear as the only reasonable method of treatment for patients with Mallory–Weiss syndrome. All known methods of endoscopic hemostasis can be divided into thermal, injection, and application techniques.

- Thermal methods include monopolar and bipolar electrocoagulation, laser photocoagulation, cryocautery of the source of bleeding, and others.
- Injection methods to stop gastroduodenal bleedings are widely used because of their availability and implementation simplicity: ε-aminocaproic acid, epinephrine, and ethanol injections. The initial hemostatic effect of injection methods is high and reaches 80.5–90% [43].
- The method of endoscopic treatment of gastroduodenal ulcers by insufflation of dry powdered gel sorbent into a defect region has become widespread in recent years. Hydrophilic granular sorbents are polymeric agents capable to expand in aqueous solutions and form soft gels [44].
- Another method to stop bleeding includes endoscopic adhesive applications with syringe barrels or cartridges: Lifusolum, Statisolum, Gastrosolum, biological adhesives MK-6, MK-8, and others. Parkhisenko injected a biological adhesive under pressure using a needleless injector, which provides reliable hemostasis by forming hemostatic infiltration in tissues and specific adhesive seals [45].

The basis of this disease is not just a tear in the layers of the gastroesophageal junction but also a syndrome that should be correctly called discontinuous-hemorrhagic. It is known that today, there are no specific methods of prediction, prevention, and treatment of discontinuous-hemorrhagic (Mallory–Weiss) syndrome, and they are therefore still to be developed.

Summary

Hyperemesis gravidarum remains a disease of diagnosis based on clinical judgment and not upon strict, well-defined diagnostic criteria. Variability in the clinical definition contributes to the difficulty in performing meta-analyses of available research and currently hyperemesis gravidarum does not have a clearly established etiology.

Recent literature points to a genetic predisposition in addition to previously studied factors such as infectious, psychiatric, and hormonal contributions. Maternal morbidity is commonly described on Wernicke encephalopathy and Mallory Weiss Syndrome a seriously complications of hyperemesis gravidarum, those entities have variety of therapeutic options.

References

1. Bacon CS. The vomiting of pregnancy. Am J Med Sci. 1898;115:680–3.
2. Boelig RC, Barton SJ, Saccone G, Kelly AJ, Edwards SJ, Berghella V. Interventions for treating hyperemesis gravidarum. Cochrane Database Syst Rev. 2016;5:1–147.

3. American College of Obstetricians and Gynecologists. Practice bulletin no. 153: nausea and vomiting of pregnancy. Obstet Gynecol. 2015;126:e12–24.
4. Ebrahimi N, Maltepe C, Bournissen FG, Koren G. Nausea and vomiting of pregnancy: using the 24-hour pregnancy-unique quantification of emesis (PUQE-24) scale. J Obstet Gynaecol Can. 2009;31:803–7.
5. Viktoriya L, et al. Hyperemesis gravidarum: a review of recent literature. Pharmacology. 2017;100:161–71.
6. Chiossi G, Neri I, Cavazzuti M, Basso G, Facchinetti F. Hyperemesis gravidarum complicated by Wernicke encephalopathy: background, case report, and review of the literature. Obstet Gynecol Surv. 2006;61(4):255–68.
7. Eboué C, Carlier-Guérin C, De La Sayette V, Grall JY, Herlicoviez M. A rare complication of vomiting in pregnancy: Wernicke's encephalopathy. J Gynecol Obstet Biol Reprod (Paris). 2006;35(8 Pt 1):822–5.
8. Thomson AD, Guerrini A, Marshall EJ. The evolution and treatment of Korsakoff's syndrome. Out of sight, out of mind? Neuropsychol Rev. 2012;22(2):81–92. https://doi.org/10.1007/s11065-012-9196-z.
9. Kaineg B, Hudgins PA. Images in clinical medicine. Wernicke's encephalopathy. N Engl J Med. 2005;352(19):e18.
10. Azim W, Walker R. Wernicke's encephalopathy: a frequently missed problem. Hosp Med. 2003;64(6):326–7.
11. Fell DB, Dodds L, Joseph KS, et al. Risk factors for hyperemesis gravidarum requiring hospital admission during pregnancy. Obstet Gynecol. 2006;107(2 Pt 1):277–84.
12. Pearce JM. Wernicke-Korsakoff encephalopathy. Eur Neurol. 2008;59:101–4.
13. Kasper B, Fauci H, Longo J. Harrison's principles of internal medicine. 16th ed: Mc Graw Hill; 2005. Wernicke's disease. Chapter 258. p. 1806–7.
14. Niebyl R. Nausea and Vomiting in 8. Pregnancy. N Engl J Med. 2010:15441550. S. Fejzo, Borzouyeh poursharif, et al.
15. Symptoms and pregnancy Outcomes Asociated with Extreme Weight Loss among women with Hyperemesis Gravidarum. J Women Heath. 2009;18:1981–7.
16. Ase V, et al. Maternal body 11. In: Composition, soking and hyperemesis gravidarum, vol. 20: Elsevier Inc; 2010. p. 592–8.
17. Chin W-C, et al. Total Parenteral Nutrition Treatment in Diabetic pregnant woman complicated with Hyperemesis Gravidarum, Taiwanese. J Obstet Gynecol. 2004;43:42–5.
18. Wilson RK, Kuncl RW, Corse AM. Wernicke's encephalopathy: beyond alcoholism. Nat Clin Pract Neurol. 2006;2:54–8.
19. Koguchi K, Nakatsuji Y, Abe K, Sakoda S. Wernickes's encephalopahy after glucosa infusion. Neurology. 2004;62:512.
20. Desjardins P, Butterworth RF. Role of mitocondrial dysfunction and oxidative stress in the pathogenesis of selective neuronal loss in Wernickes's encephalopathy. Mol Neurobiol. 2015;31:285–9.
21. Zuccoli G, Santa Cruz D, Bertolini M, Rovira A, Gallucci M, Carollo C, et al. MR imaging findings in 56 patients with Wernicke encephalopathy: nonalcoholics may differ from alcoholics. AJNR Am J Neuroradiol. 2009;30(1):171–6. https://doi.org/10.3174/ajnr.A1280. [Epub 2008 Oct 22].
22. Galvin R, Brathen G, Ivashynka A, Hillbom M, Tanasescu R, Leone MA. EFNS guidelines for diagnosis, therapy and prevention of Wernicke encephalopathy. Eur J Neurol. 2010;17(12):1.408–18. https://doi.org/10.1111/j.1468-1331.2010.03153.x.
23. Kumar D, Geller F, Wang L, Wagner B, FitzGerald MJ, Schwendimann R. Wernicke's encephalopathy in a patient with hyperemesis gravidarum. Psychosomatics. 2012;53:172–4.
24. Roseboom Tessa J, et al. Maternal 2. Characteristics largely explain poor pregnancy outcome after hyperemesis gravidarum. Eur J Obstet Gynecol Biol. 2011;156:56–9.
25. Anais L, Amandine L, et al. Metoclopramide and diphenhydramine in the treatment of hyperemesis gravidarum: effectiveness and predictors of rehospitalisation. Eur J Obstet Biol. 2009;143:43–9.

26. Petek KB, et al. Maternal 3. serum cytokine levels in women with Hyperemesis Gravidarum in the first trimester of pregnancy. Fertil Steril. 2003;79:3.
27. Ismail K, et al. Review on 4. Hyperemesis gravidarum, best practice and research clinical gastro enterology. 2007;21:755–69.
28. Kasper B, Fauci H, Longo J. Harrison's principles of internal medicine. 16th ed: Mc Graw Hill; 2005. Thiamine. Chapter 61. p. 452.
29. Thomson AD, Cook CC, Touquet R, Henry JA. The Royal College of Physicians report on alcohol: guidelines for managing Wernicke's encephalopathy in the accident and Emergency Department. Alcohol. 2002;37:513–21.
30. Onieva-Gonzalez, y col. Encefalopatía de Wernicke tras duodenopancreatectomia cefálica. Rev Esp Enferm Dig. 2011;103(11):594–6.
31. Reuker JB, Girard DE, Cooney TG. Wernicke's encephalophaty. N Engl J Med. 1985;312(16):1035–9.
32. Secci G, Serra A. Wernickes's encephalopathy: new clinical setting and recent advances in diagnosis and mangement. Lancet Neurol. 2007;6:422–55.
33. Anaforoglu I, Yildiz B, Incecayir O, Algún E. A woman with thyrotoxicosis-and hyperemesis gravidum-associated Wernicke's encephalopathty. Neuro Endocrinol Lett. 2012;33:285–9.
34. Lehmann HC, Lindenberg R, Arendt G, Ploner M. Acute axonal neuropathy and Wernicke's encephalopathy. J Neurol. 2016;253(11):1516–7.
35. Bailit JL. Hyperemesis gravidarium: epidemiologic findings from a large cohort. Am J Obstet Gynecol. 2005;193(3 Pt 1):811–4.
36. Lacroix R, Eason E, Melzack R. Nausea and vomiting during pregnancy: a prospective study of its frequency, intensity, and patterns of change. Am J Obstet Gynecol. 2000;182(4):931–7.
37. Whiteman VE, Homko CJ, Reece EA. Management of hypoglycemia and diabetic ketoacidosis in pregnancy. Obstet Gynecol Clin N Am. 1996;23(1):87–107.
38. Mallory K, Weiss S. Lesions of the cardiac orifice of the stomach produced by vomiting. JAMA. 1932;98:1353–5.
39. Buchanan GM, Franklin V. Hamman and Boerhaave syndromes – diagnostic dilemmas in a patient presenting with hyperemesis gravidarum: a case report. Scott Med J. 2014;59:e12–6.
40. Rich H. Mallory-weiss tear, vol. 795: Ferri's Clinical Advisor; 2018.
41. Ljubicic N, Budimir I, Pavic T, et al. Mortality in high-risk patients with bleeding Mallory-Weiss Syndrome is similar to that of peptic ulcer bleeding. Results of a prospective database study. Scand J Gastroenterol. 2014;49:458–64.
42. Wang C, Qin J, Zhu D. Rockall score in predicting outcomes of elderly patients with acute upper gastrointestinal bleeding. World J Gastroenterol. 2013;19(22):3466–72.
43. Sordia DG. [Endoscopic infiltration of adrenaline in treatment of gastroduodenal bleedings]. New technologies in surgery: papers of the International Surgical Congress: Rostov-on-Don; 2005. p. 243.
44. Cherednikov EF. [On the mechanism of action of gel sorbents for gastroduodenal bleedings]. Current issues of emergency medical care—reality and perspectives: abstracts of the paper. Pract Conf (Voronezh). 1996;(1):72–3.
45. Parkhisenko YA. [Treatment of ulcerous gastroduodenal bleedings with regard to the posthemorrhagic condition]: abstracts of the doctoral thesis: Voronezh; 1997. p. 43.

Part III
Endocrine

Chapter 10
Diabetic Ketoacidosis and Pregnancy

Nares-Torices Miguel Angel, Flores-Cortés Mildred Ibeth, and Hernández-Pacheco José Antonio

Box 10.1 Definitions

Diabetic ketoacidosis (DKA)	Biochemical triad; hyperglycemia, ketonemia, and metabolic acidosis with high anionic gap
Hyperglycemic hyperosmolar state (HHS)	Consists of moderate or variable degrees of clinical ketosis and alterations in consciousness can often be present without coma

Both DKA and HHS are characterized by hyperglycemia and absolute or relative insulinopenia. Clinically it can be differentiated by the severity of dehydration, ketosis, and metabolic acidosis (see Box 10.2).

N.-T. M. Angel (✉)
Medical Emergencies Specialist, Critical Medicine and Obstetric Critical Medicine Sub-specialist, National Medical Center IMSS "La Raza", México City, Mexico

F.-C. M. Ibeth
Gynecology and Obstetrics Specialist, Private Medicine, México City, Mexico

H.-P. J. Antonio
Internal Medicine Specialist, Critical Medicine and Obstetric Critical Medicine Sub-specialist, National Institute of Perinatology, México City, Mexico

C. Montufar et al. (eds.), *Obstetric Catastrophes*,
https://doi.org/10.1007/978-3-030-70034-8_10

Box 10.2 Criteria for diabetic ketoacidosis (DKA) and hyperosmolar hyperglycemic state (HHS)

Diabetic ketoacidosis (DKA)				Hyperosmolar hyperglycemic state (HHS)
	Mild	Moderate	Severe	HSS
Glycemia	>250 mg/dL	>250 mg/dL	>250 mg/dL	>600 mg/dL
pH	7.25–7.30	7.00–7.24	<7.0	>7.30
Bicarbonate mEq/L	15–18	10–15	<15	>18
Seric/urinary ketone	+	+	+	Low
Effective osmolarity	Variable	Variable	Variable	>320 mOm
GAP anion	>10	>12	>12	Variable
Mental state	Alert	Obtunded	Stupor	Stupor/coma

The triad of DKA (hyperglycemia, acidemia, and ketonemia) and other conditions with the individual components are associated. From Kitabchi and Wall [1].

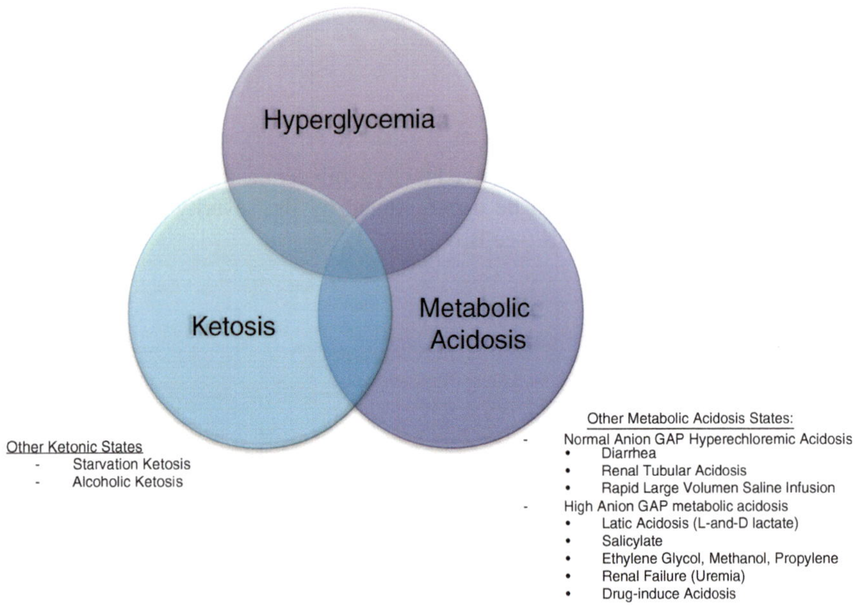

Diabetic Ketoacidosis and Pregnancy

It is a medical emergency that could present maternal and fetal morbidity and mortality. The worldwide prevalence of diabetes and pregnancy has even increased in recent years, due to the tendency of diets in high calories, decreased physical activity, and increased obesity. Factors like pregnancy in women with obesity and the genetic burden of women with a history of diabetes mellitus make women more prone to gestational diabetes in pregnancy [2].

The incidence of diabetic ketoacidosis and pregnancy is difficult to establish since there are only cases report, retrospective studies in small numbers, and review articles. The incidence of diabetes in pregnancy is between 6% and 7%. The populations with greater risk are African-Americans, Hispanic or latino descents with obesity, there is an even higher prevalence as high as 30% [3].

It is more frequent to occur in the last trimester of pregnancy and in patients with type 1 diabetes, although it can also occur in patients with type 2 diabetes, gestational diabetes, and in women who use steroids.

Lack of glucose supply at the intracellular level, lack of adequate availability of insulin, as well as elevation of hormones against regulators such as glucagon and epinephrine can produce this alteration. Glycogen stores are rapidly depleted, and gluconeogenesis becomes the main metabolic pathway. There is a greater source of glucose precursors resulting from lipolysis in excessive amounts of glycerol released into the circulation and muscle, the storage of free fatty acidosis by adipocytes decreases. During ketoacidosis high levels of glucose are present in the intravascular space, creating an osmotic gradient which results in marked diuresis, which in turn produces dehydration and hypovolemia, hydroelectrolytic alterations. By favoring acidosis, electrolytes such as sodium, potassium, and phosphorus bind to the anions of the acetoacids in the bloodstream and are excreted in the urine.

The increased oxidation of fatty acidosis resulting from insulin deficiency, as well as elevation of counterregulatory hormones, increases the production of acetyl CoA which in turn is converted by the liver into ketone bodies (beta hydroxybutyrate, acetoacetate, acetone).

Physiopathology

Ketoacidosis occurs due to a lack of insulin production, resulting from a perception of hypoglycemia, which targets cells in the liver, adipose tissue, and muscle tissue release large amounts of glucagon, worsening hyperglycemia and causing osmotic, hypovolemic, hydroelectrolyte alterations. At the level of adipose tissue, free fatty acids are released into the circulation. After their oxidation, ketonic bodies are formed, giving rise to a metabolic acidosis with a high anionic gap. Ketoacidosis binds to sodium and potassium that are excreted in the urine, resulting in alterations of K and Na+.

During pregnancy, there is an increase in the resistance of insulin by placental lactogen. Between the physiological changes in pregnancy increases the respiratory rate producing a respiratory alkalosis, so at the metabolic level to compensate there is a decrease in serum bicarbonate which decreases the body's normal damping capacity, thus predisposing the pregnant woman to diabetic ketoacidosis [4].

Diabetic ketoacidosis occurs due to insulin deficiency, generally in patients with type 1 diabetes, but it has also occurred in patients with the use of sodium glucose 2 inhibitors (SGLT-2).

Factors That Increase the Risk of Diabetic Ketoacidosis

- Pregnancy, which predisposes ketoacidosis; insulin resistance decreases insulin sensitivity by up to 56%.
- The production of antagonists of insulin in the human placental lactogen, prolactin, and cortisol, so that women in pregnancy and diabetes require higher doses as pregnancy increases.
- Progesterone levels decrease gastric emptying that produces increased absorption of carbohydrates, promoting hyperglycemia.
- Due to starvation in pregnancy, in the 2–3 trimester of pregnancy, the fetus and placenta use large amounts of maternal glucose as a source of energy, and this leads to the decrease of maternal fasting, which is associated with insulin deficiency.
- The increase in free degree acidosis that subsequently becomes ketones at the liver level (see Box 10.3) [5].

The symptoms nausea and vomiting due to increased hCG contribute to the presence of dehydration, as well as the presence of respiratory alkalosis with metabolic acidosis mechanism as compensatory metabolism decreased buffer capacity. There are also other symptoms and signs (see Box 10.4).

Box 10.3 Factors that precipitate diabetic ketoacidosis in pregnancy

Vomiting
Infection
Inadequate follow-up of treatment with insulin
Beta-sympathomimetic drugs
Use of corticosteroids
Insufficient insulin dose in pregnancy

Box 10.4 Diabetic ketoacidosis symptoms and signs

Symptoms
Polyuria Polydipsia Nausea Vomiting Abdominal pain Weakness Weight loss
Signs
Tachycardia Hypotension Dehydration Hyperventilation Kussmaul breathing Ketone breath Neurologic alterations

The patients present the following: abdominal pain, malaise, nausea, persistent vomiting, thirst, hyperventilation, tachycardia, dehydration, and polyuria. If metabolic acidosis is important, it may present alterations in the state of alertness. The diagnosis is corroborated with the following:

- Hyperglycemia>250 mg/dL
- Metabolic acidosis pH: <7.3
- Serum bicarbonate <15 mmol/L
- Ketonuria and/or ketonemia

It is important to calculate of the anion gap, which is high, patients can present acute kidney injury, hydroelectrolytic alterations mainly in potassium and serum sodium.

Metabolic acidosis with a high anion gap due ketone excess ketone (acetone, beta-hydroxybutyric acid, and acetoacetate), increased lipolysis, increased glucose levels 500 mg/dL, with osmotic diuresis, with significant decrease in intravascular volume [6].

The degree of complication of diabetic ketoacidosis is classified according to the following variables based on the degree of abnormality, which varies according to the base acid state:

- Mild acidosis: pH 7.25–7.30
- Moderate acidosis pH: 7.24–7.00
- Severe acidosis pH <7.0

Diabetic ketoacidosis in pregnant women can present even with serum glucose levels <200 mg/dL, with factors that can precipitate their presentation emesis, infection, use of sympathomimetics, tocolytic agents, and steroids [7]. At the fetal level, the presence of maternal acidemia results in alterations in the fetal heart rate, decreased variability, and/or the presence of delayed decelerations; it is important to correct maternal underlying before intervention for the fetus [8].

Hyperosmolar state generally has only mild acidosis (lactic or ketosis due to mild starvation), but with a glucose level higher than 600 mg/dL, significant dehydration and serum hyperosmolarity >320 mOsm, presented neurological alterations stupor and coma compared to the diabetic ketoacidosis [9].

The treatment of both syndromes has been quite standard; it requires the restoration of intravascular volume, correction of electrolyte deficiency, and insulin replacement. A systematic and protocolized approach to treatment has been associated with a more efficient resolution of these syndromes [10].

Laboratory and Image Studies

During pregnancy with history that during pregnancy, with a history of type 1 diabetes, predisposing factors, infection is more frequent than this complication, complementary studies are required: arterial blood gases, glycemia, ketonemia and/or ketonuria, renal function tests creatinine, urea, complete blood count, urinalysis, culture taking of possible infectious focus, chest X-ray, and electrocardiogram.

Its important to calculate the gap anion, serum osmolarity, as well as the calculation of serum Na, since upon admission the patient is found to have decreased sodium concentrations due to acute osmotic flow from the intracellular space to the extracellular space produced by the hyperglycemia, so assess the severity of sodium deficit and acute should calculate the correction of sodium. Serum potassium levels are usually elevated due to movement of intracellular potassium to the extracellular space caused by acidemia, hypertonicity, and insulin deficiency.

Euglycemic Diabetic Ketoacidosis

Diabetic ketoacidosis is defined by the presence of blood glucose of >250 mg/dL, metabolic acidosis with pH <7.3, and serum bicarbonate <15 mEq/dL, with an increase in GAP anion and the presence of ketone bodies in the blood and/or urine [11].

There are different forms of presentation that differs from the usual way for the first time described by Munro in 1973, we may have patients with glucose levels <250 mg/dL wich can presented up to 6% and patients with glucose levels <180 mg/dL in 1%. The most common causes are insulin administration and fasting [12].

The diagnosis of euglycemic diabetic ketoacidosis is a challenge since there is no significant hyperglycemia, and on the other hand there are several causes of metabolic acidosis, although we could be guided by the presence of a high anion gap. There may be different causes such as decrease in the action of insulin and increase in the production of counterregulatory hormones [13] (see Box 10.5).

The incidence of diabetic ketoacidosis in pregnant women varies between 0.5% and 3%, being more frequent in women with type 1 diabetes mellitus.

Box 10.5 Causes of euglycemic diabetic ketoacidosis

Pregnancy
Hepatic cirrhosis
Acute pancreatitis
Septicemia
Use of SGLT-2
Use of insulin pump
Drug abuse: cocaine
Use of insulin after hospital admission

SGLT-2 sodium-glucose cotransporter type2

Fetal Complications

Maternal morbidity includes acute kidney injury, acute respiratory failure, myocardial ischemia, cerebral edema, and even death. The frequency of these complications depends on the severity of the maternal condition; there is a report of cases of diabetic ketoacidosis in pregnancy with a mortality of less than 1%, with a reported fetal mortality rate of 9–36% [14, 15].

The harmful effects of diabetic ketoacidosis to the fetus are caused by the presence of ketone bodies and glucose that crosses the placental barrier. Fetal acidosis is caused by hyperglycemia, which leads to osmotic diuresis and decreased fetal intravascular volume. Fetal hyperinsulinemia increases oxygen uptake. A decrease of 2,3-DPG oxygen affinity for hemoglobin decreasing fetal oxygen availability and general hypoxemia [16].

The hydroelectrolytic alterations, mainly in potassium K, can generate maternal and fetal arrhythmias, as well as decrease in placental perfusion. Among the complications have been death and preterm delivery in women with diabetic ketoacidosis. Fetal mortality can occur between 9% and 35%. In Morrison 2017 study, factors associated with increased risk in pregnant women with diabetic ketoacidosis include premature birth, admission to NICU, and prematurity. Diabetes Ketoacidosis during pregnancy represents a risk to the fetus both at the time of the episode and following. A table identify fetal complications in women with complications with diabetic ketoacidosis pregnancies with live DKA vs. pregnancies with DKA fetal death [17].

Treatment of Diabetic Ketoacidosis

The objectives of treatment in patients with hyperglycemic crisis include the following:

1. Improvement of the circulatory volume and tissue perfusion
2. Gradual reduction of glucose and serum osmolarity
3. Correction of the electrolyte imbalance
4. Identification and rapid treatment of the cause that precipitated the crisis
5. Successful treatment of these patients requires admission to the ICU, and frequent monitoring with laboratory and clinical objectives

Patients with DKA who are alert and able to tolerate oral fluids may receive treatment fluid resuscitation and subcutaneous insulin.

The management of patients with diabetic ketoacidosis must be in the intensive care unit, administration of intravenous (IV) fluids, potassium, and insulin (See Box 10.6).

Box. 10.6 Treatment

Treatment	Plan
Maternal stabilization A. Secure airway B. Improve breathing C. Improve circulation (left lateral decubitus for maternal and fetal circulation)	Consider ICU admission; place Foley catheter, serial vital signs, I/0's Consult critical care, endocrinology, maternal fetal medicine
Fluid replacement (estimated ~ 100 mL/kg) Insulin administration Goal FSBG 150–200 in DKA	Correct 75% total deficit in first 24 h Begin with 0.9% normal saline Convert to D5–0.45% normal saline when FSBG < 250 Regular insulin via IV bolus 0.1 U/kg followed by 0.1 U/kg/h continuous
	Infusion goal reduction 20–25% over 2 h (if not increase IV infusion 1.5–2×) Continue IV insulin until acidosis and ketosis resolves
	Start SQ insulin therapy 1–2 h before stopping IV insulin
Laboratory evaluation	CMP/Mg and Phos, pH, serum ketones every 2–4 h initially Replete K+ once <5 mmol/L (goal 4–5) Replete HCO_3 if pH <6.9 with $NaHCO_3$ until pH >7.0
Identify cause	Rule out infection and other causes

CMP, comprehensive metabolic panel; DKA, diabetic ketoacidosis; FSBG, fingerstick blood glucose; ICU, intensive care unit; IV, intravenous; Phos, phosphorous; SQ, subcutaneous [22]

1. *Resuscitation with IV fluids*

Fluid administration is the first line in the treatment. Part of the fluid resuscitation is not only to improve the intravascular volume, but also the serum glucose level, and the increase in blood pressure, improve cardiac output, ensure perfusion of peripheral tissues, and facilitate the resolution of metabolic acidosis. The American Diabetes Association (ADA) guidelines and the UK, a solution of choice for the solution of sodium chloride 0.9% for immediate replacement of liquid is provided.

- 0.9% Saline solution 1000–1500 ml during the first hour.
- After the first hour, the IV fluid rate will adjust to the hemodynamic function of the patient, and the electrolyte status will be maintained between 250 and 500 ml/h in patients with heart or kidney failure and liver disease.

– After initial resuscitation, the patient may present hyperchloremic acidosis, due to the high dose of 0.9% sodium chloride solutions.
– In patients with glucose level of 200 mg/d, you should start a 5% glucose solution to continue with the infusion of insulin to resolve ketonemia, in this patients you have to avoid the hypoglycemia.

2. *Potassium replacement therapy*

Initially, patients may have elevated serum K levels. The ADA recommends adding 20–30 mEq potassium in each liter of infusion fluid when the serum potassium is below 5.2 mEq/L. The optimal rate of potassium replacement in patients with ketoacidosis diabetes should be considered important, since patients with insulin therapy promote an intracellular change of potassium. It is recommended that insulin should not be started if the serum potassium is below 3 mmol/L to avoid worsening of hypokalemia [18].

3. *Insulin IV*

The main objective of insulin in diabetic ketoacidosis is to stop lipolysis and ketogenesis. Even patients with euglycemic diabetic ketoacidosis need adequate insulin therapy to resolve ketonemia, although with the early addition of dextrose-containing fluids to avoid hypoglycemia.

Insulin should not be started until after water resuscitation and correction of hypokalemia to avoid intravascular worsening of volume or decrease in serum potassium due to changes in potassium, glucose, and extracellular water to the intracellular fluid compartment. The ADA recommends starting IV insulin at a dose of 0.14 units/kg/h or a dose based on weight of 0.1 U/kg/h after a bolus of 0.1 U/kg bolus IV. The ADA guidelines suggests reducing insulin infusion at doses of 0.02–0.05 U/kg/h at the same time as adding 5% dextrose solution IV when the central glycemia drops to less than 200 mg/dL. After administration of insulin, the ADA recommends increasing the rate of insulin infusion every hour to reduce blood at a rate of 3–4 mmol/L/h (50–75 mg/dL/h), up to concentrations of 8–11 mmol/L (150–200 mg/dL) [18–20].

4. *Use of bicarbonate*

The use of bicarbonate is controversial. Systematic review founds available evidence including 3 randomized control trials, that bicarbonate substitution is not recommended in adult patients with diabetic ketoacidosis with pH > 6.9 finding transient paradoxical worsening of ketosis and a greater need for potassium replacement in patients receiving bicarbonate. The United Kingdom does not recommend the use of bicarbonate in any patient with diabetic ketoacidosis. In patients with pH lower than 6.9, the ADA recommends the slow administration of 100 mmol (100 mEq) $NaHCO_3$ for 2 hours [21] (see Box 10.7).

Box 10.7 Management of diabetic ketoacidosis DKA in the ADA and the UK

	ADA	UK
Fluids 1 hr	0.9% sodium chloride solution for initial replacement 1000–1500 ml during the first hour	0.9% sodium chloride solution 1000 ml during the first hour
	Adjust the IV fluid rate to the patient's hemodynamic and electrolyte status. 250–500 ml/h Patient with high levels Na considers using solutions at 0.45% NaCl 5% glucose solution when serum glucose falls below 11 mmol/L (200 mg/dL)	Continue with infusion of solution 0.9% output throughout the DKA Consider the risk of hyperchloremic acidosis due to the use of large amounts of solutions with 0.9% NaCl Add 10% dextrose solution when the blood falls below 14 mmol/L (250 mg/dL)
Electrolytes Potassium	Replacement of 20–30 mmol (20–30 mEq) of potassium for each liter of infusion when serum potassium <5.2 mmol/L (<5.2 mEq/L). Recommendations: Insulin initiation is not recommended if the serum potassium is <3 mmol/L (<3 mEq/L) to avoid worsening of hypokalemia	Replacement of 40 mmol (40 mEq) in each liter of saline when the serum potassium is <5.5 mmol/L (<5.5 mEq/L) Recommendations: Insulin initiation is not recommended if the serum potassium is <3 mmol/L (<3 mEq/L) to avoid worsening of hypokalemia
Phosphate electrolytes	Routine form is not recommended	It is not recommended routinely
Insulin IV	Intravenous insulin should not be started until after the start of fluid resuscitation, correction of potassium Bolus dose of 0.14 U/kg/h or a dose of 0.1 U/kg/h and continue with 0.1 U/kg/h If there is no reduction in time of 3–4 mmol/L (50–75 mg/dL, you should increase the insulin infusion until you achieve a steady decrease in glucose	The adjustment of the intravenous insulin rate is necessary to guarantee the resolution of the DKA Administer rapid-acting insulin at a fixed dose based on weight of 0.1 U/kg/h Increase the rate of intravenous insulin every hour using direct measurement of β-hydroxybutyrate and increased insulin speed of 1 U/h to increase to achieve the goal of reducing ketones at least 0.5 mmol/L/h (5.2 mg/dL/h) if blood β-hydroxybutyrate cannot be measured, increase insulin, the infusion rate of 1 U/h spends achieve. Bicarbonate increases of >3.0 mmol. Decreased glucose>3 mmol/L/h (>50 mg/dL)
Sodium bicarbonate	It is recommended only in cases with pH <6.9.	It is not recommended routinely

ADA = recommendations in the American Diabetes Association guideline [23]; UK = recommendation in the Joint British Diabetes Societies for Inpatient Care guideline [11]

Prevention

Women with diabetes mellitus, who wish to become pregnant, should measure the risk with a preconceptional risk table, and those cases that do not have adequate metabolic control should offer a method of family planning. Women should be educated about the risks of complications during pregnancy, such as diabetic ketoacidosis. All non-diabetic pregnant women should be screened for gestational diabetes between week 24 and 28 SDG, and in women at risk (obesity, direct family history of diabetes mellitus, Hispanic race, impaired glucose metabolism), it should be done at the first consultation or before 14 weeks of gestation to identify pregestational diabetes. Diet, exercise, and strict prenatal control with determination of glucose levels, detection of urinary tract infection, vaccination in the winter season against influenza are actions that have to be carried out in patients with diabetes such as prevention of decompensation or complications. In women with preterm delivery avoid the use of tocolytic agents such as subcutaneous or oral terbutaline. Consider adjusting insulin in case of steroid use for fetal lung maturity [24].

Conclusion

Diabetic ketoacidosis is a rare but serious complication. It requires early recognition and diagnosis and adequate management to reduce the risk of maternal and fetal complications. You must enter the intensive care unit with a multidisciplinary approach and management with maternal and fetal monitoring after the viability is indicated.

References

1. Kitabchi AE, Pared BM. Cetoacidosis diabética. Med Clin North Am. 1995;79:9–37.
2. Kilvert JA, Nicholson HO, Wright AD. Ketoacidosis in diabetic pregnancy. Diabet Med. 1993;10:278–81.
3. Gestational diabetes mellitus. Practice Bulletin No. 137. American College of Obstetricians and Gynecologists. Obstet Gynecol. 2013;122:406–16.
4. Parker JA, Conway DL. Diabetic ketoacidosis in pregnancy. Obstet Gynecol Clin N Am. 2007;34:533–43.
5. Kamalakannan D, Baskar V, Barton DM, Abdu TAM. Diabetic ketoacidosis in pregnancy; 2003. p. 454–7.
6. Jacobi J. Management of Endocrine Emergencies in the ICU; 2019. https://doi.org/10.1177/0897190019834771.
7. Vyas AA, Vyas P, Fillipon NP, et al. Successful treatment of thyroid storm with plasmapheresis in a patient with MMI-induced agranulocytosis. Endocr Pract. 2010;16:673–6.
8. Abdu TAM, Barton DM, Baskar V, et al. Diabetic ketoacidosis on pregnancy. Postgrad Med J. 2003;79:934:454.
9. Gosmanov AR, Gosmanova ER, Dillard-Cannon E. Management of adult diabetic ketoacidosis. Diabetes Metab Synd Obes: Targets Ther. 2014;7:255–2.

10. Goodier CG. Endocrine Emergencies in Obstetrics. Clin Obstet Gynecol. 2019;62(2):339–46.
11. Kitabchi AE, Umpierrez GE, Miles JM, Fisher JN. Hyperglycemic crises in adult patients with diabetes. Diabetes Care. 2009;32(7):1335–43. https://doi.org/10.2337/dc09-9032. pmid:19564476
12. Munro JF, Campbell IW, McCuish AC, Duncan LJ. Euglycaemic diabetic ketoacidosis. Br Med J. 1973;2(5866):578–80.
13. Lucero P, Chapela S. Euglycemic Diabetic Ketoacidosis in the ICU: 3 Case Reports and Review of Literature. Case Rep Crit Care. 2018;2018:1–6. https://doi.org/10.1155/2018/1747850.
14. Kamalakannan D, Baskar V, Barton DM, Abdu TA. Diabetic ketoacidosis in pregnancy. Postgrad Med J. 2003;79:454–7.
15. Parker JA, Conway DL. Diabetic ketoacidosis in pregnancy. Obstet Gynecol Clin North Am. 2007;34:533–43, xii.
16. Veciana MD. Diabetes ketoacidosis in pregnancy. Seminars Perinatol. 2013;37(4):267–73.
17. Morrison FJR, Movassaghian M, Seely EW, Curran A, Shubina M, Morton-Eggleston E, et al. Fetal outcomes after diabetic ketoacidosis during pregnancy. Diabetes Care. 2017;40(7):e77–9. https://doi.org/10.2337/dc17-0186.
18. Viallon A, Zeni F, Lafond P, Venet C, Tardy B, Page Y, Bertrand JC. Does bicarbonate therapy improve the management of severe diabetic ketoacidosis? Crit Care Med. 1999;27:2690–3.
19. Glaser NS, Wootton-Gorges SL, Marcin JP, Buonocore MH, Dicarlo J, Neely EK, Barnes P, Bottomly J, Kuppermann N. Mechanism of cerebral edema in children with diabetic ketoacidosis. J Pediatr. 2004;145:164–17.
20. Green SM, Rothrock SG, Ho JD, Gallant RD, Borger R, Thomas TL, Zimmerman GJ. Failure of adjunctive bicarbonate to improve outcome in severe pediatric diabetic ketoacidosis. Ann Emerg Med. 1998;31:41–8.
21. Fisher JN, Kitabchi AE. A randomized study of phosphate therapy in the treatment of diabetic ketoacidosis. J Clin Endocrinol Metab. 1983;57:177–80.
22. Kitabchi AE, Umpierrez GE, Murphy MB, Kreisberg RA. Crisis de hiperglucemia en pacientes adultos con diabetes: una declaración de consenso de la American Diabetes Association. Cuidado de la diabetes. 2006;29:2739–48.
23. Joint British Diabetes Societies Inpatient Care Group. The management of diabetic ketoacidosis in adults. 2nd ed; 2013. http://www.diabetologists-abcd.org.uk/JBDS/JBDS_IP_DKA_Adults_Revised.pdf
24. Gabbe S, Graves C. Management of diabetes mellitus complicating pregnancy. Obstet Gynecol. 2003;102:857–68.

Chapter 11
Hypoglycemia and Pregnancy

Nares-Torices Miguel Angel, Flores-Cortés Mildred Ibeth, and Hernández-Pacheco José Antonio

Gestational diabetes mellitus (GDM) is defined as "any degree of glucose intolerance with its onset or first recognition during pregnancy" [1]

In pregnancy, maternal serum glucose levels have a direct relationship with adverse outcomes [2, 3].

Uncontrolled hyperglycemia in women with DMG is associated with maternal adverse effects and perinatal outcomes [2–4]. Optimal glycemic control in women with DMG is essential to prevent these complications, but hypoglycemia is an important complication, particularly in those patients in treatment with insulin [5–7].

The tendency to use fasting glucose target levels of 60–90 mg/dL may increase the risk of hypoglycemia [8, 9]. However, the effect of maternal hypoglycemia in pregnancy is not very clear [10, 11].

It has been found that hypoglycemia is more frequent during pregnancy compared to non-pregnant women and occurs in approximately 36–71% of pregnant women who require insulin [12, 13].

In addition, plasma glucose levels during pregnancy are almost 20% lower in normal pregnant women, in pregnant women with gestational diabetes, and in pregnant women with pre-existing diabetes compared to non-pregnant women [13, 14].

Traditionally, hypoglycemia in pregnancy has been defined as a plasma glucose level <60 mg/dL or <63 mg/dL with typical symptoms of hypoglycemia. More

N.-T. M. Angel (✉)
Medical Emergencies Specialist, Critical Medicine and Obstetric Critical Medicine Sub-specialist, National Medical Center IMSS "La Raza", México City, Mexico

F.-C. M. Ibeth
Gynecology and Obstetrics Specialist, Private Medicine, México City, Mexico

H.-P. J. Antonio
Internal Medicine Specialist, Critical Medicine and Obstetric Critical Medicine Sub-specialist, National Institute of Perinatology, México City, Mexico

C. Montufar et al. (eds.), *Obstetric Catastrophes*,
https://doi.org/10.1007/978-3-030-70034-8_11

recently, with the increased availability of continuous glucose monitoring (MCG), the term "masked hypoglycemia" has been introduced.

Masked hypoglycemia is defined as interstitial glucose levels 50 mg/dL for ≥30 min, without symptoms, detected by MCG [14].

Hypoglycemia during pregnancy can compromise both fetal and maternal well-being.

It has been hypothesized that hypoglycemia during pregnancy can potentially induce adverse effects that lead to fetal malformations, small fetuses for gestational age, and poor neuropsychiatric development.

The association between the level of hypoglycemia and diabetic embryopathy remains uncertain.

However, historical studies on DMG and studies of hyperglycemia and pregnancy (HAPO, ACHOIS) have not addressed the risk of hypoglycemia and its effect on pregnancy outcomes.

The reported incidence of hypoglycemia varies in different studies and this is because hypoglycemia can be asymptomatic, poorly recognized, or poorly informed [5–8].

An MCG profile shows the magnitude, duration and frequency of glucose fluctuations, thus providing a greater understanding of dynamic glucose than intermittent blood glucose measurements.

Masked hypoglycemia has been observed in women with DMG also treated with insulin as pregnant women without DMG. The majority (>90%) of hypoglycemia events were nocturnal (23.00–06.00 hours).

Nighttime hypoglycemia could be explained, in part, by the persistence of normal circadian rhythms for glucose [15–17].

Asymptomatic hypoglycemia with longer episodes occurred in women with DMG treated with insulin. Masked hypoglycemia was diagnosed as serum glucose less than 50 mg/dL in at least 30 min (6 consecutive values); episodes of hypoglycemia were occasionally observed mid-morning and before dinner. None of those episodes of hypoglycemia was captured capillary blood glucose test. This could be attributable to the time of the test: most episodes of hypoglycemia occurred while the subjects were asleep.

In addition, in women with DMG on insulin therapy, 40% had masked hypoglycemia and 10% of these women had glucose levels ≤40 mg/dL, suggesting a lower threshold for developing hypoglycemia.

In view of nocturnal hypoglycemia, we suggest that pregnant women take adequate time to sleep snacks to prevent hypoglycemia. The implications of low fasting glucose levels in pregnant women without DMG it may need more research in a larger population [17].

Bibliography

1. Naik D, Shyamasunder AH, Mruthyunjaya MD, Patil RG, Paul TV, Christina F, et al. Masked hypoglycemia in pregnancy. J Diabetes. 2017;9:778–86.
2. HAPO Study Cooperative Research Group. Hyperglycemia and adverse pregnancy outcomes. N Engl J Med. 2008;358:1991–2002.

3. Crowther CA, Hiller JE, Moss JR, McPhee AJ, Jeffries WS, Robinson JS. Effect of treatment of gestational diabetes mellitus on pregnancy outcomes. N Engl J Med. 2005;352:2477–86.
4. Jang HC, Cho NH, Min YK, Han IK, Jung KB, Metzeger BE. Increased macrosomia and perinatal morbidity independent of maternal obesity and advanced age in Korean women with GDM. Diabetes Care. 1997;20:1582–8.
5. Langer O, Levy J, Brustman L, Anyaegbunam A, Merkatz R, Divon M. Glycemic control in gestational diabetes mellitus: how tight is tight enough: small for gestational age versus large for gestational age? Am J Obstet Gynecol. 1989;161:646–53.
6. Blumer I, Hadar E, Hadden DR, et al. Diabetes and pregnancy; an Endocrine Society clinical practice guideline. J Clin Endocrinol Metab. 2013;98:4227–49.
7. Hernandez TL, Friedman JE, Van Pelt RE, Barbour LA. Patterns of glycemia in normal pregnancy: should the current therapeutic targets be challenged? Diabetes Care. 2011;34:1660–8.
8. Combs CA, Gunderson E, Kitzmiller JL, Gavin LA, Main EK. Relationship of fetal macrosomia to maternal postprandial glucose control during pregnancy. Diabetes Care. 1992;15:1251–7.
9. Parikh RM, Joshi SR, Menon PS, Shah NS. Intensive glycemic control in diabetic pregnancy with intrauterine growth restriction is determined to fetus. Med Hypotheses. 2007;69:203–5.
10. Persson M, Norman M, Hanson U. Obstetric and perinatal outcomes in type 1 diabetic pregnancies: a large, population-based study. Diabetes Care. 2009;32:2005–9.
11. Nielsen LR, Pedersen-Bjergaard U, Thorsteinsson B, Johansen M, Damm P, Mathiesen ER. Hypoglycemia in pregnant women with type 1 diabetes: predictors and role of metabolic control. Diabetes Care. 2008;31:9–14.
12. Yogev Y, Ben-Haroush A, Chen R, Rosenn B, Hod M, Langer O. Diurnal glycemic profile in obese and normal weight nondiabetic pregnant women. Am J Obstet Gynecol. 2004;191:949–53.
13. Murphy HR, Rayman G, Lewis K, et al. Effectiveness of continuous glucose monitoring in pregnant women with diabetes: randomized clinical trial. BMJ. 2008;337
14. Sacks DA, Chen W, Greenspoon JS, Wolde-Tsadik G. Should the same glucose values be targeted for type 1 as for type 2 diabetics in pregnancy? Am J Obstet Gynecol. 1997;177:1113–9.
15. Dalfrà MG, Sartore G, Di Cianni G, et al. Glucose variability In diabetic pregnancy. Diabetes Technol Ther. 2011;13:853–9.
16. Skyler JS. Control of diabetes during pregnancy: 1985. JAMA. 1986;255:647–8.
17. Sutherland HW, Pearson DW, Powrie JK. Management of the pregnant diabetic patients. Drugs. 1988;36:239–48.

Chapter 12
Thyroid Emergency and Pregnancy

Aura Meliza Mejia Monroy

Introduction

The thyroid is located below the larynx and on both sides and in front of the trachea. It is one of the largest endocrine glands, weighing 15–20 grams in healthy adults. The thyroid secretes two important hormones, thyroxine (T4) and triiodothyronine (T3) [1, 2]. The complete absence of thyroid secretion frequently causes metabolic decreases between 40% and 50% lower than the normal value, while excessive secretion increases the basal metabolism between 60% and 100% above its normal value [1]. Thyroid storm and myxedema coma are the severe decompensated pathological conditions of hyperthyroidism and hypothyroidism that are associated with increased morbidity and mortality. Early and accurate recognition of both conditions is necessary to initiate treatment and support measures.

This chapter focuses on the overhaul of the essential principles of clinical presentation, diagnosis, and management of both decompensated pathological conditions of hyperthyroidism and hypothyroidism, thyroid storm, and myxedema coma, respectively.

Thyroid Disease

Thyroid disease affects approximately 6% of the population, being present 4–5 times more frequently in women than in men, it is common in women of childbearing age, ranking second in women of reproductive age and is one of the most common pre-pregnancy diseases in pregnant women [3–6].

A. M. M. Monroy (✉)
General Hospital San Juan de Dios, Ministry of Public Health and Social Assistance of Guatemala, Guatemala, Guatemala

C. Montufar et al. (eds.), *Obstetric Catastrophes*,
https://doi.org/10.1007/978-3-030-70034-8_12

The most common thyroid diseases during pregnancy are hyperthyroidism and hypothyroidism. In a large percentage of patients, these diseases are recognized for the first time during pregnancy or in the postpartum period, since the signs and secondary symptoms are often confused with the physiological changes of pregnancy [3, 7].

The function of the thyroid gland suffers profound and complex effects due to hormonal changes and alterations in the metabolic demands of pregnancy.

Hyperthyroidism in pregnancy is rare, its prevalence ranges from 0.1% to 1%, and in the United States, it is 1.2%. However, with about 1 in every 500 pregnancies, pregnant women with hyperthyroidism require rigorous treatment in order to prevent maternal and neonatal complications. The thyroid storm is common in women who receive limited or no prenatal care and have medical or obstetric complications [3, 4, 8–11].

Physiology

Thyroid cells synthesize and secrete thyroglobulin to the follicles, which contains the amino acid tyrosine (the main substrate that combines with iodine to produce thyroid hormones), forming thyroid hormones within the thyroglobulin molecule. Thus, thyroxine and triiodothyronine form a part of the thyroglobulin molecule during and after the synthesis of thyroid hormones [1].

Thyroglobulin is not released into circulating blood in large quantities, but it is necessary, first, that thyroxine and triiodothyronine are excised from the thyroglobulin molecule; and subsequently, both are secreted in free form.

Under normal conditions, the hormones with metabolic activity secreted daily by the thyroid gland are in 93% thyroxine and with 7% triiodothyronine; however, over time, almost all thyroxine is converted into triiodothyronine in the tissues (biologically active form of the hormone). Both hormones have qualitatively similar functions, although they differ in the speed and intensity of the action. Triiodothyronine is four times more potent than thyroxine, although a much smaller amount is detected in the blood and its duration is shorter [1].

The regulation of thyroid hormone secretion is under the direct control of the pituitary thyroid stimulating hormone (TSH). In order to maintain a normal metabolic activity in the body, the TSH pituitary hormone stimulates all known secretory activities of the glandular thyroid cells [1].

In more than 99%, thyroxine and triiodothyronine are immediately combined with various plasma proteins synthesized by the liver, to be transported in the peripheral circulation, mainly linked to thyroxine-binding globulin and, to a lesser extent, transthyretin (formerly called prealbumin) and thyroxine-binding albumin. Under normal conditions, the linked hormone fraction is in balance with an unlinked free fraction, which represents a small amount of total circulating thyroid hormone: 0.04% for T4 and 0.5% for T3 [1, 3, 4, 6].

During pregnancy, there is an increase in thyroxine-binding globulin (TBG), beginning to increase after a few weeks of pregnancy and reaching a plateau in the middle of pregnancy 2.5 times higher than the initial value, secondary to the decrease of hepatic clearance and the estrogen-induced change in the structure of the TBG that prolongs the serum half-life [4, 6, 8].

Alterations in the total levels of thyroid hormones in pregnancy are a direct consequence of the marked increase in serum TBG levels. The levels of T4 and T3 increase during the first 20 weeks of pregnancy, reaching its plateau at 20 weeks without being modified until the end of pregnancy. Due to the 20-fold greater affinity of TBG for T4 compared to T3, changes in T4 levels are more pronounced [4, 6, 8, 12].

In normal pregnant women without thyroid disease and residing in areas with sufficient iodine supply, serum TSH levels remain stable, after the transient drop in serum TSH near the end of the first trimester in pregnancy, caused by partial suppression of TSH associated with the elevation of circulating human chorionic Gonadotropin (hCG) [4, 6, 8].

The feedback mechanism through the hypothalamic-pituitary-thyroid axis works normally in pregnant women because serum TSH levels in pregnancy remain similar to those of non-pregnant women when the iodine supply is adequate [4, 6].

Thyroid Storm

Definition

Thyroid storm is an endocrinological emergency and rare but potentially fatal hypermetabolic complication of hyperthyroidism. It is the clinical manifestation of elevated serum thyroid hormone concentrations, resulting in the extreme alteration of the usual symptoms of hyperthyroidism. In most cases, it occurs after a triggering event and is associated with high morbidity and mortality [2–4, 9, 13, 14].

The incidence of thyroid storm is estimated to occur in 1–2% of pregnancies complicated with hyperthyroidism; however, it is difficult to determine the incidence due to its rarity and the variability in the criteria for diagnosis [4, 8, 9]. The maternal mortality rate of the thyroid storm varies from 8% to 30%, so it is extremely essential to recognize and initiate timely and aggressively its management [2, 9, 13–16].

Etiology

It is unlikely that the thyroid storm is the initial manifestation of hyperthyroidism, occurring in the highest percentage of cases in women with severe untreated or undiagnosed hyperthyroidism and concurrent precipitating factors, among the factors are the following:

- Labor
- Surgical delivery
- Infections

- Thromboembolism
- Diabetic ketoacidosis
- Ischemic heart disease
- Pre-eclampsia
- Traumas
- Irregular use or cessation of antithyroid drugs

It is still not being clear yet why certain factors result in the development of thyroid storm [2, 4, 8, 9, 12–15, 17].

Clinical Presentation

The clinical manifestations of the thyroid storm can be very varied; patients can have a wide range of signs and symptoms, characterized by an altered mental state, hyperthermia, increased pulse pressure, tachycardia, and left ventricular dysfunction. Tachycardia is often out of proportion with hyperthermia; blood pressure is usually normal, although with an increased pulse pressure. There is a cardiovascular compromise (tachycardia out of proportion with fever, arrhythmia, congestive heart failure), hyperpyrexia, and changes in the central nervous system (restlessness, nervousness, change in mental status, confusion and convulsions) [2, 4, 9, 11, 14, 15, 17].

Taking into consideration that it is not evident to differentiate between severe thyrotoxicosis and thyroid storm, scales of signs and symptoms have been defined that allow us to differentiate between these two pathologies. For example, on the Burch and Wartofsky scale, the following parameters are taken:

- Thermoregulatory dysfunction
- Compromising of the central nervous system
- Gastrointestinal compromise
- Cardiovascular dysfunction
- Congestive heart failure
- Atrial fibrillation
- Precipitating event

To obtain a score higher than 45 is interpreted as highly suggestive of thyroid storm, with a score between 25 and 44 is suggestive of thyroid storm and a score of less than 25 is unlikely of thyroid storm [11, 16–18].

Diagnosis

The diagnosis of thyroid storm is essentially clinical and is based on the presence of hyperthyroidism in a patient with severe and potentially fatal manifestations; laboratory tests of thyroid function are only confirmatory [2, 8, 11, 15, 16].

The diagnosis of thyroid storm is made by a combination of laboratory biochemical tests that confirm thyrotoxicosis in a patient with the severe and life-threatening symptoms of hyperthyroidism.

Among the biochemical tests that can be found altered are suppressed TSH and elevated free T4 or in cases of thyrotoxicosis due to T3; free T4 will be low and free and total T3 will be elevated with TSH suppressed as well. In addition, there are other biochemical tests that can be altered, increasing their values over established normal levels of glycemia, calcium, alkaline phosphatase, white blood cells, and hepatic transaminases [4, 8, 15].

There are several diagnostic scoring systems that can be used to assess the likelihood of thyroid storm in patients and facilitate diagnosis. The Burch-Wartofsky scoring system is based on factors related to temperature, central nervous system effects, gastrointestinal/hepatic dysfunction, cardiovascular dysfunction, heart failure, and any precipitating history. The Akamizu criteria are similar and have also been proposed as another diagnostic scoring system in the evaluation of thyroid storm [2, 11, 16, 18].

Some other criteria for the diagnosis of thyroid storm are as follows:

1. Presence of thyrotoxicosis (elevated levels of free T3 and / or thyroxine T4) and at least one manifestation of the central nervous system (CNS) plus one of the following: fever (38 ° C or higher), tachycardia (130 beats / min or faster), congestive heart failure, or gastrointestinal / hepatic manifestations.
2. Presence of thyrotoxicosis and three or more of the manifestations previously listed that are not CNS manifestations [17].

Early recognition of the thyroid storm is essential to initiate treatment, which must be performed in an intensive care unit setting and with a multidisciplinary treatment approach.

The underlying cause of the thyroid storm should always be treated and identified and never forget that when a thyroid storm is suspected, the treatment should not be delayed regardless of whether the laboratory results have not yet been confirmed.

Management

The gold standard for the treatment of thyroid storm is primary prevention. The prevention of thyroid storm requires careful control and management of hyperthyroidism [3].

Thyroid storm treatment usually consists of multiple measures and medications directed at the various causes and effects of thyrotoxicosis, and treatment should never be delayed at the time of suspicion.

In the treatment of this endocrinological emergency, the basic aspects for the good outcome of the patient must be treated, carrying out the stabilization of the patient's clinical condition, treating the triggering cause of the process, and treating the underlying hyperthyroidism.

Patients who present thyroid storm will require intensive control, antithyroid drugs, a supplement for the systemic decompensation of a hyper metabolic state, the elimination of precipitating events and support measures.

The objectives of treatment in the thyroid storm are as follows:

1. Decrease the synthesis and secretion of thyroid hormone
2. Reduce circulating thyroid hormones and increase the concentration of TBG
3. Control the peripheral effects of thyroid hormone
4. Block the peripheral conversion from free T4 to free T3
5. Resolve the systemic manifestation and give support
6. Treat precipitating conditions [4, 16]

The basic principles in the treatment of this endocrinological emergency revolve around providing the following:

1. Supportive therapy and symptomatic treatment in critical care unit:
   - Cardiac monitoring
   - Respiratory and hemodynamic assistance
   - Measures to control hyperthermia
   - Oxygen therapy
   - Management of hypertension
   - Replacement of liquids and electrolytes
   - Antipyretics
   - Environmental cooling
   - Management of cardiac arrhythmias and heart failure
2. Management of hyperthyroidism:
   In the management of hyperthyroidism, there are several ways to approach treatment:

   Block thyroid hormone synthesis: This point is achieved through the use of thioamides and the use of iodine solutions. It should be taken into consideration that the use of iodine solutions should be after the beginning of thioamide therapy, because if used before, there is a possibility that a load of iodine to the organism, without having blocked the synthesis first, can complicate hyperthyroidism further.

   - Propylthiouracil (PTU) enteral (or through nasogastric tube if necessary), with an initial loading dose of 300 milligrams to 600 milligrams and then 150 milligrams to 300 milligrams every 6 hours.
   - Iodide is started 1 to 2 hours after administering PTU:
     - Intravenous sodium iodide 500 to 1000 milligrams every 8 hours.
     - Lugol oral iodine solution, 8 drops every 6 hours.

   Block the release of thyroid hormone already synthesized: The drug of choice is the saturated solution of iodine or lugol, which can be useful during the first 72 hours.

Block the conversion of T4 to T3 in peripheral tissues: Three medications can be used types of medications that can be used, propylthiouracil, corticosteroids such as dexamethasone, which has shown the blockade of deiodinase activity.

- Dexamethasone 2 milligrams intravenously or intramuscularly every 6 hours for four doses.
- Hydrocortisone 300 milligrams per day intravenously.
- Prednisone 60 milligrams orally.

Control adrenergic symptoms: Using beta-blockers such as propranolol is also useful for the effect of controlling the adrenergic symptoms of these patients, as could metoprolol, whose cardioselectivity could be of clinical importance in some patients.

- Propranolol can be administered (30 to 80 milligrams orally or by nasogastric tube every 4 to 6 hours or 1 to 2 milligrams / minute intravenously for 5 minutes to a total dose of 6 milligrams, followed by 1 to 10 milligrams every 4 hours intravenously). If the patient has a history of severe bronchospasm, reserpine or guanethidine may be used:
  - Reserpine: 1 to 5 milligrams intramuscular every 4 to 6 hours.
  - Guanetidin: 1 milligram / kilo orally every 12 hours.

3. The treatment of the precipitating / underlying disease is essential. Common causes, such as fever, infection, stress, pain, and others, should be treated in the fastest way [2, 4, 8, 11, 15].

There are other therapies that could be coadjutants in the medical management of the thyroid storm, such as use lithium, which inhibits the release of thyroid hormones or, in extreme cases and in refractory cases, plasmapheresis, plasma exchange, and peritoneal hemodialysis can be used to eliminate circulating thyroid hormone in patients who do not respond to conventional therapy, achieving rapid control of its levels [4, 15].

Myxedema Coma

Definition

Myxedema coma is the severe form of decompensated hypothyroidism that is potentially fatal. It is a rare disease and difficult to recognize clinically. It usually develops in a patient with previous hypothyroidism that develops a serious intercurrent disease or in a case of hypothyroidism not treated and not properly diagnosed. It is very rare to occur in pregnancy, and usually affects older patients [2, 4, 15, 19].

There is a shortage of epidemiological data in the world, with mortality rates reported from 25% to 60%, even with the adequate treatment provided [4, 14, 18].

Etiology

The most common precipitating factors of myxedema coma may include burns, trauma, surgery, severe infection, hypothermia, cardiovascular event, sepsis medications, among others. Diuretics may mask some of the myxedema features and may also aggravate the hyponatremia associated with the myxedema crisis [2, 15, 19].

The most common precipitating factors of myxedema coma may include burns, trauma, fractures, surgery, severe infection, hypothermia, cardiovascular event, medications (anesthetics, sedatives, tranquilizers, amiodarone, and lithium), sepsis, gastrointestinal bleeding, among others. Diuretics may mask some of the myxedema features and may also aggravate the hyponatremia associated with the myxedema crisis [2, 15, 19].

A precipitating factor that is frequent and not taken into consideration in myxedema coma is the suspension of thyroid medications in critically ill patients. This is possibly due to the fact that attention may focus on presenting features and precipitating factors, and associated hypothyroidism is generally ignored [2, 19].

Clinical Presentation

Most cases occur in winter, and hypothermia is a common manifestation. The clinical manifestations are similar to hypothyroidism, but of greater magnitude. Critically ill patients may develop hypothermia and altered mental status, which can lead to stupor or a frank coma. Hypothermia is the hallmark, with a body temperature as low as 21 degrees Celsius [2, 4, 15, 19].

Myxedema coma may present the following manifestations:

- Hemodynamic and driving disorders:
  - Sinus bradycardia.
  - Extended QT interval (marker of electrical instability).
  - Cardiac branch locks.
  - Decreased cardiac output.
  - Pericardial effusion, which can ultimately cause a cardiovascular collapse.
- The central nervous system can present altered responses to hypercarbia and hypoxia, and the associated respiratory muscle weakness can lead to hypoventilation and respiratory failure.
- Adrenal insufficiency can coexist and contribute cardiac abnormalities and in electrolytes.
- Other manifestations are generalized swelling of the skin and soft tissues, periorbital edema, ptosis, macroglossia, and the presence of cold and dry skin.
- The metabolism of drugs is significantly depressed. The usual doses of sedatives can lead to hypoventilation [15, 19].

The study of heart rate variability parameters also indicates that hypothyroidism leads to a state of sympathovagal imbalance, characterized by a decrease in cardiovascular and vagal sympathetic modulation [19].

Diagnosis

For the diagnosis of myxedema coma, the following should be taken into consideration:

- Clinical manifestations (previously described), among which is alteration of consciousness, hypothermia, among others
- Biochemical alterations of hypothyroidism
- Patient's history regarding hypothyroidism (not in treatment)
- Presence of precipitating factors

If the patient complies with some of the aforementioned manifestations or criteria, it indicates a high index of suspicion, and it is mandatory for the treating physician to initiate replacement therapy while confirming the results of serum TSH and T4 [2, 4, 15, 19].

In addition, you should start the active search for the presence of precipitating causes, through diagnostic tests that include the following:

- White blood cell counts
- Urine tests
- Blood cultures
- Serum electrolytes
- Serum creatinine
- Chest X-ray
- Electrocardiogram and other studies that may be necessary [4, 19]

Although the clinical picture of myxedema coma is quite atypical in critically ill patients, the diagnosis can be confirmed by thyroid function tests. TSH is typically elevated with low levels of T3 and T4; laboratory results may reveal hyponatremia, hypoglycemia, hypercapnia, and respiratory acidosis [15].

Management

The treatment of myxedema coma must be fast and multidimensional, fulfilling the following basic principles of therapy in this endocrine emergency:

1. Rapid replacement of thyroid hormones:
   - Sodium levothyroxine, loading dose of 300–500 micrograms, followed by 50–100 micrograms per day, according to age, weight, and risk of patient

complications. Oral doses of 50–200 micrograms are initiated when the patient wanders.
- Intravenous triiodothyronine can be administered as an initial bolus dose of 10–20 micrograms, followed by 10 micrograms every 4–24 hours, with gradual decrease to 10 micrograms every 6 hours.

2. Supportive therapy includes the following:

   - Management in intensive care unit
   - Cardiac monitoring

     – Electrocardiogram
     – Levels of troponin and creatine-phosphokinase (CPK) to rule out myocardial infarction
     – Monitoring of blood pressure

   - Control of central venous pressure and pulmonary capillary wedge pressure in patients with heart disease
   - Oxygen therapy
   - Non-invasive or invasive ventilation if required
   - Proper handling of liquids
   - Management of hypoglycemia and hyponatremia
   - Use of vasopressors to control hypotension
   - Empirical antibiotic therapy until the results of the cultures are known
   - Passive heating

3. Aggressive management of precipitating causes.
4. Corticosteroids:

   - Hydrocortisone 100 mg every 8 hours until the basal cortisol level is known and then titrated according to the results [2, 4, 15, 19].

It cannot be overemphasized that the precipitating factors require urgent attention with antibiotics in case of infection, hemodialysis due to associated renal insufficiency, and integral attention to multi-organ dysfunction.

In conclusion, the prognosis of a patient with thyroid storm or myxedema coma may be somber, but timely management of the symptoms of decompensated pathological conditions of hyperthyroidism and hypothyroidism, therapeutically addressing the pathophysiological, may allow the evolution to be satisfactory.

References

1. Hall J. Thyroid metabolic hormones. In: Hall JE, editor. Guyton and Hall textbook of medical physiology. 12th ed. Philadelphia: Elsevier; 2011. p. 907–19.
2. Angela M. Thyroid emergencies. J Infus Nurs. 2016;39(5):281–6.
3. Waltman P, Brewer J, Lobert S. Thyroid storm during pregnancy a medical emergency. 2004 [Access June 2019];24 (2): 74–79. Available in: http://ccn.aacnjournals.org/

4. Belfort M. Thyroid emergencies and other endocrine emergencies. In: Foley M, Strong T, Garite T, editors. Critical care obstetrics. 3rd ed. New York, NY: McGraw-Hill Companies; 2011. p. 907–19.
5. Labadzhyan A, Brent G, Hershman J, Leung A. Thyrotoxicosis of pregnancy. J Clin Transl Endocrinol. 2014;1:140–4.
6. Glinoer D. The regulation of thyroid function in pregnancy: pathways of endocrine adaptation from physiology to pathology. Endocr Rev. 1997;18(3):404–33.
7. Krassas G, Karras S, Pontikides N. Thyroid diseases during pregnancy: a number of important issues. Hormones. 2015;14(1):59–69.
8. Winkler C, Coleman F. Endocrine emergencies. In: Belfort M, Saade G, Foley M, Phelan J, Dildy G, editors. Critical care obstetrics. 5th ed. Hoboken, NJ: Wiley-Blackwell, A John Wiley & Sons, Ltd., Publication; 2014. p. 425–37.
9. Moleti M, Di Mauro M, Sturniolo G, Russo M, Vermiglio F. Hyperthyroidism in the pregnant woman: maternal and fetal aspects. J Clin Transl Endocrinol. 2019. [Access May, 2019]; 16. Available in: https://doi.org/10.1016/j.jcte.2019.100190.
10. Alexander E, et al.2017 Guidelines of the American Thyroid Association for the Diagnosis and Management of Thyroid Disease During Pregnancy and the Postpartum. Thyroid. 2017. [Access May 2019]; 27 (3). Available in: https://doi.org/10.1089/thy.2016.0457.
11. Lane A, Tarvade S. Thyroid storm causing placental abruption: cardiovascular and management complications for the Intensivist. J Intens Care Soc. 2015;16(3):247–52.
12. Soma-Pillay P, Nelson-Piercy C, Tolppanen H, Mebazaa A. Physiological changes in pregnancy. Cardiovasc J Afr. 2016;27(2):89–94.
13. Nuguyen C, Sasso E, Barton L, Mestman J. Graves' hyperthyroidism in pregnancy: a clinical review. Clin Diabet Endocrinol. 2018. [Access May, 2019]; 4(4); Available in: https://doi.org/10.1186/s40842-018-0054-7.
14. Ma Y, et al. Impending thyroid storm in a pregnant woman with undiagnosed hyperthyroidism A case report and literature review. Medicine. 2018. [Access May 2019]; 97(3). Available in: https://doi.org/10.1097/MD.0000000000009606
15. Singh Bajwa S, Jindal R. Endocrine emergencies in critically ill patients: challenges in diagnosis and management. Indian Journal of Endocrinology and Metabolism. 2012. [Access May 2019]; 16(5). Available in: https://doi.org/10.4103/2230-8210.100661
16. De Leo S, Lee S, Braverman L. Hyperthyroidism. Lancet. 2016;388(10047):906–018.
17. Sugiyama Y, et al. A case of sudden onset of thyroid storm just before cesarean section manifesting congestive heart failure and pulmonary edema. JA Clin Rep. 2017. [Access May 2019]; 3(20). Available in: http://10.1186/s40981-017-0088-3
18. Hwang W, Im D, Kim E. Persistent perioperative tachycardia and hypertension diagnosed as thyroid storm induced by a hydatidiform mole -a case report. Korean J Anesthesiol. 2014;67(3):205–8.
19. Vivek M, et al. Myxedema coma: a new look into an-old crisis. J Thyroid Res. 2011. [Access May 2019]; Available in: https://doi.org/10.4061/2011/493462

Chapter 13
Ovarian Hyperstimulation: Pathophysiology, Risk Factors, Prevention, and Management

Konstantinos Tserotas and José Luis Neyro

Introduction

The ovarian hyperstimulation syndrome (OHSS) is a syndrome comprising marked ovarian enlargement, high concentration of sex steroids, and extravascular exudate accumulation. This exudate is generated by an increased vascular permeability and massive shift of fluid and protein from the intravascular fluid and protein from the intravascular compartment to the peritoneal cavity and other compartments. The resulting depletion in intravascular volume may lead to hemoconcentration, decreased perfusion of many vital organs, and propensity for thromboembolic phenomena [1, 2].

OHSS is a potentially life-threatening iatrogenic complication of the early luteal phase and/or early pregnancy after ovulation induction (OI) or ovarian stimulation (OS) [3–6].

The worldwide popularity of assisted reproductive technology (ART) and ovulation induction/controlled ovarian hyperstimulation (COH) employed in ART for either in vivo fertilization or in vitro fertilization (IVF), in the last two decades, has been accompanied by an increase in the cases of OHSS. The incidence of severe OHSS ranges between 0.1% and 2%, and that of moderate OHSS has been reported to range between 3% and 7% of the women undergoing ovulation induction and COH by human menopausal gonadotropins (hMGs) and human chorionic gonadotropin (hCG) [2].

K. Tserotas (✉)
Servicio de Ginecología, Complejo Hospitalario "Dr. Arnulfo Arias Madrid", Caja del Seguro Social de Panamá, Ciudad de Panamá, Panamá
e-mail: ktserotas@gmail.com

J. L. Neyro
Servicio de Ginecología y Obstetricia, Universidad del País Vasco EHU-UPV, Hospital Universitario Cruces, Bilbao, Spain
e-mail: doctor@neyro.com

C. Montufar et al. (eds.), *Obstetric Catastrophes*,
https://doi.org/10.1007/978-3-030-70034-8_13

Although OHSS may occasionally occur spontaneously, the great majority of cases are due to COS in women undergoing ART [4]. Ovary enlargement is common in controlled ovarian stimulation, which could continue several months during a successful pregnancy [8].

In 1966, Drs. Melvin Taymor and Somers Sturgis described ovarian hyperstimulation. They tried to delineate the underlying etiology of this mysterious phenomenon and noted that hyperstimulation was more common in patients with polycystic ovaries. Also that hyperstimulation was dose-dependently linked with increasing doses of gonadotropins over a prolonged period of time [9]. Today we know that hCG administered for oocyte maturation is the paramount stimulus for hyperstimulation.

In the last two decades, the substitution of hCG by gonadotropin-releasing hormone agonists (GnRHas), as triggering of final follicular maturation, before ovulation and follicular aspiration, has significantly decreased the incidence and severity of OHSS in clinical practice. According to the latest European Society of Human Reproduction and Embryology report, the incidence of OHSS ranges from 0.18% to 1.40% in European countries [2]. However, OHSS is still subject to substantial underreporting.

Finally, OHSS is a diagnosis that may be unfamiliar to many emergency physicians. With the increasing frequency of in vitro fertilization procedures, this disease process is becoming more common, and patients come to the emergency room with abdominal bloating and nausea (common presenting complaints in pregnant women) and free fluid on abdominal sonogram. These findings should lead to appropriate intervention and consultation [10, 11].

The purpose of this review is to bring a complete overview of OHSS to the various professionals that deal with patients undergoing this potentially life-threatening iatrogenic complication.

Pathophysiology

Understanding the pathophysiology of this condition may aid in identifying measures to prevent its development and treat associated symptoms [3].

The hallmark of OHSS is an increase in the permeability of the capillaries with arteriolar vasodilation, resulting in a fluid shift form the intravascular space to the extravascular compartments and enlargement of ovaries [2, 7]. This fluid shift results in a state of hypovolemic hyponatremia.

Vascular endothelial growth factor (VEGF) is involved in follicular growth, corpus luteum function, angiogenesis, and vascular endothelial stimulation [3].

VEGF plays a critical role in the pathogenesis of OHSS by increasing vascular permeability [12–14]. VEGF is secreted by the granulosa cells, and human chorionic gonadotropin (hCG) stimulates its secretion. Severe OHSS is associated with higher levels of VEGF. The other suggested factors that may act directly or indirectly on the development or severity of OHSS are angiotensin II, insulin-like growth factor, epidermal growth factor, transforming growth factor alpha and beta, basic fibroblast growth factor, platelet-derived growth factor, interleukin-1B, and interleukin-6 [7]. High levels of IL-6 in the follicular fluid are predictive of OHSS [2].

The intraovarian renin-angiotensin system (RAS) is another pathophysiological mechanism implicated in OHSS. Prorenin is also generated by the ovary, placenta, and other tissues. Renin is cleaved twice to angiotensin II (AII). In parallel to the midcycle LH surge, there is a significant increase in prorenin and a second increase parallel to the midluteal progesterone (P4) [15], the latter accompanied also by a rise in active renin. Plasma prorenin also increases after hCG administration in hMG/hCG ovulation induction and COH, and follicular fluid (FF) prorenin levels in such patients are about tenfold higher than plasma prorenin concentrations after hMG/hCG stimulation [2]. Although AII is primarily a pressor agent, its ability to increase the vascular permeability and to induce angiogenesis suggests an important pathophysiological role in the accumulation of postovulatory peritoneal fluid in spontaneous cycles and in OHSS. AII also increases the capillary filtration pressure by constricting the postcapillary venules, leading to a further increase in vascular permeability. High levels of the VEGF and the RAS seem to play a role in the development of OHSS.

Early ovarian hyperstimulation syndrome occurs during luteal phase of controlled ovarian stimulation within 9 days after human chorionic gonadotropin trigger and reflects an acute consequence of this hormone on the ovaries [16].

Late ovarian hyperstimulation syndrome occurs 10 or more days after human chorionic gonadotropin trigger and reflects increased endogenous human chorionic gonadotropin levels following pregnancy [6]. Human chorionic gonadotropin stimulates granulosa-lutein cells to produce vascular endothelial growth factor which increases vascular permeability. The most severe cases are usually the late OHSS cases that occur when a pregnancy is established [6]; several predictive markers have been introduced to identify the high-risk patient profile and consequently develop preventive strategies.

Risk Factors

The prevention of OHSS is based on its prediction [6]. There is no method that can completely abolish OHSS. However, its prevention can be lifesaving and is principally preferred over its treatment. The primary risk factors for moderate to severe OHSS are young age (less than 35 years old), low body mass index, ovulation disorders or polycystic ovarian syndrome (PCOS), and history of previous OHSS (Table 13.1). Serum anti-Müllerian hormone (AMH) is a biomarker that may predict the risk of OHSS [17]. An AMH level >3.36 ng/mL was able to predict the development of OHSS (sensitivity = 90.5% and specificity = 81.3%). The antral follicle count (AFC) is also predictive of OHSS [17]. Risk increases from 2.2% in women with an AFC <24 to 8.6% with an AFC ≥24 [3].

Table 13.1 Risk factors for ovarian hyperstimulation syndrome

1. Age less than 35 years old
2. Low body mass index
3. Ovulation disorders/polycystic ovary syndrome
4. History of previous OHSS

The secondary risk factors depend on ovarian response to COS. Ultrasound monitoring and serum E2 are the vital components of surveillance for OHSS. A large number of growing follicles on the day of triggering (>14 follicles with a diameter of 11 mm) and a large number of oocytes retrieved are the risk factors for OHSS. During COS, serum estradiol monitoring is a significant predictor to control the risk of OHSS. A rapid rise in estradiol levels and serum estradiol concentrations >2500 pg/mL are important predictive factors. However, none is capable of independently forecasting OHSS [18].

Classification

The main event in the pathogenesis of OHSS is ovarian enlargement, secretion of vasoactive substances, ascites, and hypovolemia resulting from an acute extravasation of fluid into the interstitial space [18, 19]. OHSS is classified into four categories based on the severity of symptoms, signs, and laboratory findings.

1. *Mild ovarian hyperstimulation syndrome:* It is defined by the enlargement of bilateral ovaries with multiple follicular and corpus luteal cysts, measuring up to 8 cm and accompanied by abdominal bloating and mild abdominal pain.
2. *Moderate ovarian hyperstimulation syndrome:* It is characterized by the enlargement of the ovaries up to 12 cm, accompanied by abdominal bloating due to an increase in ovarian size and gastrointestinal symptoms (e.g., nausea, vomiting, and diarrhea) as well as ultrasound evidence of ascites. A rapid weight gain of over 3 kg might be the initial sign of moderate hyperstimulation.
3. *Severe ovarian hyperstimulation syndrome:* About 2% of OHSS cases are classified as severe. The severe form is described by the presence of large ovarian cysts (>12 × 12 cm), clinical ascites with or without hydrothorax, hyperkalemia, hyponatremia, hypo-osmolarity (osmolarity <282 mOsm/kg), hypoproteinemia (serum albumin <35 g/L), oliguria (<300 mL/d or <30 mL/h), creatinine, and hypovolemic shock. Hemoconcentration, high white cell count, liver dysfunction, increased blood viscosity, and thromboembolic events occur in the most severe cases [2, 18–21].
4. *Critical ovarian hyperstimulation syndrome:* It is diagnosed when there is adult respiratory distress syndrome, severe ascites or hydrothorax, hematocrit >55%, white cell count >25,000/mL, oliguria or anuria, creatinine ≥1.6 mg/dL, creatinine clearance <50 mL/min, thromboembolism, or acute respiratory distress syndrome [2, 18–21] (Table 13.2).

Table 13.2 Classification of OHSS symptoms

OHSS stage	Clinical feature	Laboratory feature
Mild	Abdominal distension/discomfort	No important alterations
	Mild nausea/vomiting	
	Mild dyspnea	
	Diarrhea	
	Enlarged ovaries	
Moderate	Mild features	Hemoconcentration (Hct >41%)
	Ultrasonographic evidence of ascites	Elevated WBC (>15,000 mL)
Severe	Mild and moderate features	Severe hemoconcentration (Hct >55%)
	Clinical evidence of ascites	WBC >25,000 mL
	Hydrothorax	CrCl <50 mL/min
	Severe dyspnea	Cr >1.6 mg/dL
	Oliguria/anuria	Na+ <135 mEq/L
	Intractable nausea/vomiting	K+ >5 mEq/L
		Elevated liver enzymes
	Low blood/central venous pressure	
	Pleural effusion	
	Rapid weight gain (>1 kg in 24 h)	
	Syncope	
	Severe abdominal pain	
	Venous thrombosis	
Critical	Anuria/acute renal failure	Worsening of findings
	Arrhythmia	
	Thromboembolism	
	Pericardial effusion	
	Massive hydrothorax	
	Arterial thrombosis	
	Adult respiratory distress syndrome	
	Sepsis	

Practice Committee of the American Society for Reproductive Medicine. Prevention and treatment of moderate and severe OHSS. Fertil Steril 2016 [3]

Preventive Strategies

Parameters Assessed Before COS (Ovarian Reserve Markers)

Basal serum follicle-stimulating hormone Follicle-stimulating hormone (FSH) regulates the cyclic recruitment of follicles, forming the basis of the menstrual cycle as it promotes the secretion of estradiol from the dominant follicle. Basal FSH level may be considered an indirect marker of the functional ovarian reserve, i.e., the number of ovarian follicles that might grow if stimulated by FSH. Ovarian reserve measures may be useful for planning ovarian stimulation protocols and counseling patients regarding risk [3].

Antral follicle count Follicles are oocytes surrounded by granulosa cells, and it is recommended that antral follicle count (AFC) be assessed between days 2 and 4 of a spontaneous menstrual cycle, in the absence of a follicle>10 mm.

Anti-Müllerian hormone Anti-Müllerian hormone (AMH) is detectable in female blood from birth and reaches its highest levels during puberty; its serum concentration declines with age, becoming undetectable after menopause. AMH is produced by the granulosa cells of pre-antral and small antral follicles, until they have reached about 6 mm in size. With continuous follicle growth, AMH expression decreases and becomes undetectable once FSH-dependent follicular growth has been initiated. AMH plays an important role in regulating the number of follicles that grow from the primordial pool. Higher values of AMH may indicate a larger cohort of smaller antral follicles, which may translate into more follicles responding to COS and a higher risk of OHSS [3, 22, 23].

Parameters Assessed During COS (Ovarian Stimulation Parameters)

Estradiol Hormone dosage, particularly serum estradiol concentration, is frequently used for monitoring COS, one reason for which is to assess the risk of OHSS as a marker of increased granulosa cell activity. Absolute high or rapidly rising values may potentially predict OHSS.

Number of larger follicles The number of follicles being stimulated during COS reflects the degree of ovarian stimulation. The greater the stimulation at the time of hCG triggering the greater the risk of OHSS. This parameter might be used to assess OHSS risk and help in deciding on the adoption of a preventive strategy.

Prediction of Moderate/Severe OHSS

During COS, OHSS may be predicted successfully by three markers of high ovarian response: estradiol levels, medium/large follicle count on the day of hCG administration, and the number of oocytes retrieved subsequent to follicle aspiration [7].

Prediction of High Ovarian Response

High ovarian response was defined as more than 15–20 oocytes retrieved. Both AMH and AFC are useful tests for predicting high response [24].

Interventions to Reduce the Occurrence of OHSS

Volume Expanders

The administration of intravenous fluid expanders immediately after oocyte retrieval improves renal function and might help in the excretion of hCG during the hours of peak concentration. It may reduce rates of modest and severe OHSS in women at high risk. There is also evidence that albumin reduces pregnancy rates [3, 5, 25].

Antagonist Protocols

Stimulation protocols utilizing gonadotropin-releasing hormone (GnRH) antagonists for ovulation suppression are associated with a lower incidence of OHSS compared with protocols that use a GnRH agonist (5.1% vs 8.9%) and constitute an alternative for the prevention of premature luteinizing hormone (LH) surges during COS. The mechanism is thought to be related to a reduction in circulating estradiol levels seen with GnRH antagonist suppression. The introduction of a GnRH antagonist in COS enables the use of shorter protocols with reduced amounts of gonadotropin. Live-birth rates were no different between groups, 22.8% vs 23.8%, respectively. Looking specifically at IVF in women with PCOS, suppression with antagonist as opposed to agonist also appears to be beneficial in this high-risk subset of patients [3, 17, 24, 26–30].

Dopamine Agonists (Several)

Cabergoline is a dopamine agonist that is suggested to successfully reduce the incidence of moderate OHSS (OR = 0.38, 95% CI = 0.19–0.78), with no significant effect on clinical pregnancy rates (RR 1.02, 95% CI 0.78–1.34) and miscarriage rates, starting on the day of hCG triggering at a dose of 0.5 mg/d for 8 days [12, 25, 31, 32].

Freeze All

The risk of OHSS among women undergoing COS is greater among those who achieve conception and is limited to cases in which exposure to hCG has occurred. One strategy to decrease hCG exposure would be to limit the use of hCG to the trigger dose only, avoiding extended exposure to the natural hCG from pregnancy, which could prolong and worsen an otherwise brief OHSS. In "freeze all" following oocyte retrieval, all oocytes/embryos are cryopreserved and, afterward, transferred in a non-stimulated cycle [14, 25, 33, 34].

Late-onset OHSS after 10 days of hCG administration is probably due to the pregnancy and not the exogenous hCG from the oocyte maturation triggering. Moreover, late-onset OHSS is probably a more severe condition responsible for longer stays in hospital. There is an increased proportion of severe cases among women with late-onset OHSS (61.2% (95% CI, 47.2–74.3%)). OHSS in women who became pregnant tended to be more severe than OHSS in the absence of pregnancy. The proportion of severe OHSS cases among those with early OHSS who did not become pregnant was 26% and hospitalized for an average of 7 days. Among those with early-onset OHSS who became pregnant, the proportion of severe cases was 46%, and they were hospitalized for 20 days, while among cases of late-onset OHSS, the proportion that were severe was 32%, and the women were hospitalized for 12 days.

Metformin for Women with Polycystic Ovary Syndrome (PCOS)

"Androgen priming" is the concept that androgens increase the ovarian response to gonadotropin stimulation by enhancing early follicular growth. By improving intra-ovarian hyperandrogenism, it is theorized that metformin can affect the ovarian response by reducing the number of non-periovulatory follicles and thereby reduce estradiol secretion. Metformin use decreases the incidence of OHSS in PCOS patients (OR 0.27, 95% CI 0.16–0.46) [35], with no difference in pregnancy rates, live-birth rates, and spontaneous abortion rates. Metformin administration was started within 4 months before the commencement of COS, and daily doses are maintained until maturation triggering with hCG, oocyte retrieval, a pregnancy test, or until 12 weeks' gestation [29].

Mild Stimulation

Lowering the dose of hCG is a strategy with conflicting results and may or may not consistently reduce OHSS in high-risk patients. Given that lowering the hCG dose is not a perfect solution, alternate strategies should be considered. But this strategy does not produce a clinically relevant difference in clinical pregnancy rate [18, 24].

Secondary Preventive Measures (Patients with an Exaggerated Response)

Interventions to Reduce the Occurrence of OHSS

Coasting or delaying human chorionic gonadotropin administration In patients in whom a dangerously high serum E2 concentration is reached or a large number of follicles are developed, hCG triggering might be delayed for several days until E2 levels decrease or plateau. After the administration of gonadotropins is stopped, mature follicles continue to grow in size for 4 days, and serum estradiol concentrations continue to increase for about 1 or 2 days. Withholding should not last more than 4 days to avoid decreasing the pregnancy rates, which would happen following longer periods of coasting [3, 25].

Cancellation of the cycle Withholding the final HCG triggering is the only definite method for prevention of OHSS. However during GnRH antagonist protocols, high estradiol levels are well tolerated [18].

Freeze All

Calcium Calcium IV infusion (10 mL of 10% calcium gluconate in 200 mL normal saline) on the day of oocyte retrieval and days 1, 2, and 3 after oocyte retrieval can decrease OHSS risk. Increased calcium is postulated to inhibit cAMP-stimulated renin secretion, which decreases angiotensin II synthesis and its subsequent effect on VEGF production with no difference in clinical pregnancies. The observed effect was not greater than that of cabergoline [3, 5].

Low-dose aspirin Increased platelet activation due to VEGF levels may lead to release of substances, such as histamine, serotonin, platelet-derived growth factor, or lysophosphatidic acid, that can further potentiate the physiologic cascade of OHSS. 100 mg aspirin from the first day of stimulation until the day of the pregnancy test may reduce the risk of severe OHSS. Some studies add prednisolone in varying doses (10 mg to 30 mg) for the same time frame with similar results [3] (Table 13.3).

Management/Treatment

Women with severe ovarian hyperstimulation syndrome require hospitalization for more careful monitoring and treatment [14]. Once OHSS is present, the treatment of OHSS is mainly supportive [36].

The clinical treatment of OHSS depends on its severity, complications, and absence or presence of pregnancy. The treatment involves dealing with electrolytic imbalance, hemodynamic changes, liver dysfunction, pulmonary manifestations, hypoglobulinemia, febrile morbidity, thromboembolic events, adnexal torsion, and neurological manifestations [18].

Spontaneous regression occurs over 10–14 days in mild to moderate cases, but it may take longer if implantation occurs. Mild degrees of OHSS do not need any special treatment [18]. Moderate OHSS may be followed up by daily telephone calls as a minimum in addition to office visits twice weekly. The evaluation consists of liver function tests, pelvic ultrasound, complete blood count, and

Table 13.3 Strategies to reduce the occurrence of ovarian hyperstimulation syndrome (OHSS) [7]

Before starting controlled ovarian stimulation:			
Low risk of high response (e.g., AMH $\leq$ 1 ng/mL and/or AFC $\leq$ 6)			
	No strategy needed		
High risk of high response (e.g., AMH $\geq$ 3 ng/mL and/or AFC $\geq$ 16)			
	Antagonist protocol recommended		
Intermediate risk or not assessed			
	Consider using antagonist protocol		
Day of triggering final follicular maturation:			
Low risk of OHSS (e.g., $\leq$10 follicles $\geq$10 mm in size and/or estradiol <1500 pg/mL)			
	No strategy needed		
High risk of OHSS (e.g., $\geq$18 follicles $\geq$10 mm and/or estradiol >3000 pg/mL)			
	When using antagonist protocol		
		Replace hCG (triggering with GnRH agonist) and freeze all	
		Freeze all is not an option	
			Cabergoline administration
			Replace hCG (triggering with GnRH agonist) and fresh embryo transfer
	When using an agonist protocol		
		Cabergoline administration and/or freeze all	
Intermediate risk of OHSS			
	Same interventions suggested for women at high risk might be employed		
Day of oocyte retrieval:			
High risk of OHSS (e.g., $\geq$15 oocytes retrieved)			
	Consider cabergoline and/or freeze all		

coagulation profile. The patients should be directed to report to the hospital in case of development of dyspnea, decrease in urine volume, or upon starting any unusual symptoms such as leg swelling, numbness, dizziness, and neurological problems.

1. Indications for admission: Patients with severe OHSS should be admitted to the hospital for treatment if they suffer from severe abdominal pain, nausea and vomiting, hemoconcentration, severe ascites, profound oliguria or anuria, decrease in blood pressure, tachypnea or dyspnea, light-headedness or syncope, electrolyte disturbances (hyponatremia and hyperkalemia), or abnormal liver function test. Careful observation of an OHSS patient is highly recommended because a mild disease may suddenly progress to the advanced stages [21].
2. Biochemical monitoring in the hospital: The laboratory results of severely affected OHSS patients are comprised of hemoconcentration (hematocrit >45%), decreased creatinine clearance (serum creatinine >1.2 and creatinine clearance

<50 mL/min), electrolyte imbalances (hyponatremia [sodium <135 mEq/L] and hyperkalemia [potassium >5.0 mEq/L]), leukocytosis (white blood cell count >15,000), and elevated liver enzymes [21, 37–39].

3. Suggestions for the assessment and monitoring of hospitalized patients with ovarian hyperstimulation syndrome:

   - Vital signs (every 2–8 hours, according to clinical status)
   - Complete physical examination (daily, avoiding bimanual pelvic examination)
   - Weight (recorded daily)
   - Abdominal circumference (at the navel, recorded daily)
   - Ultrasound evaluation of ascites and ovarian size (repeated as necessary to guide management or paracentesis)
   - Daily monitoring of fluid intake and output
   - Pulse oximetry (for patients with symptoms of pulmonary compromise)
   - Chest X-ray and echocardiogram when pleural or pericardial effusion is suspected (repeated as necessary)
   - Pregnancy test
   - Electrolytes (daily)
   - Complete blood count (daily or more often as needed to guide fluid management)
   - Liver enzymes (repeated as necessary)
   - Serum creatinine or creatinine clearance and urine specific gravity (repeated as necessary)

A. *Medical Treatment* (Table 13.4)

   1. Circulatory volume correction: The key line of treatment is to correct the circulatory volume and electrolyte imbalance. Every effort should be made

Table 13.4 Management of hospitalized OHSS patient

A. Medical Management
(a) Circulatory volume correction
(b) Electrolyte replacement
(c) Anticoagulant therapy
(d) Antibiotic treatment
(e) Diuretics
(f) Dopamine
(g) Aspiration of the ascitic fluid
(i) Abdominal paracentesis
(ii) Transvaginal aspiration
(iii) Treatment of pulmonary complications and pleurocentesis
B. Surgical Management
(a) Surgery for ruptured cysts
(b) Surgery for ovarian torsion (untwist the pedicle)
(c) Surgery for ectopic or heterotopic pregnancy
(d) Pregnancy termination

to maintain a normal intravascular volume and to conserve adequate renal function [3]. Fluids should be administered thoughtfully, in the volumes required, to retain an adequate urine output (>20–30 mL/h) and to reverse hemoconcentration. Dextrose 5% in normal saline is preferable to lactated Ringer's solution. Plasma colloid expanders may be used if necessary. The use of albumin, mannitol, dextran, HES, or fresh frozen plasma with the aim of increasing the intravascular oncotic pressure in order to maintain the intravascular volume is recommended. The advantages of HES solutions over albumin are their high molecular weight (200–1000 kDa vs 69 kDa) and a non-biological origin, lower possibility of anaphylactic reactions, and viral contaminations. A clinical trial demonstrated fewer necessary paracentesis, higher urine output, and shorter hospital stays after HES utilization for patients with severe OHSS compared to albumin [3, 40].

2. Electrolyte replacement: Salt and water restriction is not broadly advocated since sodium and water restriction does not affect the patient's weight, peripheral edema, or abdominal circumference. Hyperkalemia may lead to cardiac dysrhythmia, and acute management includes treatments that shift potassium into the intracellular space (sodium bicarbonate, insulin and glucose, and albuterol). Calcium gluconate may be used to protect the cardiac tissue against hyperkalemia. ECG signs of hyperkalemia show the need for urgent treatment with calcium gluconate. Kayexalate also may be used to remove potassium from the body slowly with the onset of action in 1–2 hours and can be administered orally or rectally as a retention enema [37–39].
3. Anticoagulant therapy: Venous thrombosis is the most significant life-threatening complication of OHSS [3, 41]. When there is a risk of thrombosis, preventive measures are indicated. The risk factors for thromboembolism in moderate to severe OHSS are as follows [42, 43]: immobilization, pressure induced by large ovaries or ascites on pelvic vessels, and hypercoagulable states due to pregnancy or high estrogen levels. The incidence of deep vein thrombosis is obviously increased in patients with Leiden factor V mutation, antithrombin III deficiency, protein C and S deficiency, and personal or familial history of thrombosis. The utilization of low-molecular weight heparin improves the risk of thrombotic complications. Enoxaparin (40 mg/d) or dalteparin (5000 IU/d) is recommended for thromboprophylaxis with easy administration and no need for monitoring. Anticoagulation is recommended for pregnant women and should be continued at least to the end of the first trimester. There are reports on late thrombosis even up to 20 weeks post embryo transfer.
4. Antibiotic treatment: The administration of antibiotics is not unusual in the treatment of OHSS because of repeated catheterizations, venipuncture, pleural drainage, and transvaginal aspiration of the ascitic fluid. Preoperative antibiotic prophylaxis is highly recommended [44].
5. Diuretics: Diuretic therapy without previous volume expansion might be harmful in as much as it may further constrict the intravascular volume and

worsen hypotension and its squeals. Diuretics may raise blood viscosity and increase the risk of venous thrombosis. The administration of diuretics is usually limited to the management of pulmonary edema [44].

6. Dopamine: Dopamine is used in oliguric patients with severe OHSS and confers a notable improvement in renal function, acting through an increased renal blood flow and the glomerular filtration rate [45].
7. Aspiration of the ascitic fluid and pleural effusion in severe ovarian hyperstimulation syndrome: The development of ascites is the hallmark of OHSS. The most common reason for hospitalization is symptoms due to ascites. Aspiration is not suggested for all patients. Paracentesis is applied via the transabdominal or transvaginal method for severe abdominal pain, respiratory compromise as shown by tachypnea and pulse oximetry, and renal compromise as demonstrated by oliguria and increased creatinine concentrations. It eliminates the vasoactive factors, such as VEGF, in the ascitic fluid, diminishes the mechanical pressure on the diaphragm, and significantly increases diuresis.

    (a) Abdominal paracentesis: Soon after the paracentesis procedure, urinary output increases together with a decrease in the patient's weight, lower extremity edema, and abdominal circumference. In addition, the creatinine clearance rate is raised following the procedure. Paracentesis decreases respiratory and abdominal distress, but since the fluid tends to return, some patients need frequent paracenteses and drainage of effusions. Ultrasonographic guidance minimizes the risk of damage to the ovaries. The percutaneous placement of a pigtail catheter may be a safe and effective alternative to multiple vaginal or abdominal paracenteses in severe OHSS patients. The monitoring of plasma proteins is necessary, and HES or human albumin should be infused whenever needed.
    (b) Transvaginal aspiration under ultrasound guidance: Transvaginal aspiration under ultrasound guidance is an effective and safe procedure. Injury to the ovaries is avoided when the puncture is performed under ultrasonic visualization. Since the pouch of Douglas is the best site for the drainage of ascites, no anesthesia is required and minimizes hospitalizations [46].
    (c) Treatment of pulmonary complications and pleurocentesis: The assessment and treatment of patients with dyspnea in severe OHSS starts with a complete physical examination, chest X-ray and ultrasound, and arterial blood gas test. It is necessary to assess any pulmonary condition that may lead to hypoxia. Severe ascites may be accompanied by hydrothorax, particularly on the right side, due to the transfer of the abdominal fluid to the chest through the thoracic duct. Paracentesis will usually be effective in the resolution of hydrothorax, and thoracentesis may be reserved for those with bilateral or severe persistent pleural effusions. Pericardial effusion rarely occurs, but if it does, drainage may be necessary by an expert physician [47, 48].

B. *Surgical Treatment*

1. Surgery for ruptured cysts: Laparotomy should usually be avoided in OHSS. When proven necessary in cases with hemorrhagic ovarian cysts, it should be done to perform hemostasis and to save the ovaries.
2. Surgery for ovarian torsion: Ovarian torsion is a rare complication of ovulation induction and leads to the loss of one or both ovaries if not diagnosed and treated surgically on time. The symptoms of ovarian torsion include severe unilateral colicky adnexal pain. Ultrasonography with Doppler flow study can be diagnostic; nevertheless, a result of a normal blood flow does not rule out ovarian torsion. The purpose of surgery is to untwist the ovarian pedicle and try to save it.
3. Surgery for ectopic or heterotopic pregnancy associated with ovarian hyperstimulation syndrome: The association between OHSS and ectopic or heterotopic pregnancy is not common, and the diagnosis needs a high index of suspicion. However, in ART cycles, due to the presence of multiple oocytes or multiple embryos and special manipulations, ectopic or heterotopic pregnancies may occur more than usual. The diagnosis of tubal pregnancy is not always possible via vaginal ultrasound examination at early stages. The presence of enlarged OHSS ovaries also obscures the vision during ultrasound scanning. Also, the presence of fluid in the pouch of Douglas is of limited diagnostic importance in the presence of ascites. All the aforementioned issues make the diagnosis difficult. However, when ectopic or heterotopic pregnancies are diagnosed, surgery is indicated in the majority of the cases.
4. Pregnancy termination: Pregnancy termination is done in extreme cases to save the mother's life. The termination of pregnancy in critical and prolonged cases is performed in order to stop hormone production and to terminate the cascade of events leading to OHSS. The termination of pregnancy has been stated to improve the clinical respiratory, cardiological, nephrological, hematological, and vascular complications.

Final Recommendations [3]

- Women with PCOS, elevated AMH values, and elevated AFC may benefit from ovarian stimulation protocols that reduce the risk of OHSS (Grade B).
- Ovarian stimulation protocols using GnRH antagonists are preferable in women at high risk of OHSS (Grade A).
- The use of a GnRH agonist to trigger oocyte maturation prior to oocyte retrieval is recommended to reduce the risk of OHSS if peak estradiol levels are high or multifollicular development occurs during stimulation (Grade A).
- Low-dose hCG co-trigger, luteal hormonal support, and cryopreservation of embryos are strategies that may improve pregnancy rates in this setting (Grade B).

- Dopamine agonist administration starting at the time of hCG trigger for several days also may be used to reduce the incidence of OHSS (Grade A).
- Additional strategies to prevent OHSS which may be helpful include the use of metformin in PCOS patients (Grade A), aspirin administration (Grade A), and cryopreservation of embryos (Grade B).
- The mainstay of OHSS treatment includes fluid resuscitation and prophylactic anticoagulation. Paracentesis or culdocentesis may be recommended for management of OHSS when a large amount of ascites is present (Grade B).

Conclusions

OHSS is a known complication of controlled ovarian stimulation. Adequate experience with ovulation induction therapy and identifying patients with known risk factors are essential in preventing OHSS [13].

Stimulation protocols should be selected that minimize the risk of OHSS. The use of GnRH antagonist protocols with a GnRH agonist (with or without low-dose hCG) to trigger final oocyte maturation of oocytes is a particularly effective strategy. Other strategies that show some benefit include the use of cabergoline and cryopreservation of all embryos rather than transfer.

If OHSS prevention strategies are not effective and a patient experiences severe OHSS, fluid resuscitation, supportive care, paracentesis, and prophylactic anticoagulation are recommended.

Nowadays, the establishment of OHSS-free clinics is feasible through careful primary evaluation of infertile couples; severe OHSS, which was deemed an iatrogenic life-threatening condition two decades ago, can now be effectively prevented and managed during the early stages [18].

References

1. Beall SA, Decherney A. The history and challenges surrounding ovarian stimulation in the treatment of Infertility. Fertil Steril. 2012;97(4):795–801.
2. Blumenfeld Z. The ovarian Hyperstimulation syndrome. Vitam Horm. 2018;107:423–51.
3. Prevention and treatment of moderate and severe ovarian hyperstimulation syndrome: a guideline. Practice Committee of the American Society for Reproductive Medicine American Society for Reproductive Medicine, Birmingham, Alabama. Fertil Steril. 2016;106:1634–47.
4. Humaidan P, Nelson SM, Devroey P, et al. Ovarian hyperstimulation syndrome: review and new classification criteria for reporting in clinical trials. Hum Reprod. 2016;31(9):1997–2004.
5. Youssef MA, Mourad S. Volume expanders for the prevention of ovarian hyperstimulation syndrome. Cochrane Database Syst Rev. 2016;(8):CD001302.
6. Papanikolaou EG, Humaidan P, Polyzos NP, Tarlatzis B. Identification of the high-risk patient for ovarian hyperstimulation syndrome. Semin Reprod Med. 2010;28(6):458–62.
7. Nastri CO, Teixeira DM, Moroni RM, et al. Ovarian hyperstimulation syndrome: pathophysiology, staging, prediction and prevention. Ultrasound Obstet Gynecol. 2015;45:377–93.

8. Shi J, Ren X, Tian Q, et al. Persistent megalocystic ovaries after ovarian hyperstimulation syndrome in a postpartum patient with polycystic ovarian syndrome: a case report. J Ovarian Res. 2018;11(1):79.
9. Feinberg EC. Ovarian hyperstimulation: past, present, and future. Fertil Steril. 2016;106(6):1330.
10. Bellapu S, Guttman J. Use of point-of-care ultrasound for the diagnosis of ovarian hyperstimulation syndrome. J Emerg Med. 2017;52(4):e101–4.
11. Madill JJ, Mullen NB, Harrison BP. Ovarian hyperstimulation syndrome: a potentially fatal complication of early pregnancy. J Emerg Med. 2008;35(3):283–6.
12. Soares SR. Etiology of OHSS and use of dopamine agonists. Fertil Steril. 2012;7(3):517–22.
13. Eskew AM, Omurtag KR. Ovarian hyperstimulation syndrome management strategies: where are we going? Minerva Endocrinol. 2018;43(1):50–6.
14. Chen CD, Chen SU, Yang YS. Prevention and management of ovarian hyperstimulation syndrome. Best Pract Res Clin Obstet Gynaecol. 2012;26(6):817–27.
15. Neyro JL, Cristóbal I, Vásquez-Awad D. Soporte de fase lútea en reproducción asistida: estado actual. REVCOG. 2018;22(1):6–13. (spanish).
16. Mai Q, Hu X, Yang G, et al. Effect of letrozole on moderate and severe early-onset ovarian hyperstimulation syndrome in high-risk women: a prospective randomized trial. Am J Obstet Gynecol. 2017;216(1):42. e1–42.e10.
17. Humaidan P, Quartarolo J, Papanikolaou EG. Preventing ovarian hyperstimulation syndrome: guidance for the clinician. Fertil Steril. 2010;94(2):389–400.
18. Jahromi BN, Parsanezhad ME, Shomali Z. Ovarian hyperstimulation syndrome: a narrative review of its pathophysiology, risk factors, prevention, classification, and management. IJMS. 2018;43(3):248–60.
19. Navot D, Bergh PA, Laufer N. Ovarian hyperstimulation syndrome in novel reproductive technologies: prevention and treatment. Fertil Steril. 1992;58:249–61.
20. Mathur R, Evbuomwan I, Jenkins J. Prevention and management of ovarian hyperstimulation syndrome. Curr Obstet Gynaecol. 2005;15:132–8.
21. Department of Health, Government of South Australia. South Australian Paediatric Clinical Guidelines: Ovarian hyperstimulation syndrome. South Australia: GoSA; 2007.
22. Broekmans FJ, Visser JA, Laven JS, et al. Anti-Mullerian hormone and ovarian dysfunction. Trends Endocrinol Metab. 2008;19:340–7.
23. La Marca A, Sighinolfi G, Radi D, et al. Anti-Mullerian hormone (AMH) as a predictive marker in assisted reproductive technology (ART). Hum Reprod Update. 2010;16:113–30.
24. Controlled Ovarian Stimulation for IVF/ICSI. ESHRE Reproductive Endocrinology Guideline Group. February 2019, pp.115–120.
25. Corbett S, Shmorgun D, Claman P, Reproductive Endocrinology Infertility Committee; Special Contributor. The prevention of ovarian hyperstimulation syndrome. J Obstet Gynaecol Can. 2014;36(11):1024–33.
26. Toftager M, Bogstad J, Bryndorf T, et al. Risk of severe ovarian hyperstimulation in GnRH antagonist versus GnRH agonist protocol: RCT including 1050 first IVF/ICSI cycles. Hum Reprod. 2016;31(6):1253–64.
27. Mascarenhas M, Balen AH. The high responder: a review of pathophysiology and outcomes during IVF treatment. Hum Fertil (Camb). 2017;20(3):155–67.
28. Alama P, Bellver J, Vidal C, Giles J. GnRH analogues in the prevention of ovarian hyperstimulation syndrome. Int J Endocrinol Metab. 2013;11(2):107–16.
29. Neyro JL, Barrenetxea G, Montoya F, Rodriguez-Escudero FJ. Pure FSH for ovulation induction in patients with polycystic ovary syndrome and resistant to clomiphene citrate therapy. Hum Reprod. 1991;6(2):218–21.
30. Perelson del Pozo I, Ruesta-Terán C, Neyro JL, et al. The impact of different ovarian stimulating protocols in artificial insemination based on the glycosylation pattern of the follicle stimulating hormone. Ginecol Obstet Mex. 2017;85(9):578–588 (spanish).
31. Ferraretti AP, Gianaroli L, Diotallevi L, et al. Dopamine treatment for severe ovarian hyperstimulation syndrome. Hum Reprod. 1992;7:180–3.

32. Baumgarten M, Polanski L, Campbell B, Raine-Fenning N. Do dopamine agonists prevent or reduce the severity of ovarian hyperstimulation syndrome in women undergoing assisted reproduction? A systematic review and meta-analysis. Hum Fertil (Camb). 2013;16(3):168–74.
33. Dahan MH, Tannus S, Seyhan A, et al. Combined modalities for the prevention of ovarian hyperstimulation syndrome following an excessive response to stimulation. Gynecol Endocrinol. 2018;34(3):252–5.
34. Mahajan N, Gupta S, Sharma S, et al. Early onset ovarian hyperstimulation despite use of segmentation approach and ovarian hyperstimulation syndrome prophylaxis. J Hum Reprod Sci. 2015;8(4):234–8.
35. Palomba S, Falbo A, La Sala GB. Effects of metformin in women with polycystic ovary syndrome treated with gonadotrophins for in vitro fertilization and intracytoplasmic sperm injection cycles: a systematic review and meta-analysis of randomized controlled trials. BJOG. 2013;120:267–76.
36. Kwik M, Karia S, Boothroyd C. RANZCOG CREI consensus statement on treatment of ovarian hyperstimulation syndrome. Aust N Z J Obstet Gynaecol. 2015;55(5):413–9.
37. Budev MM, Arroliga AC, Falcone T. Ovarian hyperstimulation syndrome. Crit Care Med. 2005;33:S301–6.
38. Alper MM, Smith LP, Sills ES. Ovarian hyperstimulation syndrome: current views on pathophysiology, risk factors, prevention, and management. J Exp Clin Assist Reprod. 2009;6:3.
39. Kumar P, Sait SF, Sharma A, Kumar M. Ovarian hyperstimulation syndrome. J Hum Reprod Sci. 2011;4:70–5.
40. Yakovenko S, Sivozhelezov V, Zorina I, et al. Prevention of OHSS by intravenous calcium. Hum Reprod. 2009;i61:24.
41. Mor YS, Schenker JG. Ovarian hyperstimulation syndrome and thrombotic events. Am J Reprod Immunol. 2014;72(6):541–8.
42. Rizk B, Meagher S, Fisher AM. Severe ovarian hyperstimulation syndrome and cerebrovascular accidents. Hum Reprod. 1990;5:697–8.
43. Fabregues F, Tassies D, Reverter JC, et al. Prevalence of thrombophilia in women with severe ovarian hyperstimulation syndrome and cost-effectiveness of screening. Fertil Steril. 2004;81:989–95.
44. Jakimiuk AJ, Fritz A, Grzybowski W, et al. Diagnosing and management of iatrogenic moderate and severe ovarian hyperstimulation syndrome (OHSS) in clinical material. Folia Histochem Cytobiol. 2007;45(Suppl 1):S105–8.
45. Zhang Q, Xia L, Gao G. A new effective method in the treatment of severe ovarian hyperstimulation syndrome. Iran J Reprod Med. 2012;10:589–94.
46. Chen CD, Chen SU, Yang YS. Prevention and management of ovarian hyperstimulation syndrome. Best Pract Res Clin Obstet Gynaecol. 2012;26:817–27.
47. Abramov Y, Elchalal U, Schenker JG. Pulmonary manifestations of severe ovarian hyperstimulation syndrome: a multicenter study. Fertil Steril. 1999;71:645–51.
48. Rinaldi ML, Spirtos NJ. Chest tube drainage of pleural effusion correcting abdominal ascites in a patient with severe ovarian hyperstimulation syndrome: a case report. Fertil Steril. 1995;63:1114–7.

Chapter 14
Iatrogenic Multiple Pregnancy

Saul Barrera and Mayka Morgan

Introduction

Multiple pregnancy is defined as the simultaneous development in the uterus of more than one fetus. The multiple pregnancy rate has increased around the world in the last three decades as a result of an increase in assisted reproduction treatment (ART) [1]. The increase in the number of in vitro fertilizations performed and the use of medications for ovarian stimulation, which may add to the gestations in late maternal ages, all together lead to an increase in these rates. More than 200,000 babies are born worldwide each year by ART, and currently, approximately 5 million babies are born as a result of all forms of conception [2].

Multiple pregnancies as a result of ART have increased worldwide in the last decade, due to increases in the treatments performed and the transfer of more than two embryos in order to improve the results and the pregnancy rate [3]. Despite the effort to limit the number of embryos to change with SET (selective embryo transfer), it has not been possible to reduce the multiple pregnancy rate, if there is a very high pressure to have the best pregnancy rates that makes this increase unacceptable for its maternal outcome and adverse perinatal [4]. The final effect is reflected in the data showing that 21.8% of all participants after TRA culminate in pregnancies with more than one fetus [5].

Consider that the most serious complication that can be generated as a result of the assisted reproduction treatments performed is the high incidence of multiple pregnancy after infertility treatments. It is well documented that multiple pregnancies have adverse obstetric outcomes and higher rates of perinatal morbidity and mortality when compared to single pregnancies [6].

S. Barrera · M. Morgan (✉)
IVI-RMA Global, Panama City, Panama
e-mail: saul.barrera@ivirma.com; mayka.morgan@ivirma.com

C. Montufar et al. (eds.), *Obstetric Catastrophes*,
https://doi.org/10.1007/978-3-030-70034-8_14

Placentation

Although the vast majority of assisted reproduction twins are dizygotic (DZ) after the transfer of two embryos, monozygotic twin pregnancies (MZ) have a direct impact on prenatal care and obstetric management of twin pregnancies after assisted reproduction treatment [7].

Monochorionic twin pregnancies are associated with a threefold increase in perinatal mortality and a tenfold increase in the occurrence of prenatally acquired neurological lesions [8]. In general, perinatal mortality is around 11% in MZ pregnancies compared with 5.0% in DC twin pregnancies [9].

In monochorionic twins we find vascular anastomoses that are the pathophysiological basis of fetal transfusional syndrome; its diagnosis and late treatment lead to 90% of fetal mortality [9].

There is a higher incidence of fetal loss before 24 weeks in the monozygotics. After 32 weeks, the risk of intrauterine fetal death is significantly higher in monozygotic than dizygotic [10].

The three configurations of monozygotic placentation (bicorionic-biamniotic, mono-ionic-biamniotic, and mono-ammonic-monoamionic) have been found after the reproduction treatments were performed. This indicates that variations in placentation occur at different times of embryonic development and by means of different mechanisms. Derom et al. (1987) were one of the first to report a twofold increase in the rate of MC after ovarian stimulation for IVF compared to 0.4% found in spontaneous twin pregnancies [11]. Subsequent studies have documented even higher rates that go between 1% and 5% of MZ twin pregnancies after IVF.

Studies published in the last decade have also confirmed that women who use mediation for ovarian stimulation have twice as many risks for developing multiple pregnancies [12]. A greater relationship has been established in the appearance of twin pregnancy in patients who are users of medication for ovarian stimulation such as clomiphene citrate when compared with patients who underwent IVF by controlling the number of embryos to be transferred [13].

The membranous diagnosis of a multiple pregnancy is very important to determine the obstetric prognosis. It has been reported that several factors, such as patient history, maternal age, ovarian stimulation, and in vitro culture condition, influence the incidence of multiple pregnancy in advanced assisted reproduction techniques. In addition, numerous reports have implicit procedures, such as micromanipulation of the pellucid zone, embryo assisted hatching, and ICSI, as factors related to multiple pregnancy.

However, other studies suggest that these factors may not be independent causes of multiple pregnancy. Although extending the culture from the cleavage stage to the blastocyst stage may increase the incidence of multiple pregnancy, a recent study suggested that blastocyst transfers are not associated with a higher rate of monozygotic twin pregnancy when controlling the quality of the embryonic cohort. Given the complexity of an multiple pregnancy event, several factors may be associated with the underlying mechanisms.

An increase in twin MZ pregnancies has been reported in patients undergoing ICSI (intracytoplasmic sperm injection). Manipulation of the zona pellucida, assisted hatching, and extended embryo culture during ICSI/preimplantation genetic diagnosis can contribute to changes in fertilized oocyte division, and these factors could explain the relatively high rates of twin and triple assisted pregnancies [14].

The higher rate of multiple pregnancy in IVF treatments is mainly due to the increase in the number of pregnancies after the transfer of multiple embryos.

In general, a recent review of the literature identified maternal age and the performance of assisted reproduction treatments as the main risk factors to enhance the appearance of monozygotic twins [15].

Maternal Complications

Medical complications are more common in women with multifetal gestations than with singleton gestations. These include hyperemesis, gestational diabetes mellitus, hypertension, anemia, hemorrhage, cesarean delivery, and postpartum depression [16].

Women with multifetal gestations have an increased incidence of hypertensive conditions associated with pregnancy. The occurrence of hypertensive complications is proportional to the total fetal number, with singletons at 6.5%, twins at 12.7%, and triplets at 20.0% [17].

One study found that ART pregnancies were at increased risk (relative risk [RR], 2.1) of developing mild or severe preeclampsia, even after controlling for maternal age and parity [18]. Hypertensive disorders of pregnancy (HDP) in cases of Multiple gestation is usually more severe, with a higher risk of HELLP syndrome, eclampsia, and disseminated intravascular coagulation, resulting in a significant increase in maternal morbidity and mortality.

The likelihood of a multifetal gestation increases with maternal age, even outside of ART use. The multiple birth ratio increases from 16.3 per 1000 live births for women younger than 20 years to 71.1 per 1000 live births for women 40 years and older [19]. Older women also are more likely to have obstetric complications irrespective of fetal number, including gestational hypertension, gestational diabetes mellitus, and abruptio placentae.

In the case of triple pregnancy, there is a 20% risk of developing preeclampsia, 30% anemia, and 35% postpartum hemorrhage. Within the latter is uterine atony, most often in twin pregnancies due to uterine distention. As a preventive measure, uterotonics are used after the first twin has exited and intravenous oxytocic infusion after vaginal and cesarean delivery.

The dilutional anemia associated with pregnancy is often aggravated by the iron deficiency generally accentuated in twins. The incidence of anemia is doubled in twin pregnancies increasing the risk of premature labor and the severity of a postpartum hemorrhage.

Mothers carrying twins are also more likely to present with pregnancy-associated nausea and vomiting and higher body mass index leading to glucose intolerance and gestational diabetes than those carrying singletons [20].

Depression is more common in mothers of multiple births than with singletons, and having more than one child per birth, whether resulting from the use of assisted reproduction treatment or not, increases psychosocial risks for the parents during pregnancy and after delivery. In IVF pregnancies, anxiety scores, but not depression scores, are higher in women with twin gestations. In particular, primiparous mothers of IVF twins are vulnerable to stress in early stages of adaptation to the maternal role and may require professional interventions [21, 22].

Intrahepatic cholestasis of pregnancy (ICP) is the most common pregnancy-specific liver disease that typically presents in the third trimester. ICP is associated with an increased risk of adverse perinatal outcomes, including spontaneous preterm delivery, meconium staining of the amniotic fluid, and stillbirth. The etiology of ICP is yet to be resolved, but genetic, environmental, and hormonal factors, including estrogen and progesterone, probably have a roll. ICP in twin pregnancies presents earlier and is characterized by higher serum levels and elevated levels of bile acids which suggest that the disease is more severe in twins and consequently the risk of fetal death may be increased compared to singletons [23].

Neonatal Outcome of Multiple Pregnancies

Multiple pregnancy is associated with increased perinatal morbidity/mortality and elevated costs to health service [24]. This is largely attributable to complications of prematurity. It is estimated that 1% of singletons, 19% of twins, and 25% of triplet and higher-order multiples are due to IVF [24].

The average gestational ages at delivery for twins, triplets, and quadruplets are 35.3, 31.9, and 29.5 weeks, respectively [25].

Women with multifetal gestations are 6 times more likely to give birth preterm and 13 times more likely to give birth before 32 weeks of gestation than women with singleton gestations. This increases a fivefold risk of stillbirth and a sevenfold increased risk of neonatal death, which primarily is due to complications of prematurity [26].

Preterm delivery results in conditions associated with prematurity like intraventricular hemorrhage, periventricular leukomalacia (PVL), necrotizing enterocolitis, retinopathy, and respiratory distress syndrome, all of them leading to long-term morbidity, like cerebral palsy and mortality [27]. Perinatal mortality risk is 4/1000 for single, 26/1000 for twins, and 63/1000 for triplets. In cerebral palsy the incidence is 2% for single, 10% for twins, and 30% for triplets [28].

Different studies evaluated if ART procedures influenced neonatal outcomes in singletons with early preterm delivery. Evidence evaluates the relationship between in vitro fertilization (IVF) and neonatal outcomes in very low birth weight preterm infants (less than 32 weeks), with no detectable difference with neonatal outcomes

[29]. Other studies with similar conclusions that fetal outcomes seem to be equal between ART and SC in early preterm neonates only see an increase in risk of C-section rate and pregnancy complications such as placenta previa which seem to be higher in the ART group [30].

Although most of the current research states that obstetric outcomes of ART twins are similar to naturally conceived twins, twin pregnancy per se significantly increases the risk of obstetric complications and perinatal mortality and morbidity [31]. Most reports suggest that the maternal and neonatal outcomes of ART twins are comparable to that of naturally conceived twins. In a systematic review of 25 studies (3437 assisted and 3429 naturally conceived twins), ART twins had similar outcomes to those naturally conceived [32]. There does not seem to be an increase in perinatal mortality between naturally conceived twins and those conceived after ART, but there appears to be a modest increase in the caesarean section rate and low birth weight in ART twins [33].

Few data exist concerning obstetric and perinatal outcome in ART triplets versus naturally conceived triplets. A small study suggested an increased rate of neonatal malformations in the ART triplets; however the study is too small for definitive conclusions.

Congenital Abnormality

Congenital abnormality (CA) is a common and complex adverse pregnancy outcome associated with perinatal or infant mortality and morbidity worldwide. Initial studies comparing babies born following IVF or ICSI with spontaneously conceived controls suggested no increase in incidence of congenital abnormalities. However, systemic reviews found an increased risk of congenital abnormalities and some birth complications in ART in comparison with normal conception [34].

Single fetuses conceived with IVF/ICSI methods are at an increased risk of developing congenital heart disease compared with those conceived spontaneously. Due to heterogeneity of ART procedures and cardiac defects, there is not conclusive evidences and required further investigation [35].

Data confirmed that multiple pregnancies of IVF/ICSI were significantly associated with the risk of developing congenital in their offspring [36]. A recent meta-analysis aimed to evaluate congenital malformations in infants conceived by assisted reproductive techniques compared with infants conceived spontaneously involving 61,815 IVF/ICSI multiple births and 204,471 spontaneous conception multiple births indicated that the multiple pregnancies generated by IVF/ICSI, when compared with those conceived naturally, were at a significantly higher risk of 18% for urogenital system malformations, 36% for chromosomal defects, and 22% for circulatory system malformations, but the remaining specific congenital abnormalities, such as cleft lip and/or palate, eye, ear, face and neck, respiratory, musculoskeletal, nervous and digestive system malformations, were similar in the two groups [37].

Decreasing the Risks of Multiples

Due to the increased perinatal and maternal risks of multiple pregnancy, it is very important to look for strategies to preventing iatrogenic multiple pregnancies. Multiple pregnancy remains the single biggest risk to the health of children born after IVF [38].

Primary forms of preventing multiple pregnancy include canceling ovulation induction cycles in which multifollicular development has increased risk. In IVF cycles limiting the number of embryos transferred is the first step in reducing multiple pregnancy rates; the complications and risks of multiple pregnancies can be reduced by implementing a strategy using elective single embryo transfer.

Single Embryo Transfer

Despite the substantial risks associated with multiple pregnancy, double embryo transfer (DET) during IVF treatment continues to be widely practiced [39]. Variation in IVF regulation worldwide has resulted in significant differences in embryo transfer practices between countries. To encourage the use of SET, the American Society for Reproductive Medicine (ASRM) [40], the British Fertility Society (BFS), and the Association of Clinical Embryologists (ACE) have all produced guidelines to assist centers to select patients eligible for eSET. These guidelines identify patients who are at the greatest risk of multiple pregnancy by using factors such as patient age and embryo quality and made specific recommendations in this groups.

Data from SART National of 2013 demonstrate that elective single-embryo transfer (eSET) in women aged <38 years have decreased rates of multiple gestation, with no significant impact on cumulative live-birth rates [41].

In women 42 years or younger, transferring a single euploid blastocyst resulted in pregnancy rates similar to transferring two untested blastocysts while dramatically reducing the risk of twins [42].

The widespread application of single embryo transfer has significantly reduced the twin pregnancy rate without any decrease in cumulative pregnancy rates. A meta-analysis of eight randomized controlled trials researching the clinical effectiveness of single embryo transfer found that the odds of a term singleton birth after elective single embryo transfer was almost five times higher than the odds after double embryo transfer (OR: 4.93; 95% CI: 2.98e8.18) [43].

Each country and clinic must establish, according to their results, the policies to implement the (eSET). Two requirements are essential for this: Optimizing selection methods of good-quality embryo is crucial and effective cryopreservation programs to ensure that the cumulative pregnancy from elective single fresh and frozen cycles is equivalent to those achieved with DETs.

Multifetal Pregnancy Reduction

Multifetal pregnancy fetal reduction is a first-trimester or early second-trimester procedure for reducing by one or more the total number of fetuses in a multifetal pregnancy [44]. It is an effort to reduce the risk associated with multiple gestation and high-order multiple gestation. Selective reduction to a twin pregnancy has been shown to reduce the risk of preterm delivery, low birth weight delivery, cesarean delivery, neonatal death, and prenatal complications comparable with that of a spontaneously conceived twin pregnancy [45].

The risk associated with reduction itself is not insignificant and correlates with the initial number of fetuses in the pregnancy, ranging from 11.1% risk of unintended loss of a healthy fetus when reducing from three or more fetuses to a 2.4% unintended loss rate when reducing from twins to a singleton [44].

In high-order multifetal pregnancy, reduction of triplets to twins is associated with a better pregnancy outcome compared with that of nonreduced triplets. Multifetal pregnancy reduction may be the appropriate alternative to reduce perinatal morbidity and mortality in trichorionic triplet pregnancies [46, 47].

Bibliography

1. Halliday JL, Ukoumunne OC, Baker HW, Breheny S, Jaques AM, Garrett C, et al. Increased risk of blastogenesis birth defects, arising in the first 4 weeks of pregnancy, after assisted reproductive technologies. Hum Reprod. 2010;25:59–65.
2. Kissin DM, Jamieson DJ, Barfield WD. Monitoring health outcomes of assisted reproductive technology. N Engl J Med. 2014;371:91–3.
3. Moini A, Shiva M, Arabipoor A, Hosseini R, Chehrazi M, Sadeghi M. Obstetric and neonatal outcomes of twin pregnancies conceived by assisted reproductive technology compared with twin pregnancies conceived spontaneously: a prospective follow-up study. Eur J Obstet Gynecol Reprod Biol. 2012;165:29–32.
4. Shevell T, Malone FD, Vidaver J, Porter TF, Luthy DA, Comstock CH, et al. Assisted reproductive technology and pregnancy outcome. Obstet Gynecol. 2005;106:1039–45.
5. Nyboe Andersen A, Goossens V, Bhattacharya S, Ferraretti AP, Kupka MS, de Mouzon J, et al. Assisted reproductive technology and intrauterine inseminations in Europe, 2005: results generated from European registers by ESHRE. The European IVF Monitoring Programme (EIM), for the European Society of Human Reproduction and Embryology (ESHRE). Hum Reprod. 2009;24:1267–87.
6. Farhi A, Reichman B, Boyko V, Hourvitz A, Ron-El R, Lerner-Geva L. Maternal and neonatal health outcomes following assisted reproduction. Reprod Biomed Online. 2013;26:454–61.
7. Tocino A, Blasco V, Prados N, Vargas MJ, Requena A, Pellicer A, et al. Monozygotic twinning after assisted reproductive technologies: a case report of asymmetric development and incidence during 19 years in an international group of in vitro fertilization clinics. Fertil Steril. 2015;103:1185–9.
8. Hillman SC, Morris RK, Kilby MD. Co-twin prognosis after single fetal death: a systematic review and meta-analysis. Obstet Gynecol. 2011;118:928–40.
9. Huber A, Hecher K. How can we diagnose and manage twin–twin transfusion syndrome. Best Pract Res Clin Obstet Gynecol. 2004;18:543–56.

10. Hack KE, Derks JB, Elias SG, Franx A, Roos EJ, Voerman SK, Bode CL, Koopman-Esseboom C, Visser GH. Increased perinatal mortality and morbidity in monochorionic versus dichorionic twin pregnancies: clinical implications of a large Dutch cohort study. BJOG. 2008;115:58–67.
11. Aston KI, Peterson CM, Carrell DT. Monozygotic twinning associated with assisted reproductive technologies: a review. Reproduction. 2008;136:377–86.
12. Kallen B, Olausson PO, Nygren KG. Neonatal outcome in pregnancies from ovarian stimulation. Obstet Gynecol. 2002;100:414–9.
13. Derom C, Leroy F, Vlietinck R, Fryns JP, Derom R. High frequency of iatrogenic monozygotic twins with administration of clomiphene citrate and a change in chorionicity. Fertil Steril. 2006;85:755–7.
14. Haimov-Kochman R, Daum H, Lossos F, Aizenman E, Werner M, Yagel S, Laufer N, Simon A, Hurwitz A. Monozygotic multiple gestation after intracytoplasmic sperm injection and preimplantation genetic diagnosis. Fertil Steril. 2009;92:44, 2037.e11–17.
15. Esfandiari N, Kapoor M, Burjaq H, Chang P, Gotlieb L, Casper RF. Monozygotic twins in infertile patients with advanced maternal age: case reports and review of the literature. Fertil Steril. 2009;92:1168.
16. Luke B, Brown MB. Contemporary risks of maternal morbidity and adverse outcomes with increasing maternal age and plurality. Fertil Steril. 2007;88:283–93.
17. Day MC, Barton JR, O'Brien JM, Istwan NB, Sibai BM. The effect of fetal number on the development of hypertensive conditions of pregnancy. Obstet Gynecol. 2005;106:927–31.
18. Lynch A, McDuffie R Jr, Murphy J, Faber K, Orleans M. Preeclampsia in multiple gestation: the role of assisted reproductive technologies. Obstet Gynecol. 2002;99:445–51.(Level II-3).
19. Martin JA, Hamilton BE, Ventura SJ, Osterman MJ, Kirmeyer S, Mathews TJ, et al. Births: final data for 2009. Natl Vital Rep. 2011;60:1–70.
20. Louik C, Hernandez-Diaz S, Werler MM, Mitchell AA. Nausea and vomiting in pregnancy: maternal characteristics and risk factors. Paediatr Perinat Epidemiol. 2006;20:270–8.
21. Jahangiri F, Hirshfeld-Cytron J, Goldman K, Pavone ME, Gerber S, Klock SC. Correlation between depression, anxiety, and nausea and vomiting during pregnancy in an in vitro fertilization population: a pilot study. J Psychosom Obstet Gynaecol. 2011;32:113–8.
22. Roca-de Bes M, Gutierrez-Maldonado J, Gris-Marŕ ınez JM. Comparative study of the psychosocial risks associated with families with multiple births resulting from assisted reproductive technology (ART) and without ART. Fertil Steril. 2011;96:170–4.
23. Batsry L, Zloto K, Kalter A, et al. Arch Gynecol Obstet. 2019; https://doi.org/10.1007/s00404-019-05247-0.
24. National Institute for Health and Care Excellence. Clinical guideline 129. Multiple pregnancy e the management of twin and triplet pregnancies in the antenatal period; 2011.
25. American College of Obstetricians and Gynecologists; Society for Maternal- Fetal Medicine. ACOG Practice Bulletin No. 144: multifetal gestations: twin, triplet, and higher-order multifetal pregnancies. Obstet Gynecol. 2014;123:1118–32.
26. Kulkarni AD, Jamieson DJ, Jones HW Jr, et al. Fertility treatments and multiple births in the United States. N Engl J Med. 2013;369:2218.
27. Elliott JP. High-order multiple gestations. Semin Perinatol. 2005;29:305e11.
28. Hansen M, Colvin Lpetterson B, et al. Twins born following assisted reproductive technology:perinatal outcome and admission to hospital. Hum Reprod. 2009;24:2321–31.
29. Al-Hathlol K. Relationship between in vitro fertilization and neonatal outcomes in very low birth weight preterm infants. Am J Perinatol. 2018;35(11):1113–8.
30. Di Tommaso M, et al. Influence of assisted reproductive technologies on maternal and neonatal outcomes in early preterm deliveries. J Gynecol Obstet Hum Reprod. 2019;48:845.
31. Fitzsimmons B, Bebbington W, Fluker M. Perinatal and neonatal outcomes in multiple gestations: assisted reproduction versus spontaneous conception. Am J Obstet Gynecol. 1998;179:1162e7.
32. Helmerhorst F, Perquin D, Donker D, Keirse M. Perinatal outcome of single- tons and twins after assisted conception: a systematic review of controlled studies. BMJ. 2004;328:261e5.

33. Joy J, McClure I, Cooke E. A comparison of spontaneously conceived twins and twins conceived by artificial reproductive technologies. J Obstet Gynaecol. 2008;28:580e5.
34. Hoorsan H, Mirmiran P, Chaichian S, Moradi Y, Hoorsan R, Jesmi F. Congenital malformations in infants of mothers undergoing assisted reproductive technologies: a systematic review and meta-analysis study. J Prev Med Public Health. 2017;50(6):347–60. https://doi.org/10.3961/jpmph.16.122.
35. Giorgione V, Parazzini F, Fesslova V, Cipriani S, Candiani M, Inversetti A, Sigismondi C, Tiberio F, Cavoretto P. Congenital heart defects in IVF/ICSI pregnancy: systematic review and meta-analysis. Ultrasound Obstet Gynecol. 2018;51:33–42.
36. Liberman RF, Getz KD, Heinke D, Luke B, Stern JE, Declercq ER, Chen X, Lin AE, Anderka M. Assisted reproductive technology and birth defects: effects of subfertility and multiple births. Birth Defects Res. 2017;109:1144–53.
37. Zan Zheng, Letao Chen, Tubao Yang, Hong Yu, Hua Wang, Jiabi Qin. Multiple pregnancies achieved with IVF/ICSI and risk of specific congenital malformations: a meta-analysis of cohort studies. Reprod Biomed Online. 2018;36(4):472–82.
38. Gelbaya T, Tsoumpou I, Nardo L. The likelihood of live birth and multiple birth after single versus double embryo transfer at the cleavage stage: a systematic review and meta-analysis. Fertil Steril. 2010;94:936e45.
39. Maheshwari A, Griffiths S, Bhattacharya S. Global variations in the uptake of single embryo transfer. Hum Reprod Update. 2011;17:107–20.
40. Practice committee of the American Society for Reproductive Medicine Practice Committee of the Society for Assisted Reproductive Technology. Criteria for number of embryos to transfer: a committee opinion. Fertil Steril. 2013;99(1):44e6.
41. Mancuso A, Boulet SL, Duran E, Munch E, Kissin DM, Van Voorhis BJ. Elec- tive single embryo transfer in women under age 38 reduces multiple birth rates, but not live birth rates in United States fertility clinics. Fertil Steril. 2016;106:1107–14.
42. Orman EJ, Hong KH, Ferry KM, Tao X, Taylor D, Levy B, et al. In vitro fertilization with single euploid blastocyst transfer: a randomized controlled trial. Fertil Steril. 2013;100:100–7.
43. McLernon D, Harrild K, Bergh C, et al. Clinical effectiveness of elective single versus double embryo transfer: meta-analysis of individual patient data from randomised trials. BMJ. 2010;341:1136e48.
44. American College of Obstetricians and Gynecologists. ACOG Committee opinion no. 553: multifetal pregnancy reduction. Obstet Gynecol. 2013;121:405–10.
45. Dodd JM, Crowther CA. Reduction of the number of fetuses for women with a multiple pregnancy. Cochrane Database Syst Rev. 2012;(10):Art. No.: CD003932. https://doi.org/10.1002/14651858.CD003932.pub2.
46. Eddleman KA, Stone JL, Lynch L, Berkowitz RL. Selective termination of anomalous fetuses in multifetal pregnancies: two hundred cases at a single center. Am J Obstet Gynecol. 2002;187:1168–72.
47. Anthoulakis C, Dagklis T, Mamopoulos A, Athanasiadis A. Risks of miscarriage or preterm delivery in trichorionic and dichorionic triplet pregnancies with embryo reduction versus expectant management: a systematic review and meta-analysis. Hum Reprod. 2017;32(6):1351–9.

Part IV
Procedures in the Critical Ill Obstetric Patient

Chapter 15
Procedures in Pregnant Women in Critical Condition

Bayardo J. Robelo-Pentzke

Radial Catheter

The complications related with any catheter placement into a blood vessel are rare, but they may be less common if the catheter is inserted in the wrist.

The small size and the closer location to the skin surface make the radial artery an ideal vascular site to prevent complications as external bleeding during arterial catheterization.

Before using the radial artery, it is advisable to test the blood supply to the hand and be sure that both ulnar and radial arteries are working; performing a modified Allen's test is the best way to proceed in this case.

A potential risk after the catheterization of the radial artery is the occlusion of the vessel as a result of a blood clot formation; if there are redundant blood supplies to the hand, there will be no issues for this hand.

Invasive blood pressure is considered the "gold standard" for arterial pressure monitoring in patients admitted to critical care units.

Arterial pressure measurement represents a mandatory step in the evaluation of patient hemodynamics because it gives primary information about the performance of the cardiovascular system and tissue perfusion [3].

Invasive arterial pressure allows a continuous monitoring and provides vascular access for obtaining blood samples (arterial blood gases and other laboratory studies). It is also indicated in patients receiving vasoactive infusions or those with fluctuating, unstable blood pressures.

An arterial catheter may be inserted into the radial, brachial, femoral, or dorsal pedis artery. The radial artery is the preferred site because of easier accessibility. The catheter is attached to a fluid-filled pressure transducer system incorporating a

B. J. Robelo-Pentzke (✉)
Hospital Dr. Rafael A. Calderon-Guardia, San José, Costa Rica

C. Montufar et al. (eds.), *Obstetric Catastrophes*,
https://doi.org/10.1007/978-3-030-70034-8_15

flush system to maintain patency. An attached transducer senses arterial pressure and converts the pressure signal to a waveform on the bedside monitor.

The waveform reflects pressure generated by the left ventricle during systole and diastole, and the monitor displays the corresponding numerical values.

The technique is performed usually in the radial artery of the non-dominant arm after determining the permeability of the radial and ulnar arteries in such arm using Allen's test; in case the patient is unconscious or is not cooperating, the verification of patency is recommended with Doppler sonography or pulse oximetry.

In case that any of these arteries are not patent, it is not recommended to make a puncture of these vessels in this hand; proceed with the evaluation of the arterial circulation at the contralateral hand.

Indications

- Administration of drugs
- Catheter insertion for coronography
- Continuous and invasive monitorization of the arterial pressure
- To get serial blood arterial samples for gasometry

Contraindications

- Raynaud syndrome
- Thromboangiitis obliterans
- Arterial insufficiency
- Infection at the puncture site
- Arterial lesions next to the puncture site
- Severe alterations in coagulation

Technique Description

With the patient's hand in a supine position and dorsiflexion, proceed to clean the area and make antisepsis of the skin; drape the zone, and palpate the pulse in the radial artery one or two centimeters above the wrist between the styloid apophysis of the radius and the flexor radial muscle tendon. Apply local anesthesia to the skin, insert the arterial cannula distal to the palpated radial artery with an angle between 30° and 45°, slowly advance the cannula through the artery until blood is drawn in a pulsatile way, introduce the rest of the cannula with an angle between 10° and 15°, remove the guide from the cannula pressing the artery, and close the cannula. Make the fixation of the cannula with skin stiches and adapt the system for pressure monitoring [2].

Removal of the Arterial Line

Rationale

The arterial line should be removed if:

- The arterial line is no longer required for close blood pressure monitoring and/or blood samples.
- If there are any sign of infection and phlebitis or if the line is no longer functioning well.
- When the patient has signs of sepsis and the intensive care unit team has decided to replace all lines [4].

Proceed to cut the stiches and gently remove the cannula from the radial artery keeping pressure to permit cloth formation at the site of puncture; once there is no risk of bleeding, use a compressive bandage, and verify the correct circulation to the hand.

Central Venous Catheters

A central venous catheter is a catheter with a tip that lies within the proximal third of the superior vena cava, the right atrium, or the inferior vena cava. Catheter can be inserted through a peripheral vein or a proximal central vein, most commonly the internal jugular, subclavian, or femoral vein.

Central venous cannulation is considered the procedure, which facilitates resuscitation, nutritional support, and long-term vascular access between other uses like access for giving drugs, access for extracorporeal blood circuits, and hemodynamic monitoring and interventions. As all invasive procedures, it is not free of complications; knowledge of surface and deep anatomy minimizes complications.

Between these complications are infection, thrombosis, bleeding, vascular occlusion, and other mechanical complications that usually occur during insertion and are intimately related to the anatomic relationships of the central veins. Overall complications may rate 15% [1]. That is why anatomic surface landmarks are useful to orient the deep course of cannulating needle tracts.

Nowadays, the real-time ultrasound visualization enhances the safety of internal jugular and femoral venous cannulation and also offers the axillary vein as a visible alternative of blind subclavian approaches.

To prevent infections is mandatory always considering strict attention to antisepsis and sterile technique.

The most frequent procedure used to establish central venous cannulation is the called Seldinger technique, it was introduced in the early 1950s as an innovation, and Trendelenburg position for internal jugular and subclavian cannulation allows gravity to enhance central venous filling, making the venous puncture more successful and minimizing the air embolus risk. The collapse of the vein increases the risk of back wall puncture and potential intra-arterial placement of the devices.

Incorrect placement of the catheter tip increases mechanical and thrombotic complications, but the ideal location of the catheter tip depends on the indications for catheterization and the site of insertion. No single catheter tip position is ideal for all patients.

Once the catheter is introduced, in general, the correct place to ubicate its tip is at the junction of the superior vena cava with the right atrium, at this place, there is a high blood flow that prevents thrombosis and arrhythmias from catheter irritation of the atrial wall. The surface landmark corresponding to this position is the angle of Louis of the sternum. On the control chest X-ray, this point corresponds to the right tracheobronchial angle; high placement of the catheter tip in the superior vena cava increases the risk of thrombosis; and it is recommended that long-term catheters should be placed precisely under fluoroscopy and the position of short-term central lines should be confirmed with a chest X-ray.

The understanding of the correct underlying vein trajectory is critical to prevent potential injuries to the venous sidewalls to be punctured by a wide-bore and stiff dilator. Vascular injury may lead to life-threatening hemorrhage or cardiac tamponade.

With the right internal jugular and left subclavian approaches, the veins respectively take straight and gently curving trajectories to the superior vena cava. The right subclavian vein takes a near right angle turn into the superior vena cava, and the left internal jugular vein has two turns, one into the brachiocephalic vein and a second into the superior vena cava. All these are points for potential injury when passing the catheter or the dilator [1].

That is why dilators are used only to develop a subcutaneous tract, they should be advanced to the level of the adventitial vein surface but never in to the vein, and the depth at which the vein was accessed with the venipuncture should be kept in mind as the maximal distance the dilator could be inserted.

Ultrasound Visualization

Given the superficial location of the central veins at the sites of venipuncture, a high-frequency probe of 7.5 MHz creates optimal images. Ultrasound-directed techniques for insertion are now the standard of care. Ultrasound-guided placement results in lower failure rates, reduced complications, and faster access compared with landmark technique. Subclavian cannulation remains a blind technique; the use of ultrasound has improved outcomes for internal jugular vein cannulation and is considered a current standard of care for cannulation at this site.

The site of insertion depends on several factors: indication for insertion, predicted duration of use, previous line insertion sites (where veins may be thrombosed or stenosed), and presence of relative contraindications. Potential contraindications to central venous catheterization are coagulopathy, thrombocytopenia, ipsilateral hemothorax or pneumothorax, vessel thrombosis, stenosis or disruption, infection overlying the insertion site, and ipsilateral indwelling central vascular devices.

Internal Jugular Vein Approach

The internal jugular vein is often the access of choice for central venous cannulation, because of its superficial location, easy ultrasonic visualization, and straight course to the superior vena cava on the right side [1].

There are three percutaneous approaches to the internal jugular vein: anterior, central, and posterior. The essential surface anatomy is comprised between the borders of Sedillot's triangle, which limits are:

- The sternal head of the sternocleidomastoid muscle medially
- The clavicular head of the sternocleidomastoid laterally
- The superior border of the medial third of the clavicle inferiorly

Central Approach

For the central approach, cannulation begins with cutaneous puncture at the superior apex of Sedillot's triangle. The internal jugular vein lies immediately posterior to the apex of this anatomic triangle with a frequency of 97% on the right and 79% on the left and is thus relatively superficial in location, 1.0–1.5 cms beneath the cutaneous surface; be careful, at this point there is the risk of puncture of the pulmonary apex and the carotid artery.

Posterior Approach

For the posterior approach, the needle is placed at the posterior border of the sternocleidomastoid muscle at a point one-third of the way from the sternoclavicular joint to the mastoid process; the sternal jugular vein crosses the sternocleidomastoid muscle at this point and is a useful landmark. The needle is advanced toward the ipsilateral sternoclavicular joint at an angle of 30°–40° off the skin.

Anterior Approach

In the anterior approach, the cutaneous puncture site is at the medial border of the sternocleidomastoid at the level of the cricoid cartilage; the needle tip should pass medial to the sternocleidomastoid directed 30°–45° posteriorly from a coronal plane and 15°–45° laterally from a sagittal plane.

The internal jugular vein generally lays anterolateral to the carotid artery; the vein may also lay directly anterior to the artery predisposing to arterial puncture. Rarely, the internal jugular vein lays medial to the carotid artery. The palpation of carotid artery diminishes internal jugular vein diameter. Trendelenburg position should be employed whenever feasible; the head should be rotated to the contralateral side only so far as to provide access to the neck.

Anatomic complications during the central venous cannulation are puncture or cannulation of the internal carotid artery and pneumothorax.

Carotid puncture is avoided by preventing medial angulation of the needle as it passes bellow the cutaneous surface and also by staying high in Sedillot's triangle.

Ultrasonography images visually differentiate the internal jugular vein and common carotid artery, facilitate venipuncture rather than arterial puncture, guard against through-and-through puncture of the internal jugular vein, and prevent deep passage of a needle into deep cervical and thoracic structures.

Ultrasound images through Sedillot's triangle will demonstrate the carotid artery and internal jugular vein as two sonolucent circles. The artery is recognized as the smaller in diameter, noncompressible vessel with a visible pulsation. Real-time ultrasound guidance has been shown to improve the technical efficiency and efficacy of internal jugular venous cannulation and to decrease the frequency of arterial punctures; sonographic guidance has also decreased the frequency of hematomas, hemothorax, and pneumothorax [5].

Subclavian Cannulation

The subclavian cannulation is long favored by surgeons, may be associated with fewer infectious complications, and remains accessible after localized thrombosis of the internal jugular vein. The incidences of pneumothorax, hemothorax, and thrombosis are equivalent to the jugular approach. The enhanced safety of ultrasound in the internal jugular position increases interest in sonographically assisted cannulation of the axillary vein as an alternative. Any advantage of this technique over landmark-guided subclavian cannulation remains unproven.

There are two approaches for subclavian venipuncture technique: infraclavicular and supraclavicular.

Infraclavicular Subclavian Approach

The operator stands on the side to be cannulated, and the patient should be placed in the Trendelenburg position to maximize venous filling of the vein and minimize risk of air embolus.

The goal of subclavian venipuncture is to pass a needle inferior to the clavicle and superior to the first rib to access the subclavian vein as it courses over the first rib. The appropriate course of the needle passes immediately beneath the junction of the medial one-third and lateral two-thirds of the clavicle. The appropriate point for cutaneous puncture lays 1–2 cms inferior and lateral to the clavicular transition point.

A cutaneous puncture site closer to the clavicle creates difficulty maneuvering the needle beneath the clavicle. More medial cannulation may be impeded by calcification of the costoclavicular ligament. As the needle is advanced, it must remain absolutely parallel to the floor; if the needle is directed posteriorly, the risk of pneumothorax is greatly increased.

Alternative landmark is the deltoid tuberosity of the clavicle, which is palpable as an anterior projection laying roughly at the junction of the lateral one-third and medial two-thirds of the clavicle. The cutaneous puncture site in this case is placed 1.5 cm inferior to the medial border of this landmark, and the needle is advanced toward the sternoclavicular joint and sternal notch.

Supraclavicular Subclavian Approach

The essential landmark for this approach is the junction of the lateral border of the clavicular head of the sternocleidomastoid with the clavicle. The point for cutaneous puncture lays 1 cm superior and 1 cm lateral to this junction. Between the junctions of the sternocleidomastoid with the clavicle is the clavicle sternocleidomastoid angle. The cannulation needle tip is angled posteriorly 5°–15° off a coronal plane and advanced along a line that bisects the clavicular sternocleidomastoid angle. This will lead to subclavian venipuncture between the clavicle and the anterior scalene muscle.

An aspect to take in mind is that the more medially the catheter enters the vein, the more anteriorly it will lie within the acute angle formed between the clavicle and first rib. The more anteriorly the catheter lies, the more likely it will be compressed as the costoclavicular angle closes with upright position. With a relatively lateral venipuncture, the catheter will pass through the wider, posterior point of this triangular space, rendering compression with arm abduction less likely than if the catheter lies in a more anterior position. As a consequence of this compression of the catheter, at this point it may be transected, creating a catheter embolus that may be asymptomatic in 24% of cases. Most commonly, in 56% of cases without transection, it may present as catheter malfunction; less frequent symptoms include arrhythmias, pulmonary complaints, and sepsis; this is called pinch-off syndrome [1].

Complications

- Subclavian arterial lesion.
- Direct brachial plexus injury or compression neuropathy caused by hematoma
- Lesion of structures in posterior relationship with the subclavian vein as the phrenic nerve (located medially of the anterior scalene muscle) and the internal mammary artery and the apical pleura

Pneumothorax is avoided by keeping the needle and syringe absolutely parallel to the floor at the moment of the puncture.

Axillary Vein Cannulation

The axillary vein and artery can be easily visualized with ultrasound more laterally on the chest wall, anterior to the lateral clavicle. The axillary vein can be recognized as a compressible structure lying anterior to the noncompressible, pulsating axillary artery.

Ultrasound-guided cannulation of the axillary vein may prove to be a safer technique than blind subclavian cannulation, especially for those operators without extensive experience with other approaches.

Femoral Cannulation

This technique was first described for Moncrief in 1958 [8].

It is a procedure that may be favored during emergent resuscitation when procedures such as endotracheal intubation and cardiac compressions limit concurrent access to the internal jugular vein and subclavian vein.

The venipuncture is performed below the inguinal ligament; this runs from the pubic tubercle medially to the anterosuperior iliac spine laterally. The femoral artery bisects this ligament, and the femoral vein is immediately medial to it.

Cutaneous puncture is performed approximately 1 cm medial to the point of maximal pulsation of the femoral artery; it can be facilitated by real-time ultrasound localization. Make sure that the puncture is below the level of the inguinal ligament; above this ligament is the external iliac vein, which becomes a deep retroperitoneal structure making it difficult to place pressure on the insertion site if bleeding occurs.

The femoral vein catheters are associated with higher rates of infection and thrombosis than subclavian or internal jugular vein catheters [1].

The compression for the inferior vena cava when the gravid uterus is in advanced stage, difficult a rapid and high flow infusion during an emergency, nevertheless the femoral vein access even may be useful.

Therefore, the femoral vein is considered the third choice for central catheterization and is used only when other approaches are not feasible, for example, during cardiopulmonary resuscitation; nevertheless, the femoral vein may be collapsed in such a patient, making cannulation quite challenging. Ultrasound may be a useful adjunct in the placement of femoral catheters. The femoral vein is a typically larger caliber, compressible structure anteromedial to the femoral artery, which should be noncompressible and pulsatile.

Pericardiocentesis

The most frequent etiology of pericardial effusion is neoplastic; generally lung or breast tumors are involved. Its diagnosis is simple, there are minimum complications in evacuation, and the means and actual monitorization allow to make pericardiocentesis in optimum conditions.

Pericardial effusions result as incremental in the quantity of liquid inside the pericardial cavity that exceeds its capacity of reabsorption, increasing the intrapericardial pressure; it may cause tachycardia, hypotension, paradoxical pulse, and an increase on central venous pressure; this is called cardiac tamponade. When instauration is slow, it can be tolerated by the patient; if the instauration is rapid, even small quantities of liquid can cause hemodynamic collapse.

The diagnosis is clinical and is reinforced by echocardiography, showing diastolic collapse of the right cavities of the heart, occasionally collapsing also the left cavities.

To drain this liquid with pericardiocentesis is the gold standard, it must be performed urgently or in a programed way, and it depends on the hemodynamic situation of the patient. The increase in invasive diagnostic and therapeutic techniques has favored iatrogenic pericardial effusion, which is secondary in etiology.

Pericardiocentesis is not a technique free of risk, its mortality can reach even 4%, and this risk improves where the procedure is performed under echocardiography control, besides adequate monitorization of the arterial pressure and the cardiac rhythm [6].

The pericardiocentesis procedure consists of the puncture of the pericardial cavity through the chest wall to proceed with the extraction of the pericardial fluid for diagnosis and/or therapeutic option when this liquid is under tension.

The normal pericardium is a fibroelastic membrane composed of connective tissue surrounding the external surface of the heart, the roots of the greatest arteries, and the union of the cavas and pulmonary veins with the respective atrium. It is formed by two layers, the visceral pericardium that covers the surface of the heart and the parietal serosa layer, less than two millimeters thick. Between these two layers, there is a virtual space with approximately 30 ml of liquid, which under normal conditions is clear; its function is to lubricate, contributing to the normal sliding between both layers of pericardium during cardiac movements.

Pericardium has mechanical functions: these are to limit the ventricular filling to prevent excessively acute dilatation of the cardiac chambers, to distribute the pressure between both ventricles and atrium, and to facilitate the cardiac movements during systole and diastole. It also makes the function of a ligament because it is anchored to other thoracic structures.

The first pericardiocentesis with echocardiographic control was made in 1978, at Mayo Clinic; this procedure may cause complications like myocardial injury, lesion to coronary arteries, gas embolism, pneumothorax, arrhythmias, lesions to intra-peritoneal organs, and lesions to esophagus with mediastinitis and pericarditis [7].

The classical presentation of cardiac tamponade is called Beck's triad and consists of:

- Jugular distention
- Decrease in cardiac sounds
- Absence of peripheral pulse

This triad is present in less than 30% of cases. Other signs of cardiac tamponade may be paradoxical pulse, that is, a decrease in systolic pressure more than 10 mmHg during normal inspiration, decrease in size of electrocardiographic complexes, and Kussmaul sign, which consist of increase in jugular venous distention during inspiration.

Between the indications of pericardiocentesis are:

- To confirm a pericardial effusion
- To infuse therapeutic agents like antibiotics, cytostatic, and sclerosing materials
- To insufflate air for image diagnosis
- To drain cardiac tamponade

Between the contraindications we may say:

- Avoid puncture when skin lesions are present.
- When the cause of cardiac tamponade is traumatic and pericardial effusion is present with hemodynamic instability.
- Myocardial rupture.
- Aortic dissection.
- Severe hemostatic disorder.

Pericardiocentesis Technique

There are two frequent approaches, the subxiphoid, also called Marfan technique and the parasternal technique.

The puncture must be made easily, keeping continuous suction through the syringe and trying to feel the sensation when the pericardial membrane is overcome.

Subxiphoid Technique

This approach is not recommended in case of patients in advanced stage of pregnancy because of the obstacle gravid uterus, which may be compromised during the subxiphoid approach making it difficult.

Place the patient in supine decubitus, with his head 30° over the horizontal plane; the electrocardiographic monitoring is important to detect arrhythmias. The target point is located between the angle formed by the xiphoid process and the seventh left rib; it is mandatory to clean and make antisepsis of the skin and drape the zone, apply local anesthesia, and make the puncture with a needle in a 30° angle with direction to the right shoulder keeping constant suction until you get pericardial effusion. One way to confirm you are in the pericardial space is infusing air and the contrast on the echocardiographic screen is observed. Insert a wire guide through the needle, remove the needle and then introduce the draining catheter over the wire guide, confirm the presence of liquid sucking once again, and keep the catheter with a firm stitch to the skin.

Parasternal Technique

This approach is recommended in case of advanced pregnancy. Observe the same recommendations regarding the preparation of the patient; the target point in this case is located in the fifth left intercostal space, 2 cm outside the sternal border, to avoid damage to the internal thoracic artery and veins. Make the puncture with the needle directed in anteroposterior and caudal direction, from right to left through the cardiac apex, keeping constant suction until get the pericardial fluid. Insert a wire guide trough the needle and then remove the needle introducing later a pericardial catheter over the wire guide and proceed to suture the catheter with a firm stitch to the skin.

The extracted liquid must be analyzed with cytology, cell count, hematocrit, Gram stain, Ziehl-Neelsen stain, bacteriological cultures, mycotic cultures and Koch bacillus culture, PCR (polymeric chain reaction), and ELISA.

The appropriate moment to remove the pericardial catheter will be determined for the characteristics of the liquid and the amount of pericardial effusion drained in a period of 24 hours. If the quantity of liquid drained is less than 100 milliliters, it will be safe to remove the catheter.

Removing the catheter is made simply by cutting the stitch that was fixed to the skin and applying a compressive apposite.

Thoracentesis

This procedure, also known as pleural puncture, the same as pericardiocentesis is useful for diagnosis and in many cases it can be therapeutic. The objective is to drain air or liquid from the pleural cavity.

Clinical exam and analysis of the pleural effusion could determine the etiology, depending on its nature: exudate or transudate.

As in any other invasive procedures, it is necessary to evaluate risk vs. benefit of the procedure. The experience of the operator and the correct evaluation of the presence of air or liquid by physical exam, chest X-ray, and ultrasonography are very important; discard blood anomalies with coagulation and thrombosis prior to the procedure.

Indications

- Pneumothorax evacuation.
- Pleural effusion analysis to determine if it is an exudate or a transudate, blood, pus, lymph, etc.
- Evacuate pleural effusion to improve the breathing condition.

Contraindications

There are no absolute contraindications; precaution is advised in the following cases:

- Critical respiratory dysfunction
- Severe hemodynamic instability
- Severe deficiency in coagulation
- Concomitant use of mechanical ventilation

Thoracentesis Technique

Patient position could be seated, in lateral decubitus (in case of advanced pregnancy, left lateral decubitus is advised), or supine decubitus with elevation of the head 30° over the horizontal plane if not contraindicated. Monitoring the patient physiological parameters is essential.

In case of pneumothorax, the target site recommended for puncture is on the second intercostal space at the middle-clavicle line over the rib to avoid damage to the subcostal vessels and nerves. Nevertheless, any of the target sites used for liquid evacuation may be appropriate.

In case of liquid evacuation, the target point must be located in the middle-axillar or anterior-axillar line, at the sixth or fifth intercostal space; this last is preferred in case of advanced gravid uterus present or when there is an abnormal elevation of the diaphragm with the increased risk of damage to other abdominal organs. The use of the anterior-axillar line is preferred to avoid muscles like pectoral major or latissimus dorsi; this approach is highly recommended.

The procedure must be made with previous cleaning of the skin with antiseptic solutions, drape of the site, and local anesthesia application to the chest wall. It is important to introduce the anesthetic agent suctioning to avoid any intravascular administration; once you get pleural liquid, apply more anesthesia in the parietal pleura as it will prevent unnecessary pain to the patient.

The introduction of the trocar needle must be made at the intercostal space over the rib to avoid the vascular-nervous intercostal structures located at the inferior border of the rib, keeping suction until liquid is obtained, introduce the catheter through the trocar, remove the trocar, and adapt the catheter to a three-way device for suction of the liquid, which must be collected to laboratory and bacterial tests. Try to do the evacuation slowly and no more than 1500 ml to prevent pulmonary edema post expansion. Fix the catheter to the chest wall with a secured stitch, and finally, adapt the catheter to a collecting recipient with negative pressure or a water seal to a suction system.

The analysis of the liquid must include:

- Cytology
- Cell count and differential
- Hematocrit
- pH, proteins, LDH, amylase, glucose, and lipids
- Gram stain
- Ziehl-Neelsen stain
- Bacterial cultures for Koch bacillus, viruses, and fungi
- Determination of PCR

Complications

- Intense pain
- Air embolus
- Hemothorax
- Lesion to other organs (lung, heart, liver, bowel, diaphragm, nerves, and vascular system)
- Pneumothorax
- Lung rapid expansion syndrome with pulmonary edema
- Persistent cough

The appropriate moment to remove the pleural catheter will be determined also by the characteristics of the liquid drained and the amount produced in a period of 24 hours. If less than 250 milliliters of a clear liquid were drained in that period, it will considered safe to remove the catheter.

To remove the catheter, cut the fixing stitch, and gently ask the patient to breathe deeply to fill the thoracic space with the lungs; keeping in such way the pleural space collapsed is necessary to hold this inspiratory maneuver to remove with a rapid movement the catheter from the pleural cavity; this will prevent a pneumothorax formation. Finally proceed to close the puncture site with a compressive apposite.

In case the patient is unconscious and in mechanical-assisted ventilation, make the procedure of removing the pleural catheter during the inspirational phase using the positive pressure of the ventilator to keep the pleural space collapsed and the lungs expanded.

Appendix

We can't leave without mention a relative recent and useful procedure utilized in the support of hemorrhage control while in an intensive care unit environment. Cardiovascular collapse during hemorrhage is the cause of death unless blood flow is maintained to the heart and brain.

There is a minimal invasive technique using a balloon catheter to temporarily occlude large vessels giving time to an adequate and definitive surgical approach and control. This procedure is called resuscitative endovascular balloon occlusion of the aorta (REBOA). It consists of placing an endovascular balloon in the aorta to control hemorrhage and to augment afterload in traumatic arrest and hemorrhagic shock states such as aortic aneurysm surgery, gastrointestinal bleeding, trauma, and postpartum hemorrhage [9].

In the past, to get this same effect, the aortic cross-clamping was used through thoracotomy or laparotomy, causing more physiological disturbance and higher rates of complications with less rates of technical success than REBOA.

As all invasive procedures, REBOA has indications and contraindications and is performed through a peripheral access in the common femoral artery using Seldinger technique to introduce the balloon catheter using a 12 Fr sheath inserted into the abdominal or thoracic aorta to control noncompressible torso or pelvic hemorrhages.

Like all medical procedures, there are risks associated with the REBOA technique; however, in the setting of severe pelvic hemorrhage, the benefit of traditional control with pelvic packing and/or internal iliac ligation can be augmented by REBOA placing prior to these measurements as abridge to hemostasis. It is a less-invasive procedure and permits earlier intervention prior to cardiovascular collapse, using less blood product transfusions with their inherent risks, and less stress on cardiac function, decreasing secondary brain injury giving more chance to survival.

For this kind of procedure to be used in widespread practice, a better understanding of the potential complications that can arise in all stages must be well recognized [9].

Conclusion

This is a brief guide in the use of some procedures employed frequently in intensive care unit environment with critical patients.

The advent of new technologies like ultrasound and monitoring systems has made these kinds of procedures easier and safer, giving confidence to the operator and reducing the multiple complications expected in all invasive medical techniques.

Despite the benefits of central venous lines to patients and clinicians, more than 15% of patients will have a catheter-related complication [10].

The knowledge of the surface anatomy and its relationship with the deep organs and structures involved in the process is very important to facilitate and keep this standard of safety for the patient.

New techniques and approaches in the management of critical patients are constantly emerging, and we must be open-minded.

References

1. Bannon MP, Heller SF, Rivera M. Anatomic considerations for central venous cannulation for central venous cannulation. Risk Manag Healthc Policy. 2011;4:27–39.
2. Balaji NR, Shah PB. Radial artery catheterization. Circulation. 2011;124:e407–8.
3. Antonelli M, Levy M, Andrews PJ, Chastre J, Houdson LD, Manthous C, et al. Hemodynamic monitoring in shock and implications for management. International consensus conference. Paris, France, 27–28 Apr. 2006. Intensive Care Med. 2007;33:575–90.
4. Liverpool Hospital. Intensive Care Unit (I. C. U.) guideline; arterial lines monitoring and management. [Internet]. Approved by: I. C. U. Medical Director. Publication date: [Cited 2014 Dec.]. Available from: http://www.aci.health.nsw.gov.av.
5. Troianos CA, Jobes DR, Ellison N. Ultrasound guided cannulation of the internal jugular vein. A prospective randomized study. Anesth Analg. 1991;72:823–6.
6. Ridruejo SR, Zalba EB. Pericardiocentesis en una unidad de cuidados intensivos. An Med Interna (Madrid). 2005;22:275–8.
7. Tsang TS, Freeman WK, Sinak LJ, Seward JB. Echocardiographically guided pericardiocentesis: evolution and state-of-the-art technique. Mayo Clinic Proc. 1998;73:647–52.
8. Diaz H. Manual de procedimientos invasivos en medicina intensiva y emergencias. 1a. ed. Olivos: Marketing & Research. 2014. E-Book. [Internet.]. Available from: www.intramed.net.
9. Smith RN, Nolan JP. Central venous catheters. BMJ. 2013;347:f6570.
10. Ribeiro M, Feng C, Nguyeng A, Rodrigues V, Bechara G, et al. The complications associated with Resuscitative Endovascular Balloon Occlusion of the Aorta (REBOA). World J Emerg Surg. 2018;13:20. Available from: https://doi.org/10.1186/513017-018-0181-6

Chapter 16
Extracorporeal Membrane Oxygenation in Pregnancy

Tal E. Sandler and Shaun L. Thompson

Introduction

Since its inception in the 1950s by John Gibbon, extracorporeal membrane oxygenation has improved our ability to facilitate and augment oxygenation, ventilation, and cardiac support in critically ill patients [1]. Technological advancements improved ECMO utilization and are now considered to play a major role in acute respiratory failure, cardiac arrest, and shock states. Additionally, pre-hospital applications have successfully been implemented, to include management of cardiovascular collapse secondary to pulmonary embolism, airway obstruction leading to refractory hypoxemia, overdoses, and hypothermia, to name a few [3]. The combination of ECMO technology and advancements in critical care has allowed for favorable survivability with decrease in morbidity [4]. As access to ECMO services has increased worldwide and with improvements in cannulation methods and equipment, early use has been well defined in the literature. Specialty population whom may benefit from ECMO, such as obstetric patients, have little evidence in regard to overall utilization and favorability [2]. This chapter will focus on describing disease processes in pregnancy and peripartum period that may benefit from ECMO. In addition, considerations regarding pharmacology, physiology, and complications that the pregnant patient may pose while utilizing ECMO will be discussed.

T. E. Sandler · S. L. Thompson (✉)
University of Nebraska Medical Center, Department of Anesthesiology, Division of Critical Care Medicine, Omaha, NE, USA
e-mail: slthomps@unmc.edu

C. Montufar et al. (eds.), *Obstetric Catastrophes*,
https://doi.org/10.1007/978-3-030-70034-8_16

Basics of ECMO

Extracorporeal membrane oxygenation is defined as extravascular cardiopulmonary life support. Blood is drained from the venous system, circulated by a mechanical pump through an oxygenator (also known as membrane lung), and returned back into systemic circulation (venous versus arterial). Oxygenation and carbon dioxide elimination is accomplished through passive diffusion and determined by flow rate and rate of countercurrent flow (sweep), respectively [3]. Depending on the indication for ECMO, there are two types of ECMO that are utilized. First is veno-venous (VV) ECMO, and this is utilized in order to replace lung function in states of refractory respiratory failure. The other variant is veno-arterial (VA) ECMO and is implemented in states of cardiogenic shock or combined cardiopulmonary failure. The nomenclature of VV or VA ECMO indicates which vessels are cannulated in order to drain blood from the patient to the membrane lung and then back into the patient into either the venous (VV) or arterial (VA) system. Indications for VV ECMO include refractory hypoxia and hypercarbia despite maximal medical and ventilator support, status asthmaticus, pneumonia, anterior mediastinal masses, and most commonly acute respiratory distress syndrome [5]. Indications for VA ECMO include cardiac failure following myocardial infarction, acute chronic heart failure, acute heart failure including postpartum cardiomyopathy, pulmonary embolism, amniotic fluid embolism, and refractory ventricular tachycardia [5].

Circuit Design

The ECMO circuit is based on the cardiopulmonary bypass circuit utilized in the operating room for open heart surgical procedures. Large bore cannulas, typically 19–25 French, are placed in either the femoral vein or artery via percutaneous approach. This site is typically chosen due to need for rapid placement and also due to favorable size of vessels to accommodate the large cannula. Other configurations that can be utilized are femoral/internal jugular access for both VV and VA ECMO and use of a dual lumen cannula for VV ECMO which is placed in the internal jugular vein.

Once cannulas are in place, they are attached to large bore polyvinylchloride (PVC) tubing that is typically 3/16 to ½ inch in diameter. Large bore cannulas and tubing are utilized in order to reduce resistance to flow based on the Law of Laplace [5]. This tubing will bring blood to the membrane oxygenator, or membrane lung, via a centrifugal pump. The first half of the membrane lung is utilized for temperature regulation in order to maintain the body temperature at 37° C. The second stage of the membrane lung allows for oxygenation and carbon dioxide removal via passive diffusion as stated above. Figure 16.1 is a cross section of a membrane lung and shows the separation of these two halves.

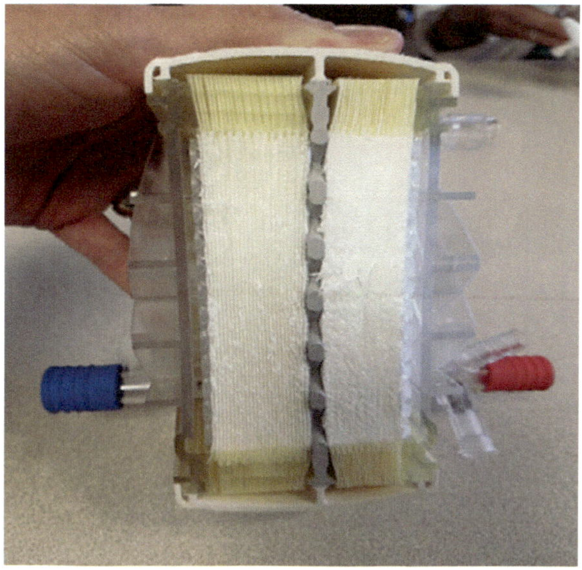

Fig. 16.1 Cross section of the membrane lung. The first half of the membrane lung is utilized for temperature management to maintain normothermia. The second half is where diffusion of gases occurs across concentration gradients. Blood enters the left side of the membrane lung, denoted by the blue plug. Blood exits the membrane lung and back to the patient on the right side, denoted by the red plug. (Image courtesy of Shaun Thompson, MD)

Centers have the ability to customize the ECMO circuit according to the intended patient population. Additional components of modern ECMO circuits include pressure monitors, hemoglobin and oxyhemoglobin saturation monitors, and pump speed monitoring. Circuit bridge/access connectors are available for the ability to conduct lab draws and give the ability to add inline renal replacement therapy [6, 7]. Figure 16.2 shows a photograph of an ECMO circuit in use.

Type of Pumps

Newly designed ECMO circuits utilize centrifugal pumps to provide suction away from the patient and return blood following gas exchange in the membrane lung. Centrifugal pumps have largely replaced previous utilized roller pumps due to their smaller size, durability, and ability to be used for prolonged circulation while avoiding complications such as mechanical hemolysis [6, 7]. The centrifugal pumps used in modern ECMO machines are magnetically levitated and driven which help to reduce mechanical shear forces on red blood cells to minimize damage and hemolysis [8]. Use of magnetically driven pumps also decreases friction and reduces the production of heat [9]. Because of these technical improvements, these pumps have been shown to be safely used for long periods of time allowing extended runs on ECMO if necessary [8, 9].

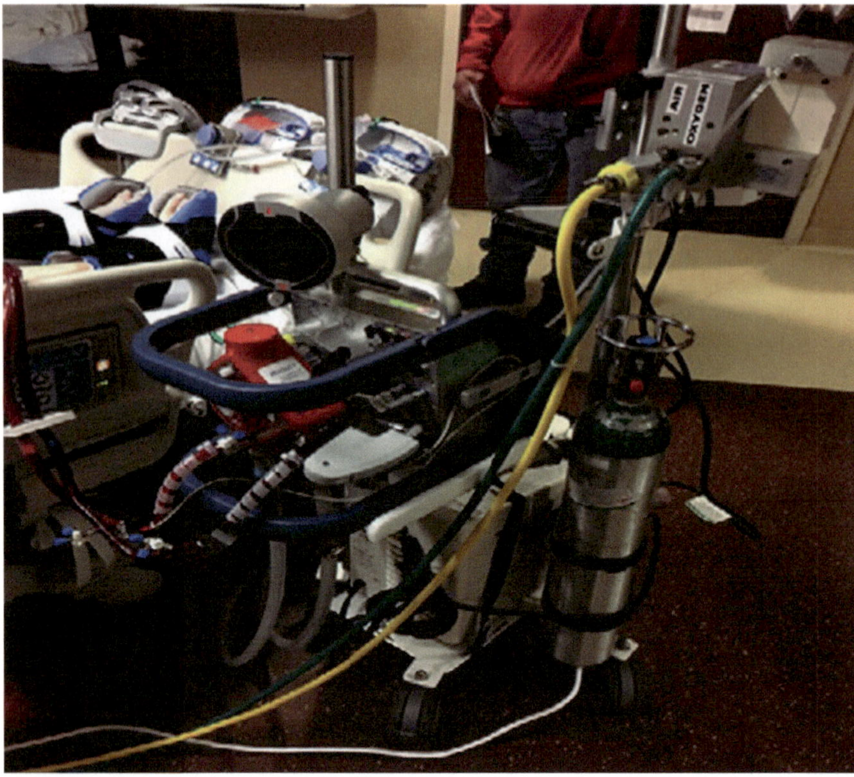

Fig. 16.2 ECMO circuit: components of the ECMO circuit are seen in this photo. The membrane lung is encased in plastic that is red in color in this picture. Drainage and return cannula are marked with blue and red tape, respectively, on the left side of the photo. (Photo courtesy of Dan Johnson, MD and used with permission)

Membrane Oxygenator (Membrane Lung)

As noted, the ECMO circuit provides gas exchange, independent of the patient's lung, through an oxygenator membrane. Through the years, oxygenators were composed of different types of biomaterials including silicone rubber and polypropylene hollow fibers. Newer membranes surfaces are often made from polymethylpentene, polyvinylchloride, or polyurethane which provide efficient gas exchange with low resistance to flow. Polymethylpentene (PMP) membranes are more commonly used currently because of their low resistance to flow, optimal gas exchange with a smaller needed surface area, and minimization of plasma leakage that decreases efficiency of the membrane lung [8]. The surface area of the oxygenator membrane and the path of blood mixing determine the capacity for gas exchange. Ultimately, blood and gas flow occur in counter-current direction allowing for the gas exchange to happen by passive diffusion through the membrane against concentration gradients [6, 7].

Cannulas

Multiple cannulas are available that can be selectively chosen for the individual patient, based on body size, with sizes ranging from 6Fr to 51Fr. In order to avoid luminal occlusion, cannulas are manufactured with wire reinforcements. Fenestrations are added to the flexible tip of jugular and femoral venous drainage cannulas to maximize flow, while return cannulas have either a single port or a short fenestrated tip.

Many cannulas are coated with heparin in order to limit the potential development of thrombus in the cannula. Systemic heparin is also given during cannulation, and these steps are vital to perform as thrombosis of the cannula can be life-threatening and possibly fatal if the patient is completely reliant upon ECMO for survival [5].

It is imperative to properly choose the correct size and configuration to ensure efficient and optimal performance of the circuit [6].

Veno-Venous ECMO

VV ECMO is utilized for respiratory support when cardiac function is preserved. Cannulation can be performed in a few ways and depends on the urgency of the situation at the time of implementation of ECMO. For rapid deployment, percutaneous insertion of cannulas into the femoral veins bilaterally can be performed [5]. Other orientations that can be utilized include a drainage cannula in the femoral vein with a return cannula in the internal jugular vein and dual lumen cannulas which are placed in the internal jugular vein. In all cannulation scenarios, blood is removed via the vena cava and returned to the right atrium [3]. Figure 16.3 shows schematic examples of ECMO cannulation positions for VV ECMO.

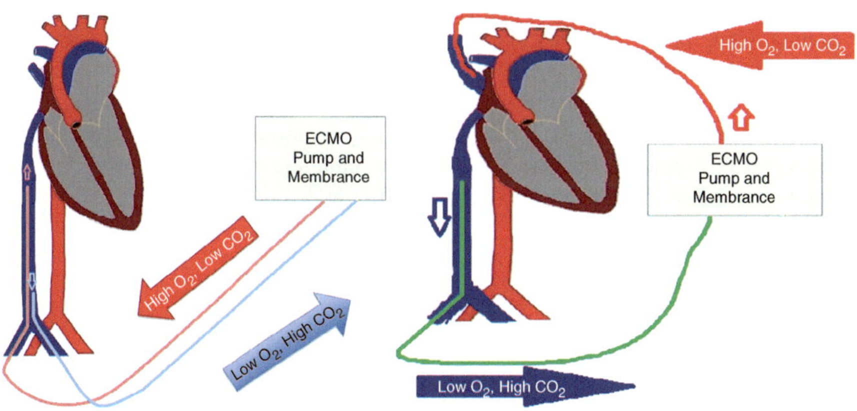

Fig. 16.3 Configurations of veno-venous extracorporeal membrane oxygenation. Drainage cannula is positioned in the distal portion of the IVC with the return cannula positioned in the proximal portion of the IVC close to the right atrium. Another configuration would be if the return cannula was introduced through the internal jugular vein with the cannula terminating in the right atrium (B). (Image courtesy of Walker Thomas, MHPTT, FASE, RDCS and used with permission)

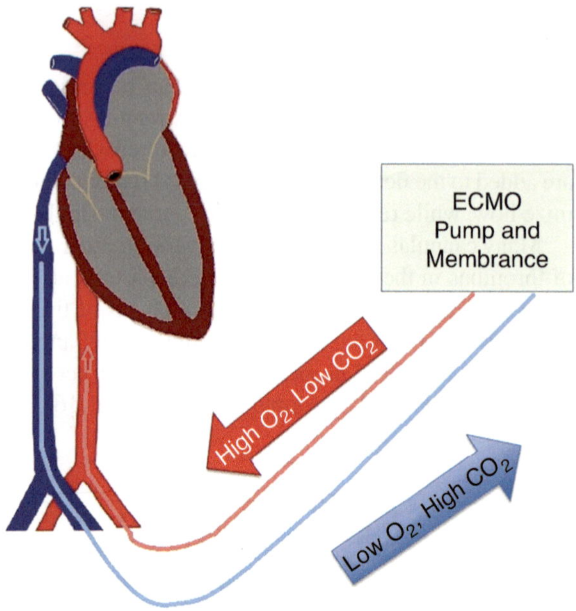

Fig. 16.4 Configuration of veno-arterial extracorporeal membrane oxygenation. Drainage cannula is positioned in the proximal portion of the IVC close to the cavo-atrial junction with the return cannula positioned in the abdominal aorta. (Image courtesy of Walker Thomas, MHPTT, FASE, RDCS and used with permission)

Veno-Arterial ECMO

VA ECMO is utilized in situations of cardiac failure or combined cardiorespiratory failure. The circuit is configured parallel to the heart and lung. Similar to VV ECMO, cannula placement is performed with percutaneous access and advancement of cannulas over guidewires into the respective vessels. Blood is drained from the venous system and returned to the arterial system bypassing the heart and lung. Cannulation strategy includes access of the femoral vein (most common) with return via the femoral, axillary, or carotid arteries [3]. The most common cannulation scenario in adults requiring VA ECMO support is femoral vein/femoral artery access due to the emergent nature that is typically required if this form of support is necessary [5]. Figure 16.4 shows a schematic of cannulation strategy for VA ECMO if the femoral arteries were utilized for cannulation.

Ultrasound Guidance for Cannulation

Echocardiography has been successfully utilized as a tool to aid in cannulation [10–14]. Both transthoracic and transesophageal echocardiography allow for guidewire visualization within the inferior vena cava (IVC) and aorta [10, 11]. This ensures and reduces the chances of extravascular cannula placement [14]. Moreover, cannula position can be verified prior to initiating and also during ECMO support for optimal results [10–14]. Echocardiography of the heart should also occur prior to placement onto ECMO in order to verify or exclude cardiac dysfunction as failure to do so may result in improper implementation of VV ECMO if cardiac failure exists [10–14].

Contraindications to Implementation of ECMO

Absolute contraindications include futility of care in cases where an exit strategy is unlikely such as patients not candidates for durable mechanical support or transplantation. Other examples of contraindications include metastatic cancer, severe brain injury, unrepaired aortic dissection, chronic severe organ dysfunction, and unwitnessed cardiac arrest [5]. Relative contraindications include advance age, severe obesity, severe peripheral vascular disease, morbid obesity, and contraindication for anticoagulation [5]. Multidiscipline consultation with intensivist, cardiologist, cardiac surgeon, and pulmonologist is recommended prior to initiating support [5].

Pregnancy and Peripartum Complications

Acute Respiratory Failure

Pregnancy is associated with multiple physiological and anatomical changes that affect the respiratory system. The parturient experiences decrease in functional residual capacity and an increase in minute ventilation secondary to increase in respiratory rate, leading to overall increase in PaO2 (~105 mmHg) and a lower PaCO2 (~30 mmHg) compared to the nonpregnant state of health. Compensatory metabolic acidosis (HCO3 ~18) occurs in response to the respiratory alkalosis. The overall affect causes a right shift of the hemoglobin-dissociated curve reducing the affinity of maternal hemoglobin to oxygen and enabling transfer of oxygen to the fetus. While these changes are crucial to the survivability of the fetus, they can be deleterious to the parturient as they are predisposed to states of acidosis such as in respiratory failure [15].

Etiology of respiratory failure is similar to the non-obstetric patient; these include reactive airway disease, pulmonary infections, and ARDS secondary to sepsis, trauma, pancreatitis, and multiple blood transfusions [16]. The risk of pulmonary infection is increased in the parturient secondary to changes in immunity. Downregulation of cell-mediated immunity occurs in response to allow tolerance of the paternal-derived fetal antigens predisposing the pregnant woman to increased complications [17]. Viral infections such as the previously reported influenza outbreak in the late 2000s proved that pregnancy is an independent risk factor for respiratory complications such as ARDS. Other pregnancy-related causes of ARDS are illustrated in Table 16.1 [17].

Table 16.1 Disease states in pregnancy that can cause ARDS [2, 16, 20]

Acute respiratory failure cause in the obstetric population
Preeclampsia-induced pulmonary edema
Chorioamnionitis
Acute fatty liver of pregnancy
Obstetric hemorrhage
Tocolytic-induced pulmonary edema
Amniotic fluid embolism
Septic abortion
Retained products of conception
Aspiration

While respiratory failure is uncommon, mortality associated with ARDS is increased compared to the non-obstetric patient (24–39%) [16]. Therefore it is crucial that the clinician has an understanding of the physiological respiratory changes in order to manage these patients appropriately.

Initial management includes identification of cause, maternal supportive care, and fetal monitoring for signs of distress, although conservative management approaches, such as invasive mechanical ventilation, should be utilized promptly, if needed. The 2009 influenza pandemic paved the way for the application of ECMO in refractory hypoxemic states. Multiple case reports have been published in the successful use of ECMO in both pregnant and postpartum patients. Multicentered reports from France, Australia, and New Zealand have described the use of ECMO with favorable survival rate similar to general population [16].

Massive Pulmonary Embolism

The hypercoagulable state of pregnancy increases the risk of thromboembolic complications. It is reported that pulmonary embolism has an incidence of 1 in 3000 and is considered to be the most common cause of maternal mortality in the developing world [18]. Treatment for hemodynamically stable pulmonary embolism has been well described, while that of massive and unstable pulmonary embolism is not well defined in pregnancy. Current guidelines indicate that thrombolytic therapy is a relative contraindication in the obstetric patient but has been described [19]. The use of ECMO is not fully supported given limited evidence. Review of the literature illustrates a limited number of utilizations of ECMO in hemodynamically unstable patients (pregnant and postpartum) with favorable maternal and fetal survivability [20].

Cardiac Arrest

Cardiac arrest is a rare event in pregnancy. The reported incidence is 1 in 12,000 admission for delivery in the United States. Outcomes are dependent on etiology, with a relatively good prognosis as survival rate has been reported up to 58% [21]. Pregnancy is associated with cardiovascular changes as early as 6 weeks, which needs to be well understood in order to manage cardiac arrest. Heart rate increases 20–30% with an associated increase in cardiac output by 30–50%. Plasma volume expansion is noted up to 50% at term. These physiological changes are adaptive to supply oxygen and nutrition to the growing fetus. As the uterus enlarges, aorto-cava compression can occur, decreasing preload, leading to relative hypotension and bradycardia [21].

Management of cardiac arrest differs in the obstetric population. While standard ACLS is implemented, the obstetric team should promote left uterine displacement, remove all fetal monitors, and prepare for emergency caesarean delivery within 4 min of resuscitative efforts if return of spontaneous circulation (ROSC) is not successful [21]. If ROSC is achieved, then the reported survivability is favorable. ECMO utilization as a bridge to recovery has been utilized post ROSC, but data is limited into overall benefit [20].

Cardiomyopathy

Peripartum cardiomyopathy is described as the development of heart failure, of undetermined etiology, during the last month of pregnancy or within 5 months postpartum. Incidence is very low, affecting less than 0.1% of the obstetric population. Risk factors include advanced age, preeclampsia, gestational hypertension, multiparity, substance abuse, and cardiovascular comorbidities [22]. As described in the cardiac arrest section, multiple physiological changes occur during pregnancy that affect the cardiovascular system. The overall increase in intravascular volume and cardiac output causes a transient but reversible left ventricular hypertrophy (LVH) [21, 22]. Although not completely understood, this increase in LVH and inflammation, autoimmune response, and/or genetic predisposition to peripartum cardiomyopathy are believed to be contributing factors. Outcomes can vary, with mortality rates varying from 4% to 80% [22]. While medical treatments include standard heart failure therapy, ECMO has been described in case reports as bridge to recovery versus advance therapies such as assist devices/transplant [22].

ECMO in the Obstetrical Patient

Initiating ECMO support for cardiopulmonary failure in the obstetric patient is rare and uncommon. To date, evidence in the overall benefit and utility of ECMO is based on individual case reports. Comprehensive literature review focusing on ECMO utilization and pregnancy, albeit limited, concludes that ECMO can be relatively safe and effective as a bridge to recovery of the mother with limited adverse consequence to the fetus [23]. Survivability has been reported up to 77% for mothers and 65% for fetuses [23]. Multiple centers are successfully implementing ECMO in this special population with positive results, although research and analysis need to be completed in order to implement pregnancy-related guidelines for ECMO administration.

Cannulation Strategy

Strategy for cannulation should be individualized for each patient. Currently, no defined protocol is described in the literature for the obstetric population. Cannulation in the femoral vessels may prove to be difficult secondary to the gravid uterus [24]. Additionally, flow limitation can occur secondary to aorto-caval compression. The procedure list must take these factors into account when planning the ECMO configuration and cannulation sites. Placing the patient in a slight left lateral decubitus in order to displace the gravid uterus off the inferior vena cava may be of benefit as it will maintain venous return.

Ultrasound and echocardiography have important roles in the cannulation of any patient onto ECMO support. To evaluate the vessels to be cannulated, ultrasound can be performed to estimate size of the vessels in order to verify that the cannulas to be used will be accommodated and are the appropriate size for the vessels to be used for cannulation [10].

Echocardiography can then be employed to verify guidewire placement into the IVC and SVC for VV ECMO and into the IVC and aorta for VA ECMO [10, 11, 14]. Once guidewire placement is verified to be correct, the cannulas can be placed. Appropriate positioning of the cannulas is paramount in order to supply proper support to the patient. For VV and VA ECMO, the multistage drainage cannula should lie in the IVC below the level of the right atrium [10, 11, 25]. Figure 16.5 shows a transthoracic echocardiographic image of a drainage cannula in proper position below the level of the right atrium.

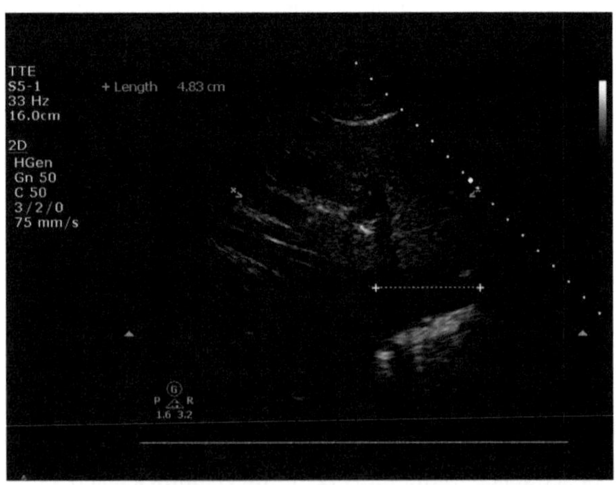

Fig. 16.5 Echocardiographic visualization of cannula/wire: the tip of the cannula shown 4.8 cm from the right atrium in proper position

The return cannula for VV ECMO should terminate at the level of the right atrium with flow directed toward the tricuspid valve [10, 11, 25]. Color Doppler can be used to verify proper flow of both the drainage and return cannula [11, 25]. The return cannula can be difficult to visualize with ultrasound as the tip of the cannula terminates in the distal aorta or proximal iliac artery.

Anticoagulation

Once ECMO has been initiated, anticoagulation needs to be started in order to avoid clot formation in the membrane, circuit, or patient. Given the artificial nature of the cannula, upregulation of the coagulation cascade and immune response occurs once blood contacts the non-endothelialized surface of the circuit [26]. The effect may be compounded secondary to the prothrombotic state of pregnancy. Approaching anticoagulation choice for the obstetric population requires balancing type of anticoagulant and benefit versus risk to the mother and fetus. In non-obstetric patients, unfractionated heparin is the most commonly used anticoagulant given the rapid onset and reversal and ease of monitoring effect [26]. This can be translated to the obstetric population. Unfractionated heparin is noted to be a large molecule that does not cross the placenta [27]. Maternal adverse effects include osteoporosis, if used long term, and heparin-induced thrombocytopenia. Although uncommon, low-molecular-weight heparin, well tolerated in the pregnancy, has been described in case reports as an agent to prevent thrombosis while on ECMO [26, 27]. Both unfractionated heparin and low-molecular-weight heparin can be safely used while breastfeeding [28]. Novel agents, such as direct thrombin inhibitors (argatroban and bivalirudin), have little data available into their safety profile during pregnancy. Case reports have been published with use, without adverse effects [29].

Sedation

While sedation may be required to facilitate cannulation, once ECMO has been initiated, sedation is not essential to tolerate the circuit. If the use of sedation is necessary, choice of sedative requires a balance of benefit versus risk to the mother and fetus, as noted in the anticoagulation section. Recent studies suggest that the use of opioids, hypnotics, anxiolytic, and sedatives does not have deleterious effects on fetal development [22] with the exception of benzodiazepines [30]. Conversely, meta-analysis review shows conflicting results in overall teratogenicity of benzodiazepine; overall consensus suggest to avoid use in the first trimester secondary to the potential cause of cleft lip or palate [30, 31].

Complications

The most common complication related to ECMO utilization is hemorrhage, estimated in 20–33% of patients [26]. One study of pregnant patient and ARDS, during the 2000s N1H1 pandemic, concluded that there is no significant difference in bleeding in pregnant or postpartum patients who require ECMO compared to women of similar age. Another potential concern is the development of thrombi and thromboembolic events given the hypercoagulable state of pregnancy, warranting the use of anticoagulation [32, 33]. Associated complications may occur during cannulation, as noted previously, secondary to the gravid uterus. Late pregnancy may cause aorto-cava compression, affect pre-load and limiting flow, and therefore require more aggressive fluid administration resulting in possible fluid overload [24].

Hypoxemia can still occur in patients requiring VV or VA ECMO and in a pregnant patient can cause serious issues not only for the mother but also for the fetus [20]. Recirculation is a phenomenon unique to VV ECMO and occurs when oxygenated blood returned to the patient is taken back immediately by the drainage cannula prior to entering the patient's circulation [34–36]. This is typically remedied by repositioning the cannulas in order to allow adequate distance between the cannulas [36]. Other things that can increase recirculation include high intrathoracic pressures, intracardiac pressures, or intra-abdominal pressures [34, 36]. If pathology exists that results in these situations, it should be addressed and treated immediately. In the case of pregnancy, the gravid uterus may not allow adequate venous return, so left uterine displacement may be needed in order to allow adequate drainage to allow proper flow to support the patient [20].

Other causes of hypoxemia besides recirculation on VV ECMO include anemia, improper flow settings to meet patient demands, and increased oxygen consumption by the patient not only due to critical illness but also due to the extraction by the fetus [5, 20, 34, 35]. Treatment of this includes increasing flow on the ECMO circuit, blood transfusion to increase oxygen-carrying capacity, deepening of sedation, and possible paralysis. Worst case scenario would be a transition from VV to VA ECMO to provide systemic delivery of oxygenated blood to the patient [5, 20, 34–36].

Hypoxia can occur on VA ECMO as well and is caused when oxygenated blood from the ECMO circuit mixes with deoxygenated coming from the patient's lungs that may not be fully participating in gas exchange [35]. This is known as "North-South syndrome" or "Harlequin syndrome." Treatment of this is typically accomplished by increasing flow on the ECMO circuit in order to move the "mixing zone" between oxygenated blood from the circuit and deoxygenated blood from the patient in the aorta closer to the innominate artery on the right side in order to assure that oxygenated blood is being distributed to all areas [5, 35].

Lastly, equipment failure should be ruled out if hypoxia persists despite optimization of the cannulas and patient parameters. The membrane lung performance can be measured by looking at pre- and post-membrane blood oxygenation [5]. If the pre- and post-membrane oxygenation values are similar, then the membrane lung may need to be replaced.

Despite the aforementioned complications, ECMO can be considered as a safe treatment option for the obstetric population that suffer from respiratory and/or cardiac failure [20].

Conclusion

Rescuc modality for pulmonary or cardiopulmonary failure in the obstetric population is emerging in practice. Multiple case reports have been published in regard to the safe and successful use of ECMO in both pregnancy and the peripartum period. Despite no consensus on guidelines or treatment protocols, centers of excellence who are well versed in ECMO should continue to pave the way in research, thereby promoting ECMO as a practical option for the obstetric population.

References

1. Mosier JM, et al. Extracorporeal membrane oxygenation (ECMO) for critically ill adults in the emergency department: history, current applications, and future directions. Crit Care. 2015;19:431.
2. Pacheco LD, Saade GR, Hankins GDV. Extracorporeal membrane oxygenation (ECMO) during pregnancy and postpartum. Semin Perinatol. 2018;42(1):21–5.
3. Makdisi G, Wang IW. Extra corporeal membrane oxygenation (ECMO) review of a lifesaving technology. J Thorac Dis. 2015;7(7):E166–76.
4. Peek GJ, et al. CESAR: conventional ventilatory support vs extracorporeal membrane oxygenation for severe adult respiratory failure. BMC Health Serv Res. 2006;6:163.
5. Brogan TV, Lorusso R, MacLaren G, Peek G. Extracorporeal life support: the ELSO red book, vol. 5. 1st ed; 2017.
6. Lequier L, et al. Extracorporeal membrane oxygenation circuitry. Pediatr Crit Care Med. 2013;14(5 Suppl 1):S7–12.
7. Van Meurs K, Peek G, Zwischenberger JB. ECMO extracorporeal cardiopulmonary support in critical care, vol. 290. Ann Arbor: Extracorporeal Life Support Organization; 2005.
8. Palanzo D, et al. Evolution of the extracorporeal life support circuitry. Artif Organs. 2010;34(11):869–73.
9. Palanzo DA, et al. Choosing a pump for extracorporeal membrane oxygenation in the USA. Artif Organs. 2014;38(1):1–4.
10. Donker DW, et al. Echocardiography in extracorporeal life support: a key player in procedural guidance, tailoring and monitoring. Perfusion. 2018;33(1_suppl):31–41.
11. Doufle G, et al. Echocardiography for adult patients supported with extracorporeal membrane oxygenation. Crit Care. 2015;19:326.
12. Kapoor PM. Echocardiography in extracorporeal membrane oxygenation. Ann Card Anaesth. 2017;20(Supplement):S1–3.
13. Peris A, et al. Clinical significance of echocardiography in patients supported by venous-venous extracorporeal membrane oxygenation. J Artif Organs. 2015;18(2):99–105.
14. Platts DG, et al. The role of echocardiography in the management of patients supported by extracorporeal membrane oxygenation. J Am Soc Echocardiogr. 2012;25(2):131–41.
15. Mehta N, et al. Respiratory disease in pregnancy. Best Pract Res Clin Obstet Gynaecol. 2015;29(5):598–611.
16. Duarte AG. ARDS in pregnancy. Clin Obstet Gynecol. 2014;57(4):862–70.

17. Lapinsky SE. Acute respiratory failure in pregnancy. Obstet Med. 2015;8(3):126–32.
18. Sultan AA, et al. Risk factors for first venous thromboembolism around pregnancy: a population-based cohort study from the United Kingdom. Blood. 2013;121(19):3953–61.
19. Kearon C, et al. Antithrombotic therapy for VTE disease: antithrombotic therapy and prevention of thrombosis, 9th ed: American College of Chest Physicians Evidence-Based Clinical Practice Guidelines. Chest. 2012;141(2 Suppl):e419S–96S.
20. Sharma NS, et al. Modern use of extracorporeal life support in pregnancy and postpartum. ASAIO J. 2015;61(1):110–4.
21. Kikuchi J, Deering S. Cardiac arrest in pregnancy. Semin Perinatol. 2018;42(1):33–8.
22. Hamdan R, et al. Peripartum cardiomyopathy, place of drug therapy, assist devices, and outcome after left ventricular assistance. J Crit Care. 2017;37:185–8.
23. Moore SA, Dietl CA, Coleman DM. Extracorporeal life support during pregnancy. J Thorac Cardiovasc Surg. 2016;151(4):1154–60.
24. Grasselli G, et al. Use of extracorporeal respiratory support during pregnancy: a case report and literature review. ASAIO J. 2012;58(3):281–4.
25. Frenckner B, Broman M, Broome M. Position of draining venous cannula in extracorporeal membrane oxygenation for respiratory and respiratory/circulatory support in adult patients. Crit Care. 2018;22(1):163.
26. Mulder MMG, Lance MD. ECMO and anticoagulation: a comprehensive review. Neth J Crit Care. 2018;26(1):6–13.
27. Gibson PS, Powrie R. Anticoagulants and pregnancy: when are they safe? Cleve Clin J Med. 2009;76(2):113–27.
28. Bates SM, et al. American Society of Hematology 2018 guidelines for management of venous thromboembolism: venous thromboembolism in the context of pregnancy. Blood Adv. 2018;2(22):3317–59.
29. Young SK, et al. Successful use of argatroban during the third trimester of pregnancy: case report and review of the literature. Pharmacotherapy. 2008;28(12):1531–6.
30. Walton NKD. Anaesthesia for non-obstetric surgery during pregnancy. Contin Educ Anaesth Crit Care Pain. 2006;6:83–5.
31. Neuman G. Safety of procedural sedation in pregnancy. J Obstet Gynaecol Can. 2013;35(2):168–73.
32. Alshawabkeh L, Economy KE, Valente AM. Anticoagulation during pregnancy: evolving strategies with a focus on mechanical valves. J Am Coll Cardiol. 2016;68(16):1804–13.
33. Saad AF, et al. Extracorporeal membrane oxygenation in pregnant and postpartum women with H1N1-related acute respiratory distress syndrome: a systematic review and meta-analysis. Obstet Gynecol. 2016;127(2):241–7.
34. Abrams D, Bacchetta M, Brodie D. Recirculation in venovenous extracorporeal membrane oxygenation. ASAIO J. 2015;61(2):115–21.
35. Alexis-Ruiz A, et al. Hypoxia and complications of oxygenation in extracorporeal membrane oxygenation. J Cardiothorac Vasc Anesth. 2019;33(5):1375–81.
36. Montisci A, et al. Management of refractory hypoxemia during venovenous extracorporeal membrane oxygenation for ARDS. ASAIO J. 2015;61(3):227–36.

Chapter 17
Nutrition in the Critically Ill Obstetric Patient

Alfredo A. Matos and Kirenia Petterson

Physiological Changes of the Pregnant Woman

Pregnancy generates important physiological and anatomical changes, which involve the cardiovascular, respiratory, hematological, renal, gastrointestinal, and endocrine systems, which are also related to the nutritional aspect (Table 17.1) [1–5]. All these changes are necessary to allow the adaptation and survival of the mother and the fetus until the moment of delivery, including the puerperium and lactation. In addition to these changes, there is an increase in physical (body composition) and metabolic demands (increase in caloric requirement), which warrants a rigorous follow-up during the different stages of pregnancy [6]; the follow-up and monitoring becomes a challenge, since the physical and biochemical variables change constantly. Therefore, knowledge of the variants occurring during pregnancy is essential to be able to interpret the clinical findings in an individualized manner and to define in a timely manner pathophysiological conditions that lead the patient to a critical condition that endangers the life of both the mother and the fetus [5, 6].

A. A. Matos (✉)
Enteral and Parenteral Nutrition, Head of Surgery Intensive Care Unit, Hospital Social Security Complex, Panama City, Republic of Panama

K. Petterson
Nutritionist and Dietitian, Enteral Therapy and Parenteral Nutrition, Intensive Care Unit, Hospital Social Security Complex, Panama City, Republic of Panama

C. Montufar et al. (eds.), *Obstetric Catastrophes*,
https://doi.org/10.1007/978-3-030-70034-8_17

Table 17.1 Changes in pregnancy related to nutrition

Cardiovascular	Hematological	Renal	Gastrointestinal	Body composition	Metabolic
Increased cardiac output (50%)	Increase in coagulation factors	Increase in renal blood flow (50%)	Hypomotility	Weight gain (fetus, placenta, uterus, breasts, and extracellular fluids)	Increase in oxygen consumption
Increase of heart rate (20%)	Increase on red blood cell	Increase of glomerular filtration (50%)	Decreased gastric emptying	Increase in fat reserves	Increase in metabolic rate/ increase in caloric requirements
Decrease in systemic vascular resistance (20%)	Dilution anemia	Increased clearance of creatinine, glucose, urea, and protein	Gastroesophageal reflux	Increase in total body water (6–9 L)	Alterations in insulin sensitivity
			Constipation		Increase in leptin concentrations

Body Composition

Physiological and metabolic changes lead to gestational weight gain, which involves an increase in maternal and fetal body mass, as well as placental tissue growth, and increased amniotic fluid and blood volume [7, 8].

Although there are many methods and tools to perform the evaluation of body composition, many of these are not applicable in pregnancy, and it is necessary to make adjustments in some cases to be able to use them. Regardless of the usefulness of the methods and tools, pre-pregnancy weight and control of weight gain are recognized as important factors in the prevention of risks during pregnancy and in adequate fetal development [4, 7, 9].

Gestational Weight Gain (GWG)

GWG is a complex biological process and is influenced not only by the maternal metabolism and physiological changes of pregnancy but also by placental metabolism. The placenta functions as an endocrine organ, also as a barrier and as a transporter of substances between the mother and the fetus. Therefore, the placenta plays a preponderant role, not only in the transport of nutrients to the fetus but also in the maintenance of homeostasis, through the secretion of hormones [4].

As pregnancy progresses, water, minerals, proteins, and fats are deposited in the fetus, placenta, and amniotic fluid, representing 35% of the GWG. The development of uterus and breast tissue, as well as extracellular fluid, blood, and adipose tissues, contributes to the maternal component and represents approximately 65% of GWG [8].

Excessive weight gain during pregnancy has been associated with an increase in complications such as gestational diabetes, preeclampsia, and eclampsia among others, and, on the other hand, a below-expected increase has been linked to increased perinatal morbidity [10].

Due to the increasing population of women who become pregnant with overweight and obesity at conception, the Institute of Medicine (IM) published in 2009 the reference guidelines for weight gain in pregnancy according to the body mass index (BMI) pregestational which was used to ensure adequate weight gain and prevent the mentioned complications [7] (Table 17.2).

The fat-free mass and the fat mass, considered important in the nutritional evaluation, are measured by different techniques with a certain degree of difficulty in the pregnant woman, which will be detailed later.

The fat-free mass (proteins) accumulates mainly in the fetus (42%), uterus (17%), blood, placenta, and mammary glands, while the fat mass accumulates in greater quantity in the fetus.

Evaluation of Body Composition

In the critically ill pregnant, it may be even more difficult to evaluate the body composition, so it is necessary to study the likely alternatives that bring us closer to a clearer diagnosis.

The measurement of skinfold thickness provides an estimate of subcutaneous fat deposits. The sum of the folds in different anatomical points serves to estimate total

Table 17.2 Weight gain according to pregestational IMC

Category	IMC pregestational	Total weight gain range		Weekly weight gain in the second and third trimester per week		Total weight gain in twin pregnancy	
		Lbs	Kg	Lbs	Kg	Lbs	Kg
Underweight	<18.5	28–40	12.7–18.2	1 (1–1.3)	0.7	–	–
Normal weight	18.5–24.9	25–35	11.2–15.9	1 (0.8–1)	0.5	37–54	16.8–24.4
Overweight	25–29.9	15–25	6.8–11.3	0.6 (0.5–0.7)	0.3	31–50	14.1–22.7
Obese	<39	11–20	4.5–9.0	0.5 (0.4–0.6)	0.25	25–42	11.3–19.1

subcutaneous fat. It is considered a safe, practical, and easy method; however, it requires training and experience from the evaluator to achieve precise measurements. A stretch of the skin occurs in the pregnant woman, which can interfere with the proper measurement. According to the studies of Taggart et al., there are changes in the thickness of the skinfolds (suprailiac, scapular, costal, bicipital, knee, and thigh) between week 10 and 30 of gestation. They also found that the crease of the thigh presented minor changes, only until weeks 30–38, in relation to the other anatomical sites. A greater amount of subcutaneous fat was also found in the uniparous mothers than in the multiparous [11]. Similar observations were reported by Pipe et al.; they used the sum of four anatomical sites (triceps, biceps, subscapular, suprailiac); fold increases were observed until weeks 36–38 due to increased fat gains in the suprailiac fold area [12].

In general, the anthropometric measures in critically ill patients are not useful, due to the lack of precision generated by the presence of edema, bed rest, and difficulty in performing the measurement among other limiting factors [13].

Bioimpedance, which is also considered a safe method, is based on the conductivity of electric current that is determined by the amount of water contained in the biological tissue. Tissues with high water content (muscle) are more conductive than tissue with less water content (bone, fat). Therefore, the volume of conductive tissue can be calculated from the resistance of the electrical signal throughout the body. An estimate of total body water is also allowed [14, 15]. Taking into account that in pregnant women the volume of liquid increases, and that it depends largely on the hydration states, which is very variable, this method can be unreliable to estimate the content of fat-free mass and fat mass.

According to the most recent 2016 guidelines from the American Society for Parenteral and Enteral Nutrition (ASPEN) [13], more objective imaging methods should be used to evaluate the body composition and nutritional status of critical patients such as computed axial tomography (CAT), magnetic resonance, and ultrasound, among others, recognizing that some are not very available.

Some studies have been done using magnetic resonance imaging to assess body composition. These investigations consider that magnetic resonance is highly promising with respect to body composition analysis in pregnant women, and it will be essential to advance in the understanding of changes in fat distribution, especially the accumulation of abdominal fat [16, 17]. However, MRI also presents certain limitations, among them the cost and, on the other hand, the discomfort of the reduced physical space and the positions that must be adopted during the study.

Ultrasound can be used not only to assess fetal growth but also to evaluate subcutaneous and visceral fat. It has been correlated with the measurements obtained from skinfolds, to evaluate subcutaneous fat with the advantage of eliminating the error generated by skin tightening [18]. In relation to visceral fat, it has been validated with CAT measurements and has been correlated with risk factors and metabolic effects [19]. Ultrasound images of adipose tissue thickness are limited to a single body area and are not the reflection of total body fat; therefore, further studies will be necessary to make more accurate estimates. Other studies in critically ill patients profile ultrasound as a useful tool for identifying the decrease in muscle thickness at different anatomical points, within which the most used is the rectum femoral muscle; however, at the moment there is no standardized technique, but it allows us to identify progressive changes in muscle wear and to follow up with periodic measurements in the same patient without generating higher costs and risks [20–22]. In the obstetric critical patient, it could also become an indicator of muscle catabolism and monitoring of nutritional therapy.

Nutritional Requirements During Pregnancy

Calories

Given this new situation, women need a greater calorie intake in the different stages since there is an overload in the functioning of some organs and maternal systems throughout pregnancy. This increase in caloric requirements will change depending on the gestation trimester in which it is found and the previous nutritional status, avoiding both excessive and low weight gain, since both situations can alter the development of pregnancy. From the hormonal point of view, two well-defined phases are presented: the phase of anabolism during the first half of pregnancy where there is a greater influx of progesterone and aldosterone and the catabolism phase, during the second half of pregnancy, where the placental lactogen, cortisol, estrogen, and deoxycorticosterone have their effect on the pregnant woman. During the phase of anabolism, there will be an increase in maternal weight due to the formation of greater deposits of fat, minerals, proteins, and fluids. In the catabolism phase there is a greater placental growth and an increase in the use of proteins and stored energy in the form of glycogen and fat that will be delivered to the growing embryo through the placenta, with different types of transport, in simpler ways (free fatty acids, glucose, and amino acids) [23]. Leptin also appears to be a determining factor in the metabolic adaptations of pregnancy. Maternal leptin concentrations increase in week 12 of pregnancy and have a significant positive correlation with maternal body fat (increased fat oxidation), changes in insulin sensitivity during pregnancy, and an increase in basal metabolic rate.

The energy recommendations for the pregnant woman are based on the resting metabolic rate (RMR), the thermal effect of the food, the physical activity, plus an additional caloric intake necessary for the formation of maternal tissues and fetal growth during pregnancy.

According to the recommended dietary intake (RDI), it is suggested that every pregnant woman consume the energy requirement at rest calculated by the Harris-Benedict formula, plus an extra intake of 340 calories during the second trimester and 452 calories during the third trimester [24]. The new European Guidelines for Nutritional Medical Therapy in Critical Patients recommend indirect calorimetry as the best method for calculating energy requirements [25]. It would also be the best method for the critical pregnant patient.

According to the recommendations of the American Dietetic Association (ADA), during the first trimester of pregnancy, it is not recommended to increase the energy supply unless the woman is underweight prior to pregnancy [26].

For women who are overweight and obese prior to pregnancy, the caloric intake should not be increased during the first trimester. The current energy patterns of the Institute of Medicine suggest an increase of 450 kcal/day and an additional 350 kcal/day during the second and third quarters, respectively [24]. There is considerable individual variability; therefore, the best assessment of adequate energy intake is the monitoring of gestational weight gain and fetal growth [4]

Proteins

Amino acids are necessary for tissue production (maternal and fetal), expansion of maternal blood volume, and fluid balance. They are fundamental for the development of organs and synthesis of enzymes; its deficiency can affect fetal growth and cause damage to DNA and RNA, as well as affect enzymatic processes [4, 8, 9].

It is recommended that every pregnant woman increase her protein intake, since it has been estimated that in the second and third trimester about 21 g of proteins are deposited daily in maternal, fetal, and placental tissues. During pregnancy, the woman synthesizes from 925 to 950 g of proteins for the replacement and elimination of proteins in the fetus uterus, mammary glands, skeletal muscle, as well as for the growth of the fetus [9].

The current literature suggests a daily minimum of proteins during pregnancy of approximately 1 g/kg to meet maternal and fetal demands [4]. According to the RDI, the protein requirement for healthy pregnant women is 71 g per day, without making any differences in age and weight nor establish extra contributions during the different trimesters or weeks of pregnancy [24].

In the critically ill patient, an increase in protein catabolism has been identified, measured by negative nitrogen balances and by progressive decrease in muscle mass, depending on the degree of inflammation generated by the pathophysiological condition [26].

As already mentioned, during the second half of pregnancy occurs a catabolic phase with a flow of nutrients to the placenta and the fetus. This condition, expected in pregnancy, which involves increasing protein calorie intake, suggests that in critical conditions the protein intake could be even higher than in a healthy pregnant woman.

The guidelines of the American Society for Parenteral and Enteral Nutrition (ASPEN) and the European Society of Parenteral and Enteral Nutrition (ESPEN) on critical patient nutrition do not define the contribution of proteins for the critical obstetric patient specifically [13, 25]. These guidelines, in general, suggest for the critical patient a protein contribution between 1.2 and 2.0 g/kg/day and, under more specific conditions such as kidney disease on dialysis or obesity (BMI >40), can increase up to 2.5 g/kg/day considering that the hypercatabolic state increases the protein demands; however, it is not well defined if this amount is adequate for a pregnant woman, since as we have mentioned there is a progressive weight gain and the calculation of proteins using these recommendations could be excessive if it was done according to the current weight at any stage of pregnancy.

Carbohydrates

The intake of carbohydrates will depend, among other things, on serum glucose levels and therapeutic goals. The metabolism of carbohydrates should be monitored closely, since during pregnancy there is a significant risk of developing insulin resistance due to hormonal factors; on the other hand, a low intake of carbohydrates could cause ketosis [26].

The RDI for carbohydrates is 175 g per day and 28 g of fiber per day [24]. It suggests a carbohydrate intake between 55% and 65% of the estimated calories, and in case of gestational diabetes, a distribution between 40% and 45% is considered adequate [27].

Fat

The Institute of Medicine recommends 20–35% of calories from fat. For the type of fat, emphasis is placed on the sources of essential fatty acids linoleic and α-linolenic acid, as well as on choline [7]. The amounts of essential fatty acids available to the fetus depend on the maternal diet and must include 13 g/day of omega-6 fatty acids and 1.4 g/day of omega-3 fatty acids.

It has been theorized that optimum inflammatory and thrombotic homeostatic states result from a balance between omega-3 and omega-6, with ideal diets that have an omega-6/omega-3 ratio of 1–2:1. A deficiency in omega-3 results in a prothrombotic and proinflammatory state that has been associated with an increased risk of cardiovascular and inflammatory diseases [28].

An in vitro test of single pregnancies and twins showed that the concentration of docosahexaenoic acid (DHA) in the membrane of fetal erythrocytes was directly related to maternal concentration and that a lower concentration of omega-3 was associated with an increase in rigidity of the membrane and an increase in the resistance to flow. In this study, the average concentration of DHA in erythrocytes was significantly lower in twin pregnancies, which led the authors to conclude that the fetal demand of DHA in multiple pregnancies cannot be satisfied with the typical dietary intake [29].

The World Health Organization advises the administration of marine oil supplements during pregnancy, which has been evaluated as a possible method to prevent prematurity and eclampsia and also to increase birth weight. And it currently recommends 300–500 mg per day of omega-3 (such as DHA and eicosapentaenoic acid) in an effort to promote fetal mental development and early childhood.

Lipids are an important component of TPN in the pregnant patient for the following reasons:

1. They are an excellent energy source.
2. Essential fatty acids are used for fetal fat deposition, brain development, myelination, and pulmonary surfactant synthesis.
3. The metabolism of fatty acids requires less oxygen and produces less carbon dioxide than glucose metabolism.
4. Most of the solutions available on the market are a suspension of chylomicrons of precursors of arachidonic acid and essential fatty acids in a base of safflower or soybean oil. Emulsions are available in concentrations of 10% and 20%. The infusion is usually limited to 12 h per day, because chylomicrons can remain in

maternal circulation up to 8–10 h. After administration Critically ill patient nutritional requirements fat and due to concern about possible bacterial contamination from emulsion to perfusion, the "waiting time" is prolonged. Since the placenta transport of fatty acids are mainly by passive diffusion, a high maternal fetal concentration gradient is necessary to ensure adequate lipid transfer. Deficiency of essential fatty acids usually requires 4 weeks or more of nutritional depletion to develop clinically. Hypertriglyceridemia and ketosis are important complications of lipid use that must be sought and corrected. Initial concerns about premature delivery and placental infraction of fat embolism have not materialized with concentrations commonly used for TPN (i.e., 30–40% of total calorie requirements).

Micronutrients

Micronutrients, trace elements and vitamins, have numerous functions that they usually exert in combination: they are essential for the metabolism of carbohydrates, proteins, and lipids, for immunity and antioxidant defense, for endocrine function, and for DNA synthesis, gene repair, and signaling cells.

Oxidative stress, defined as an imbalance between the increase of reactive oxygen and nitrogen species and endogenous antioxidant mechanisms, is observed in severe critical care conditions that require mechanical ventilation, such as septic shock, severe pancreatitis, ARDS, and traumas: this is associated with damage to proteins and cell membrane lipids. The levels of antioxidant micronutrients, such as vitamins C and E and minerals such as zinc, copper, and selenium, under conditions of metabolic stress decrease below the reference ranges [27].

The requirements of micronutrients in pregnant women are also increased, especially those that have a participation in the development of the neural tube of the fetus, the synthesis of new tissues, DNA, and RNA.

The ASPEN and ESPEN guidelines also do not mention the contribution of micronutrients in critically ill obstetric patient. They provide a micronutrient contribution according to the daily intake recommendations. These recommendations for the pregnant woman can be found in Table 17.3.

Malnutrition

The prevalence of malnutrition in critically ill patients ranges from 38% to 78%. Malnutrition worsens clinical outcomes and has a negative impact on the recovery of the disease, which is why the high prevalence of malnourished patients is so worrisome [30]. Figures range from 65% to 75% [31, 32] according to recent studies.

Malnutrition is an independent risk factor for nosocomial infections in hospitalized patients, so the management of malnutrition from admission can theoretically help to prevent infections associated with health care. Evidence also shows that pre-existing malnutrition influences post-discharge outcomes, including mortality

Table 17.3 Recommended daily ingestion of micronutrients in the pregnant

Micronutrients	Requirements	Functions
Folate	600 mcg por día	Neural tube formation
Pyridoxine (B6)	1.9 mg por día	Coenzyme for maternal energy metabolism
Cobalamine (B12)	2.6 mcg per day	Metabolism of maternal folate, tissue synthesis, DNA, and RNA
Vitamin A	770 mcg per day	Cell differentiation and tissue development of the fetus
Calcium	1000 mg (19–50 years)1300 mg (14–18 years)	Bone mineralization of the fetus
Iron	27 mg per day	Synthesis of hemoglobin, expansion of maternal blood volume
Zinc	11 mg/day (19–50 years)12 mg/day (14–18 years)	DNA synthesis and enzyme cofactor
Potassium	4.7 g/day	Transmission of nerve impulses. Greater intracellular cation
Sodium	1.5 g/day	Transmission of nerve impulses. Greater extracellular cation

and re-entry rates. Early recognition of malnutrition, nutritional intervention, and monitoring of compliance with protein calorie targets can reduce complications, length of hospital stay, and re-entry rates, while reducing the overall cost of care [33].

The prevalence of malnutrition in the critical obstetric patient is still unknown, but we presume that the hypermetabolism and hypercatabolism characteristic of the critical illness added to the increase in the caloric and protein needs of pregnancy and to the barriers that limit the adequate contribution of the nutritional therapy in a critically ill patient, leading to an increased risk of malnutrition in the pregnant woman and therefore at increased risk of complications related to it, which will affect not only the mother but also the fetus.

Hemodynamic Instability

Circulatory shock is defined as a lack of adequate tissue perfusion that would allow appropriate nutrient and oxygen supply to the tissue beds to maintain homeostatic cellular functional mechanisms. Several mechanisms lead to circulatory shock, and understanding the cause and subsequent consequences of circulatory shock is important to determine which treatment modalities are needed to counter the negative sequelae of circulatory shock. Some of these treatment modalities are specific to the cause of the shock state, whereas others, such as nutrition, are universal. Controversy surrounding the appropriate form and timing of nutrition support of the patient with circulatory shock continues. Clinical studies have demonstrated improvements in outcomes related to the administration of enteral nutrition to critically ill patients; however, in patients with ongoing circulatory shock, the timing of enteral nutrition is of concern based primarily on several anecdotal reports in the literature of complications stemming from feeding the gut.

The question is whether patients with low flow states have altered intestinal perfusion

That leads to limited nutrient absorption efficiency and whether this increases the risks related to enteral feeds.

One of the complications of pregnancy is the patient with obstetric hemorrhage of multiple causes that can carry out a hemodynamic instability or patients with septic shock. Any pathological alteration that carries out a hemodynamic instability is also considered [34, 35].

The intestinal mucosa has three pathophysiological mechanisms that make it highly susceptible to hypoperfusion during states of shock [36]. The first is the countercurrent mechanism, the mechanism that allows the absorption of nutrients, but a short circuit occurs between the arterial branch that carries oxygen to the villus and the venous branch that extracts carbon dioxide from the villus. A shunt occurs, and the oxygen progressively crosses from the arterial side to the venous side, reaching little oxygen to the tip of the villus, but it is sufficient for the epithelial cells of the tip of the villus to survive. However, in shock situations, the shunt is higher, and the amount of oxygen that reaches the tip of the villus is much lower and leads to cellular apoptosis of the tip of the villus. The second mechanism is that the arterial vessels leave at 90° angle toward the villus; in states of shock the red blood cells, because of the hyperdynamic state, are few that they turn 90° to enter to the villus carrying oxygen. The third mechanism is that there is a contraction of the arterial precapillary sphincters during shock by the action of the sympathetic system and all this favors ischemia in the villi and intestinal mucosa during shock states, which would worsen if the patient received complete nutrition in shock leading to non-occlusive intestinal ischemia [37].

During circulatory shock, there is a redistribution of blood flow attributable to factors that cause vasoconstriction or vasodilation. In cases of hypovolemia, where the effective circulating blood volume is reduced, vasoconstriction causes a reduction of blood flow from the skin, skeletal muscles, and the gut. Severe hepatosplanchnic vasoconstriction can occur, even before systemic abnormalities are noticed. There is intense vasoconstriction of the superior mesenteric artery in this case, which may represent disordered auto regulation because it occurs despite normal systemic blood pressures. GI ischemia usually only occurs when the flow is reduced to <50% from basal values. With hepatosplanchnic vasoconstriction, blood flow is unevenly distributed. The small intestine is at a higher risk than the colon because of a countercurrent exchange mechanism at the base of the villi.

Another aspect that should be considered is the effect and dose of vasopressor that the pregnant patient is receiving, regardless of the cause of the shock [38].

Table 17.4 shows the different effects on blood flow to the intestinal mucosa and Table 17.5 shows that dose of vasopressor contraindicates enteral and parenteral nutrition.

Table 17.4 Vasopressor agents and splanchnic perfusion

Agent	Effect
Norepinephrine	In septic shock: increases gastric pHi, increases splanchnic perfusion Hypovolemia: decreases mucosal blood flow
Epinephrine	Decreases splanchnic blood flow
Vasopressin	In sepsis: with severe hypotension, increases arterial pressure (causes intestinal vasoconstriction, may cause severe gastric mucosal acidosis) Enhances pressor response to catecholamines
Dopamine	In septic shock: decreases gastric pHi, increases oxygen delivery. Causes precapillary vasoconstriction with diversion of blood flow away from gut mucosa
Dobutamine	Increases GI mucosal blood flow Increases gastric pHi

pHi intramucosal pH, *GI* gastrointestinal

Table 17.5 Candidates for enteral nutrition

Yes Enteral nutrition	Patients should be considered for EN with monitoring of GI tolerance if hemodynamically stable on: Norepinephrine 5 mcg/min or less, and/or Epinephrine 5 mcg/min or less, and/or Vasopressin 0.04 units/min or less, and/or Dopamine 10 mcg/Kg/min or less, and/or Milrinone 0.375 mcg/Kg/min Thorough assessment completed of premorbid medical conditions and nutritional history
No Enteral nutrition	Any hemodynamically unstable patient Those with active bleeding requiring ongoing transfusions A mean arterial blood pressure consistently <60 mmHg An increasing requirement for vasoactive agents Those requiring massive fluid resuscitation A low flow state as a result of cardiac pump failure Known critical stenosis in the mesenteric vasculature Patients on: Norepinephrine >5 mcg/min Epinephrine >5 mcg/min Vasopressin >0.04 Units/min Dopamine >10 mcg/kg/min Milrinone >0.375 mcg/kg/min

Preeclampsia – Eclampsia

Hypertensive disorders during pregnancy, according to the WHO [39], are an important cause of severe morbidity, long-term disability, and increased mortality among mothers and their babies. The majority of deaths due to preeclampsia and eclampsia are preventable through the provision of timely information. Preeclampsia is defined as the onset of hypertension and proteinuria after the 20th week of pregnancy. It is usually accompanied by edema, but it is not necessary for them to be diagnosed. It is a characteristic disease characteristic of pregnancy from which symptoms can be treated, but it is only cured with the completion of it and if not properly treated it can cause serious complications for both the pregnant woman and the fetus [40]. In the pregnant, it can be complicated evolving to an eclampsia, or it can manifest itself with the severe syndrome of HELLP syndrome, but also in the form of cerebral hemorrhages, acute pulmonary edema, renal failure, CID, etc. which explain that it is one of the four major causes of maternal mortality even in developed countries.

Current thinking about preeclampsia characterizes the reduction in perfusion as stage 1 of preeclampsia, which is proposed to be a two-stage disease. Stage 2 is the maternal syndrome. Although recognized by hypertension and proteinuria, preeclampsia is much more than these two changes. A predominant pathophysiological feature is reduced perfusion of virtually all organs that is due to vasoconstriction, microthrombi formation, and reduced circulating plasma volume. The vasoconstriction is secondary to an increased sensitivity of the vasculature to any pressor agent. Activation of the coagulation cascade produces microthrombi. The reduced plasma volume, reflecting an endothelial leak with fluid loss from the intravascular compartment, further compromises perfusion. These abnormalities precede clinically evident disease by weeks to months and have led to the suggestion that a primary target in preeclampsia is the vascular endothelium. This hypothesis has been extensively supported by both old and new data [41–43].

Abundant data from the past 10 years not only indicate endothelial dysfunction in preeclampsia but also demonstrate that alterations in function antedate clinically evident preeclampsia. This supports the concept that endothelial dysfunction may be causally important in the disorder.

Nitric oxide is a potent endothelium-derived vasodilator [44], and defective synthesis of nitric oxide has been documented in preeclampsia [45]. The main site of production of nitric oxide is nitric oxide synthase in endothelial cells, which uses circulating L-arginine as a substrate. Hence, the local availability of this amino acid may be critical to the endothelial adaptive regulatory mechanisms opposing the vasoconstrictors in preeclampsia. L-arginine is considered to be a semi essential amino acid because under increased demands endogenous synthesis is not sufficient to fulfill requirements. Moreover, pregnancy has been reported to be a state of relative arginine deficiency [46], imposed by the increased formation of nitric oxide, supporting the adaptive vasodilatation of pregnancy, and use of L-arginine by the fetus. Preeclampsia is also associated with increased concentrations of factors that inhibit nitric oxide production. Concentrations of asymmetric dimethyl arginine, a competitive inhibitor of nitric oxide synthase, are raised in women with preeclampsia.

Concentrations of soluble fms-like tyrosine kinase 1, which antagonizes vascular endothelial growth factor dependent activation of nitric oxide synthase, have also been shown to be increased in preeclampsia [47]. Endoglin, which impairs activation of nitric oxide synthase mediated by transforming growth factor-β, is also increased [48].

Vadillo-Ortega et al. [49] conducted a prospective double-blind, placebo-controlled study. They included 228 women with 14–32 weeks of pregnancy with preeclampsia who received arginine + antioxidant vitamins every day (Arg: 6.6 g + Vit C 500 mg + Vit E 400 UI + Folate 400 μg). 222 pregnant patients to the placebo group. Finding that the study group had a lower incidence of preeclampsia. Other studies have found the same findings [50–52].

Ways for Nutrition Therapy

The recommendation is that patients should be fed orally, and if this is not possible, the enteral route should be used through a tube to the stomach or intestine. If the intestine cannot be used, then resort to the parenteral route (TPN) [25].

The critical obstetric patient can rarely receive food orally. The majority of these patients require an enteral or parenteral route. The enteral route has sufficient advantages over the parenteral route (Table 17.6) [53]); however, there are critical pregnant patients who cannot receive enteral nutrition and must receive parenteral nutrition (TPN). (Table 17.7). As an example; in case of being a patient weighting 70 kg the calculation of the NPT that the patient requires is shown Table 17.8.

Table 17.6 Advantages of enteral nutrition on the parenteral

Always first choice
More physiological
Preservation of mucosal architecture
Preservation of gut-associated lymphoid tissue (GALT)
Preservation of hepatic immune function
Preservation of pulmonary immune function
Reduction of inflammation
Reduction of antigenic leak from gut
Interference with pathogenicity of gut organisms
Less hyperglycemia
Requires less trained personnel
Less infections
Less expensive

Table 17.7 Indications of parenteral nutrition critic pregnant patient

Non-functional gastrointestinal tract
Impossible to access the digestive tract
Inability to use the gastrointestinal tract
Intestinal obstruction
Peritonitis
Intractable vomiting
Severe diarrhea
High-output enterocutaneous fistula
Severe malabsorption
Maternal malnutrition
Weight loss >1 Kg/week for 4 weeks consecutively
Total weight loss of 6 Kg or failure to gain weight

Table 17.8 Calculation of NPT (volume and calories) for pregnant patient moderately critical catabolic – 70 Kg weight

1. Protein: 1.5 g/Kg = 1.5 × 70 = 105 g/day Using 10% amino acids (10 g/100cc) = 1050cc
2. Carbohydrates: 6.0 g/Kg = 6 × 70 = 420 g/day Using Dextrose 50%(50 g/100cc) = 840cc
3. Lipids: 0.8 g/Kg = 0.8 × 70 = 56 g/day Using SMOF Lipid 20% (20 g/100cc) = 280cc
4. Additives (electrolytes, vitamins, trace elements) = 80cc (total between 50 and 80cc)
Now the 4 volumes are added and passed every hour by central vein
Total volume: 2250cc/24 h = 94cc/h
It starts at 100% ie 85cc/h
Corresponds to the following contribution of calories
Protein: 4 Kcal × 105 g = 420 Kcal
Dextrose: 3.4 Kcal × 420 g = 1428 Kcal (72% non-protein calorie)
SMOF Lipid: 10.0 Kcal × 56 g = 560 Kcal (28% non-protein calorie)
Total: 2408 Kcal/70 g = 34 Kcal/Kg/day

Monitoring and Complications of Total Parenteral Nutrition

Compared to enteral or hypocaloric oral nutrition, the use of PN (parenteral nutrition) is not associated with increased mortality, overall frequency of complications, or longer length of hospital stay (LOS) [54]. The risk of PN complications (e.g., refeeding syndrome, hyperglycemia, bone demineralization, catheter infections) can be minimized by carefully monitoring patients and the use of nutrition support teams particularly during long-term PN. Occurring complications are, e.g., the refeeding syndrome in patients suffering from severe and malnutrition with the initiation of refeeding or metabolic, hypertriglyceridemia, hyperglycemia, osteomalacia and osteoporosis, and hepatic complications including fatty liver, non-alcoholic fatty liver disease, cholestasis, cholecystitis, and cholelithiasis [55]. Efficient monitoring in all types of PN can result in reduced PN-associated complications and reduced costs. Water and electrolyte balance, blood sugar, and cardiovascular function should regularly be monitored during PN. Regular checks of serum electrolytes and triglycerides as well as additional monitoring measures are necessary in patients with altered renal function, electrolyte-free substrate intake, lipid infusions, and in intensive care patients [56, 57]. The metabolic monitoring of patients under long-term PN should be carried out according to standardized procedures. Monitoring metabolic determinants of bone metabolism is particularly important in patients receiving long-term PN. Markers of intermediary, electrolyte, and trace element metabolism require regular checks.

Once the NPT begins, it requires strict follow-up monitoring (Tables 17.9 and 17.10).

Table 17.9 Recommendations for monitoring TPN in hospitalized patients

Parameter	Initial frequency	Frequency when more stable
Body weight	Daily	Every other day
Inputs and outputs	Daily	Daily
Vital signs	3–4 times daily	1–2 times daily
Serum electrolytes	Daily	2–3 times weekly
BUN, creatinine	Daily	2–3 times weekly
Blood glucose	4–6 times day	Daily
Triglycerides	Daily	Weekly
Liver function test	Daily	Weekly
Complete blood count	Daily	Weekly
Albumin, prealbumin	Weekly	Weekly
Nitrogen balance	Weekly	Weekly

Table 17.10 Complications of total parenteral nutrition

Mechanical problems	
Insertion	
Air embolus	
Pneumothorax, hemothorax, chylothorax, hydrothorax	
Hemorrhage	
Dislodgement	
Thrombosis of vein	
Phlebitis	
Metabolic problems	Infection
Hyperglycemia, hypoglycemia	Fungus
Altered renal function	Gram-positive bacteria
Essential fatty acid deficiency	Gram-negative bacteria
Electrolytes and vitamin excesses and deficiencies	
Trace mineral deficiencies	
Hyperlipidemia	

Enteral nutrition is often insufficient, or occasionally contraindicated, in critically ill patients and results in growing energy and protein deficit. The cost benefit of using early parenteral nutrition in patients with short-term relative contraindications to enteral nutrition has been reported. In selected patients supplemental parenteral nutrition has been associated with a decreased risk of infection, a reduced duration of mechanical ventilation, and a shorter stay in the ICU [58].

Pregnant patients less catabolic, who do not tolerate enteral route, could benefit from peripheral parenteral nutrition as an excellent option.

Peripheral parenteral nutrition is an alternative to total parenteral nutrition and is a complement to enteral nutrition and the oral route. Progress in catheter design and materials, infusion techniques, and an improved knowledge of the optimal nutriments has made peripheral parenteral nutrition a safe, efficient, and useful method to treat patients over certain periods of time [59, 60].

References

1. Trikha A, Singh PM, et al. The critically ill obstetric patient – recent concepts. Indian J Anaesth. 2010;54:421–7.
2. Kaur M, Singh P, Trikha A. Management of critically ill obstetric patients: a review. J Obstet Anaesth Crit Care. 2017;7(1):3–12.
3. Price LC, Slack A, Nelson-Piercy C. Aims of obstetric critical care management. Best Pract Res Clin Obstet Gynaecol. 2008;22(5):775–99.
4. Tang B, Tang MJ, Phelan JP. Nutritional support. In: Phelan JP, Pacheco LD, Foley MR, editors. Critical care obstetric. 6th ed. Oxford: Wiley Blackwell; 2019. p. 265–72.
5. Tan EK, Tan EL, et al. Alterations in physiology and anatomy during pregnancy. Best Pract Res Clin Obstet Gynaecol. 2013;27(6):791–802.
6. Carlin A, Alfirevic Z, et al. Physiological changes of pregnancy and monitoring. Best Pract Res Clin Obstet Gynaecol. 2008;22:801–23.
7. Rasmussen KM, Yaktine AL, Institute of Medicine (U.S.). Committee to Reexamine IOM Pregnancy Weight Guidelines. Weight gain during pregnancy : reexamining the guidelines. Washington, DC: National Academies Press; 2009. 854 p.
8. Lammi-Keefe CJ, Couch SC, Kirwan JP. Handbook of nutrition and pregnancy. 2nd ed. Cham: Humana Press; 2018. XLIII, 445 p.
9. Cox S. Weight gain during pregnancy. J Midwifery Womens Health. 2003;48(3):229–30.
10. Guelinckx I, Devlieger R, Beckers K, et al. Maternal obesity: pregnancy complications, gestational weight gain and nutrition. Obes Rev. 2008;9(2):140–50.
11. Taggart NR, Holliday RM, Billewicz WZ, Hytten FE, Thomson AM. Changes in skinfolds during pregnancy. Br J Nutr. 1967;21(2):439–51.
12. Pipe NG, Smith T, Halliday D, Edmonds CJ, Williams C, Coltart TM. Changes in fat, fat-free mass and body water in human normal pregnancy. Br J Obstet Gynaecol. 1979;86(12):929–40.
13. McClave SA, Taylor BE, Martindale RG, et al. Guidelines for the provision and assessment of nutrition support therapy in the adult critically ill patient: Society of Critical Care Medicine (SCCM) and American Society for Parenteral and Enteral Nutrition (A.S.P.E.N.). J Parenter Enter Nutr. 2016;40(2):159–211.
14. Prado CMM, Heymsfield SB. Lean tissue imaging: a new era for nutritional assessment and intervention LST assessment by most commonly used. JPEN J Parenter Enteral Nutr. 2014;38:940–53.
15. Mundi MS, Patel JJ, Martindale R. Body composition technology: implications for the ICU. Nutr Clin Pract. 2019;34(1):48–58.
16. Sohlstrom A, Kabir N, Sadurskis A, Forsum E. Body composition and fat distribution during the first 2 weeks of gestation in ad lib.-fed and energy-restricted rats. Br J Nutr. 1994;71(3):317–33.
17. Takahashi K, Ohkuchi A, Furukawa R, et al. Establishing measurements of subcutaneous and visceral fat area ratio in the early second trimester by magnetic resonance imaging in obese pregnant women. J Obstet Gynaecol Res. 2014;40(5):1304–7.
18. Armellini F, Zamboni M, Rigo L, et al. The contribution of sonography to the measurement of intra-abdominal fat. J Clin Ultrasound. 1990;18(7):563–7.
19. Bartha JL, Marin-Segura P, Gonzalez-Gonzalez NL, et al. Ultrasound evaluation of visceral fat and metabolic risk factors during early pregnancy. Obesity. 2007;15(9):2233–9.
20. Connolly B, MacBean V, Crowley C, et al. Ultrasound for the assessment of peripheral skeletal muscle architecture in critical illness: a systematic review. Crit Care Med. 2015;43:897–905.
21. Tillquist M, Leung R, Kutsogiannis D. Bedside ultrasound is a practical and reliable measurement tool for assessing quadriceps muscle layer thickness. J Parenter Enter Nutr. 2014;38(7):886–90.
22. Mourtzakis M, Wichmeyer P. Bedside ultrasound measurement of skeletal muscle Bedside ultrasound measurement of skeletal muscle. Curr Opin Clin Nutr Metab Care. 2014;17:389–95.

23. Dunnihoo D. Fundamentals of gynecology and obstetrics. Philadelphia: JB Lippincott; 1990. p. 164–76.
24. Institute of Medicine, Food and Nutrition Board. Dietary reference intakes for energy, carbohydrate, fiber, fatty acids, cholesterol, protein and amino acids. Washington: National Academies Press; 2002.
25. Singer P, Blaser AR, Berger MM, et al. ESPEN guideline on clinical nutrition in the intensive care unit. Clin Nutr. 2019;38:48–79.
26. Gómez E, Reyes AL. Planificación dietética en el embarazo. En: Terapia Nutricia Médica en Ginecología y Obstetricia, Sección II, Parte IV. Editorial McGrawHill; 2011, p. 162–77.
27. Sharma K, Mogensen KM, Robinson MK. Pathophysiology of critical illness and role of nutrition. Nutr Clin Pract. 2019;34(1):12–22.
28. Genuis S, Schwalfenberg GK. Time for an oil check: the role of essential omega-3 fatty acids in maternal and pediatric health. J Perinatol. 2006;26:359–65.
29. McFadyen M, Farquharson J, Cockburn F. Maternal and umbilical cord erythrocyte omega-3 and omega-6 fatty acids and haemorheology in singleton and twin pregnancies. Arch Dis Child Fetal Neonatal Ed. 2003;88:F134–8.
30. Lew CCH, Yandell R, Fraser RJL, Chua AP, Chong MFF, Miller M. Association between malnutrition and clinical outcomes in the intensive care unit: a systematic review. JPEN J Parenter Enteral Nutr. 2017;41(5):744–58.
31. Mogensen KM, Robinson MK, Casey JD, et al. Nutritional status and mortality in the critically ill. Crit Care Med Dic. 2015;43:2605–15.
32. Vallejo KP, Mendes CM, Matos AA, et al. Current clinical nutrition practices in critically ill patients in Latin America: a multinational observational study. Crit Care. 2017;21:227.
33. Schneider SM, Veyres P, Pivot X, et al. Malnutrition is an independent factor associated with nosocomial infections. Br J Nutr. 2004;92(1):105–11.
34. Lollar D, Collier B, et al. Nutrition therapy in shock. Curr Surg Rep. 2016;4:42.
35. De Aguilar-Nascimento JE, Dock-Nascimento DB, Bragagnolo R. Role of enteral nutrition and pharmaconutrients in conditions of splanchnic hypoperfusion. Nutrition. 2010;26(4):354–8.
36. Cresci G, Cúe J. The patient with circulatory shock: to feed or not to feed? Nutr Clin Prac. 2008;23(5):501–9.
37. Bourcier S, Oudjit A, Goudard G, et al. Diagnosis of nonocclusive acute mesenteric ischemia in the intensive care unit. Ann Intensive Care. 2016;6(1):112.
38. Turza KC, Krenitsky J, Sawyer RG. Enteral feeding and vasoactive agents: suggested guidelines for clinicians. Pract Gastroenterol. 2009;78(September):11–22.
39. WHO recommendations for prevention and treatment of pre-eclampsia and eclampsia. ©World Health Organization, 2011.
40. Roberts JM, Balk JL, Bodnar LM, et al. Nutrient involvement in preeclampsia. J Nutr. 2003;133:1684S–92S.
41. Mignini LE, Villar J, Khan KS. Mapping the theories of pre-eclampsia: the need for systematic reviews of mechanisms of the disease. Am J Obstet Gynecol. 2006;194:317–21.
42. Sibai B, Dekker G, Kupferminc M. Pre-eclampsia. Lancet. 2005;365:785–99.
43. Meher S, Duley L. Interventions for preventing pre-eclampsia and its consequences: generic protocol. Cochrane Database Syst Rev. 2005;2:CD005301.
44. Rees DD, Palmer RM, Moncada S. Role of endothelium-derived nitric oxide in the regulation of blood pressure. Proc Natl Acad Sci U S A. 1989;86:3375–8.
45. Morris N, Eaton BM. Nitric oxide, the endothelium, pregnancy and pre-eclampsia. Br J Obstet Gynaecol. 1996;103:4–15.
46. Savvidou MD, Hingorani AD, Tsikas D, et al. Endothelial dysfunction and raised plasma concentrations of asymmetric dimetylarginine in pregnant women who subsequently develop preeclampsia. Lancet. 2003;361:1511–7.
47. Maynard SE, Min JY, Merchan J, et al. Excess placental soluble fms-like tyrosine kinase 1 (sFlt1)may contribute to endothelial dysfunction, hypertension, and proteinuria in preeclampsia. J Clin Invest. 2003;111:649–58.

48. Venkatesha S, Toporsian M, Lam C, et al. Soluble endoglin contributes to the pathogenesis of preeclampsia. Nat Med. 2006;12:642–9.
49. Vadillo-Ortega F, Perichart-Perera O, Espino S, et al. Effect of supplementation during pregnancy with L-arginine and antioxidant vitamins in medical food on pre-eclampsia in high risk population: randomised controlled trial. BMJ. 2011;342:d2901.
50. Germain AM, Valdez G, Romanik MC, et al. Letter to the editor: evidence supporting a beneficial role for long term L-arginine supplementation in high-risk pregnancies. Hypertension. 2004;44:e1.
51. Staff AC, Berge L, Haugen G, Lorenzen B, et al. Dietary supplementation with L-arginine or placebo in women with pre-eclampsia. Acta Obstet Gynecol Scand. 2004;83:103–7.
52. Neri I, Monari F, Sgarbi L, et al. L-arginine supplementation in women with chronic hypertension: impact on blood pressure andmaternal and neonatal complications. J Matern Fetal Neonatal Med. 2010;23:1456–60.
53. Seres DS, Valcarcel M, Guillaume A. Advantages of enteral nutrition over parenteral nutrition. Ther Adv Gastroenterol. 2013;6(2):157–67.
54. Thibault R, Pichard C. Parenteral nutrition. World Rev Nutr Diet. 2013;105:59–68.
55. Sobotka L, Camilo ME. Basics in clinical nutrition: Metabolic complications of parenteral nutrition. e-SPEN. 2009;4:e120–2.
56. Hon K, Bihari S, Holt A, et al. Rate of catheter-related bloodstream infections between tunneled central venous catheters versus peripherally inserted central catheters in adult home parenteral nutrition: a meta-analysis. JPEN J Parenter Enteral Nutr. 2019;43:41.
57. Mirtallo J, Canada T, Johnson D, et al. Safe practices for parenteral nutrition. JPEN J Parenter Enteral Nutr. 2004;28:S39.
58. Berger MM, Najate A, Pichard C. Parenteral nutrition in intensive care patients: medicoeconomic aspects. Curr Opin Clini Nutr Metab Care. 2018;21:223–37.
59. Gura KM. Is there still a role for peripheral parenteral nutrition? Nutr Clin Pract. 2009;24(6):709–17.
60. Sugrue D, Jarrel AS, Kruer R, et al. Appropriateness of peripheral parenteral nutrition use in adult patients at an academic medical center. Clin Nutr ESPEN. 2018;23:117–21.

Part V
Surgical Emergencies

Chapter 18
Blunt Trauma

Inês Mourato Nunes and António Gandra d'Almeida

Introduction

Trauma is the most common cause of non-obstetric death among pregnant women [1].

Motor vehicle accidents, domestic or intimate partner violence, and falls account for most cases of blunt trauma during pregnancy [1, 2].

Trauma affects 6–8 percent of pregnancies [3]. A 2013 systematic review of studies on trauma in pregnancy reported the following prevalence of blunt trauma causes [4]:

- Domestic violence – 8307/100,000 live births
- Motor vehicle crash – 207/100,000 live births
- Falls – 49/100,000 live births

Evaluation of the pregnant patient with major trauma presents unique challenges since the presence of a fetus means two patients are potentially at risk, both of which require evaluation and management.

The management of a pregnant trauma patient warrants consideration of several issues specific to pregnancy such as alterations in maternal physiology and anatomy, exposure to radiation and other possible teratogens, the need to access fetal well-being, and conditions that are unique to pregnancy and are related to trauma (Rh immunization, placental abruption, and preterm labor) [5].

I. Mourato Nunes (✉)
Hospital das Forças Armadas, Lisboa, Portugal

Hospital de Cascais, Alcabideche, Portugal

A. Gandra d'Almeida
Education and Simulation Coimbra Militar Health Center, Coimbra, Portugal

Head of Education of CSMC, Coimbra, Portugal

C. Montufar et al. (eds.), *Obstetric Catastrophes*,
https://doi.org/10.1007/978-3-030-70034-8_18

It requires a multidisciplinary team approach involving trauma surgeons, emergency medicine physicians, obstetricians, neonatologists, nursing staff, and technicians.

Physiological changes related to pregnancy occur in virtually all systems and are caused by both hormonal and mechanical factors. These normal changes need to be considered when evaluating the status of pregnant trauma victims [6].

Pertinent changes in major organ systems are detailed in previous chapters.

Initial Evaluation and Management of Major Trauma

As previously mentioned the assessment of a pregnant trauma patient in the ER may require the involvement of a multidisciplinary team that may include an emergency physician or trauma specialist, an obstetrician, a neonatologist, an anesthetist, and skilled nursing staff. The pregnant patient should be fully assessed, as is a nonpregnant patient, with a thorough history, examination, laboratory tests, imaging studies, and invasive diagnostic procedures as indicated. In addition, special attention should be given to fetal evaluation when gestational age is ≥23 weeks and to trauma complications that are unique to pregnancy such as placental abruption [5].

Seriously injured trauma victims are occasionally unable to communicate with the primary caregiver. And as some women may not be aware of their pregnancy status, every injured female of childbearing age should be considered pregnant until proven otherwise [5].

The initial assessment of an acutely injured pregnant woman should include securing airway, ensuring breathing, and maintaining adequate circulation. The most important lifesaving primary interventions might include intubation and controlling severe external bleeding. So the assessment should start with the ABCDE approach.

Airway

The pregnant patient has a greater risk for airway management problems and difficult intubation than the nonpregnant patient [7]. Weight gain, respiratory tract mucosal edema, decreased functional residual capacity, reduced respiratory system compliance, increased airway resistance, and increased oxygen requirements are pregnancy-induced changes that place the injured pregnant woman at risk for failure to maintain a patent airway and secured ventilation [6].

Injured pregnant women with an unsecured airway are at increased risk for aspiration of gastric contents. Gastric emptying is delayed in pregnancy, and pregnant women should be considered to have a full stomach for up to 24 h after their last meal [8].

Breathing

Marked increases in basal oxygen consumption and extreme sensitivity of the fetus to maternal hypoxia mandate supplemental oxygen by a nasal cannula, mask, or endotracheal tube to all pregnant trauma patients to maintain oxygen saturation above 95% [6].

We must be aware that the displacement of the diaphragm during pregnancy the thoracostomy tube, when indicated, must be placed one to two intercostal spaces higher than usual [9].

Circulation

The heart rate increases by 15% during pregnancy. Tachycardia and hypotension, typical of hypovolemic shock, may appear late in the pregnant trauma patient because of her increased blood volume [10]. During pregnancy, maternal vital signs and perfusion may be preserved at the expense of uteroplacental perfusion, delaying the occurrence of signs of hypovolemic shock. Not uncommonly, noticeable alterations in vital signs occur only after significant blood loss that may have already diminished uteroplacental perfusion. In these instances, an atypical or abnormal fetal heart rate pattern, in addition to indicating impending fetal hypoxemic injury or even death, may be the first indicator of significant maternal hypovolemia due to hemorrhage [5].

Administration of fluids and blood products during resuscitation should proceed according to standard trauma protocols. Nevertheless, some modifications should be made in the pregnant trauma victim [5].

The uteroplacental vasculature is highly responsive to vasopressors, and their administration may decrease placental perfusion. In cases of maternal hypotension, vasopressors should be avoided unless the patient is unresponsive to replenishment of intravascular volume by fluid administration [11]. Bicarbonate should be used with caution, because rapid correction of maternal acidosis can reduce the compensatory hyperventilation.

Care must be taken to avoid supine hypotension in the pregnant trauma patient after mid-pregnancy. Compression of the vena cava by the uterus can cause up to 30% reduction in cardiac output. The displacement of the uterus off of the inferior vena cava and abdominal aorta enhances maternal venous return and cardiac output and consequently improves uterine perfusion. This can be achieved either by placing the patient in the left lateral position or by manual displacement of the uterus while the injured patient is secured in the supine position. The latter may allow more effective chest compressions while cardio-pulmonary resuscitation is in progress. A third option is to use a backboard for lateral tilt with secured spine in suspected spinal injuries. Fetal risks from maternal defibrillation are small, especially if all fetal monitors have been removed [5].

In the setting of acute blood loss necessitating immediate administration of blood products in a pregnant trauma patient, O-negative blood should be transfused in order to avoid Rh sensitization in Rh-negative women until type-specific or cross-matched donor blood becomes available [5].

All body parts of the pregnant trauma patient should be exposed and thoroughly examined.

The abdomen should be carefully evaluated because serious injuries may involve the gravid uterus as well as other abdominal organs. An abnormal distension may be a sign of intra-abdominal hemorrhage or perforation of hollow viscus.

The uterus should be assessed for fundal height, shape, hypertonus, and tenderness. Tenderness over the uterus is an important sign suggestive of abruption of the placenta. Irregularities on the abdomen may represent fetal body parts in cases of traumatic uterine rupture. In these cases, rapid response of the medical team can significantly reduce maternal and fetal risks, and urgent obstetrical consultation is recommended [12].

Vaginal examination should be performed for cervical dilatation, effacement, fetal presentation, and station. However, in cases of vaginal bleeding after 23 weeks, speculum or digital vaginal examination should be deferred until placenta previa is excluded by an ultrasound scan. A speculum examination should be performed to assess for vaginal bleeding, pooling of amniotic fluid, cervical dilatation, vaginal or cervical lacerations, and expulsion of gestational tissue [3].

In a pregnant patient ≥23 weeks' gestation, fetal heart rate monitoring should be initiated as soon as possible. This may require having staff from the maternity visit the unit where the pregnant woman is receiving care for her injuries. For those <23 weeks' gestation, a brief assessment of fetal viability is adequate. Continuous monitoring of oxygen saturation is advised since maternal desaturation may compromise oxygenation of the fetus. Oxygen supplementation should be given to increase oxygen saturation [3].

Complementary diagnostic tests should be performed to complete maternal assessment.

Radiographic Studies

Plain radiographs of the cervical spine, chest, and pelvis are first-line radiological studies [13]. Clinicians are often reluctant to order imaging studies for pregnant patients out of concern about fetal exposure to ionizing radiation. Ionizing radiation has the highest teratogenic potential during the period of organogenesis (5–10 weeks), with an increased risk of miscarriage before this period. After 10 weeks, radiation is more likely to produce growth restriction or CNS effects than teratogenic changes [14]. Fetal exposure from the radiological examinations used in the evaluation of pregnant trauma patients presents a very low risk to the developing fetus [14]. Radiation exposure with a cumulative dose of >5–10 rads (50–100 mGy) is associated with an increased risk of fetal malformation or CNS effects, limited usually to a gestational age <18 weeks [14]. Concerns about fetal exposure to radiation should not preclude or delay any indicated radiological evaluation. CT studies are associated with increased fetal radiation exposure depending on the body part being scanned, the gestational age, the number and thickness of slices, and the equipment used. With abdominal CT during the third trimester, the fetal exposure is around 3.5 rads, which is still under the threshold for fetal damage [15]. Use of gadolinium-based contrast agents has shown fetal toxicity in animal studies, though no adverse effects have been reported in human fetuses [16]. Their use can be considered when the maternal benefit outweighs potential fetal risks.

Laboratory Tests

In pregnant patients there are alterations in the normal range of laboratory values as previously described. Special attention is paid to fibrinogen values that are often more than 4 g/L during pregnancy; therefore the normal values of 2.5–3 g/L for a non-pregnant patient may actually signify mild hypofibrinogenemia, and levels below 2 g/L may indicate disseminated intravascular coagulation, a frequent comorbidity of significant placental abruption. D-dimer is often positive and therefore is of little value in the diagnosis or exclusion of venous thromboembolism. Normal range for the partial pressure of CO_2 is decreased during pregnancy to 27–32 mmHg; thus normal non-pregnant values of 40 mmHg may result from mild hypoventilation. Serum creatinine levels are decreased during pregnancy to 50–60 μmol/L, and even a value as low as 90 μmol/L may be abnormal.

Abdominal Ultrasound

FAST is a useful aid for the detection of intraperitoneal fluid in pregnant trauma patients with suspected intra-abdominal injury. The sensitivity of FAST in detecting intraperitoneal fluid in pregnant blunt trauma patients was 83% in a study that reviewed 127 pregnant trauma patients [17]. FAST is an easy and rapid modality that has the added advantage of avoiding fetal exposure to ionizing radiation; it should therefore be part of the secondary survey in pregnant patients with major trauma [3].

Diagnostic Peritoneal Lavage (DPL) and Laparotomy

DPL is a very rapid and sensitive test with sensitivity of 96–100% for detection of traumatic intra-abdominal injury. The main disadvantages are that it does not provide information about specific organ damage and abdominal injuries that can be managed conservatively following CT would require operative intervention based upon DPL.

For these reasons, among patients with abdominal trauma, diagnostic peritoneal lavage has been almost entirely replaced by ultrasound and multidetector helical CT scanning. CT identifies specific organ injury, evaluates the retroperitoneum as well, and is less invasive than DPL.

The procedure may be necessary in some cases, such as in hypotensive patients with equivocal results on FAST examination and multiple potential sources of blood loss, and in resource-poor settings where advanced imaging is unavailable.

The open lavage technique is preferable over a blind needle insertion in the pregnant patient in order to minimize uterine injury. When significant abdominal blood is detected, an exploratory laparotomy with a midline incision superior to the uterine fundus is recommended [18].

Pregnancy Evaluation and Management After Initial Maternal Stabilization

Fetal Assessment

Assessment of a viable fetus (≥23 weeks gestational age) should be initiated immediately following or in parallel with the physical examination of the stabilized mother since it has been shown that most placental abruptions occur shortly after the insult [19]. It's essential to know the estimated gestational age for appropriate interpretation of tests for fetal viability and well-being. Electronic monitoring of the fetal heart rate should be initiated on viable fetuses (≥23 weeks) as soon as possible. With a confirmed pre-viable fetus, it may be sufficient to demonstrate the presence of fetal cardiac activity.

The objectives of the fetal assessment are identification of impending hypoxemic fetal injury or death as a result of uteroplacental compromise or placental abruption; detection of trauma-related complications of pregnancy such as placental abruption, preterm delivery, and spontaneous rupture of the membranes; evaluation of the degree of maternal-fetal hemorrhage and resultant fetal anemia; delineation of fetal injuries; and identification of compensated maternal hypovolemia first manifested by decreased placental perfusion [5].

Monitoring of Fetal Heart Rate and Uterine Activity

Electronic fetal monitoring (EFM) allows assessment of fetal well-being and uterine activity, with abnormality of being predictive of potential obstetrical complications such as placental abruption, fetal hypoxic injury, or fetal death.

Maternal hypovolemic shock can reduce uterine perfusion, and this can be further compounded by visceral vasoconstriction [5]. Placental abruption can further reduce transplacental oxygenation. A combination of these factors can lead to fetal hypoxemic injury. Compromised fetal perfusion and oxygenation usually present with abnormalities in the fetal heart rate pattern and may also be the first sign of maternal hemodynamic compromise, before [20].

The duration of fetal monitoring following maternal trauma remains disputed. A prospective study of pregnant trauma patients that had EFM for a minimum of 4 h suggested that 4 h of monitoring was a sensitive method of predicting immediate posttraumatic adverse obstetrical outcomes, as placental abruption [21]. Another retrospective study of 271 pregnant patients suggested monitoring for at least 24 h only for a selected group of patients at high risk for fetal demise, preterm labor, and placental abruption [22]. This high-risk group consisted of patients involved in motorcycle, pedestrian, or high-velocity collisions, those ejected from motor vehicles and patients demonstrating maternal tachycardia, abnormal fetal heart rate pattern, and high injury severity scores.

This suggests hospitalization and intermittent fetal heart rate and uterine activity monitoring by EFM for 24 h for patients with uterine tenderness, significant abdominal pain, vaginal bleeding, a contraction frequency of more than once per 10 min during a monitoring period of 4 h, rupture of the membranes, atypical or abnormal fetal heart rate pattern (fetal tachycardia, bradycardia, or decelerations), high-risk mechanism of injury (motorcycle, pedestrian, high-speed crash), or serum fibrinogen <200 mg/dL [5].

Monitoring for 4 h is sufficient to rule out major trauma-related complications in low-risk patients without the abovementioned risk factors [5].

Prevention of Rh Alloimmunization and Evaluation of Maternal-Fetal Hemorrhage (MFH)

Traumatic placental injury can result in maternal-fetal hemorrhage that occurs in 10–30% of pregnant trauma patients [23].

This rare complication of trauma is usually clinically evident, with fetal demise, abnormal fetal heart rate pattern (bradycardia or recurrent decelerations), or abrupt fetal anemia and cardiac failure. The quantification of the amount of fetal blood cells in the maternal circulation enables the obstetric care provider to roughly estimate the degree of transplacental hemorrhage. This may be important in prevention of Rh alloimmunization in Rh-negative mothers [24].

The Rh antigen is well developed by 6 weeks' gestation, and only a 0.001 mL of fetal blood can cause sensitization of the Rh-negative mother, leading to sensitizing MFH. Therefore, anti-D IgG should be given to all Rh-negative pregnant trauma patients. A single dose of 300 mg, administered within 72 h of injury, provides protection against sensitization for up to 30 mL of fetal blood in the maternal circulation [25]. The feto-placental blood volume is estimated to be 120 mL/kg of fetal weight. In most cases of traumatic maternal-fetal hemorrhage, the estimated volume of fetal blood in the maternal circulation is less than 15 mL, and in more than 90% of cases it is less than 30 mL [24].

A novel approach for detecting MFH, using flow cytometry as a simpler, more objective, and more precise alternative to the KB method, has been advocated, but as this test is not available in most medical facilities and its added value is still being investigated, we cannot recommend its routine use at this time [26].

The universal use of KB testing for all pregnant trauma patients, regardless of their Rh status, had been advocated by some, hypothesizing that the magnitude of MFH reflects severity of injury and therefore would be predictive of trauma-related obstetrical complication such as preterm labor [27].

Ultrasound Evaluation

Ultrasonography is a rapid, noninvasive, valuable tool in the assessment of pregnant trauma patients. Performing an obstetrical ultrasound scan is essential and should be done urgently in cases where the gestational age cannot be determined with certainty and need for delivery is anticipated based on an atypical or abnormal fetal heart rate pattern or suspicion of placental abruption. However, it is not sensitive in diagnosing placental abruption, missing between 50% and 80% of them. In the setting of trauma, EFM is a more sensitive tool not only to rule out a placental abruption but also for assessment of fetal well-being as compared to ultrasound [21].

Nevertheless, ultrasound is an important adjunctive to the physical examination and fetal assessment tests. Ultrasonography may assist in determination of gestational age; demonstration of fetal cardiac rate and rhythm; placental localization and exclusion of placenta previa; assessment of amniotic fluid volume; cervical length assessment; fetal well-being (biophysical profile); detection of fetal anemia by peak systolic flow velocity in the middle cerebral artery; delineation of possible fetal injury; and confirmation of fetal demise [5].

Therefore, an obstetrical ultrasound examination is recommended in all cases of significant maternal trauma that are admitted for monitoring for more than 4 h, as a complement of EFM.

Obstetrical Complications of Trauma

Placental Abruption

Placental abruption occurs in 5–50% of maternal trauma, being its major complication and the most common cause of fetal death in cases of blunt trauma [21]. It results from the difference in physical properties of the relatively inelastic placental tissue versus the elastic myometrium; significant abruption of the highly vascular uteroplacental interface can mediate rapid maternal and in some cases fetal exsanguination. Most abruptions occur within 2–6 h after the injury and almost all of them with 24 h of injury [19].

Typical findings include abdominal pain, uterine tenderness, uterine contractions or hypertonicity, vaginal bleeding, preterm labor, or an atypical or abnormal EFM tracing. Specific sonographic findings are uncommon; retroplacental hematoma is seen in 2–25% of abruptions. Treatment should never be delayed for ultrasound confirmation because ultrasonography is not reliable in diagnosing placental abruption [5]. Abruption, occult or concealed, may lead to major maternal bleeding and consumption coagulopathy with thrombocytopenia, prolonged coagulation tests, and hypofibrinogenemia [28].

Although severe placental abruption can be lethal to the fetus, a timely and prompt caesarean section may result in considerable survival rates of up to 75% [29]. Delay in recognition of non-reassuring fetal status, in such cases, was accountable for 60% of potentially preventable perinatal deaths. In cases of a nonviable fetus, vaginal birth is preferable [5].

Uterine Rupture

Post-trauma uterine rupture is rare (0.6% of all maternal injuries), seen more frequently with a scarred uterus or with direct abdominal impact during the latter half of pregnancy and 75% involve the fundal area. The degree of rupture may vary from complete avulsion of the uterus to serosal hemorrhage and abrasions. Symptoms and signs suggestive of uterine rupture include maternal shock, abdominal distension, irregular uterine contour, palpable fetal parts, sudden abnormal fetal heart rate pattern, ascent of fetal presenting part, and peritoneal irritation (abdominal rigidity, guarding and tenderness) [5]. Maternal mortality has been described with traumatic uterine rupture, and fetal mortality is almost universal. It is the cause of MVC-related perinatal death in 17.5% of the cases [30]. Suspected uterine rupture with maternal and/or fetal comprise should prompt urgent laparotomy to control bleeding and facilitate resuscitation [5].

Preterm Labor

Traumatic injury during pregnancy can result in preterm labor through several mechanisms, such as placental abruption, premature rupture of membranes, and prostaglandin production secondary to extravasation of blood at the placental margin [31].

Signs of preterm labor should be sought in every patient with a viable fetus, using EFM to assess regularity and frequency of contractions. If risk of preterm delivery is high because of preterm labor or preterm premature rupture of membranes, steroids and neonatology consultation should be considered. In many cases, iatrogenic preterm delivery may be indicated to improve fetal or maternal outcome [5].

Direct Fetal Injury

Direct fetal injury is seen in less than 1% of blunt maternal trauma, because maternal soft tissues, uterus, and amniotic fluid serve to diminish the force delivered to the fetus. Most of the mechanisms involve the fetal skull and brain, as deceleration injury of an unengaged head or fetal skull fracture resulting from the fracture of the maternal pelvis in late gestation with an engaged fetal head [32–34].

Perimortem Caesarean Section

A perimortem caesarean section is rare, and it is recommended for viable fetus (≥23 weeks, or fundal height 2 or more fingerbreadths above the umbilicus) and should be performed no latter than 4 min following maternal cardiac arrest. Delivery within 5 min carries the best chance of fetal and maternal survival [35].

Prolonged resuscitation is not recommended if no pulse can be obtained, and the uterus should be emptied to increase the likelihood of successful maternal resuscitation and a healthy infant [5].

References

1. Grossman NB. Blunt trauma in pregnancy, 2004. Am Acad Family Phys. 2004;70(7):1303–10.
2. Kuo C, Jamieson DJ, ML MP, Meikle SF, Posner SF. Injury hospitalizations of pregnant women in the United States, 2002. Am J Obstet Gynecol. 2007;196(2):161, e1.
3. Huls CK, Detlefs C. Trauma in pregnancy. Semin Perinatol. 2018;42(1):13–20.
4. Mendez-Figueroa H, Dahlke JD, Vrees RA, Rouse DJ. Trauma in pregnancy: an updated systematic review. Am J Obstet Gynecol. 2013;209(1):1.
5. Jain V, Chari R, Maslovitz S. Guidelines for the management of a pregnant trauma patient. J Obstet Gynaecol Can. 2015;37(6):553–74.
6. Irwin RS, Lilly CM, Mayo PH, Rippe JM. Irwin & Rippe's intensive care medicine. 8th ed. Philadelphia: Wolters Kluwer; 2012.
7. Suresh MS, Wali A. Failed intubation in obstetrics: airway management strategies. Anesthesiol Clin North Am. 1998;16:477–98.
8. Ramsay G, Paglia M, Bourjeily G. When the heart stops: a review of cardiac arrest in pregnancy. J Intensive Care Med. 2013;28:204–14.
9. Tsuei BJ. Assessment of the pregnant trauma patient. Injury. 2006;37(5):367–73.
10. Norwitz ER, Robinson JN. Pregnancy-induced physiologic alterations. In: Belfort MA, Saade GR, Foley MR, Phelan JP, Dildy GA, editors. Critical care obstetrics. 5th ed. Malden: Wiley-Blackwell; 2010. p. 30–52.
11. Sperry JL, Minei JP, Frankel HL, West MA, Harbrecht BG, Moore EE, et al. Early use of vasopressors after injury: caution before constriction. J Trauma. 2008;64:9–14.

12. Rothenberger D, Quattlebaum FW, Perry JF Jr, Zabel J, Fischer RP. Blunt maternal trauma: a review of 103 cases. J Trauma. 1978;18:173–9.
13. American College of Surgeons Committee on Trauma. Trauma in women. In: Advanced trauma life support for doctors: student course manual. 8th ed. Chicago: American College of Surgeons; 2008. p. 259–68.
14. Puri A, Khadem P, Ahmed S, Yadav P, Al-Dulaimy K. Imaging of trauma in a pregnant patient. Semin Ultrasound CT MR. 2012;33:37–45.
15. De Santis M, Di Gianantonio E, Straface G, Cavaliere AF, Caruso A, Schiavon F, et al. Ionizing radiations in pregnancy and teratogenesis: a review of literature. Reprod Toxicol. 2005;20:323–9.
16. Patel SJ, Reede DL, Katz DS, Subramaniam R, Amorosa JK. Imaging of pregnant patient for nonobstetric conditions: algorithm and radiation dose considerations. Radiographics. 2007;27:1705–22.
17. Goodwin H, Holmes JF, Wisner DH. Abdominal ultrasound examination in pregnant blunt trauma patients. J Trauma. 2001;50:689–93.
18. Nagy KK, Roberts RR, Joseph KT, Smith RF, An GC, Bokhari F, Barrett J. Experience with over 2500 diagnostic peritoneal lavages. Injury. 2000;31(7):479.
19. Shah KH, Simons RK, Holbrook T, Fortlage D, Winchell RJ, Hoyt DB. Trauma in pregnancy: maternal and fetal outcomes. J Trauma. 1998;45:83–6.
20. Hoff WS, D'Amelio LF, Tinkoff GH, Lucke JF, Rhodes M, Diamond DL, et al. Maternal predictors of fetal demise in trauma during pregnancy. Surg Gynecol Obstet. 1991;172:175–80.
21. Pearlman MD, Tintinalli JE, Lorenz RP. A prospective controlled study of outcome after trauma during pregnancy. Am J Obstet Gynecol. 1990;162:1502–10.
22. Curet MJ, Schermer CR, Demarest GB, Bieneik EJ 3rd, Curet LB. Predictors of outcome in trauma during pregnancy: identification of patients who can be monitored for less than 6 hours. J Trauma. 2000;49:18–24.
23. Hull SB, Bennett S. The pregnant trauma patient: assessment and anesthetic management. Int Anesthesiol Clin. 2007;45(3):1–18.
24. Goodwin TM, Breen MT. Pregnancy outcome and fetomaternal hemorrhage after noncatastrophic trauma. Am J Obstet Gynecol. 1990;162:665–71.
25. Fung Kee Fung K, Eason E, Crane J, Armson A, De La Ronde S, Farine D, et al. Prevention of Rh alloimmunization. J Obstet Gynaecol Can. 2003;25:765–73.
26. Porra V, Bernaud J, Gueret P, Bricca P, Rigal D, Follea G, et al. Identification and quantification of fetal red blood cells in maternal blood by a dual-color flow cytometric method: evaluation of the Fetal Cell Count kit. Transfusion. 2007;47:1281–9.
27. Weintraub AY, Leron E, Mazor M. The pathophysiology of trauma in pregnancy: a review. J Matern Fetal Neonatal Med. 2006;19:601–5.
28. Doan-Wiggens L. Trauma in pregnancy. In: Benrubi GI, editor. Obstetric and gynecologic emergencies. Philadelphia: Lippencott; 1994. p. 57–76.
29. Ananth CV, Berkowitz GS, Savitz DA, Lapinski RH. Placental abruption and adverse perinatal outcomes. JAMA. 1999;282:1646–51.
30. Kvarnstrand L, Milsom I, Lekander T, Druid H, Jacobsson B. Maternal fatalities, fetal and neonatal deaths related to motor vehicle crashes during pregnancy: a national population-based study. Acta Obstet Gynecol Scand. 2008;87:946–52.
31. Sperry JL, Casey BM, McIntire DD, Minei JP, Gentilello LM, Shafi S. Long-term fetal outcomes in pregnant trauma patients. Am J Surg. 2006;192:715–21.
32. Van Hook JW. Trauma in pregnancy. Clin Obstet Gynecol. 2002;45:414–24.
33. Fries MH, Hankins GDV. Motor vehicle accidents associated with minimal maternal trauma but subsequent fetal demise. Ann Emerg Med. 1989;18:301–4.
34. Palmer JD, Sparrow OC. Extradural haematoma following intrauterine trauma. Injury. 1994;25:671–3.
35. Katz VL, Dotters DJ, Droegemueller W. Perimortem cesarean delivery. Obstet Gynecol. 1986;68:571–6.

Chapter 19
Adynamic Ileus: Intra-abdominal Hypertension Syndrome

Juan Carlos Barrientos Rojas

Intra-abdominal Hypertension Syndrome

Introduction

Actually, significant advances in the understanding of intra-abdominal hypertension syndrome (IAHS) have now been made, creating even the World Society of Abdominal Compartment Syndrome (WSACS), in 2013, and they update their consensus definitions and clinical practice guidelines. However, their low recognition is observed in the obstetric patient and therefore as this phenomenon could influence pregnancy. From this, it is important to analyze the impact on the maternal and perinatal results of IAHS, as well as to question the application in pregnancy of the form of intra-abdominal pressure (IAP) measurement and its values, considering the physiological variants of the obstetric patient, also its possible relationship with the development of maternal complications such as preeclampsia, eclampsia, and fetal disorders [2] (Table 19.1).

There are conditions that predispose the development of intra-abdominal hypertension: acidosis, hypothermia, polytransfusion, coagulopathy, sepsis, hepatic dysfunction, mechanic ventilation, pneumonia, pregnancy, obesity, etc. (Table 19.2).

Prolonged shock, ischemia/intestinal reperfusion, and excessive administration of crystalloids establish the genesis of the abdominal compartment syndrome.

Massive resuscitation with crystalloids increases intra-abdominal pressure, establishing a positive feedback with greater visceral edema and a negative feedback with a deterioration of cardiac preload that requires greater contribution of crystalloids. The volume loading increases the hydrostatic pressure of mesenteric capillaries and decreases the oncotic pressure of the plasma. This promotes a flow

J. C. Barrientos Rojas (✉)
Head of the Critical Obstetrics Unit, Gynecology and Obstetrics Department, Hospital General San Juan de Dios, University of San Carlos de Guatemala, Guatemala City, Guatemala

C. Montufar et al. (eds.), *Obstetric Catastrophes*,
https://doi.org/10.1007/978-3-030-70034-8_19

Table 19.1 Causes of intra-abdominal hypertension

Spontaneous	Postoperatory	Posttraumatic	Iatrogenic	Chronic
Peritonitis Intra-abdominal Abscess Broken aortic aneurysm Pneumoperitoneum to tension Pancreatitis Mesenteric venous thrombosis Intestinal obstruction	Peritonitis Intra-abdominal abscess Ileus Gastric dilation Intra-abdominal hemorrhage Damage control surgery	Hemoperitoneum Visceral edema post resuscitation	Massive fluid resuscitation Very high PEEP Laparoscopic surgery Anti-shock suit Pelvic abdominal packing Abdominal closure to tension	Ascites Tumor Dialysis Pregnancy Obesity

Table 19.2 Final 2013 Consensus Definitions of the WSACS – The Abdominal Compartment Society

Adult consensus definitions (ACS, abdominal compartment syndrome; APP, abdominal perfusion pressure; IAH, intra-abdominal hypertension; IAP, intra-abdominal pressure; MAP, mean arterial pressure)
Definitions
1. IAP is the steady-state pressure concealed within the abdominal cavity
2. The reference standard for intermittent IAP measurements is via the bladder with a maximal instillation volume of 25 ml of sterile saline
Diagnosis
3. IAP should be expressed in mmHg and measured at end expiration in the supine position after ensuring that abdominal muscle contractions are absent and with the transducer zeroed at the level of the midaxillary line
4. IAP is approximately 5–7 mmHg in critically ill adults
5. IAH is defined by a sustained or repeated pathological elevation in IAP greater than 12 mmHg
6. ACS is defined as a sustained IAP more than 20 mmHg (with or without an APP less than 60 mmHg) that is associated with new organ dysfunction/failure
7. IAH is graded as follows:
Grade I, IAP 12–15 mmHg
Grade II, IAP 16–20 mmHg
Grade III, IAP 21–25 mmHg
Grade IV, IAP >25 mmHg
8. Primary IAH or ACS is a condition associated with injury or disease in the abdominal pelvic region that frequently requires early surgical or interventional radiological intervention
9. Secondary IAH or ACS refers to conditions that do not originate in the abdominopelvic region
10. Recurrent IAH or ACS refers to the condition in which IAH or ACS redevelops following previous surgical or medical treatment of primary or secondary IAH or ACS
11. APP = MAP – IAP
12. A polycompartment syndrome is a condition where two or more anatomical compartments have elevated compartmental pressures

Table 19.2 (continued)

13. Abdominal compliance is a measure of the ease of abdominal expansion, which is determined by the elasticity of the abdominal wall and diaphragm. It should be expressed as the change in intra-abdominal volume per change in IAP
14. The open abdomen is one that requires a temporary abdominal closure due to the skin and fascia not being closed after laparotomy
15. Lateralization of the abdominal wall is the phenomenon where the musculature and fascia of the abdominal wall, most exemplified by the rectus abdominus muscles and their enveloping fascia, move laterally away from the midline with time [1]

of fluids into the interstitium. The increase in interstitial pressure initially increases the lymphatic flow; however, the increase in intra-abdominal pressure produces a lymphatic compression that limits the discharge of the interstitial fluid. Additionally, it produces an obstruction to the venous flow, with the consequent increase in hydrostatic capillary pressure and fluid flow.

The best way to prevent this pathology is the early recognition of patients who are at risk and to establish interventions aimed at minimizing the development of intra-abdominal hypertension.

These decisions should be made during laparotomy and involve choices related to the decision to complete an operation due to major physiological alterations (hypothermia, acidosis, and coagulopathy) and method of closing the abdominal wall.

Obstetric hemorrhage, preeclampsia-eclampsia, and sepsis are the main causes of maternal mortality in the world, and 90% occur in developing countries, being considered those that survive as severe maternal morbidity, requiring critical care between 1% and 3%, which face health professionals who are not familiar with maternal and fetal physiology combined with a critical illness. Therefore, the impact of IAP is not recognized under these physiological conditions of the pregnant women [3].

From an intensive care unit (UCI), study that IAH is present in 38% of patients upon admission and is an independent predictor of mortality and the overall prevalence of IAH reached 59% and 8% for ACS. Therefore, monitoring IAP is becoming a standard of care in ICU, especially for patients admitted with respiratory failure, increased abdominal contents, or massive fluid resuscitation [1].

An obstetrician, in 1913, Paramore, on IAHS, "there is almost no recognition or appreciation of their presence, influence and management in pregnancy and peripartum period" [4]. The recognition through monitoring of the IAP allows early detection and at the same time performs interventions to prevent the development of IAHS, which can be presented prepartum, peripartum, or postpartum; therefore efforts should be directed to populations where there is little understanding, as the obstetric patient, since pregnancy is a possible event in almost half of the world population at some point in life [5]. There is uncertainty regarding whether the standardized values on IAP are applicable in pregnancy, due to hormonal, cardiovascular, hemodynamic changes or the mechanical effect of compression of the uterus in crescendo that exerts on the pelvic vasculature, and at the same time generates an increase on IAP, which is completely physiological in a healthy woman. However, in those who have comorbidities, genetic predisposition, or some factor triggering IAHS, these physiological variants can dramatically impact negatively on fetal and maternal development, triggering catastrophic complications.

Normal Physiology in Pregnancy

It is important to understand the normal physiological variants that occur in all organs and systems of the organism during pregnancy, as a principle of adaptability and support, allowing fetal intrauterine growth and development for a limited time.

The average weight gained during pregnancy is approximately 12.5 kg, of which the uterus contributes approximately 1 kg and the amniotic fluid, the placenta, and the fetus with approximately 5 kg. To accommodate this growth, the hormone relaxin allows greater laxity of the ligaments, allowing uterine growth. It increases the thoracic cage on its anteroposterior and transverse diameters; likewise it raises the diaphragm forward caudal, diminishing the functional residual capacity (CRF) in 20%. The tidal volume (Vt) increases generating a 45% increase in alveolar ventilation per minute, resulting in general respiratory alkalosis, which is compensated by the reduction of serum bicarbonate to 20 mEq/L and a total basal buffer capacity of 5 mEq/L. Oxygen consumption (V02), gas exchange, and acid-base status are affected by factors including the growth of the placental fetus unit, progesterone levels, and carbon dioxide production (CO2). The VO2 increases 15–20%. These changes make the obstetric patient more vulnerable to hypoxemia and acidemia, who does not have enough reserve.

It also increases the plasma volume by 50%, generating dilutional anemia, and increases blood circulation by 40%. Cardiac output (CO) increases 30–50% and uterine flow increases ten times. After 20 weeks of gestation, the uterus generates a mechanical effect of aorto-cava obstruction in the supine position and results in supine hypotension syndrome, explained by the limitation of venous return to compensate the cardiovascular circulatory system. Compensatory vertebral, paravertebral, epidural, and ovarian collateral circulation is generated. IAP could exacerbate aorto-cava compression and maintain a cause-effect relationship [6].

The growing uterus and fetus occupy most of the abdominal cavity as pregnancy progresses; this effect causes an increase in IAP, particularly in the third trimester; however this is gradual throughout gestation, allowing it to adapt; the organ dysfunction that is normally seen in non-obstetric critical patients is not frequently observed in the pregnant woman because the change in the IAP is not acute, but it is gradual; otherwise the placental uterine perfusion would be affected [7].

Pathogenesis

Theories suggest that IAH/ACS often develops as a result of two physiological phases, which together sequentially produce a self-perpetuating process called "acute intestinal distress syndrome" [8]. In the first phase, resuscitation of patients in shock induces bowel ischemia-reperfusion injury [9]. This "acute bowel injury" results in release of pro-inflammatory mediators into the peritoneum and systemic circulation, leading to neutrophil priming, increased intestinal wall permeability, extravasation of fluid into the bowel wall and mesentery, translocation of intestinal bacteria, and absorption of bacterial endotoxin [10].

In the second phase, the resultant abdominal visceral edema leads to IAH, which compresses intra-abdominal lymphatic and results in a progressive decrease in bowel wall perfusion, mucosa-to-serosa intestinal necrosis, a further increase in bowel wall permeability, and heightened bacterial translocation/endotoxin absorption and release of pro-inflammatory mediators and induces multiorgan dysfunction syndrome [11].

This highlights that alternate definitions and management strategies may be needed for other patient populations, including pregnant women [12]. Lozada et al. recently proposed management algorithm, definition, and classification of peripartum intra-abdominal hypertension and abdominal compartment syndrome, defined an IAH in pregnancy as a sustained or repeated pathological elevation in IAP ≥14 mm Hg, and defined ACS in pregnancy as a sustained IAP >25 mm Hg that is associated with new organ failure/dysfunction [13].

The grade I can be considered as normal, without negative repercussions. In grade II the need for surgical treatment is based on the clinical condition of each patient. In the absence of oliguria, hypoxemia, or severe elevations in airway pressure, no treatment is warranted; however patients with this degree of IAP require close observation. The majority of patients with grade III IAP require abdominal decompression. All patients with a grade IV IAP require abdominal decompression.

The abdominal compartment syndrome (ACS) should be suspected in those patients with a tight abdomen, distended, with elevated IAP, those with signs of low cardiac output, increased pressure in the right atrium and pulmonary capillary pressure, hepatic hypoperfusion, hyperbilirubinemia, metabolic acidosis and refractory lactic acidosis, oliguria refractory to volume administration, splanchnic hypoperfusion (increase of intramucosal PCO2 by gastric tonometry), increase in respiratory work, increase in peak and plateau pressure in mechanically ventilated patients, progressive hypoxemia, hypercapnia, and elevated ICP. There may be edema in the lower limbs and tendency to deep vein thrombosis.

Risk Factors

IAP should be measured whenever a patient has one or more risk factors for IAH; these included obesity (OR 5.1), sepsis (OR 2.38), abdominal infection (OR 2.49), abdominal surgery (OR 1.93), post-laparotomy (OR 5.72), pancreatitis (OR 4.73), hepatic failure/cirrhosis (OR 2.07), gastrointestinal bleeding (OR 3.37), ileus (OR 2.05), liver dysfunction (OR 2.25), APACHE score (OR 1.6 per point increase), base deficit (OR 1.15), acidosis (OR 1.93), vasopressor use (OR 2.33), shock (OR 4.68), hypotension (OR 2.12), central venous pressure (OR 1.3 per mmHg), positive end-expiratory pressure >10 cmH2O (OR 2.41), respiratory failure (OR 1.87), acute respiratory distress syndrome (OR 3.61), mechanical ventilation (OR 6.78), fluid balance (OR 5.22), fluid collections (OR 2.01), and fluid resuscitation (OR 2.17 crystalloid or colloid >3.5 l) [1, 14].

Intra-abdominal Pressure in Pregnancy

Clinical examination is insufficient for detecting raised IAP. There is a little information about intra-abdominal pressure in pregnancy; however it is summarized in Table 19.3 [18]:

There is no evidence to suggest that is necessary to measure IAP in uncomplicated pregnancies or in chronic conditions such as obesity, liver disease with ascites, tumors, or another condition that increases the risk of IAHS; the decision to measure IAP in pregnancy, is based on the clinical presentation, using the established standard measures [19].

The best evidence concerning IAP in pregnancy was obtained through rectal manometer on primarily primigravid inmates in 1913 [4]. However, Al-Khan and colleagues published more contemporary IAP intravesical measurements in 100 healthy term parturient obtained under spinal anesthesia just prior to

Table 19.3 Intra-abdominal pressure mean in pregnancy

Author	Year	n	Gestation	Position during IAP measurement	IAP mean (mmHg)	Comments
Paramore [4]	1913	24	6 months to term	Supine; left side; knee chest; standing	Range 15–44	Rectal manometer; ambulatory subjects
Cupeert et al. [7]	2008	40	Term	Supine; left lateral	Not reported	Elective CS under spinal anesthesia
Sugerman [29]	2011	5	39 weeks	Supine; left lateral decubitus	25 ± 3; 23 ± 3	Under methods; likely ambulatory patients
Al-Khan et al. [16, 54]	2011	100	36–41 weeks	Leftward tilt	22 ± 2.9	Elective CS; unspecific leftward tilt; 50 ml saline instilled in bladder; under reference point
Chun et al. [30]	2012	20	38–40 weeks	Supine; leftward tilt	10 ± 4.7 8.9 ± 4.9	Elective Cs under spinal anesthesia, leftward tilt 10°

IAP mean means intra-abdominal pressure, *n* number, *CS* cesarean section

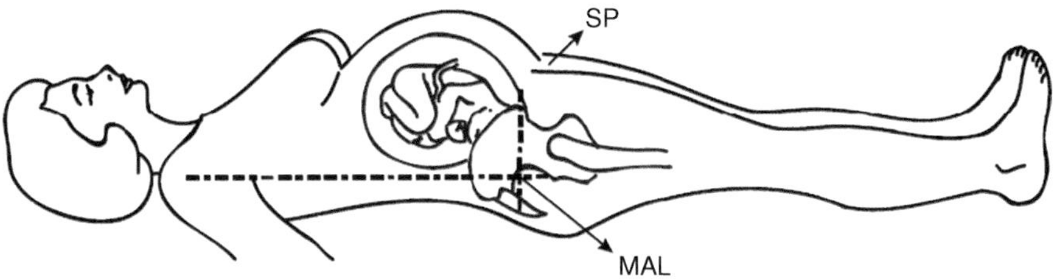

Fig. 19.1 Anatomic reference of the zero point for the measure of IAP. (Reproduced from [21], which is an open access article that permits unrestricted use of the article contents in any medium provided the work is properly cited)

commencement of elective CS. They found the median IAP in leftward tilted position to be 22 ± 2.9 mmHg (rage 15–29 mmHg), pressures actually in the threshold range for ACS if organ failure were also present. Postoperatively, after neonatal delivery, the IAP dropped significantly to a median IAP of 16 mmHg (range 11–24 mmHg) [20].

What is really is that the value of IAP increases during pregnancy, and it has been suggested that pregnancy is associated with chronically elevated IAP (10–15 mmHg), like obesity [20]; therefore, the mother should adapt to this increase in pressure; otherwise it could have maternal and fetal involvement in the development of pregnancy. Patients with a significant increase in IAP and organ dysfunction should be managed medically and/or surgically.

The measurement of the IAP should be carried out according to the recommendations of the WSACS, in totally supine position, through a catheter to the bladder, instilling 25 ml of saline solution and performing the measurement at the end of expiration, with a relaxed abdomen and measurement at the level of the midaxillary line along the iliac crest [21] (Fig. 19.1).

Current consensus guidelines on defining and measuring IAP are based on the non-pregnant population. Measurement every 4–6 h is probably adequate for patients at risk developing IAH or ACS. It is probable that the measurement through the standard method, through the bladder, is altered by the pressure exerted by the uterus on it and its relationship with the pelvis, and maybe a lateral inclination would help the measurement bias. Nevertheless, more specific research is needed for its evaluation in this population group [22, 23]. There is evidence using 10–15° left lateral tilt, for the measure of IAP [24]. The ignorance of the behavior of the IAHS in the pregnancy potentiates the risk of delay in the diagnosis and catastrophic scenarios, increasing maternal morbidity and mortality.

Systemic Consequences of the Elevated IAP

The IAHS/ACS is not limited to the intra-abdominal organs. In normal conditions, the value of intra-abdominal pressure is similar to the atmospheric pressure; when the volume of the abdominal contents increases, the pressure also increases proportionally. The consequence of this elevation is a decrease in hepatic, splanchnic, and renal perfusion by compression of the vascular beds. Intra-abdominal hypertensions are transmitted to the pleural and pericardial space, increasing the juxta-cardiac pressure and thus preventing ventricular filling. It also elevates the left ventricular afterload and redistributes the blood flow away from the abdomen; consequently, cardiac output decreases, increasing the pressure in the right atrium and at the pulmonary capillary level, that is, hemodynamically similar to cardiac tamponade.

The cephalic displacement of the diaphragm increases intrathoracic pressure; as a consequence there is a decrease in venous return (with IAP 10 mmHg), increase in peripheral vascular resistance, reduction in compliance and cardiac contractility due to the direct compressive effect of chest pressure on the heart, and decrease in cardiac output. The venous return of the lower extremities is also compromised as the flow of the inferior vena cava slows, and consequently there is predisposition to the formation of peripheral edema and deep vein thrombosis.

Compression to the pulmonary parenchyma results in an increase in the final pressure of inspiration (PIM) in mechanically ventilated alveolar atelectasis patients and alterations in the transport of oxygen through the alveolar capillary membrane increasing the intrapulmonary shunt; as a result progressive hypoxemia, hypercapnia, and respiratory acidosis ensue.

On the wall of the entire gastrointestinal tract, ischemia is produced by reduction of mesenteric blood flow, with intra-abdominal pressure of 10 mmHg, evidenced by gastric tonometry. Reduction in pancreatic and splenic blood flow has also been documented.

As a result bacterial translocation, release of free oxygen radicals, and vasoactive mediators potentially producing systemic inflammatory response syndrome (SRIS), sepsis, and multiple organ failure (FOM) ensue.

Abdominal hypertension significantly reduces renal blood flow, by direct compression to the cortex, reversing the medullary cortical renal flow, in addition to the direct mechanical effect on the renal artery and veins. In general, oliguria occurs with intra-abdominal pressure between 15 and 20 mmHg, anuria when the IAP exceeds 20 mmHg, generating acute renal failure due to direct hypoperfusion [25].

Acute abdominal compartment syndrome (ACS) also leads to neuronal ischemic damage due to decreased cerebral blood flow and intracranial hypertension by several mechanisms, among which is mentioned a reduction in cardiac output with reduction in cerebral perfusion pressure. In addition to this, increase in intrapleural pressure as a consequence of intra-abdominal hypertension, the pressure of the large intrathoracic venous vessels increases, which reduces the central venous return and, as a consequence, intracranial pressure rises. The harmful effects on perfusion and intracranial pressure are evident when the IAP exceeds 25 mmHg (Box 19.1).

Box 19.1 Systemic Consequences of Increased Intra-abdomial Pressure

Cardiovascular system Difficulty in evaluating the preload Increase in pulmonary arterial occlusion pressure Increase in central venous pressure Decrease in transmural filling pressure Increase in extravascular lung water Increase in pulse pressure variations Decrease in the volume of the end of the diastole VD Decrease in cardiac minute volume Decreased venous return Increase in systemic vascular resistance Increased risk of venous thrombosis and PTE Variable heart rate Variable effect on blood pressure Increase in pulmonary arterial pressure Decrease in compliance VI	*Respiratory system* Increase in intrathoracic pressure Increase in pleural pressure Increase of the PEEP car Decrease in functional residual capacity Decrease in all lung volumes Increase in peak pressure in the airway Increased plateau pressure in the airway Decrease in dynamic compliance Decrease in static compliance Increase in $PaCO_2$ Decrease in PaO_2 and PaO_2/FiO_2 Increased ventilation of the dead space Increase in pulmonary shunt Increase in lower inflection point Difficulty in weaning the respirator Increased alveolar inflammation
Liver system Decreased hepatic arterial flow Alveolar edema Decreased blood portal flow Increase collateral portal flow Decreased glucose metabolism Decreased mitochondrial function Increase in renal vascular resistance	*Renal system* Decrease in renal filtration pressure Decrease in lactate clearance Decrease in filtration gradient Decreased renal blood flow Decrease in diuresis Compression of the renal vein Ureter compression Increase in antidiuretic hormone
Gastrointestinal system Decrease in abdominal perfusion pressure Decreased celiac blood flow Decreased mucosal blood flow Mesenteric venous compression Decrease in intramucosal pH Increase in intestinal permeability Increase in bacterial translocation Increase in pCO_2 mucosa and CO_2 gap Increase in variceal and gastric bleeding Increase in peritoneal adhesions Failure of enteral nutrition	*Abdominal wall* Decrease in compliance Decreased blood flow of the rectus muscles Decrease blood flow of the rectus Complications of operative wounds Incisional hernias
Endocrine system Release of pro-inflammatory cytokines	*Central nervous system* Increased intracranial pressure Decrease in cerebral perfusion pressure
Multiorgan failure syndrome	

IAHS and Preeclampsia

Preeclampsia, a heterogeneous condition, and hypoperfusion syndrome characterized by vasospasm and endothelial damage, which manifests with arterial hypertension and proteinuria after 20 weeks of gestational age, are one of the main causes of maternal and perinatal morbidity and mortality, with multisystemic involvement: hematologic alteration, HELLP syndrome (hemolysis, elevated hepatic enzymes, and thrombocytopenia) hepatic and renal dysfunction, neurological sequel, retinal detachment, headache, stroke and seizures, cardiovascular disease, growth restriction (IUGR), and other abnormalities [26].

Its etiology is incomplete; however the hypothetical model consists of an abnormal placentation during the trophoblastic invasion during the second trimester of pregnancy, generating placental ischemia and release of toxic angiogenic factors, leading to endothelial dysfunction and inflammation [26, 27]. The diagnosis of IAHS in the peripartum is a challenge, because the IAP is not routinely measured, except in very obvious conditions, which leads to poor recognition in the obstetric patient, in addition to some similarities with the multisystemic manifestations of preeclampsia.

Since the 1900s, researchers suggested that decompensated IAH could be a possible etiological factor in the development of preeclampsia, hypothesizing that the nulliparous and muscular women were prone to abdominal wall muscle tone resulting in elevated IAP, compromising the perfusion of the intra-abdominal viscera [28].

There is a relationship of IAP and preeclampsia, indicating that IAHS plays a central role in the initiation of the multisystemic cascade of limited perfusion and inflammation associated with the different manifestations of preeclampsia and in the progression of the severity of the disease, and also speculated that obstruction of venous return from IAHS, especially limiting abdominal perfusion pressure due to increased pressure, resulted in decreased perfusion to organs such as the kidneys and placenta, generating the activation of the renin-angiotensin-aldosterone system, raising the levels of the latter, generating arterial hypertension and placental ischemia-necrosis, and impacting fetal growth and development, since IAHS slows uterine flow which results in compensatory fetal hypertension [29]. Because of this, it is important to consider the measurement of IAP in critical maternal conditions such as preeclampsia-eclampsia.

This relationship suggests that the most frequent time of presentation of preeclampsia is the third trimester, precisely when there are higher levels of IAP, and the established cure for preeclampsia is the interruption of pregnancy, which would lead to reduction of the IAP and improvement of the patient. However, these conclusions must be verified with further investigations.

Management of SHIA/SCA

There are not enough research and recommendations based on evidence for the management of intra-abdominal hypertension in pregnancy, for which the recommendations raised by WSACS in 2013 should be considered (Table 19.4). The IAP

Table 19.4 Final 2013 WSACS – The Abdominal Compartment Society Consensus Management Statements

Recommendations
1. We recommend measuring IAP when any known risk for IAH/ACS is present in a critically ill or injured patient [grade 1C]
2. Studies should adopt the trans-bladder technique as the standard IAP measurement technique [not GRADED]
3. We recommend use of protocolized monitoring and management of IAP versus not [grade 1C]
4. We recommend efforts and/or protocols to avoid sustained IAH as compared to inattention to IAP among critically ill or injured patients [grade 1C]
5. We recommend decompressive laparotomy in cases of overt ACS compared to strategies that do not use decompressive laparotomy in critically ill adults with ACS [grade 1D]
6. We recommend that among ICU patients with open abdominal wounds, conscious and/or protocolized efforts be made to obtain an early or at least same-hospital-stay abdominal fascial closure [grade 1D]
7. We recommend that among critically ill/injured patients with open abdominal wounds, strategies utilizing negative pressure wound therapy be used versus not [grade 1C]
Suggestions
1. We suggest that clinicians ensure that critically ill or injured patients receive optimal pain and anxiety relief [grade 2D]
2. We suggest brief trials of neuromuscular blockade as a temporizing measure in the treatment of IAH/ACS [grade 2D]
3. We suggest that the potential contribution of body position to elevated IAP be considered among patients with, or at risk of, IAH or ACS [grade 2D]
4. We suggest liberal use of enteral decompression with nasogastric or rectal tubes when the stomach or colon are dilated in the presence of IAH/ACS [grade 1D]
5. We suggest that neostigmine be used for the treatment of established colonic ileus not responding to other simple measures and associated with IAH [grade 2D]
6. We suggest using a protocol to try and avoid a positive cumulative fluid balance in the critically ill or injured patient with, or at risk of, IAH/ACS after the acute resuscitation has been completed and the inciting issues have been addressed [grade 2C]
7. We suggest use of an enhanced ratio of plasma/packed red blood cells for resuscitation of massive hemorrhage versus low or no attention to plasma/packed red blood cell ratios [grade 2D]
8. We suggest use of PCD to remove fluid (in the setting of obvious intraperitoneal fluid) in those with IAH/ACS when this is technically possible compared to doing nothing [grade 2C]. We also suggest using PCD to remove fluid (in the setting of obvious intraperitoneal fluid) in those with IAH/ACS when this is technically possible compared to immediate decompressive laparotomy as this may alleviate the need for decompressive laparotomy [grade 2D]
9. We suggest that patients undergoing laparotomy for trauma suffering from physiologic exhaustion be treated with the prophylactic use of the open abdomen versus intraoperative abdominal fascial closure and expectant IAP management [grade 2D]
10. We suggest not to routinely utilize the open abdomen for patients with severe intraperitoneal contamination undergoing emergency laparotomy for intra-abdominal sepsis unless IAH is a specific concern [grade 2B]
11. We suggest that bioprosthetic meshes should not be routinely used in the early closure of the open abdomen compared to alternative strategies [grade 2D]

(continued)

Table 19.4 (continued)

No recommendations
1. We could make no recommendation regarding use of abdominal perfusion pressure in the resuscitation or management of the critically ill or injured
2. We could make no recommendation regarding use of diuretics to mobilize fluids in hemodynamically stable patients with IAH after the acute resuscitation has been completed and the inciting issues have been addressed
3. We could make no recommendation regarding the use of renal replacement therapies to mobilize fluid in hemodynamically stable patients with IAH after the acute resuscitation has been completed and the inciting issues have been addressed
4. We could make no recommendation regarding the administration of albumin versus not, to mobilize fluid in hemodynamically stable patients with IAH after acute resuscitation has been completed and the inciting issues have been addressed
5. We could make no recommendation regarding the prophylactic use of the open abdomen in nontrauma acute care surgery patients with physiologic exhaustion versus intraoperative abdominal fascial closure and expectant IAP management
6. We could make no recommendation regarding use of an acute component separation technique versus not to facilitate abdominal fascial closure

ACS abdominal compartment syndrome, *IAH* intra-abdominal hypertension, *IAP* intra-abdominal pressure, *ICU* intensive care unit, *PCD* percutaneous catheter drainage
Reproduced from [3], which is an open access article that permits unrestricted use of the article contents in any medium provided the work is properly cited

is increased in pregnancy; however the pregnant woman develops mechanisms that allow her to adapt to the gradual increase of the IAP [30].

Targeting an abdominal perfusion pressure (APP) – defined as the difference between mean arterial pressure (MAP) and IAP – of greater than 60 mmHg has been sometimes been proposed as a resuscitation endpoint more predictive of outcome than IAP, but this is not universally accepted, and treatment strategies should probably focus on mitigating IAH rather than driving up MAP [31].

Medical management strategies included [32] sedation/analgesia and neuromuscular blocking agents that increase abdominal wall compliance, evacuation of intraluminal gastrointestinal contents with nasogastric/rectal tubes and prokinetic agents, and optimization of fluid administration decreasing fluid balance after the acute resuscitation phase, use of vasoactive medications may facilitate restoration of abdominal and systemic perfusion with lower resuscitation fluid volumes than have been traditionally required, thus reducing the risk of secondary or recurrent ACS. Removal of restrictive bandages or surgical release of restrictive burn scars or scar tissue may improve abdominal wall compliance. Evacuation of intra-abdominal space-occupying lesions, paracentesis, and large-volume (>1 L) removal of ascites or hematoma have been documented to significantly decrease IAP in a variety of disease processes. Evacuation of other intra-abdominal contents as with delivery of a gravid uterus is presumed (but not proven) to provide some benefit.

Since head-of-bed elevation and patient flexion significantly increase IAP, as documented above, temporary repositioning of a patient to a supine position may provide some transient benefit in decreasing IAH. Pharmacologic diuresis and/or removal of fluid with continuous renal replacement therapies (RRT) resulting in net ultrafiltration has been suggested to have a significant impact on IAP [33].

Damage control surgery has increased the survival of patients with severe insults; however, a group of these salvaged patients develop devastating complications as a result of an abdominal compartment syndrome. Several clinical studies have shown a clear association of ACS with multiorgan failure. It is admitted up to a third of patients who require damage control surgery and can develop an ACS; these patients present an elevated risk of IAH because they commonly require massive resuscitation with crystalloids and transfusions due to sustained hemorrhagic shock and intra-abdominal tamponade, which are independent risk factors for the development of ACS.

Damage control resuscitation should be adopted in managing of patients with significant hemorrhage, like in obstetric population, as it has been associated with a lower incidence of ACS and higher primary fascial closure, correcting coagulopathy, acidosis, and hypothermia [33].

Percutaneous catheter drainage is a minimally invasive option suggested to decrease IAP in those with IAH/ACS among patients with burns or pancreatitis with intraperitoneal fluid collections [34].

If ACS cannot be prevented with medical or surgical management strategies or treated with percutaneous catheter drainage, guidelines recommend urgent decompressive laparotomy and also recommended negative pressure wound therapy devices be used for temporary abdominal closure [1].

Some indications of open abdomen are respiratory deterioration at the time of closure, contamination or fecal peritonitis, hemodynamic instability at the time of closure, massive intestinal edema, hypothermia, tension closure, multiple intra-abdominal injuries, planned reoperation, and intra-abdominal tamponade.

After decompressive laparotomy, if the abdominal fascia is unable to be closed, some methods have been proposed to include Bogota bag, negative pressure peritoneal therapy, the Wittmann patch (Starsurgical, Burlington, Wisconsin, USA), progressive closure of a synthetic patch sutured between the fascial edges, dynamic retention using sutures or the Abdominal Reapproximation Anchor device (Canica Design Inc., Almonte, Ontario, Canada), and vacuum-assisted wound closure (VAC) and mesh-mediated fascial traction [1].

The spectrum of surgical management of IAH/ACS includes surgical prevention of IAH/ACS; abdominal decompression (via laparotomy or a minimally invasive fasciotomy); temporary abdominal closure; management of the open abdominal wound in the ICU; avoidance of wound complications, including deep soft tissue infections, abdominal abscesses, enteroatmospheric fistulae, and complex ventral hernia; staged abdominal reconstruction (reducing and closing the abdominal defect over time); or, as a last resort, use of a planned ventral hernia (an open abdominal wound that is allowed to granulate and covered with skin flaps or a split-thickness skin graft) with plans for delayed abdominal wall reconstruction [33].

Adynamic Ileus in Obstetrician

Introduction

Ileus is a pathophysiologic state of inhibited motility in the gastrointestinal tract due to a physical/anatomic obstruction in the lumen (obstructive ileus) or due to cessation of smooth muscle motor activity in the small intestine and colon (adynamic/paralytic/functional). Several myogenic, neurogenic, and humoral factors are suspected to play independent or collective roles in the basic mechanism of the development of paralytic ileus under these conditions. Paralytic ileus is more common, and its management is aimed at the causative or accompanying illness.

In obstetric patients is frequently, and the physiologic changes of pregnancy must be considered in the diagnosis and management. A team approach is necessary to optimize the care of the pregnant patient with gastrointestinal complications.

Definition

Paralytic ileus is a clinical syndrome due to acute and transient disturbance of the transportation of the content of intestinal lumen due to cessation of smooth muscle motor activity in the small intestines and colon, with the potential to return to normal. Paralytic ileus usually does not have a clear mechanism, is complex, and is not clearly understood.

The definition and nosology of these entities is confusing because of an incomplete understanding of the pathophysiology and application of different meanings to the same term (Box 19.2).

Box 19.2 Definitions of Disorders with Impaired Transit of Intestinal Contents

- *Mechanical obstruction*: severely impaired transit of intestinal contents because of intrinsic luminal obstruction or extrinsic compression
- *Ileus*: severe functionally impaired transit of intestinal contents because of decreased peristaltic activity of the gastrointestinal tract in the absence of mechanical obstruction
- *Colonic pseudo-obstruction*: severe functionally impaired transit of colonic contents and massive dilatation of the colon, in the absence of mechanical obstruction, because of uncoordinated, nonperistaltic, or attenuated colonic muscle contractions

Pathogenesis/Pathophysiology

The main function of intestines is to supply water, electrolyte, and nutrients to the body. Approximately 85% of chyme, consisting of 8 L of fluid, nutrients, vitamins, and minerals, is absorbed in the small intestines, while the remaining chyme, mainly consisting of fluid and electrolyte, is absorbed in the colon.

As chyme enters the intestines from the gaster, the proximal portion of the walls of the small intestines is stretched, which causes local concentric contraction at specific intervals along the intestines.

This segmental contraction repeatedly divides chyme each minute, causing progressive mixing of solid food particles and the secretions of the small intestines. Simultaneously, there is also a peristaltic wave that pushes the chime toward the anus with a speed of 0.5–2 cm/s. This peristaltic movement could arise from any part of the small intestines, far more rapidly at the duodenum compared to at the terminal ileum. Thus, under normal conditions, 3–5 h is required for chyme to reach the ileocecal sphincter from the pylorus. Concentric contraction also takes place in the colon, while at the same time there is contraction of the three collections of longitudinal colon muscles on three longitudinal bands known as the teniae coli.

This collective contraction causes the stimulated portion of the colon to bulge like a sac, so-called haustration. This haustral contraction occurs every hour and lasts for 30 s, causing the content to blend. This slow yet persistent haustral contraction is the main force that pushes the chyme from the ileocecal sphincter to the transverse colon, in the cecum and ascending colon. From the transverse colon to the sigmoid, a peristaltic-like motion of the bowel, known as mass movement, replaces the haustral contraction as the thrust forces for bowel content. As it moves through the colon toward the anus, the fluid chyme gradually becomes more solid, until only approximately 80–200 cc of fluid remains in the feces [35].

Progesterone prepares the body for pregnancy by relaxing smooth muscles, which is particularly important in the expanding uterus but also affects the gastrointestinal tract. Progesterone relaxes the lower esophageal sphincter and decreases gastric motility, which increases the frequency of heartburn, gastroesophageal reflux, and nausea during pregnancy. The slowing of gastric motility also leads to constipation, with resultant abdominal pain [16]. The functional changes that occur with the enlarging uterus may mechanically limit colonic emptying which probably is the main reason for symptomatic constipation in late term. There is also a significant increase in water and sodium absorption secondary to the increased aldosterone levels during pregnancy, leading to reduced stool volume and prolonged colonic transit time [17].

The small intestine exhibits decreased motility during pregnancy. Lawson noted that the mean small bowel transit time significantly increased during each trimester (first trimester, 125 ± 48 min; second trimester, 137 ± 58 min; third trimester, 75 ± 33 min) and decreased back to normal levels postpartum. This increased transit time is related to elevations in progesterone levels during normal pregnancy and may contribute to the increased symptoms of constipation in late pregnancy [36].

The pathophysiology of postoperative ileus is multifactorial. An important factor is activation by surgical trauma of the macrophages residing in the tunica muscularis external of the bowel wall. These cells release cytokines that induce the activation of further pro-inflammatory cells and their migration to the site of injury. Next, other antiperistalsis cytokines (including interleukin-6 and TNF-alpha) are released, along with neuropeptides and nitric oxide. The full clinical picture of postoperative ileus ensues, with inflammation of the tunica muscularis external of the entire gastrointestinal tract [37].

Etiology

Ileus most commonly occurs in the postoperative period, where it is recognized as an obligatory physiologic response to abdominal surgery, with small intestine motility recovering after 0–24 h, gastric motility recovering at 24–48 h, and colonic motility recovering at 48–72 h [38].

Many conditions could cause cessation of smooth muscle motor activity in the small intestines and colon, such as sepsis and peritonitis, as a side effect of certain medications; hormonal imbalance because secretin, vasoactive intestinal polypeptide (VIP), and glucagon that inhibit the intestinal peristalsis; electrolyte imbalance; and bowel ischemia due to hypoperfusion, blood-borne toxins, as well as disturbances in oxygen supply and surgery related with increased plasma catecholamine due to postoperative stress [39].

Opiates administered for postoperative analgesia are common contributing factors. Opiates profoundly inhibit gastrointestinal motility and delay recovery from postoperative ileus. Other implicated medications include anticholinergic drugs, calcium-channel antagonists, antihistamines, and various psychotropic agents, such as phenothiazines and tricyclic antidepressants [40].

Pregnancy may complicate most gastrointestinal diseases, and gastrointestinal symptoms are extremely common in the pregnant patient. Most of these symptoms are a manifestation of normal altered physiology in which changes occur both functionally and anatomically. These changes may cause new symptoms, worsen preexisting disease, or mask potentially deadly disease. A lack of experience in dealing with these symptoms can have devastating effects. The physician must be able to distinguish whether these symptoms are those of normal pregnancy or a potentially life-threatening complication such as preeclampsia.

Acute [41] colonic pseudo-obstruction (ACPO) or Ogilvie's syndrome is adynamic ileus of the colon and may occur after delivery. It is a clinical and radiological picture of acute obstruction of the colon in the absence of mechanical obstruction, leading to massive colonic dilatation. ACPO can lead to significant maternal morbidity (hypovolemia, electrolyte imbalance, cecal ischemia, cecal perforation) and mortality. If the diameter of the cecum is ≥9 cms, then there is a significant risk of bowel perforation and urgent referral for decompression is necessary (the diameter is normally up to 7.5 cm). Endoscopic colonic decompression may be needed if the colon dilates to more than 12 cm. Intravenous infusion of 2 mg of neostigmine results in prompt decompression in patients not responding to conservative measures, but should be restricted to use in the postpartum period. Endoscopy is an important and safe tool in the evaluation of gastrointestinal symptoms during pregnancy [42]. The main manifestation of this syndrome is progressive abdominal distention. Most patients (80%) complain of abdominal pain and of nausea and vomiting (60%), while many also have fecal retention or diarrhea (45%). Physical examination typically reveals abdominal tympanums and, usually, audible bowel sounds on auscultation. If peritoneal signs or fever are present, bowel ischemia and perforation must be ruled out. Ogilvie's syndrome is a diagnosis of exclusion, and the initial evaluation should include an abdominal CT scan to rule out other conditions, particularly mechanical ileus or intestinal paralysis due to other intra-abdominal or retroperitoneal disease [43].

Intestinal obstruction is relatively rare in pregnancy but is the second most common non-obstetric abdominal emergency. The incidence is one in 3000 pregnancies. It is extremely rare in early pregnancy but begins to increase between the fourth and fifth month of gestation when the uterus changes from a pelvic organ to an abdominal organ. The peak incidence of bowel obstruction occurs in the eighth month when the fetal head descends into the pelvis, but it may also occur during delivery or the puerperium when a sudden change in uterine size may shift abdominal anatomic relationships. There is no relation between maternal age or parity and the risk of intestinal obstruction. Treatment of intestinal obstruction frequently is surgical, and it is probably the delay in diagnosis and treatment that accounts for the overall maternal mortality rate of less than 6% and fetal loss of 20–30% noted in some studies [44].

Clinical Presentation

Ileus presents with abdominal distention and with abdominal pain that is typically mild and poorly localized. Variable features include hypoactive or absent bowel sounds, lack of passage of flatus and stool, intolerance of oral intake, and nausea and emesis.

Physical examination reveals a distended, tympanic abdomen; hypoactive bowel sounds; and mild, diffuse abdominal tenderness. The patient may exhibit signs of dehydration, such as tachycardia, orthostatic hypotension, poor skin turgor, and dry mucous membranes [45].

Laboratory tests should include routine serum electrolytes, creatinine, blood urea nitrogen, complete blood count, liver function tests, and amylase, lipase, and magnesium levels. Abdominal x-ray may be required to confirm colonic dilatation (large bowel >6 cm, cecum >9 cm).

Treatment and Management

There is no single effective means of preventing or treating postoperative ileus. General measures include intravenous fluid resuscitation and correction of electrolyte abnormalities. Underlying conditions should be identified and aggressively treated: antibiotics for sepsis and discontinuation of drugs that promote an ileus [46, 47]. Supportive measures are given, including nil per os, a nasogastric tube, a decompressive rectal tube, correction of electrolyte disturbances, and discontinuation of constipating drugs [48]. Patients traditionally received nothing by mouth until resolution of the ileus, recognized by passage of flatus or stool, but this treatment harms the nutritional status, thereby potentially decreasing postoperative wound healing and immunologic function. Recent studies suggest that early enteral feeding is safe, decreases the duration of postoperative ileus, and decreases the hospital stay (Box 19.3) [48]:

Gum chewing is an inexpensive and safe method to promote gut motility and resolve a postoperative ileus through vagal and enteric hormonal stimulation (sham feeding), but randomized studies have shown variable efficacy [49].

Gum chewing has been reported to enhance the intestinal function recovery after cesarean section.

Ten RCTs with a total of 1659 women were included in a meta-analysis. Gum chewing provided significant benefits in reducing the time to first passage of flatus, first defecation, first bowel sound, first bowel movement, and the length of hospital stay [50]. Other study included 372 women randomized; chewing gum significantly improved intestinal recovery with faster onset of bowel movements, first audible intestinal sounds, passage of flatus, and passage of stool ($p = 0.0001$). It was associated with significantly shorter duration of hospital stay and parenteral therapy duration ($p = 0.0001$). Abdominal distension, vomiting, and ileus postoperatively were significantly higher in non-chewing gum groups. Neither paralytic ileus nor side effects were recorded with gum use. They conclude that chewing gum, within 2 h postoperatively, is a simple, safe, and well-tolerated intervention that can boost rapid intestinal recovery and shorten hospital stay after planned cesarean deliveries.

Early ambulation does not reduce the duration of postoperative ileus but does decrease complications from prolonged immobility. Postoperative nasogastric

Box 19.3 Initial Management Is Conservative and Should Focus On the Following

- Analgesia (avoid opiate analgesics)
- Antiemetics
- Nothing by mouth to rest bowel
- IV fluids and fluid balance monitoring
- As maintenance only need to consider losses/insensible losses, thus up to 4 L per day
- Ensure adequate VTE prophylaxis

decompression is no longer routinely recommended, because of numerous negative clinical trials and the increased risks of pulmonary atelectasis, pneumonia, or pyrexia with a nasogastric tube. A nasogastric tube is, however, selectively recommended for severe gastric dilatation or protracted vomiting [15].

None of the routinely used prokinetic drugs (neostigmine, metoclopramide, erythromycin) or laxatives have been found in meta-analyses to shorten the duration of postoperative ileus (level Ia evidence) [43].

It may be necessary, particularly in cases of ileus or intractable constipation, to switch the opioid to a combined preparation (e.g., oxycodone + naloxone [level Ib evidence], naloxone being a peripheral opioid antagonist with a high first-pass effect) or to add on a peripheral opioid antagonist (subcutaneous methylnaltrexone or oral naloxegol [level Ib evidence]).

A meta-analysis confirmed the efficacy of neostigmine 2 mg i.v. in the treatment of Ogilvie's syndrome: successful treatment (flatus, defecation, reduction of abdominal circumference) was documented 30 min after the injection in 90% of patients ($p < 0.001$, number needed to treat [NNT] = 1) (level Ia evidence) [51]. On the other hand, there is no evidence for the efficacy of other drugs, such as methylnaltrexone or erythromycin [52].

If pharmacotherapy brings no improvement in 2–3 days, endoscopic deflation and insertion of a decompressive tube in the right hemicolon are recommended (level IIa evidence) [53].

References

1. Kirkpatrick AW, Roberts DJ, De Waele J, Jaeschke R, Malbrain ML, et al. Intra-abdominal hypertension and the abdominal compartment syndrome: update consensus definitions and clinical practice guidelines from the World Society of the Abdominal Compartment Syndrome. Intensive Care Med. 2013;39: 1190–1206; Malbrain ML, Chiumello D, Pelosi P, Bihari D, Innes R, et al. Incidence and prognosis of intra-abdominal hypertension in a mixed population of critically ill patients: a multiple-center epidemiological study. Crit Care Med. 2005; 33: 315–322.
2. Chun R, Kirkpatrick AW. Intra-abdominal pressure, intra-abdominal hypertension, and pregnancy: a review. Ann Intensive Care. 2012;2(Suppl 1):S5.
3. Zeeman GG. Obstetric critical care: a blueprint for improved outcomes. Crit Care Med. 2006; 34: S208–214; American College of Obstetricians and Gynecologist. AGOG Practice Bulletin No. 100: critical care in pregnancy. Obstet Gynecol. 2009; 113: 443–450.
4. Paramore RH. The intra-abdominal pressure in pregnancy. Proc R Soc Med. 1913;6:291–334.
5. Balogh ZJ, Martin A, van Wessem KP, King KL, Mackay P, Havill K. Mission to eliminate postinjury abdominal compartment syndrome. Arch Surg. 2011;146:938–43.
6. Pelosi P, Quintel M, Malbrain ML. Effect of intra-abdominal pressure on respiratory mechanics. Acta Clin Belg. 2007;62(Suppl 1):78–88; Gaiser R. Physiologic changes of pregnancy. In: Chestnut D, Polley L, Tsen L, Wong C., editors. Chestnuts obstetric anesthesia: principles and practice. 4th ed. Philadelphia: Mosby Elsevier; 2009:15–26; Bahi D. Relaxin: a pleiotropic hormone. Gen Pharmacol. 1997; 28:13–22.
7. Cuppett C, Wilson A, Janoo J, Bringman J, Toffle R. Effect of BMI on intra-abdominal pressure measurement in the third trimester of pregnancy. Am J Obstet Gynecol. 2008; 199: S151.

8. Malbrain ML, Vidts W, Ravyts M, et al. Acute intestinal distress syndrome: the importance of intra-abdominal pressure. Minerva Anestesiol. 2008; 74: 657–673; Malbrain ML, De Laet I. AIDS is coming to your ICU: be prepared for acute bowel injury and acute intestinal. Intensive Care Med. 2008; 34(9): 1565–9.
9. Carr JA. Abdominal compartment syndrome: a decade of progress. J Am Coll Surg. 2013;216:135–46.
10. Diebel LN, Dulchavsky SA, Brown WJ. Splanchnic ischemia and bacterial translocation in the abdominal compartment syndrome. J Trauma. 1997;43:852–855; Biffl WL, Moore EE, Zallen G, et al. Neutrophils are primed for cytotoxicity and resist apoptosis in injured. Surgery. 1999;126(2):198–202.
11. Leng Y, Zhang K, Fan J, et al. Effect of acute, slightly increased intra-abdominal pressure on intestinal permeability and oxidative stress in a rat model. PLoS One. 2014;9:e109350; Kirkpatrick AW, Roberts DJ, De Waele J, et al. Is intra-abdominal hypertension a missing factor that drives. Crit Care.2014;18(2):124.
12. Sawchuck DJ, Wittmann BK. Preeclampsia renamed and reframed: intra-abdominal hypertension in pregnancy. Med Hypotheses. 2014;83:619–32.
13. Lozada MJ, Goyal V, Levin D, et al. Management of peripartum intra-abdominal hypertension and abdominal compartment syndrome. Acta Obstet Gynecol Scand. 2019;98(11):1386–97.
14. Holodinsky JK, Roberts DJ, Ball CG, et al. Risk factors for intra-abdominal hypertension and abdominal compartment syndrome among adult intensive care unit patients: a systematic review and meta-analysis. Crit Care. 2013;17: R249; Roberts DJ, Bobrovitz N, Zygun DA, et al. Indications for use damage control surgery and damage control interventions in civilian trauma patients: a scoping review. J Trauma Acute Care Surg. 2015;78:1187–1196; Roberts DJ, Bobrovitz N, Zygun DA, et al. Indications for use of thoracic, abdominal, pelvic, and vascular damage control interventions in trauma patients: a content analysis and expert appropriateness rating study. J Trauma Acute Care Surg. 2015;79:568–579.
15. Waldhausen JH, Shirmer BD. The effect of ambulation on the recovery from postoperative ileus. Ann Surg 1990. 2012(6): 671–7; Cheatham ML, Chapman WC; Key SP, et al. A meta-analysis of selective versus routine nasogastric decompression after elective laparotomy. Ann Surg. 1995;221(5): 469–76; Reasbeck PG, Rice ML, Herbison GP. Nasogastric intubation after intestinal resection. Surg Gynecol Obstet. 1984;158(4):354–8.
16. Augustin G, Maierovic M. Non-obstetrical acute abdomen during pregnancy. Eur J Obstet Gynecol Reprod Biol. 2007;131(1):4–12.
17. Colonic transit in rats: effects of ovariectomy, sex steroid hormones, and pregnancy. Am J Physio. 1986; 251:46; Everson GT. Gastrointestinal motility in pregnancy. Gastroenterol Clin North Am. 1992;21:751–776.
18. Kirkpatrick AW, Brenneman FD, McLean RF, et al. Is clinical examination an accurate indicator of raised intra-abdominal pressure in critically injured patients? Can J Surg. 2000; 43:207–211; Sugrue M, Bauman A, Jones F, et al, Clinical examination is an inaccurate predictor of intra-abdominal pressure. WorJd J Surg. 2002;26:1428–1421.
19. De Keulenger BL, De Waele JJ, Powell B, Malbrainn ML. What is normal intra-abdominal pressure and how is it affected by positioning, ¿body mass and positive end-expiratory pressure? Intensive Care Med. 2009;35:969–97.
20. Malbrain ML, Cheatham ML, Kirkpatrick A, Sugrue M, Parr M, De Waele J, Balogh Z, Leppaniemi A, Olverra C, Iyatury R, et al. Results from the international conference of experts on intra-abdominal hypertension and abdominal compartment syndrome. I. Definitions. Intensive Care Med. 2006;32:1722–32.
21. Cheatham ML, Malbrain ML, Kirkpatrick A, Sugrue M, Parr M, De Waele J, Balogh Z, Leppaniemi A, Olivera C, Iyatury R, et al. Results from the international conference of expert on intra-abdominal hypertension and abdominal compartment syndrome II. Recommendations. Intensive Care Med. 33(6):951–62.
22. Staelens ASE, Van Cauwelaert S, Tomsin K, Mesens T, Malbrain MLN, et al. Intra-abdominal pressure measurements in term pregnancy and postpartum: an observational study. PLoS One. 2014;9(8):e104782.

23. Kinsella SM. Lateral tilt for pregnant women: why 15 degrees? Anesthesia. 2003;58: 835–836; Bamber JH, Dresnes M. Aortocaval compressión in pregnancy: the effect of changing the degree and direction of lateral tilt on maternal cardiac output. Anesth Analg. 2003;97: 256–258.
24. International Journal of Obstetric Anesthesia. 2012;21: 135–139.
25. Shelly MP, Robinson AA, Hesford JW. Haemodynamic effects following surgical release on increased intraabdominal pressure. Br J Anesth. 1987;59(6): 800–805; Celoria G, Steingrub. Dawson JA. Oliguria from high intra-abdominal pressure secondary to ovarian mass. Crit Care Med. 1987;15(1): 78–79.
26. Silasi M, Cohen B, Karumanchi SA, Rana S. Abnormal placentation, angiogenic factors, and the pathogenesis of preeclampsia. Obstet Gynecol Clin N Am. 2010;37:239–53.
27. Contreras F, Foiullioux C, Bolivar A, Betancourt MC, Colmenares Y, Rivero M, Israili Z, Velasco M. Endothelium and hypertensive disorders in pregnancy. Am J Ther. 2003;10:415–22.
28. Paramore RH. Eclampsia and its incidence [abstract]. Proc R Soc Med. 1992;15: 14–16; Muller JP, Dillemans M, Crombach C, Missant C, Sels A. On the abdominal pressure volume relationship. Inter J Anesthesiol. 2009; 21(1).
29. Sugerman HJ. Hypothesis: preeclampsia is a venous disease secondary to an increased intra-abdominal pressure. Med Hypothesis. 2011;77:841–9.
30. Chun R, Baahirzada L, Tiruto C, Kirkpatrick AW. Measurement on intra-abdominal pressure in term pregnancy: a pilot study. Int J Obbstet Anesth. 2012;21:135–9. https://doi.org/10.1016/j.ijoa.2011.10.010.
31. Cheatham ML, White MW, Sagraves SG, et al. Abdominal perfusion pressure: a superior parameter in the assessment of intra-abdominal hypertension. J Trauma. 2000;49(4):621–6; discussion 6–7.
32. De Laet I, Hoste E, Verholen E, et al. The effect of neuromuscular blockers in patients with intra-abdominal hypertension. Intensive Care Med. 2007; 33(10): 1811–4; Cheatham ML, Safcsak K. Percutaneous catheter decompression in the treatment of elevated intra-abdominal pressure. Chest. 2011; 140(6): 1428–35; Malbrain ML, Marik PE, Witters I, et al. Fluid overload, de-resuscitation, and outcomes in critically ill or injured patients: a systematic review with suggestions for clinical practice. Anesthesiol Intensive Ther. 2014; 46(5): 361–80.
33. Roberts DJ, De Waele J, Kirkpatrick AW, et al. Intra-abdominal hypertension and the abdominal compartment syndrome. In O'Donnell JM, Flavio N, editors. Surgical intensive care medicine. 3rd ed. Switzerland; Springer International Publishing; Cheatham ML. Non-operative management of intra-abdominal hypertension and abdominal compartment syndrome. World J Surg. 2009; 33(6): 1116–1122; Cheatam ML. Abdominal compartment syndrome. Curr Opin Crit Care. 2009;15(2): 154–162.
34. Oullet JF, Leppaniemi A, Ball CG, et al. Alternatives to formal abdominal decompression. Arn Surg. 2011;77(Suppl 1):S51–7.
35. Guyton CA. Gastrointestinal physiology. In: Textbook of medical physiology. 9th ed. Philadelphia: W.B. Saunders company; 1996. p. 793–812.
36. Lawson M, Kern F Jr, Everson GT. Gastrointestinal transit time inhuman pregnancy: prolongation in the second and third trimester followed by post-partum normalization. Gastroenterology. 1985;89:996–9.
37. Vilz O, Wehner S, Pantelis D, Katff JC. Immunomodulatory aspects in the development, prophylaxis and therapy for postoperative ileus. Zentralbl Chir. 2014;139:434–44.
38. Condon RE, Cowles VE, Ferraz AA, et al. Human colonic smooth muscle electrical activity during and after recovery from postoperative ileus. Am J Physiol. 1995;269(3 Pt 1): G408–17; Livingston EH, Passaro EP Jr. Postoperative ileus. Dig Dis Sci. 1990;35(1):121–32.
39. Jones RS, Schimmer BD. Intestinal obstruction, pseudoobstruction and ileus. In: Gastrointestinal disease: pathophysiology, diagnosis and management, vol 1, 4th ed. Philadelphia: WB. Saunders company; 1989, p. 369–80; Summers RW, Lu CC. Approach to the patient with ileus and obstruction, In: Textbook of gastroenterology, vol I, 2nd ed. Philadelphia: JB. Lippimcott Company; 1995, p. 756–812; Kumar D. Obstruction of small and large bowel and ileus. In: Gastroenterology clinical science and practice, vol 2, 2nd ed. London: WB. Saunders Company; 1993, p. 1033–44; Jones RS. Intestinal obstruction. In:

textbook of Surgery: the biological basis of modern surgical practice. 15th ed. Philadelphia: WB. Saunders Company; 1993, p. 915–23.
40. Kurz A, Sessler DI. Opioid-induced bowel-dysfunction: pathophysiology and potential new therapies. Drugs. 2003; 63(7): 640–71; Fallon MT, Hanks GW. Morphine, constipation and performance status in advanced cancer patients. Palliat Med. 1999;13(2):159–60.
41. Vanagunas A. GLob.libr. Women's med., 2008 (ISSN: 1756-2228).
42. Siddall J, Inkster H. Maternity guidelines-bowel complications after CS inc, Paralytic ileus (GL796) June 2018 NHS foundation trust.
43. Ogilvie WH. William Heneage Ogilvie 1887–1971. Large-intestine colic due to sympathetic deprivation. A new clinical syndrome. Dis Colon Rectum. 1987;30:984–7.
44. Kilpatrick CC, Monga M. Approach to the acute abdomen in pregnancy: Obstet Gynecol Clin N Am. 2007;34:389–402; Meyerson S, Holtz T, Ehrinpreis M et al. Small bowel obstruction in pregnancy. Am J Gastroenterol. 1995;90:299–302.
45. Batke M, Cappell MS. Adynamic ileus and acute colonic pseudo-obstruction. Med Clin Am. 2008;92:640–70.
46. Moore FA, Feliciano DV, Andrassy RI, et al. Early enteral feeding, compared with parenteral, reduces postoperative septic complications: the results of a meta-analysis. Ann Surg. 1992;216(2): 172–83; Binderow SR; Cohen Sm, Wexner SD, et al. Must early postoperative oral intake be limited to laparoscopy? Dis Col Rectum. 1994; 37(6):584–9; Carr CS, Ling KD, Boulos P, et al. Randomized trial of safety and efficacy of immediate postoperative enteral feeding in patients undergoing gastrointestinal resection. Br Med J. 1996; 312(7035): 869–71; Koretz RL, Avenell A, Lipman TO, et al. Does enteral nutrition affect clinical outcome? A systematic review of the randomized trials. Am J Gastroenterol. 2007; 102(2): 412–29; Shilder JM, Hurteau JA, Look KY, et al. A prospective controlled trial of early postoperative oral intake following major abdominal gynecologic surgery. Gynecol Oncol. 1997; 67(3):235–40.
47. Acute colonic pseudo-obstruction after cesarean section. The Obstetrician an Gynecologist. 2006;8:207–13.
48. Vilz TO, Stoffels B, StraBburg C, Schil HH, Kalff JC. Ileus in adults -pathogenesis, investigation and treatment. Dtsch Arztebl Int. 2017;114:508–18.
49. Matros E, Rocha F, Zinner M, et al. Does gum chewing ameliorate postoperative ileus? Results of prospective, randomized, placebo-controlled trial. J Am Coll Surg. 2006;202(5):773–8.
50. Wen Z, Shen M, Wu C, Ding J, Mei B. Chewing gum for intestinal function recovery after cesarean section: a systematic review and meta-analysis. BMC Pregnancy Childbirth. 2017;17(1): 105; Altraigev A, Ellaithv M, Atia H, Abdelrehim W, Abbas AM; Asiri M. J Matern Fetal Neonatal The effect of gum chewing on the return of bowel motility after planned cesarean delivery: a randomized controlled trial. Medicine. 2018:1-8.
51. Valle RG, Godoy FL. Neostigmine for acute colonic pseudo-obstruction: A meta-analysis. Ann Med Surg (Lond). 2014;3:60–4.
52. Pereira P, Djeudjj F, Leduc P, Fanget F, Barth X. Ogilvie's syndrome acute colonic pseudo-obstruction. J Visc Surg. 2015;152:99–105.
53. Geller A, Peterson BT, Gostout CJ Endoscopic decompression for acute colonic pseudo-obstruction. Gastrointest Endosc. 1996;44:144–50; De Giorgio R, Knowles CH. Acute colonic pseudo-obstruction. Br J Surg. 2009;96:229–39.
54. Al-Khan A, Shah M, Altabban M et al. Measurement of intra-abdominal pressure in pregnant women at term. J Reprod Med. 2011;56:53–7.

Chapter 20
Burn Management in Pregnancy

Sofia Santareno and António Gandra d'Almeida

Introduction

The estimated incidence of burns is 2.6/100,000 person-years in the non-obstetric patient, compared to 0.17/100,000 person-years in the general population [1, 2]. Burns may occur from motor vehicle collisions, fires within a closed space, electrical accidents, or chemicals [3]. Most pregnancy-associated burns in the USA occur accidentally at home (hot water, open flames); electrical and chemical burns are rare [4]. This number is low in the developed countries, so there is lack of information in order to standardize the clinical decision making for practice guidance. Most of the case reports come from undeveloped countries, where the access to the best healthcare is even harder [5–8].

Maternal-Fetal Considerations

Pregnancy itself leads to neurological and endocrine changes (activated renin-angiotensin-aldosterone system [9], increased level of cortisol and adrenaline) [10, 11]. Pregnancy-induced hypertension [12, 13] and gestational diabetes [14] are not uncommon; it is reasonable to presume that severe burns might worse these pathologies [15]. The hemodynamic changes in the pregnant burn patient also have specific characteristics – the cardiac output and volume of circulating blood starts to increase

S. Santareno (✉)
Plastic Surgery Department, Burn Unit of University Hospital of Northern, Lisbon, Portugal

The Dr Pure Clinic, Lisbon, Portugal

A. G. d'Almeida
Head of Education of CSMC, Porto e Região, Portugal

The Dr Pure Clinic, Lisbon, Portugal

C. Montufar et al. (eds.), *Obstetric Catastrophes*,
https://doi.org/10.1007/978-3-030-70034-8_20

from 6 to 8 weeks and gradually reaches a peak at 32–34 weeks of gestation, with an increase of 30–45% in total volume (average 1.5 L) [15]. Maternal blood pressure and respiratory rate return to baseline as pregnancy approaches the term [16]. Two to three weeks after delivery, the cardiac output and circulating blood volume are gradually restored [17].

Burns in pregnant patients pose a high challenge to emergency management. First, the mechanism of injury in burns differs significantly from other forms of trauma – direct thermal injury; inhalation injury to the airway; accumulation in the maternal bloodstream of toxic substances released by combustion, such as carbon monoxide or cyanide; or dissipation of electrical current [3]. Second, the anatomic and physiologic changes related to the pregnancy make the treatment of these patients more complex: not only the calculation of the TBSAB should take in consideration the extent of the expanded abdominal skin but also the increased edema of the oropharynx and larynx which lowers the threshold for intubation when an inhalation injury is suspected [3]. In pregnant patient, the supine position may cause inferior vena cava compression and significant hypotension [16].

Lastly, the fetus is the challenge, because, in pregnancy, trauma has little effect on maternal morbidity and mortality. [16]. Fetal injuries are not typically direct injuries, but rather secondary to maternal adaptive changes (loss of airway, changes to uterine blood flow, loss of oxygen dissociation, or toxicity from cyanide). There are some rare cases of direct injury to the fetus through severe thermal or electrical injury. Fetal survival is dependent on maternal survival [18].

It is widely recognized that the effect of burns on fetal and maternal survival is detrimental, and there is a relationship between the percentage of maternal TBSAB and maternal and fetal mortality, as well as premature delivery [19]. Maternal odds of death increase by 8% for every 1% in TBSAB ($P < 0.001$; 95% confidence interval, 5.5–12.7%), after adjustment for the trimester of pregnancy [20]. Furthermore, for an additional increase in mother's TBSAB, the odds of fetal death are increased by 1.9% (0.99–1.04%) adjusted for maternal death. It has been reported that maternal and fetal mortality rates approach 50% when 40–60% of a mother's TBSAB [21, 22]. For the pregnant burned patient with TBSAB of 60% or greater, maternal and therefore fetal survival become progressively less likely and rare when higher than 90% [20]. Fortunately, burns greater than 40% TBSAB are infrequent. There is no statistical association between maternal ($P = 0.650$) and fetal mortality ($P = 0.707$) and the surgical treatment of wounds [20].

In the last 20 years, there have been some cases of maternal survival with burns exceeding 60% of TBSAB [20]; this may be explained by the improvement of health assistance and the sensibility for this special condition. Most of the recent publications listed sepsis as the main cause of maternal death [5, 6, 23–26], due to hypovolemic shock with respiratory failure [27]. Other reports stated the inhalation injury as the second most important factor after TBSAB in determining fetal and maternal mortality [2, 7]. In case of fetal death, it is more frequent within a week of the initial injury [16].

Guidelines

Acute Management Guidelines

A pre-hospital communication before the transference of such patients is advisable, so that a multidisciplinary, collaborative team (general surgeon, plastic surgeon, emergency/intensive care doctor, obstetrician, pneumologist, and/or ophthalmologist) is available at the emergency room and an operating room is ready in case of need.

At the emergency room, we recommend the *Advanced Trauma Life Support* principles of ABCDE for an efficient and standardized approach of these patients [28]. Basic information regarding the accident context is collected – burn etiology, burn context, open or closed environment, time, previous measures and medications, past medical history including pregnancy health status (gestational hypertension, gestational diabetes, or other combined diseases [19]), usual medication, allergies, past immunization, and estimated body weight. Rarely, some patients attempt suicide through self-immolation; the clinician should also be concerned about the possibility of maltreatment. The burn history should be matched with the burn pattern. Lifesaving measures for the burn patient include establishing airway control, stopping the burning process, and gaining intravenous access with fluid resuscitation [28]. Evaluation of the mother and fetus is recommended to occur simultaneously, not sequentially [3].

A – The priority is the establishment of a patent and trustable *airway* [29]. If an inhalation injury is suspected (observe if face or neck burns, singeing of the eyebrows and nasal vibrissae, carbon deposits in the mouth or nose, erythema in the oropharynx, hoarseness, explosion context), the airway patency is mandatory, either by close monitoring or elective intubation with lower threshold (if needed prior to transport) [28, 30, 31]. Stridor is an indication for immediate endotracheal intubation [28]. Evidence also suggests less time available for intubation after the administration of the paralytic for general anesthesia, because oxygen saturation decreases more quickly [20]. In some cases, a surgical airway may be required [28]. The ventilator settings must consider the 30–50% tidal volume increase and the mild respiratory alkalosis of the pregnant state [32]. Also, an evaluation of the carboxyhemoglobin (CO) levels is undertaken. On the other hand, the diagnosis of cyanite (CN) poisoning is difficult and should be based on a high suspicion level regarding the accident set, the altered mental status, signs of inhalation injury, severe lactic acidosis, and venous blood with high oxygenation content [20].

B – Secondary, the *breathing* quality must be assessed. Breathing concerns arise from hypoxia (inadequate ventilation due to circumferential chest burns or thoracic trauma), carbon monoxide poisoning, and smoke inhalation injury (inhalation of carbon particles and toxic products of combustion, such as CN). The respiratory rate and peripheral oxygen saturation must be evaluated. An initial chest X-ray and arterial blood gas should be attained in case inhalation injury is suspected [28]. The maternal acidosis may predict the fetal outcome [16].

Supplemental 100% oxygen with or without intubation is advisable. If the patient's hemodynamic condition allows and spinal injury has been excluded, elevation of the head and chest by 30 degrees helps to reduce neck and chest edema. In case of a full-thickness burn of the anterolateral chest wall that leads to severe restriction of the chest wall motion, even in the absence of a circumferential burn, chest wall escharotomy may be required [28].

C – Thirdly, the *circulation status* should be addressed. Blood pressure, heart rate, and auricular body temperature measurements are mandatory. The peripheral pulses should be evaluated and the temperature of the limbs as well, especially in case of suspicion of a circumferential burn. Blood pressure assessment may be difficult or unreliable in severe burned patients, but monitoring of hourly urinary output can reliably assess circulating blood volume (in the absence of osmotic diuresis like in glycosuria). An indwelling urinary catheter and two peripheral venous accesses of at least 16 gauge, preferably in the upper limbs, should be inserted [28]. The initiation of invasive monitoring is performed only if absolutely required [33]. Positioning of the patient in a 15-degree left lateral tilt helps to prevent vena cava compression and may be better with a mechanical wedge [34, 35].

Blood tests and serologies should be collected (burn unit protocol) as well as a urinary sample. Kleihauer-Betke is not necessary [16].

D – The next step is the evaluation of *disabilities* through a quick neurologic evaluation of the mother – Glasgow Coma Scale, pupillary light response, and focal neurologic exam – and the evaluation of the fetus well-being through cardiotocographic monitoring (CTM) as soon as possible [16, 20, 28]. If the fetus is viable, CTM monitoring should be at least for 4 hours, even after a minor trauma [16].

If pregnancy history is unavailable, the correct evaluation of the gestational age by the obstetric team is mandatory (measurement of the physical indexes of the fetus – biparietal diameter, head circumference, and height of the femur using B-mode ultrasound – or fundal height measurement) [15, 20]. An early ultrasonographic evaluation may also diagnose free intraperitoneal fluid [16].

The obstetric team should also evaluate the presence of vaginal bleeding or discharge, rule out broken fetal membranes, if cervix is closed/opened, and the presence of uterine contractions and/or fetal movements [15]. The best indicator of maternal health can be the initial fetal health. If premature labor is present, tocolytic therapy should be undertaken in consultation with the obstetrician, because tocolytics can cause delirious effects upon the fluid distribution [16, 36].

E – *Exposure* of all the body surface should be performed. Any indirect signs for major bleeding. Necessary radiographs should not be withheld at any period of gestation; radiation after the 20th week of gestational age is safe [16].

The initial *evaluation* of the TBSAB is usually completed by the emergency department physician, using the rule of nines – the anterior compartment chest, abdomen, and each leg account for 9% of the total body surface area, the genitalia is 1%, and the face and each arm are 4.5%. These numbers are the same on the posterior aspect of the body, without an equivalent for the genitalia. The palmar surface (including the fingers) of the patient's hand represents approximately 1% of the patient's body surface [28]. This traditional rule underestimates the protuberance of the gravid abdomen. Only second (partial-thickness) or third (full-thickness) degree burns are considered in the calculation of TBSAB.

Extra care is provided with priority of stopping the burn process: nonadherent clothes and jewelry are carefully removed, dry chemical powders are brushed off, and the involved surface areas are rinsed with copious amount of warm tap water [28]. Burns are covered with Vaseline gauze, compresses, and light ligatures [15]. The patient is covered with warm, clean, dry linen to prevent hypothermia [28].

Aggressive resuscitation of the mother is the best management for the fetus, since fetal outcome is directly related to maternal outcome. Early and aggressive intravenous fluid administration is the most important measure, because fluid loss and utero-placental hypoperfusion are most likely in the first 12 hours after a major burn [36].

Generally, patients with greater than 20% TBSAB must undergo formal fluid resuscitation, calculated with the *Parkland* formula (4 mL/kg of lactated *Ringer*'s solution for each percentage of estimated TBSAB over the first 24 hours, the first half over the first 8 hours, followed by the second half over the next 16 hours) [37]. There is no evidence basis to guide the fluid resuscitation for a pregnant burn patient, though it appears reasonable to increase resuscitation volumes by 30%, given the same volume increase in total body water for pregnancy and a concurrent increase in maternal cardiac output of 43% (to the uterus, placenta, and breasts) [21, 38]. Furthermore, if by any chance, a delivery is undertaken within the first 24 h, the fluid management should be recalculated after it [15]. There are special situations such as inhalation injuries where patients may benefit from an extra 30% increase in fluid resuscitation [33]. The least amount of fluid required should be used to maintain adequate urine output (a urinary catheter should be placed to ensure urine output of at least 0.5 ml/kg/hour early in the course of therapy) [39]. Achieving balance in the fluid management is an art. On the one hand, overhydration must be avoided, since it may result in pulmonary edema and acute respiratory distress syndrome [40]. On the other, even mild dehydration can often trigger preterm contractions via release of vasopressin from the posterior pituitary and concurrent release of small amounts of oxytocin [41]. Also, the release of cytokines and inflammatory mediators such as prostaglandins from damage to the epidermis can interact with the uterus and also cause contractions to ensue [42].

Fetal Considerations and Outcome

Fetal outcome is inextricably linked to maternal outcome, and as such, appropriate maternal therapy should minimize or prevent fetal demise and limit injury. However, this correlation is not 100%. Continuous fetal monitoring should be commenced as soon as possible when the pregnancy is estimated to be 24 or more weeks in gestational age. Waiting for the clear indication for delivery provided by a category 3 tracing may be waiting too long to undertake expedient delivery. The cumulative data available demonstrate a maternal mortality of 35% or greater at a TBSAB of 55% with an associated fetal mortality risk of 30% or greater [20].

Within the context of ensuring the survival of the neonate, if the mother has sustained a burn greater than 50% TBSA and gestational age is over 24 weeks, urgent (as early as possible) delivery should be performed. This will improve maternal pulmonary mechanics, prevent fetal distress, and increase the fetus survival chances. If the fetus is still immature, data is lacking to support a deferred delivery in order to administer fetal lung maturation corticosteroids [15, 20, 22]. However, in cases with burns of less than 55%, continuing with resuscitative measures along with continuous fetal monitoring and administration of steroids is a reasonable approach; however until then, the fetus is under the risk of drug toxicity due to the treatment strategies [15, 20]. In this second case, continuous fetal monitoring should be continued for the first 48 hours following the burn during fluid resuscitation and the most likely time for the fetoplacental unit to fail.

Fetal implications for loss may be worse when the mother suffers inhalation injury at the time of burn because fetal deaths were reported in association with TBSAB as little as 13% during the second trimester.

In cases of maternal burn patients with inhalation injury, due to the risk of fetal asphyxia as described earlier, the authors recommend expedient delivery of a viable infant and early maternal intubation. We are unable to provide a specific TBSAB at which this should take place as our data lack the power needed to make such a conclusion [20].

Figure 20.1 is a proposed algorithm that may be used for the triage and management of pregnant burn patients.

Subacute Management

We recommend that after the initial maternal fetal-perinatal evaluation and management have been assured, these patients should be transferred to a burn center. After the acute phase of resuscitation, early skin grafting is undertaken within the

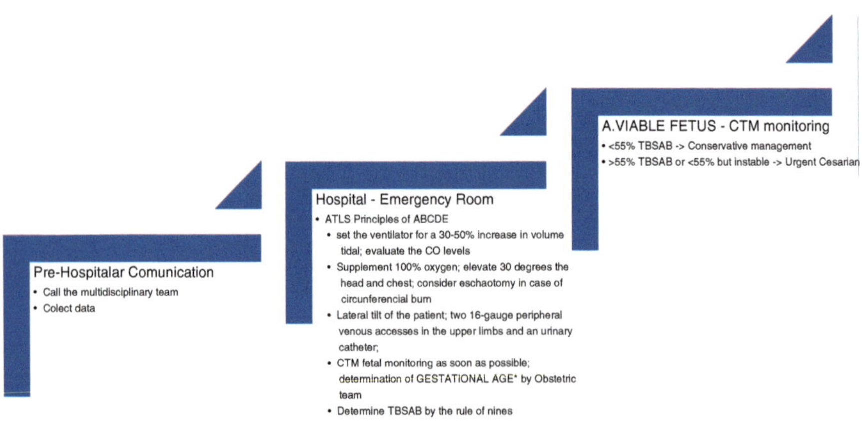

Fig. 20.1 Algorithm for the triage and management of pregnant burn patients

first 48 hours of burn injury or as early as possible. This approach, also advisable in the general population, has shown to be safe for both mother and fetus and to decrease the mortality [25]. Two studies provided evidence that conservatively treated patients had a 25% mortality rate versus only 3% in the aggressively treated surgical group (early eschar excision and skin grafting), with the rates of abortion, stillbirth, preterm delivery, and term delivery not statistically different [24, 43]. This intervention should be done in collaboration and consultation with an obstetrician because the need for emergent delivery could arise during surgery.

In case autologous skin graft is unavailable, there are no data on the safety of synthetic grafts. We highlight the idea of the utilization of the autologous amnion as a temporary skin substitute if delivery is undertaken.

General Support

These patients may be admitted for prolonged time. All patients with a major burn (greater than 20% TBSA) should be managed at a burn center, in concert with burn and obstetric consultants [16]. The obstetrician gynecologist is usually a consultant and not the primary care provider. Above 23 weeks of gestational age, frequent fetal surveillance is advisable – daily NST testing (24–26 weeks) and either frequent NST or biophysical profile testing (after 26 weeks) [20].

During prolonged hospitalization, chemical and mechanical deep venous thrombosis prophylaxis is recommended (as the hypercoagulable state of pregnancy coincides with immobilization in these victims) [44]. Gastric ulcer prophylaxis using an H2 blocker or proton pump inhibitor is also safe and recommended. Although controversial, systemic antibiotic prophylaxis is advisable by some authors to prevent sepsis, in opposition to the general burn population [45]. The US Food and Drug Administration (FDA) has classified the antibiotics into five grades (A, B, C, D, X) according to the possible side effects for the fetus. Penicillins, macrolides, cephalosporins, lincomycin, and clindamycin belong to grade B drugs, which are safe for pregnant women and could be used during pregnancy. Quinolones, itraconazole, and fluconazole belong to grade C drugs, and animal experiments have revealed negative influences on the fetus; therefore, they are selected only when potential benefits exceed potential risks [15]. Additionally, tetanus toxoid and immunoglobulin can be administered safely in pregnancy when indicated [16].

The dressings should be changed every 2 days [15]; the burns should be cleaned with chlorohexidine soap and physiologic water and then a Vaseline gauze and a topical antibiotic agent; amikacin is not advisable since it has reported teratogenic effects [20]. Care must be taken with silver sulfadiazine, since it can be absorbed from the wounds: the average $Ag +$ concentration in the blood reaches 190 ng/mL at 10 days after application for patients with <35% TBSA and deposits into the liver and kidneys [46]; on the other hand, absorption of sulfonamides is related to kernicterus [15].

Oral feeding is preferred with dietitian adjustments for the increased metabolic demands of pregnancy. The second option is enteral feeding with promotility agents such as erythromycin which may be used to counteract the depressive effects of progesterone and/or some analgesic medications on gastric motility.

We emphasize the importance of stabilizing the burned patient's airway and delaying extubation if there is evidence or risk of laryngeal edema from an inhalation injury. Specific medications to be used for induction, paralysis, and anesthesia can be in accord with institutional practices for obstetric patients undergoing surgery [20].

The mother may suffer from some complications that may impact fetal outcome. In the case of severe sepsis, delivery of the fetus is recommended because it will allow the use of aggressive antibiotics and improve the immunocompromised state of pregnancy. On the other hand, the stress of hypovolemia from the burn, increased metabolic demand during healing and vasodilation secondary to severe sepsis, and increased metabolic activity pose risks to the fetus, which likely outweigh any benefits from pregnancy continuation [20].

Fetal intervention must be weighed against the risk to maternal health, although performing a perimortem cesarean within 4 minutes of cardiac arrest may improve maternal and possibly fetal outcomes [3].

Special Considerations

Inhalation Injury

In pregnant patients, survival is correlated with carboxyhemoglobin (COHb) levels and not with the PaO2/FIO2 ratio as in non-pregnant [47]. Carbon monoxide crosses the placental barrier and affects the fetus [48, 49]. Furthermore, fetal levels of CO can reach levels up to 15% higher than those of the mother, causing several adverse effects, most importantly on the oxygen dissociation curve – it increases the hemoglobin's affinity for oxygen which results in fetal hypoxemia that may be reflected in fetal hear rate tracings [20]. The highest levels of CO are detectable on the fetal side 4 hours after the exposure [50]. Current recommendations define CO poisoning as COHb greater than 10% and define severe poisoning as levels greater than 20–25% [51]. Adverse fetal outcomes are usually seen when COHb levels exceed greater than 48%; there is increased fetal sensitivity to CO poisoning as gestation progresses [52]. It is also important to consider CN poisoning (closed-space fires, nylon and polyurethane combustion) because it can lower the threshold for lethal CO poisoning [52, 53]. CN causes dysfunction at the mitochondrial level with inhibition of the cytochrome oxidase chain, which leads to lactic acidosis.

An inhalation injury (suspected when there is soot in airway) worsens the outcomes even at low TBSAB, so early intubation is mandatory [20].

The treatment for inhaled CO poisoning (level over 10%) is 100% oxygen non-rebreather mask for at least 6 hours (reduces the half-life of CO more effectively in the mother than in the fetus) [54]. Hyperbaric oxygen can also be considered if available in the same hospital and only if the patient is stable.

Suspicion of CN poisoning (closed-space fires) should be managed with hydroxocobalamin Cyanokit® (pregnancy category C, approved by the FDA in October 2010), which is superior to the traditional CN antidote, since it does not produce methemoglobin [52, 55]. Hydroxocobalamin is the only antidote safe enough to use in a pregnant patient, and its ability to cross the placental barrier is well documented.

Electrical Burns

There are few reports on this kind of injury during pregnancy. Most home-based electrical burns are low voltage (110 or 220 V), so the injury remains superficial. However, with higher-voltage currents (lightning strikes, transmission cables), there can be serious burn, secondary traumatic injuries, and pregnancy loss [22, 56].

The physical properties of electrical lead to unique trauma, since the energy is conducted through the least-resistant tissues (mainly the bone, nerves, and vessels) and exits most often through a ground limb. Within its path, the energy may alter the electrical conduction of the heart and/or damage the bones, muscles, and blood vessels with thrombosis and/or produce nerve damage. The skin itself may not reflect the real extent of the internal injury. Patients frequently need fasciotomies [28].

A study reported a 94% live birth rate in electrical burns, concluding that neonatal outcome is usually unaffected [57]. The internal pathway of the electrical current is important, since if it goes from an upper to a lower limb and includes the uterus, it may be more harmful.

Rhabdomyolysis and cardiac dysrhythmias are possible complications. Rhabdomyolysis results in myoglobin release which can cause acute renal failure; if the patient's urine is dark, sign of myoglobinuria, fluid administration should be increased to ensure a urinary output of 100 ml/hour. Metabolic acidosis should be corrected by maintaining adequate perfusion [28].

In case of this type of injury, we advise an electrocardiogram and a Holter monitor to detect any maternal arrhythmias, which may require chest compression; a cardiology consultation should be scheduled as soon as possible in case of any arrhythmic episode. If there are no arrythmias within the first few hours of injury, monitoring is not necessary [28].

Immediately after the event, a nonstress test (NST) or Doppler ultrasonography should be undertaken to evaluate fetal status; these should be repeated 2 weeks later. It is also recommended a full neurological examination 2 weeks after [57, 58].

Chemical Burns

Chemical burns are influenced by duration of contact, concentration of the chemical, and amount of the agent. Alkali burns are generally more serious than acid burns, since the first penetrate more deeply.

There is no data regarding chemical burns in pregnant patients. We recommend the general approach of this pathology in the non-pregnant population.

In every case, the National Center for Poisoning should be immediately contacted by telephone. Rapid removal of the chemical and immediate attention to wound care are essential. If some dry powder is still present on the skin, clean it away before irrigating with water. Otherwise, immediately flush away the chemical with large amounts of water, for at least 20–30 minutes. Alkali burns require longer irrigation. Neutralizing agents should not be used, since they can cause an exothermic reaction with further damage. Alkali burns to the eye require continuous irrigation during the first 8 hours. A small catheter may be fixed in the palpebral sulcus for irrigation. Some specific chemical burns (hydrofluoric acid) require special care.

Conclusion

TBSAB independently predicts maternal and fetal mortality. However, further analysis demonstrates that maternal death is linked to fetal death and that TBSAB mediates this relationship via its effect on the mother. Evidence of fetal compromise suggests that maternal compensatory mechanisms are failing and that the mother is in significant danger as well. The most common causes for maternal death listed within these studies in descending order of frequency were sepsis/sepsis-related complications, respiratory failure, and shock.

Successful maternal and perinatal outcomes depend greatly on the quality and timeliness of aggressive emergent care. The critical points for emergent management of a burned pregnant patient include the following: (1) assure the airway patency and consider early intubation if inhalation injury is present; (2) rapid assessment of burn severity and TBSAB calculation; (3) determine gestational age; (4) if TBSAB is 20% or greater, aggressive fluid resuscitation; (5) continuous fetal heart rate monitoring if at equal to or greater than 24 weeks' gestational age; (6) if TBSAB is 55% or greater and fetus over 24 weeks' gestation, consider urgent cesarean; (7) early excision and skin grafting; (8) delivery if sepsis develops; (9) deep venous thrombosis, gastric ulcer, and antibiotic prophylaxis; and (10) continuous pregnancy or postpartum/postoperative care.

References

1. Mendez-Figueroa H, Dahlke JD, Vrees RA, Rouse DJ. Trauma in pregnancy: an updated systematic review. Am J Obstet Gynecol. 2013;209(1):1–10.
2. Maghsoudi H, Samnia R, Garadaghi A, Kianvar H. Burns in pregnancy. Burns. 2006;32(2):246–50.
3. Huls CK, Detlefs C. Trauma in pregnancy. Semin Perinatol. 2018;42(1):13–20.
4. American Burn Association.National Burn Repository annual report. 2012. Available at: http://ameriburn.org/NBR_annualreports.php. Accessed April 1 2014.

5. Mabogunje OA. Burns injuries during pregnancy: an African series. J Natl Med Assoc. 1990;82:641–4.
6. Rezavand N, Seyedzadeh A. Maternal and Foetal outcome of burns during pregnancy in Kermanshah, Iran. Ann Burns Fire Disasters. 2006;19(4):174–6.
7. Karimi H, Momeni M, Momeni M, Rahbar H. Burn injuries during pregnancy in Iran. Int J Gynaecol Obstet. 2009;104:132–4.
8. Mokube JA, Verla VS, Mbome VN, Bitang AT. Burns in pregnancy: a case report from Buea Regional Hospital, Cameroon. Pan Afr Med J. 2009;3:21.
9. Smith A, Barclay C, Quaba A, Sedowofia K, Stephen R, Thompson M, et al. The bigger the burn, the greater the stress. Burns. 1997;23:291–4.
10. Rainey WE, Rehman KS, Carr BR. Fetal and maternal adrenals in human pregnancy. Obstet Gynecol Clin N Am. 2004;31:817–35.
11. Hussein W, Lafayette RA. Renal function in normal and disordered pregnancy. Curr Opin Nephrol Hypertens. 2014;23:46–53.
12. Wanderer JP, Leffert LR, Mhyre JM, Kuklina EV, Callaghan WM, Bateman BT. Epidemiology of obstetric-related ICU admissions in Maryland: 1999–2008*. Crit Care Med. 2013;41: 1844–52.
13. Burlingame J, Horiuchi B, Ohana P, Onaka A, Sauvage LM. The contribution of heart disease to pregnancy-related mortality according to the pregnancy mortality surveillance system. J Perinatol. 2012;32:163–9.
14. Berger H, Crane J, Farine D, Armson A, De La Ronde S, Keenan-Lindsay L, et al. Maternal-fetal medicine committee, executive and Council for the Society of obstetricians and Gynaecologists of Canada. Screening for gestational diabetes mellitus. J Obstet Gynaecol Can. 2002;24:894–912.
15. Shi Y, Zhang X, Huang BG, Wang WK, Liu Y. Severe burn injury in late pregnancy: a case report and literature review. Burns Trauma. 2015;3:2.
16. Shah AJ, Kilcline BA. Trauma in pregnancy. Burns Trauma. 2015;3:2.
17. Chen H. Normal puerperium and lactation. In: Zhuang Y, editor. Modern obstetrics. 2nd ed. Beijing: Science Press; 2009. p. 173. In Chinese.
18. Parikh P, Sunesara I, Lutz E, Kolb J, Sawardecker S, Martin J. Burns during pregnancy: implications for maternal-perinatal providers and guidelines for practice. Obstet Gynecol Surv. 2015;70(10):633–43.
19. Polko LE, McMahon MJ. Burns in pregnancy. Obstet Gynecol Surv. 1998;53:50–6.
20. Parikh P, et al. Burns during pregnancy: implications for maternal-perinatal providers and guidelines for practice. Obstet Gynecol Surv. 2015;70(10):633–43.
21. Akhtar MA, Mulawkar PM, Kulkarni HR. Burns in pregnancy: effect in maternal and fetal outcomes. Burns. 1994;20:351–5.
22. Rayburn W, Smith B, Feller I, et al. Major burns during pregnancy: effects on fetal Well-being. Obstet Gynecol. 1984;63:392–5.
23. Cheah SH, Sivanesartnam V. Burns in pregnancy—maternal and fetal prognosis. Aust N Z J Obstet Gynaecol. 1989;29:143–5.
24. Jain ML, Garg AK. Burns with pregnancy—a review of 25 cases. Burns. 1993;19:166–7.
25. Prasanna M, Singh K. Early burn wound excision in "major" burns with "pregnancy": a preliminary report. Burns. 1996;22:234–7.
26. Chama CM, Na'Aya HU. Severe burn injury in pregnancy in Northern Nigeria. J Obstet Gynaecol. 2002;22:20–2.
27. Subrahmanyam M. Burns during pregnancy—effect on maternal and foetal outcomes. Ann Burns Fire Disasters. 2006;19:177–9.
28. Advanced trauma life support (ATLS®): the ninth edition. J Trauma Acute Care Surg. 2013;74(5):1363–6.
29. Hamel MS, Anderson BL, Rouse DJ. Oxygen for intrauterine resuscitation: of unproved benefit and potentially harmful. Am J Obstet Gynecol. 2014;211:124–7.
30. Madnani DD, Steele NP, de Vries E. Factors that predict the need for intubation in patients with smoke inhalation injury. Ear Nose Throat J. 2006;85:278–80.

31. Kuczkowski KM, Reisner LS, Benumof JL. Airway problems and new solutions for the obstetric patient. J Clin Anesth. 2003;15:552–63.
32. Taylor JW, Plunkett GD, McManus WF, et al. Thermal injury during pregnancy. Obstet Gynecol. 1976;47:434–8.
33. Dai NT, Chen TM, Cheng TY, et al. The comparison of early fluid therapy in extensive flame burns between inhalation and noninhalation injuries. Burns. 1998;24:671–5.
34. Fields JM, Catallo K, Au AK, et al. Resuscitation of the pregnant patient: what is the effect of patient positioning on inferior vena cava diameter? Resuscitation. 2013;84:304–8.
35. Cluver C, Novikova N, Hofmeyr GJ, et al. Maternal position during caesarean section for preventing maternal and neonatal complications. Cochrane Database Syst Rev. 2013;3:CD007623.
36. LAvery J, Staten-McCormik M. Management of moderate to severe trauma in pregnancy. Obstet Gynecol Clin N Am. 1995;22(1):69–90.
37. Pham TN, Cancio LC, Gibran NS, American Burn Association. American Burn Association practice guidelines burn shock resuscitation. J Burn Care Res. 2008;29:257–66.
38. Clark SL, Cotton DB, Lee W, et al. Central hemodynamic assessment of normal term pregnancy. Am J Obstet Gynecol. 1989;161(6 pt 1):1439–42.
39. MacKinnon DP, Lockwood CM, Williams J. Confidence limits for the indirect effect: distribution of the product and resampling methods. Multivariate Behav Res. 2004;39:99.
40. Saffle JI. The phenomenon of "fluid creep" in acute burn resuscitation. J Burn Care Res. 2007;28:382–95.
41. Antunes-Rodrigues J, de Castro M, Elias LL, et al. Neuroendocrine control of body fluid metabolism. Physiol Rev. 2004;84:169–208.
42. Stage AH. Severe burns in the pregnant patient. Obstet Gynecol. 1973;42:259–62.
43. Bartle EJ, Sun JH, Wang XW. Burns in pregnancy. J Burn Care Rehabil. 1988;9:485–7.
44. James A. Committee on practice bulletins—obstetrics. Practice bulletin no. 123: thromboembolismin pregnancy. Obstet Gynecol. 2011;118:718–29.
45. Vaizey C, Jacobson M, Cross F. Trauma in pregnancy. Br J Surg. 1994;81:1406–15.
46. Fox CL Jr. Silver sulfadiazine–a new topical therapy for Pseudomonas in burns. Therapy of Pseudomonas infection in burns. Arch Surg. 1968;96:184–8.
47. Yang HT, Yim H, Cho YS, et al. Investigation of relationship between inhalation injury assessment and prognosis in burn patients. J Korean Surg Soc. 2011;81:1–9.
48. Ginsberg MD, Myers RE. Fetal brain damage following maternal carbon monoxide intoxication: an experimental study. Acta Obstet Gynecol Scand. 1974;53:309–17.
49. Caravati EM, Adams CJ, Joyce SM, et al. Fetal toxicity associated with maternal carbon monoxide poisoning. Ann Emerg Med. 1988;17:714–7.
50. Longo LD. The biological effects of carbon monoxide on the pregnant woman, fetus and newborn infant. Am J Obstet Gynecol. 1977;129:69–103.
51. Olson K, Smollin C. Carbon monoxide poisoning (acute). BMJ Clin Evid. 2008;2008:2103.
52. Norman CA. Halton DM. Is carbon monoxide a workplace teratogen? A review and evaluation of the literature. Ann Occup Hyg. 1990;4:335–47.
53. Eckstein M, Maniscalco PM. Focus on smoke inhalation—the most common cause of acute cyanide poisoning. Prehosp Disaster Med. 2006;21:s49–55.
54. A registry for carbon monoxide poisoning in New York City. Hyperbaric Center Advisory Committee Emergency Medical Service, City of New York. J Toxicol Clin Toxicol. 1988;26:419–41.
55. Norris JC, Moore SJ, Hume AS. Synergistic lethality induced by the combination of carbon monoxide and cyanide. Toxicology. 1986;40:121–9.
56. Reess WD. Pregnant woman struck by lightning. Br Med J. 1965;1:103–4.
57. Einarson A, Bailey B, Inocencion G, et al. Accidental electric shock in pregnancy: a prospective cohort study. Am J Obstet Gynecol. 1997;176:678–81.
58. Pierce MR, Henderson RA, Mitchell JM. Cardiopulmonary arrest secondary to lightning injury in a pregnant woman. Ann Emerg Med. 1986;15:597–9.

Chapter 21
Drowning and Near-Drowning Management During Pregnancy

Judy Enamorado, Felix Parra, and Ezio Villegas

Introduction

Every year, drowning accounts for at least 500,000 deaths worldwide, including 4000 fatalities in the United States [1, 2]. In highly developed countries, the highest incidence of drowning is seen in children younger than 5 years of age and in persons 15 to 24 years of age. Reports from many parts of the world have emphasized that drowning is a leading cause of cardiac arrest in children and adolescents. Nonfatal drowning events may occur several hundred times as frequently as reported drowning deaths [3, 4].

Terminology

At the 2002 World Congress on Drowning held in Amsterdam, a group of experts suggested a new consensus definition for drowning in order to decrease the confusion over the number of terms and definitions that have appeared in the literature. This was named the "Utstein style" [5].

J. Enamorado (✉)
National Cardiopulmonary Institute, Tegucigalpa, Honduras

F. Parra
Antofagasta University Hospital and Antofagasta University, Antofagasta, Chile

E. Villegas
Obstetrics and Gynecological University Hospital Guayaquil, Guayaquil, Ecuador

C. Montufar et al. (eds.), *Obstetric Catastrophes*,
https://doi.org/10.1007/978-3-030-70034-8_21

Drowning

Drowning is a process resulting in primary respiratory impairment from submersion/immersion in a liquid medium. Implicit in this definition is that a liquid/air interface is present at the entrance of the victim's airway, preventing the victim from breathing air. The victim may live or die after this process, but whatever the outcome, the patient has been involved in a drowning incident [5].

Near Drowning

Near drowning has been defined as a "survival, at least temporarily, after suffocation by submersion in water" [6]. It usually refers to a critical aquatically predicament resolved by successful water rescue, definition implying certain recovery once the victim is removed from the water. However, this was not always the case; patients regaining consciousness after near drowning had subsequently died due to aspiration pneumonia, even though no apparent clinical signs could be found on the initial physical examination [1].

Nevertheless, it has also been used to describe patients who subsequently died from drowning. This usage has led to uncertainty about the meaning of the term. Therefore, an international group with scientific expertise in the field of drowning research that was supported by the European Resuscitation Council and the American Heart Association encouraged the abandonment of the "near-drowning" term that was considered to generate confusion [5].

Epidemiology

Drowning remains a significant worldwide public health concern, ranking as the third leading cause of unintentional injury death and accounting for 7% of all injury-related deaths [7, 8].

In the United States, from 2009 to 2019, 1539 deaths occurred in the female population (15–49 years), due to accidental drowning and submersion. No reports have been established in terms of pregnancy deaths due to drowning events [9].

Conditions Predisposing to Drowning

There are numerous clinical conditions that can lead to a drowning incident: seizures; arrhythmias, especially ventricular, torsades de pointes with long QT interval; coronary artery disease; depression; cardiomyopathy, dilated or hypertrophic obstructive; hypoglycemia; hypothermia; intoxication; alcohol and illicit drugs abuse; hyperventilation prior to a shallow dive; or trauma [8]. The most frequent cause of drowning in women is trauma.

Pathophysiology

The drowning sequence (fatal and nonfatal) typically begins with a period of panic, loss of the normal breathing pattern, breath-holding, air hunger, and struggle by the victim to stay above the water [2, 3]. In some cases, there is a primary loss of consciousness, and the victim stops after swimming underwater, floats on the surface, then becomes motionless, and quietly disappears [10]. Reflex inspiratory efforts eventually occur, leading to hypoxemia by either aspiration or reflex laryngospasm that occurs when water contacts the lower respiratory tract. Subsequently, hypoxemia affects every organ system, especially the brain, with deleterious effects and outcomes.

Aspiration of water results in decreased lung compliance, ventilation perfusion mismatching, and intrapulmonary shunting, leading to hypoxemia that causes diffuse organ disfunction due to tissue hypoxia [11].

The effects of tissue hypoxia in every organ go as follows.

Pulmonary: the aspiration of fluid results in different levels of hypoxemia, leading to noncardiogenic pulmonary edema, immediate drop in arterial pO_2, respiratory acidosis, and acute respiratory distress syndrome (ARDS) [3, 12] due to an effect of the water washing out surfactant and increase in plasma catecholamines. After inhalation of water, movement of fluid should occur along any osmotic gradient between alveolar spaces and plasma, depending on the osmolarity concentration in the water (freshwater or saltwater inhalation) [10].

Pulmonary edema in freshwater drowning has been attributed to various factors, including altered surfactant properties, altered pulmonary capillary permeability, neurogenic pulmonary edema, and forceful inspiration against a closed glottis. There are some reports in which 10–15% of drowning victims not aspirate water [10].

Respiratory insufficiency can develop rapidly o progressively; chest radiography can show localized or diffuse infiltrates. If the hypoxemia is severe, it can precipitate unconsciousness and immediate death due to cardiac arrest [10].

Neurologic: During the first minutes of submersion, the brain is deprived of oxygen. With cardiovascular compromise, cerebral blood flow falls, resulting in ischemic injury. The degree of hypoxic-ischemic damage varies in different regions of the brain; vascular end zones, the hippocampus, insular cortex, and basal ganglia are particularly susceptible [13]. The primary hypoxic-ischemic injury is irreversible, and the main aim of cerebral resuscitation is prevention of secondary neuronal damage [2]. Hypoxemia can develop neuronal damage, cerebral edema, and cranial hypertension. Approximately 20% of nonfatal drowning victims suffer from irreversible neurologic damage [14].

Cardiovascular: there are numerous of different arrhythmias seen in nonfatal drowning victims. These include from sinus tachycardia, sinus bradycardia, and atrial fibrillation to ventricular and fatal arrhythmias, especially in patients with congenital long QT syndrome in which swimming or diving can precipitate these events [15]. The cardiovascular effects seen with drowning and aspiration of water are not dependent on the tonicity of the aspirated fluid, but are the direct result of anoxia.

Acid-base and electrolytes: significant electrolyte imbalances usually are not seen, except in cases where drowning occur in highly sea saltwater. Hypermagnesemia has been described after seawater aspiration, possibly due to both ingestion and aspiration [16]. Metabolic and respiratory acidosis is often observed.

Renal: acute renal failure can develop due to acute tubular necrosis secondary to hypoxemia, shock, hemoglobinuria, or myoglobinuria [17, 18].

Coagulation: coagulopathy and hemolysis can occur, but is very rare [19].

Hypothermia: development of hypothermia is very common in immersion victims and can facilitate aspiration. When body temperature drops below 35 °C, muscular incoordination and weakness occur, which can interfere with swimming [20]. At temperatures below 30 °C, unconsciousness can occur, and the myocardium becomes irritable. Atrial fibrillation can be present, and in core temperatures below 28 °C, ventricular fibrillation is likely [10].

Management

Prompt removal for the water and effective initial resuscitation are of the utmost importance [10].

Assessment of the drowning victim should proceed using the "DRABC" algorithm: danger (to rescuer, bystanders, and casualty), response (of the casualty), airway, breathing, and circulation [10].

The initial management for pregnant women who suffered a drowning event is the same that corresponds to an adult patient, and the only change in treatment consists in the way of CPR is performed if necessary or evaluate the need for urgent delivery of the product through emergency cesarean procedure.

The management can be divided into three phases: prehospital care, emergency department care, and inpatient care.

- *Prehospital care:* the initial approach in victims who suffered drowning is rescue and immediate resuscitation to achieve restoration of spontaneous circulation. The patient should be removed onto a dry platform as quickly as possible. If it is feasible, extraction from the water should be in the horizontal position. Gravitational drainage of water and secretions from the upper airway by placing the patient in a head-down position (if possible) may be beneficial, but should not delay the institution of CPR [10]. Cardiopulmonary resuscitation should be determined as soon as possible. The best outcomes for both mother and fetus are likely to be achieved by successful maternal resuscitation. *The best care of the unborn fetus is optimal care for the mother* [21].

  Patient position has emerged as an important strategy to improve quality of CPR and resultant compression force and cardiac output. The gravid uterus can compress the inferior vena cava, impending venous return, thereby reducing stroke volume and cardiac output. Aortocaval compression can occur for singleton pregnancies at approximately 20 weeks of gestational age, at about the time the fundus is at or above the umbilicus. Manual lateral uterine displacement (LUD) effectively relieves aortocaval pressure in patients with hypotension [22]. It is very important to not delay the removal of the victim from the water. Ventilation is the first priority in CPR rather than chest compressions in drowning victims, and rescue breathing should begin as soon as the rescuer reaches shallow water or a stable surface. If the patient does not respond to the delivery of two rescue breaths that make the chest rise, the rescuer should immediately begin performing high-quality chest compressions according to standard BLS guidelines.

Cervical spinal cord injury is uncommon in nonfatal drowning victims, unless there are clinical evidence of injury or a concerning mechanism. According to the AHA Guidelines for Advanced Cardiac Life Support (ACLS), routine cervical spine immobilization can interfere with essential airway management and is not recommended [22, 23].

Life-threatening arrhythmias can be present in drowning victims; these are treated according ACLS protocols. Pulses may be very weak and difficult to palpate in the hypothermic patient with sinus bradycardia or atrial fibrillation; a careful search for pulses should be performed for at least 1 minute before initiating chest compressions in the hypothermic patient because these arrhythmias require no immediate treatment.

The Heimlich maneuver or other postural drainage techniques to remove water from the lungs are of no proven value, and rescue breathing should not be delayed in order to perform these maneuvers. If it is necessary in pregnant women, this maneuver has to be performed different than the classic; the rescuer places their hand in the center of the chest to compress, rather than in the abdomen [22, 24, 25].

High-flow supplemental oxygen should be administered to spontaneously breathing patients by face mask; apneic patients should be intubated.

Attempts at rewarming hypothermic patients with a core temperature < 33 °C should be initiated, either by passive or active means available.

– *Emergency department management:* the patient should be transferred as soon as possible to a hospital; prehospital resuscitative efforts should be continued and the airway secured.

Once the patient is admitted to the emergency room, continuous measurement of vital signs including oxygen saturation, end-tidal CO_2 cardiac telemetry via monitor, and clinical reassessment has to be performed. The obstetrics team also should be notified to attend immediately to evaluate the patient and the fetus status.

A trauma evaluation should be performed and appropriate imaging studies obtained as indicated.

Wet clothing should be removed and rewarming initiated in hypothermic patients. Methods include passive and active external rewarming and active internal core rewarming.

In symptomatic patients who do not require immediate intubation, supplemental oxygen should be provided to maintain the SpO_2 above 94 percent. Respiratory support provided by noninvasive ventilation via CPAP (continuous positive airway pressure) or BiPAP (bi-level positive airway pressure) could be useful to improve oxygenation [19].

Indications for intubation include the following: cardiorespiratory arrest, Glasgow Coma Scale (GCS) below 8 points, or evidence of neurological deterioration or inability to protect the airway, paO_2 below 60 mm Hg or oxygen saturation (SpO_2) below 90 percent despite high-flow supplemental oxygen [19].

Initial resuscitation efforts of the pregnant patient should focus on a secure protected airway and removal of blood flow obstruction caused by the gravid uterus [21]. Bag valve mask ventilation with supplemental oxygen is recommended before intubation attempts due to faster desaturation in pregnant patients. Endotracheal intubation should occur as soon as possible while maintaining cricoid pressure. Verification of endotracheal placement should be performed by colorimetric carbon dioxide detection of waveform capnometry. An orogastric tube must be placed right after endotracheal intubation to relieve gastric distension, which occurs from passive passage of fluid and is common in nonfatal drowning patients [21].

Smaller ventilatory volumes should be used given the diaphragm elevation and increased potential for gastric insufflation due to decreased lower esophageal sphincter tone. Aspiration of large volumes of fluids with submersion is rare, but increased inspiratory and positive end-expiratory pressure (PEEP) may be required to achieve adequate ventilation and oxygenation due to pulmonary edema or acute lung injury. The beneficial use of pulmonary surfactant has been documented in case reports of freshwater drowning and may be considered.

Displacement of the gravid uterus away from the inferior vena cava and aorta likely improves hemodynamics beyond 20 weeks of gestation using a one- or two-handed technique. This allows the patient to remain supine for other procedures including chest compressions and intubation. If manual displacement is not successful, tilting the patient 30° to the left from supine using blanket rolls or a commercially available wedge should be attempted [21].

Preparation for emergent cesarean delivery should be made as soon as cardiac arrest is identified in pregnant patient. Deliveries performed within 5 minutes of arrest of the mother result in the highest survival rates for infants above 24 to 25 weeks of gestational age. Early delivery may also benefit the successful resuscitation of the mother. Removing the fetus allows for decompression of the inferior vena cava and abdominal aorta, allowing for improved venous return and cardiac output in the mother. Obstetric or surgical consultants should be contacted for definite management after resuscitation if not already present for the perimortem cesarean section [21].

- Patient disposition: most nonfatal drowning victims are hospitalized because of the severity of illness or concern for clinical deterioration.

  Symptomatic patients should be admitted to a monitored setting until symptoms and physiologic disturbances resolve. Routine laboratory tests such as blood counts, renal and liver function, electrolytes, coagulation studies, and arterial blood gases if respiratory or circulatory failure develops are reasonable to carry out in the symptomatic pregnant women, and a complete study of the fetus itself including fetal Doppler and ultrasound is mandatory in this cases.

Asymptomatic patients should be closely observed for approximately 8 hours and admitted if any deterioration occurs [26, 27].

- *Inpatient management*: symptomatic patients require hospitalization for supportive care and treatment of organ-specific complications.

Neurologic injuries: the two major determinants of neurologic outcomes are the neurologic state of the patient at the time of evaluation and the duration of loss of consciousness. Therefore, therapeutic measures should be headed to prevent secondary neurologic injuries due to ongoing ischemia, cerebral edema hypoxemia, acidosis, fluid and electrolyte imbalances, and seizure activity.

Different actions can be performed in order to achieve an adequate neurocritical care including the following: the head of the bed should be elevated to 30 degrees if potential cervical spine injuries have been excluded [28], and for patients in imminent danger of cerebral herniation, hyperventilation may be used acutely as a temporizing measure to reduce intracranial pressure blood volume. Prolonged hyperventilation should be avoided because it can cause vasoconstriction, decreasing cerebral blood flow and worsening cerebral ischemia. Seizure activity, which increases cerebral oxygen consumption and blood flow, should be aggressively controlled. Neuromuscular blocking agents should be avoided because it can mask neurological examination. Euglycemia should be targeted avoiding hypo- or hyperglycemia due to their harmful effects on the brain. Normothermia is preferable than hyperthermia as it increases cerebral metabolic demands and lowers the seizure threshold. Indication for therapeutic hypothermia in nonfatal drowning patients remains unclear due to insufficient data to support its use [29].

Respiratory failure or infection: chest radiograph in nonfatal drowning patients should be only indicated if respiratory failure is detected or there is clinical worsening of oxygenation, hypercarbia, or increased respiratory distress. The chest radiograph is almost invariably abnormal and typically shows bilateral infiltrates, which cannot a priori be differentiated from any other cause of pulmonary edema. Chest CT reveals patchy or diffuse airspace consolidation. Pneumomediastinum and interstitial emphysema have been observed after near drowning on CT scan [10]. Special caution in pregnant women with less than 20 weeks of gestation due to effects of radiation; however if it is necessary, a protective leaded vest is mandatory. Bronchospasm is frequent and is treated similarly to acute asthma using inhaled beta-adrenergic agonists [29]. The routine use of systemic glucocorticoids or prophylactic antibiotics is not recommended due to lack of evidence. Antibiotics should be used only in cases of clinical pulmonary infection or if the victim was submerged in grossly contaminated water. If pneumonia follows nonfatal drowning, a high suspicion for waterborne pathogens, such as *Aeromonas*, *Pseudomonas*, and *Proteus*, must be maintained. There is no evidence that the use of diuretics can improve outcome, and fluid management should be designed to maintain hemodynamic stability and an adequate urine output [29].

More severely affected patients may require general supportive care to maintain oxygenation or an adequate cerebral perfusion pressure.

Mechanical ventilatory strategies are similar to those employed in other types of acute lung injury, including protective ventilation, using tidal volumes between 6 and 8 ml/Kg, plateau pressures below 30 cm of water, and inspiratory oxygen fraction to target an oxygen saturation between 88 and 92 percent, and in cases of respiratory distress syndrome, the use of high PEEP is mandatory to keep alveolar units open. For refractory hypoxemia, a simple intervention is prone positioning.

Patients requiring respiratory support have a high risk (around 50%) of bacterial or fungal pneumonia.

Hypotension: patients with hypothermia can have significant hypovolemia and hypotension due to a decreased antidiuretic hormone production [29].

Encephalopathy: general supportive measures should be directed toward maintenance of cerebral oxygenation. Increased intracranial pressure (ICP), due to cerebral vasodilatation, may be a concern if permissive hypercapnia is used to treat ARDS. Provided pulmonary gas exchange is adequate to allow it, maintenance of normocapnia is recommended. Seizures should be appropriately treated. Neither corticosteroids nor barbiturates coma have been shown to be efficacious [10].

Metabolic control: it is recommended that in the near-drowned patient, blood glucose should be frequently monitored and normoglycemia maintained.

Outcome

Depends on duration of submersion and the duration and severity hypoxia. In one study correlating the severity of respiratory involvement with mortality, citing 93% mortality for those presenting in arrest (emerg med clin).

Factors associated with poor outcome are duration of submersion >5 minutes (most important), time to effective life support >10 minutes, resuscitation duration >25 minutes, age > 14 years, Glasgow Coma Scale <5, ventricular tachycardia or fibrillation on initial electrocardiogram (ECG), fixed and dilated pupils on initial evaluation, persistent apnea and requirement of cardiopulmonary resuscitation in the emergency department, and arterial blood pH < 7.1 upon presentation [29].

Predictors of poor outcome in clinical imaging like magnetic resonance were brain edema, basal ganglia T2 hypersensitivity, elevated brain lactate, or depressed N-acetylaspartate or creatine levels [10].

Suspected drug or alcohol abuse preceding the drowning was associated with a bad outcome (defined as death or survival with severe neurologic sequelae).

References

1. Papa L, Hoelle R, Idris A. Systematic review of definitions for drowning incidents. Resuscitation. 2005;65:255–64.
2. Salomez F, Vincent JL. Drowning: a review of epidemiology, pathophysiology, treatment and prevention. Resuscitation. 2004;63:261.
3. Bierens JJ, Knape JT, Gelissen HP. Drowning. Curr Opin Crit Care. 2002;8:578.
4. Orlowski JP. Drowning, near-drowning, and ice-water drowning. JAMA. 1988;260:390.
5. Idris AH, Berg RA, Bierens J, et al. Recommended guidelines for uniform reporting of data from drowning: the "Utstein style". Circulation. 2003;108:2565.

6. Modell JH. Drown versus near-drown: a discussion of definitions. Crit Care Med. 1981;9:351–2.
7. Szpilman D, Sempsrott J, Webber J, Hawkins SC, Barcala-Furelos R, Schmidt A, et al. 'Dry drowning' and other myths. Cleve Clin J Med. 2018;7:529–35.
8. Dowd MD. Dry drowning: myths and misconceptions. Pediatr Ann. 2017;46(10):e354–7.
9. World Health Organization. World Health Organization Global Report on Drowning. Available at http://www.who.int/violence_injuryprevention/global_report_drowning/final_report_full_web.pdf. 2014.
10. Moon R, Long R. Drowning and near-drowning. Emerg Med. 2002;14(4):377–86.
11. Battaglia JD, Lockhart CH. Drowning and near-drowning. Pediatr Ann. 1977;6:270.
12. DeNicola LK, Falk JL, Swanson ME, et al. Submersion injuries in children and adults. Crit Care Clin. 1997;13:477.
13. Ibsen LM, Koch T. Submersion and asphyxial injury. Crit Care Med. 2002;30:S402–8.
14. Gonzalez-Rothi RJ. Near drowning: consensus and controversies in pulmonary and cerebral resuscitation. Heart Lung. 1987;16:474.
15. Rivers JF, Orr G, Lee HA. Drowning. Its clinical sequelae and management. Br Med J. 1970;2:157.
16. Cohen DS, Matthay MA, Cogan MG, et al. Pulmonary edema associated with salt water near-drowning: new insights. Am Rev Respir Dis. 1992;146:794–6.
17. Fandel I, Bancalari E. Near-drowning in children: clinical aspects. Pediatrics. 1976;58:573.
18. Bonnor R, Siddiqui M, Ahuja TS. Rhabdomyolisis associated with near-drowning. Am J Med Sci. 1999;318:201.
19. Layon AJ, Modell JH. Drowning: update 2009. Anesthesiology. 2009;110:1390.
20. Tipton M, Eglin C, Gennser M, et al. Immersion deaths and deterioration in swimming performance in cold water. Lancet. 1999;354:626–9.
21. Ferguson JD, De Guzman J. Cardiac arrest in special populations. Emerg Med Clin N Am. 2012;30:169–78.
22. Lavonas EJ, Drennan IR, Gabrielli A, et al. Part 10: special circumstances of resuscitation: 2015 American Heart Association guidelines update for cardiopulmonary resuscitation and emergency cardiovascular care. Circulation. 2015;132:S501–18.
23. Vanden Hoek TL, Morrison LJ, Shuster M, et al. Part 12: cardiac arrest in special situations: 2010 American Heart Association guidelines update for cardiopulmonary resuscitation and emergency cardiovascular care. Circulation. 2010;122:S829.
24. Schmidt AC, Sempsrott JR, Hawkins SC, et al. Wilderness medical society practice guidelines for the prevention and treatment of drowning. Wilderness Environ Med. 2016;27:236.
25. Rosen P, Stoto M, Harley J. The use of the Heimlich maneuver in near drowning: Institute of Medicine report. J Emerg Med. 1995;13:397.
26. Pratt FD, Haynes BE. Incidence of "secondary drowning" after saltwater submersion. Ann Emerg Med. 1986;15:1084.
27. Causey AL, Tilelli JA, Swanson ME. Predicting discharge in uncomplicated near-drowning. Am J Emerg Med. 2000;18:9.
28. Sarnaik AP, Preston G, Lieh-Lai M, Eisenbrey AB. Intracranial pressure and cerebral perfusion pressure in near-drowning. Crit Care Med. 1985;13:224.
29. Chandy D, Weinhouse G. Drowning (submersion injuries). In: Danzl D, editor. Uptodate, Waltham Mass.: 2019. https://www.uptodate.com/contents/drowning-submersion-injuries?search=drowning&source=search_result&selectedTitle=1~79&usage_type=default&display_rank=1. Accessed December 19, 2019.

Chapter 22
Acute Spinal Cord Compression in Pregnant Woman

Sabrina Da Re Gutiérrez, Jorge Sinclair Ávila, Jorge E. Sinclair De Frías, and Maily Velasco Miranda

Introduction

Epidural spinal hematoma (ESH) is a consequence of spinal neurosurgical procedures, but its appearance during pregnancy, postpartum, or in the general population is rare [4] and can cause permanent damage to pregnant women [15].

Bidzinski described the first case of spontaneous ESH in a 26-year-old woman with a 6-month pregnancy that suddenly presented severe interscapular pain and weakness in the lower limbs that evolved to paraplegia within the hour after the onset of symptoms [3].

On the other hand, acute subdural spinal hematoma (SDSH) was described by Shiller et al. In 1948 as a complication of hemophilia [12], it is a rare pathology, associated with high morbidity and mortality [9, 11], and it is less frequent than ESH and that cerebral subdural hematoma [2]. Mortality ranges from 1.3%; however, morbidity can reach 28% [9].

In both pathologies (ESH and SDSH), it is important to make an accurate diagnosis and timely treatment, to avoid irreversible neurological damage that may occur [11], maximizing the probability of treatment success [1]. According to Popov

S. Da Re Gutiérrez (✉)
Critical and Intensive Care Medicine, Maternal and Child Hospital, Caja Nacional de Salud (CNS), La Paz, Bolivia

J. S. Ávila
Critical Medicine, UCI Hospital Pacifica Salud/Johns Hopkins Medicine, Faculty of Medicine University of Panama, Panama City, Panamá

J. E. Sinclair De Frías
Santo Tomas Hospital, Faculty of Medicine University of Panama, Panamá City, Panamá

M. V. Miranda
Gynecological Obstetric and Pediatric University Hospital, Guayaquil, Ecuador

C. Montufar et al. (eds.), *Obstetric Catastrophes*,
https://doi.org/10.1007/978-3-030-70034-8_22

et al., approximately 15% of acute spinal cord injuries occur in women of childbearing age [8].

In the United States, more or less 1000 new spinal cord injuries are reported per year in women between 16 and 30 years, deserving that pregnancies in this group have a multidisciplinary management [7]. However, the incidence of traumatic spinal cord injuries at the gestation stage is low [6].

Definition

The SDSH is defined as the presence of bleeding in the subdural spinal space, while the ESH is the presence of bleeding in the epidural or epidural space.

Etiology

According to Beer et al., the causes of spinal hematomas can be classified in [2]:

1. *Traumatic*:
   - Typical vertebral hemangioma: secondary to blunt trauma that produced epidural hematoma [1]
   - Atypical vertebral hemangioma: minimal trauma fracture that produced anterior epidural hematomas [1]
2. *Iatrogenic*: After epidural anesthesia, lumbar puncture or spinal surgery (the frequency of epidural hematoma after spinal surgery is low compared to that inherent in epidural anesthesia where 1: 220,000 cases are described) [1].
3. *Spontaneous*: By anticoagulant therapy, vascular malformation, spinal artery aneurysm, neoplasia [5, 11], eclampsia, hemorrhagic diathesis, leukemia, thrombocytopenia, hemophilia, cryoglobulinemia, polycythemia, and systemic lupus erythematous. Rare causes of SDSH include chronic renal failure, fibromuscular dysplasia, cystic fibrosis, and rhabdomyolysis [9, 11].

   Another cause of ESH mentioned in the literature is extramedullary hematopoiesis that occurs in patients with myelosclerosis and thalassemia, although its occurrence is rare [9].

   Pereira, in his description of 151 patients with acute nontraumatic spontaneous SDSH, determined that 46% received anticoagulant therapy or had some coagulopathy secondary to a hematological disorder [9]. In another review by Domenicucci et al., regarding 106 patients with acute spontaneous SDSH, 54% of the cases were associated with hemorrhagic disorder and 14% with iatrogenic causes [9].

Pathogenesis

Anatomical Memory

The spinal cord runs through the medullary canal and extends from the great occipital hole to the thoracic 12 or lumbar 1 vertebrae where it ends as a horsetail (cauda equina) and from there continues the filum terminale to the coccyx.

The epidural space is between the dura and the periosteum of the spinal canal. The subarachnoid space is between the pia mater and arachnoid, is a real space, and contains cerebrospinal fluid, while the subdural space is virtual in physiological conditions and becomes a true space in pathological conditions [1].

According to Lazorthes, cited by Alvarez et al., "Arterial irrigation of the medulla is provided by 31 root arteries that can be divided into the root arteries in the strict sense (ending in the spinal roots or the dura, without reaching the medulla), the radiculopial arteries (which reach the arachnoid) and the radiculomedular arteries (which are solely responsible for the supply of arterial blood to the marrow and of which there are only seven or eight in the human body)" [1]. The most transcendental artery at the cervical thoracic level C1-T2 is the cervical enlargement artery, while at the thoracic level T2-T8 there is little blood supply (demonstrated by arteriography) being this, an area susceptible to ischemia. At the thoracolumbar level T9-S5 "is the great root artery that in 75% of people runs along one of the anterior spinal roots from T9 to T12; in 10% of one of the spinal roots of L1 or L2, and in 15% of one of the spinal roots of T5-T8" [1].

Pathogenesis of Spontaneous ESH

The evidence shows that this type of hematoma is of rare presentation [4].

The epidural space is a compartment with negative pressure composed of the vertebral venous system and with a blood flow dependent on both thoracoabdominal pressure changes and hydrostatic factors [4].

It is inferred that the susceptibility of epidural spinal veins to "congestion during pregnancy" [4] and the "sharp increase in epidural spinal vein pressure" contribute to the formation of SEH.

Also, the aorto-cava compression suffered by pregnant women, especially after the second trimester, would prevent adequate venous return causing greater congestion of the spinal veins of the epidural space.

Another theory for the existence of spontaneous SEH proposes that "... the abnormal development of veins, [in] areas of small local resistance (*locus minoris resistentiae*)..." [4], more structural changes of the vessels secondary to the increase in progesterone and estrogen during the third trimester of pregnancy can contribute to the formation of spontaneous SEH.

Pathogenesis of Spontaneous ESH

It is postulated that bleeding at this level is secondary "…to the rupture of the vessels within the spinal subarachnoid space after a rapid increase in intrathoracic or intra- abdominal pressure" [9], profuse "...bleeding within the subarachnoid space" [9] that breaks into the subdural space, causing SDSH.

Another possibility is also the rupture of small extra arachnoid vessels found along the dural surface [9].

Pathogenesis of Subarachnoid Spinal Hematoma (SASH)

The presence of hematoma in the subarachnoid space is secondary to the rupture of the root vessels parallel to each nerve root, knowing that there is no irrigation in this space [1].

Pathogenesis of Intramedullary Hematoma

This type of bleeding may be secondary to tumors or vascular malformations [13].

Pathogenesis of Traumatic Cause Spinal Edema

Spinal cord edema may be related to motor deficit and trauma severity. Rowland et al., cited by Saadoun and Papadopoulos state that cell edema that occurs between 2 and 48 hours after acute spinal cord injury coincides with secondary ischemia [10].

Spinal cord injury can be accompanied by both cytotoxic spinal edema secondary to the increase of water in the intracellular space through an intact spinal cord barrier and vasogenic edema due to the accumulation of water in the interstitial space that occurs in the site of spinal barrier injury [10].

The spinal subarachnoid space is larger than the cerebral. There are no hard edges around the spinal cord and the ability to "(…) expand the spinal cord in its circumference only at the site of the lesión" would be the conditions that would allow for the existence of more space to accommodate the edema of the spinal cord [10].

In this regard, the formation of spinal edema involves water channel proteins "expressed in plasma cell membranes that typically increase the osmotic permeability of the plasma cell membrane between 5 and 20 times" [10] called aquaporins. The first aquaporin was described in 1988 by Peter Agre. There are currently 13 types of aquaporins; of all of them, aquaporin 4 (AQP4) and 9 (AQP9), are found at the level of the spinal cord. On the point, in a medullary compression model performed in mice, Saadoun and Papadopoulos showed that the deletion of aquaporin 4 decreases the formation of edema in the spinal cord [10]. Once the spinal edema was formed, the water would be removed through the white matter tracts by an independent route of AQP4.

Therefore, the removal of AQP4 after a spinal cord injury would decrease the formation of cytotoxic edema without interfering with the elimination of edema.

Signs and Symptoms

Acute spinal cord injury may be due to ischemic damage or primary mechanical injury [7].

Acute spinal cord injury causes loss of sympathetic innervation with a preponderance of parasympathetic effects such as bradycardia, hypotension, decreased cardiac output, and dry and warm skin that contributes to heat loss with the consequent hypothermia. All this can generate fetal suffering [8]. In addition, peripheral vasodilation due to parasympathetic effect causes neurogenic shock that may persist for 1–3 weeks [7].

Signs and symptoms will also vary depending on the level of the injury. Thus, spinal cord lesions above T1 are accompanied by tetraplegia, bradycardia (which can be manifested with the Valsalva maneuver, position changes, aspiration of tracheal secretions, or increased intrathoracic pressures as an effect of the vagal stimulus, causing bradycardia secondary to activation of the vagus nerve), and – infrequent – autonomic dysreflexia [7]. Hypothermia occurs due to inappropriate loss of heat through the skin due to peripheral vasodilation.

In contrast, lesions below T1 but above T6 cause paraplegia and symptoms/signs of hyperreflexia or autonomic dysreflexia characterized by limb spasticity, respiratory distress, nasal congestion, symmetrical or asymmetric pupillary dilation, blurred vision, body redness above the level of the lesion [7], systemic arterial hypertension, tachycardia and/or tachyarrhythmia, sweating, headache, piloerection, profuse sweating chest pain, tremor, anxiety, nausea, seizures, intracerebral hemorrhage, and neurological deficit including death [8]. Systemic arterial hypertension may also be a response to angiotensin [7].

Dysreflexia can cause "uteroplacental vasoconstriction, fetal hypoxemia and fetal bradycardia" [7].

Verduyn performed a review of "33 women with spinal cord injuries, who had a total of 50 deliveries" [14], of the 33 cases, 15 cases (45%) suffered a car accident. The 33 women were divided into 2 groups, those with lesions above T6 and another group with lesions below T6, determining that lesions above T6 presented hyperreflexia or autonomic dysreflexia in 22 of the 27 women [14].

Cases of spontaneous SDSH are accompanied by severe pain in the posterior thorax with radicular signs, motor, sensory, and autonomic dysfunction, as well as urinary retention [9].

Domenicucci et al., cited by Rettenmaier et al., determined the presence of "motor deficits in 57% of patients, spinal pain in 45% of patients, root pain in 22% of patients and paraesthesia" [9], in addition to sphincter dysfunction and headache (2017).

Less frequently, central cord syndrome, hemiparesis, and initially only headache with stiff neck [9]) may occur.

Another review by Henry et al. determined the presence of acute pain in the interscapular region, followed by paresthesia and neurological motor and/or sensory deficits, complete or incomplete paraplegia or tetraplegia, and Brown-Sequard syndrome. He described that the time between the presence of pain and the onset of neurological deficit was 60.3 hours (range: 1–336 hours) [4].

Cervical or cervicothoracic ESH cause cervical or interscapular pain. If the spinal hematoma is in the middle thoracic level, there is chest pain, and those located in the thoracic-lumbar region have pain in the posterior thorax that can radiate to the buttocks and lower extremities.

Numbness and weakness are indicators of progressive loss of motor and sensory function below the spinal hematoma site [4].

It should not be forgotten that pregnant women can present – normally – low back pain; however this is not accompanied by motor or sensory neurological deficit nor is it acute onset [4].

Pregnant women, due to spinal injury, can trigger labor with painless cervical contraction and dilation until they reach labor [8].

Diagnosis

The diagnostic technique and the decision of the applied therapy of the pregnant woman implies intense debate for the safety of the fetus.

Bone Scans

Although the risk of "exposure of the fetus to radiation in the third trimester" is low, it should be avoided if possible (2018).

Myelography

Myelography was the study most used before 1991 for the diagnosis of spontaneous SDSH. Subsequently, he highlighted magnetic resonance as a gold standard [9].

CT Scans

Computed tomography (CT) can identify hyperacute epidural hematoma that is characterized as having a crescent, hyperdense shape. Over time the hematoma becomes isodense and its identification can be difficult [1].

Magnetic Resonance

Magnetic resonance imaging is the study considered gold standard for the detection of spinal hematomas.

If there is a suspicion of ESH or SDSH, an MRI should be performed using ionizing radiation, as no effects have been reported on "fetal growth and development (...)" [4].

"... Spinal magnetic resonance angiography is 88% sensitive, 90% specific with a Positive predictive value of 88% and a negative predictive value of 90% for the detection of spinal dural arterial venous fistulas" [9] or venous malformations.

The characteristics of the spinal hematoma change over time [1]:

Hematoma hyperacute:

- T1: iso-hypointense
- T2: hyperintense (due to intracellular oxyhemoglobin)

Acute hematoma:

- T1: slightly hypo/isointense (because of "deoxyhemoglobin in hypoxic erythrocytes"; deoxyhemoglobin in hypoxic erythrocytes")
- T2: hypointense (secondary to "progressive concentration of erythrocytes, blood clot retraction and fibrin production")

Early subacute hematoma:

- T1: hyperintense (due to "oxidation of deoxyhemoglobin to methemoglobin")
- T2: hypointense due to "intracellular methemoglobin"

Late subacute hematoma:

- T1: hyperintense.
- T2: hyperintense. This is due to "extracellular methemoglobin after lysis of red blood cells."

Chronic hematoma:

- T1: hypointense
- T2: hypointense. Secondary to "hemosiderin and ferritin in macrophages"

The contrast medium used in magnetic resonance imaging can cause a peripheral enhancement that is attributed to the hyperemia of the dura mater; on the other hand, the central enhancement may be due to extravasation of the contrast due to vascular barrier injury [1].

Angiography

Spinal angiography is a diagnostic technique that allows to locate the vascular malformation, whose suspicion would have aroused the previous magnetic resonance study [1].

Differential Diagnosis

Pereira [7] and Álvarez et al. [1] state that the differential diagnosis is made in relation to:

- Preeclampsia/eclampsia
- Infectious diseases (e.g., spinal abscess)
- Vascular malformations
- Pathological fractures associated with tumor
- Intervertebral disc herniation
- Transverse myelopathy
- Cauda equina syndrome
- Anterior spinal artery syndrome

Treatment

The proper diagnosis plus timely treatment are of the utmost importance to avoid irreversible and permanent neurological injury. It is necessary to evaluate each particular case, requiring multidisciplinary management.

Aorto-cava compression of the uterus can cause supine hypotension itself that can be avoided by placing the pregnant woman in the left lateral recumbency or using a wedge-shaped cushion [6] to displace the uterus to the left side.

For Alvarez et al., pregnant patients with small spinal hematomas without neurological deficit or with mild deficit benefit from conservative treatment. On the other hand, those pregnant women with installed neurological deficit should receive surgical treatment for spinal hematoma drainage [1].

Regarding the type of anesthetics for spinal surgery, Pedabelle et al. report using propofol in induction and rocuronium bromide for intubation. The anesthesia was maintained with isoflurane and propofol mixed with ketamine (5:1), to avoid arterial hypotension, in addition to oxygen and air. No nitrous oxide was used to avoid the increased risk of intracranial hemorrhage in the premature fetus [6].

The treatment and rehabilitation of traumatic cervical spine injury in the third trimester of pregnancy is a challenge because of the inherent risks to the mother and the fetus.

Pedaballe et al. reported three cases of spinal injury in pregnant women during the second trimester of pregnancy, obtaining good results through early surgery and allowing the pregnancy to continue, compared to three cases of women with advanced pregnancy who received counseling treatment and who had an unfavorable result for the mother and fetus [6].

Emergency non-obstetric surgery from the second trimester of pregnancy is safe due to better tolerance to procedures under general anesthesia, although if necessary, non-obstetric surgery can be performed in any trimester of pregnancy. However, we must anticipate the evolution towards preterm birth [6].

The study by Groen et al., cited by Henry et al., conducted with 330 non-pregnant patients with SEH, demonstrated good results with SEH, drainage within 36 hours in patients with complete deficit, and within 48 hours in cases with incomplete deficit.

The surgery for the drainage of SEH should be performed early (without interrupting the pregnancy), thus improving the functional state of the mother and allowing the pregnancy to continue until it reaches its end. On the contrary, if there is a fetal risk, an emergency caesarean section should be performed [4].

Jea et al. recommend the prone position (...) in the form of L (...) in relation to the lateral or sitting position [4]. Options for the treatment of SDSH include surgical drainage and percutaneous or conservative drainage. In case of mild deficit, the pregnant woman can receive conservative treatment, but if the motor or sensory deficit is severe, the surgical drainage of the hematoma should be performed [9].

Compression of the spinal cord secondary to extramedullary hematopoiesis was described in 1954 for the first time by Gatto et al. It is more common in men between and 45 years. The existence of hematopoietic tissue in the spinal canal is preferably located in the middle of the lower region of the spine [9]. These patients may require surgical decompression, blood transfusion, and even radiotherapy. Rettenmaier et al. report that patients treated with radiotherapy with a moderate dose of 10 to 30 Gray (Gy) had a remission of the complete neurological deficit by 75%, while 25% had a partial improvement. However, for pregnant women, radiotherapy is contraindicated and can benefit from "blood transfusions that could decrease red blood cell production and suppress extramedullary hematopoietic mass (…) improving cord compression symptoms" [9], with recovery at approximately 2 weeks. Through transfusions, a hematocrit of 30% is sought [9].

Neurogenic Shock

Neurogenic shock management is based on fluid administration: dobutamine to improve cardiac output and vasopressors [8].

Autonomic Dysreflexia

In the case of autonomic dysreflexia that causes an increase in blood pressure, the use of sodium nitroprusside, ganglionic blocking agents such as trimethaphan and mecamylamine, alpha-1 adrenergic blockers such as terazosin or guanethidine, and peripheral vasodilators such as hydralazine or nifedipine may be alternatives [7].

Thromboprophylaxis

Pregnancy predisposes a hypercoagulable state with a 4 to 5 times greater risk of developing thromboembolism. In this regard, prophylaxis with low molecular weight heparin (i.e., Clexane 60 mg/day subcutaneously in the thigh) can be performed, being careful not to administer it in the abdomen [6].

Treatment of Traumatic Spinal Cord Edema

The patient with spinal cord edema of a traumatic cause does not benefit from the administration of corticosteroids. The corticosteroid can be used in edema of tumor origin and in case of fetal lung maturation due to prematurity.

Agents such as hypertonic saline and mannitol are not used in spinal edema [10].

Surgical treatment is based on the stabilization of the spine with bone reduction without opening the dura; therefore, it is possible that the elevated pressure of the inflamed intraparenchymal cord at the site of the injury against the surrounding dura will continue [10].

Complications

- *Urinary tract infection*: Present in 35% during pregnancy due to urinary catheter, neurogenic bladder [7].
- *Constipation*: It is necessary to administer a diet rich in fiber and, if necessary, stool softener [7].
- *Pressure sores*: The factors that contribute to its appearance are immobilization and obesity [7].
- *Impaired lung function*: Especially in pregnant women with lesions above T5, which may require mechanical ventilatory support. Baseline vital capacity control and then serial controls are recommended [7].
- *Anemia*: Consequence of iron deficiency, folate deficiency, and/or renal failure.
- *Thromboembolism*: Pregnancy predisposes to a state of hypercoagulability with a 4 to 5 times greater risk of developing thromboembolism [6].

- *Autonomic dysreflexia*: It was described by Head and Riddoch during World War I, in 1917, and affects up to 85% of patients with spinal cord injury above T6. It is more common after cervical lesions than thoracic lesions (60% vs. 20%, respectively) [7].

Conclusion

1. The medullary compression of a pregnant woman, whether spontaneous or traumatic, is an emergency and must be treated by a multidisciplinary team determining the best options for the mother and the fetus, according to each case.
2. The evidence shows that spinal compression due to hematoma that causes severe motor or sensory deficit should receive surgical treatment.
3. Medullary compression due to small hematoma that causes mild deficit can receive conservative treatment. On the point, we report our experience with the case of a 41-year-old pregnant woman with severe preeclampsia and HELLP syndrome, undergoing caesarean section, which after regional anesthesia evolved with headache 3/10, lower limb paraplegia, and hypoesthesia with level sensitive T4. Practiced as a new anamnesis in the intensive care unit (ICU), the patient said she had pain in the neck and central region of the posterior thorax, in the hours before the caesarean section. Simple brain CT showed HSA and simple lumbar spine discarded spinal cord compression and/or lumbar occupancy, so dorsal cervical magnetic resonance was requested evidencing blood in subarachnoid space in addition to T4-T5 intramedullary bleeding. Upon admission to the ICU, the patient presented flaccid paraplegia with myotactic reflex of the lower extremities and hypoesthesia with a T4 sensory level, without bladder sphincter control (neurogenic bladder). After evaluation by neurosurgery, conservative behavior was decided without surgery. On day 20 of hospitalization, he presented paraparesis of the right lower limb 3/5 and the lower left limb 2/5. After 28 days of hospitalization, the paraparesis of the right lower limb improved to 4/5, and from the left to 3/5, and ½ hypoesthesia in T6. The new magnetic resonance control at 29 days after hospitalization showed intramedullary hematoma resolution and subarachnoid hemorrhage. The patient was discharged from hospital to follow physiotherapy sessions.

Bibliography

1. Alvarez PU, Ascencio JL, Riaño MF. Hematomas espinales. Revista Colombiana de Radiología. 2012;24(1):3640–7.
2. Beer M, Eysink M, Hille K. Spontaneous spinal subdural hematoma. Neurologist. 2017;22(1):34–9.
3. Bidzinski J. Spontaneous spinal epidural hematoma during pregnancy. J Neurosurg. 1966;24(6):1017.

4. Henry J, Messerer M, Thomas VD, Morandil X, Hamlatl A. Nontraumatic spinal epidural hematoma during pregnancy: diagnosis and management concern. Spinal Cord. 2012;50:655–60.
5. Morandi X, Riffaud L, Chabert E, Brassier G. Acute nontraumatic spinal subdural hematomas in three patients. Spine. 2001;26(23):E547–51.
6. Pedaballe A, Chhabra H, Tandon V, Chauhan P, Rachna V. Acute traumatic cervical spinal cord injury in a third-trimester pregnant female with good maternal and fetal outcome: a case report and literature review. Spinal Cord Ser Cases. 2018;4:93.
7. Pereira L. Obstetric management of the patient with spinal cord injury. Obstet Gynecol Surv. 2003;58(10):678–86.
8. Popov I, Ngambu F, Mantek G, Rout C, Moodley J. Acute spinal cord injury in pregnancy: an illustrative case and literature review. J Obstet Gynaecol. 2003;23(6):596–8.
9. Rettenmaier L, Holland M, Abel T. Acute, nontraumatic spontaneous spinal subdural hematoma: a case report and systematic review of the literature. Hindaii. Case Rep Neurol Med. 2017;2017:1–12.
10. Saadoun S, Papadopoulos M. Aquaporin-4 in brain and spinal cord oedema. Neurosicencie. 2010;168:1036–46.
11. Seizeur R, Ahmed S, Simon A, Basson G, Forlodou P. Acute non- traumatic spinal subdural haematoma: an unusual aetiology. J Clin Neurosci. 2009;16:842–3.
12. Shiller F, Neligan G, Budtz-Oslen O. Surgery in haemophilia a case of spinal subdural haematoma producing paraplegia. Lancet. 1948;27:842–5.
13. Varela P, Gonzales J, Regeuira M, Martinez P, Azevedo E. Hematomas espinales: la apoplejía espinal. Neurologia. 2010;25(2):96–103.
14. Verduyn W. Spinal cord injured women, pregnancy and delivery. Paraplegla. 1986;24:231–40.
15. Wang P, Tang Xin X, Lan H, Chen C, Liu B. Spontaneous cervical epidural hematoma during pregnancy: case report and literature review. Eur Spine J. 2011;20(2):176–9.

Chapter 23
Envenomations: Snakes Bites and Scorpion Stings

Ariatna Arlennys Aguilera Valderrama

Snakebites

Epidemiology

Poisoning by snakebites is a problem of great importance in public health worldwide especially in the regions of tropical forests in Africa, Asia, and Latin America. Reptile bites are rarely seen cases in emergency departments, but the prevalence is relatively higher in rural areas. In the past, it was estimated that mortality from venomous snakebite was around 25%; due to the availability of antivenom and advances in emergency and critical care, in those days, mortality rates are less than 0.5% [1].

The incidence of snakebites, regardless of the species involved, varies from country to country and between regions in a country, depending on factors as diverse as climate, ecological parameters, biodiversity, distribution of venomous snakes, human population density, economic activities, and types of dwellings, among others [2].

Estimates of snakebites range from 1.2 million to 5.5 million annually with envenomation occurring in 420,000 to 1,841,000 resulting in 20,000 to 94,000 deaths [3]. Other estimates suggest that more than 150,000 deaths may occur annually [4].

In Europe snakebites are relatively rare and the one involved belong to the family Viperidae represented in Europe by a few species that are not among the most poisonous; however in Britain there are approximately 200 hospitalizations annually from bites of snakes, but no deaths have been reported since 1975. On the other hand, countries such as France, Switzerland, Spain, and Italy have a very low incidence of snakebites [4].

A. A. Aguilera Valderrama (✉)
Critical Care Obstetrician, Department of Obstetrics and Gynecology, Division of Obstetrics Critical Care, Caja de Seguro Social, Panama City, Panama

C. Montufar et al. (eds.), *Obstetric Catastrophes*,
https://doi.org/10.1007/978-3-030-70034-8_23

In Africa scorpion stings are the most frequent events, and the snakebites are underestimated by health authorities over all because the information system is inaccurate. The wrong organization of health services in many countries complicates the management of patients and represents the great variation in the mortality rate [4]. In Asia there is a wide variation in the incidence of accidents according to human activities, and taking into consideration the snake species that participate in Japan, the general incidence of snakebites is about 1 case per 100,000 people so that the mortality rate of cases is less than 1% and the global mortality is approximately 0.5 per 100,000 population [4].

In this order in Canada and the United States with a population of approximately 270 million people, the annual incidence of snakebites on everything in the United States is like that observed in Europe. It has been estimated that 45 thousand of snakebites occur each year in North America, of these around 10,000 are caused by poisonous species, 6500 require medical intervention, and approximately 15 people bitten die every year [4].

In Latin America, the overall incidence of snakebite envenoming ranges from 5 to 62 cases/100,000 population per year, depending on the country (roughly corresponding from 130,000 to 150,000 cases in the whole region, with an estimated number of 2300 deaths) [5, 6]. A large number of cases, especially in Costa Rica, Nicaragua, Honduras, Panama, Colombia, Venezuela, and Ecuador, are inflicted by *Bothrops asper*, where it is responsible for 50–80% of the snakebites [7].

Panama presents the highest incidence of snakebites in the region (54–62 cases/100,000 population; 2000 bites per year), mostly by *Bothrops asper*, that is a whereas the incidence and total number of cases per year in other countries vary. These species belong to the family of Viperidae; there is another type of snake family Elapidae which are also called pit vipers; this snake venom is mainly neurotoxic, whereas Viperidae snake venom is mainly hematotoxic [7].

Effects of the Snake Venom

Snake venoms are primarily composed of mixtures of proteins and polypeptides with various properties. Many proteins have enzymatic activities, whereas others produce toxic cellular effects. Actions of snake venoms can be broadly classified as inflammatory, cytotoxic, neurotoxic, and hemotoxic; it depends on the type of snake; in some species, specific venom fractions block neuromuscular transmission, leading to ptosis, respiratory failure, and other neurologic effects. It causes local tissue injury, systemic vascular damage, hemolysis, fibrinolysis, and neuromuscular dysfunction, terminating with a combination of local and systemic endpoints. It may quickly alter blood vessel permeability, leading to loss of plasma and blood into the surrounding tissue and causing hypovolemia. It may also consume fibrinogen and platelets, causing a coagulopathy. The severity of poisoning, following snakebite, therefore, varies [10].

The cardinal signs of poisoning are the presence of one or more fang marks, localized pain, and progressive edema extending from the bite site. Other early symptoms and signs are nausea and vomiting, weakness, oral numbness or tingling of the tongue and mouth, tachycardia, dizziness, hematemesis, hematuria, thrombocytopenia, and fasciculations. In general, swelling becomes apparent within 15–30 min, but in some cases, it may not start for several hours. In severe cases, edema may progress to involve an entire limb within an hour. In less severe cases, edema may progress over a 1- to 2-day period [10].

The severity of these poisonings is very variable, and their evaluation is a fundamental element in the design of an adequate treatment. This severity depends on several factors, among which are:

- The amount of poison inoculated Viperidae species generally inoculates larger volumes of venom than the other species, thus causing higher-risk accidents.
- The anatomical site of the bite; accidents in the head and trunk tend to be more severe than bites in the extremities.
- Weight and height, as well as general physiological state, of the person bitten; for example, bites in children tend to get complicated frequently, partly due to the small volume of distribution that allows the poison to act more quickly at the systemic level.

There is a clinical gradation of snakebites envenoming that summarize next [8].

Grade	Envenomation	Skin findings	Symptoms	Laboratory abnormalities
I	None	Erythema or 1 inch of edema, puncture wounds	None	None
II	Minimal	Erythema within first 12 hr. or 1–5inch of edema	None	None
III	Moderate	Erythema within first 12 hr. or 6–12 inch of edema	Nausea, vomiting, paresthesias metallic taste, and fasciculations fibrinogen<100 mg/dl	Platelets<90,000/uL Protrombine time > 14 s Creatinine kinase>500–1000 U/L
IV	Severe	Potential compartment syndrome	Shock, life-threatening bleeding Renal failure, respiratory difficulty Altered mental status Abnormal coagulation parameter and massive bleeding	

Effects on Obstetrics Patient

The obstetric patient, unlike another group of patients, represents an important challenge for physicians engaged in critical care for clear reasons; it is well-known that pregnant patients have their own physiological changes in different systems, and since it is unknown whether they suffer major or minor changes due to bite poisoning, which must be mentioned in the obligatory concern for fetal well-being, and the singular type of disorder, in this case be a victim of a snakebite.

At the hematological system, a pregnant woman is compensated by a state of hypercoagulability, increasing the risk of deep venous thrombosis in pregnant women. Factors VII, VIII, and X and especially plasma fibrinogen increase after the third month of gestation. A decrease in the platelet count that occurs at the end of pregnancy (20%) does not alter the bleeding time; however, platelet function is increased in response to epinephrine, arachidonic acid, collagen, and adenosine; so it is not unusual to see platelet levels around 150,000. Plasminogen is increased, but the plasminogen activator is decreased as a result of its sequestration at fibrin deposition sites. The anticoagulant activity decreases due to a decrease in S protein concentrations and the resistance of activated protein C; and an alteration of fibrinolysis is seen. The increase in the D-dimer and the thrombin-antithrombin complex indicate an increase in the pro-coagulant state; we do not know if this characteristic is a protective factor to counteract the effect of the poison once inoculated [11].

At the renal system, evident changes have shown its function, showing glomerular filtration which is increased by up to 50% during pregnancy and this may be due to multiple causes, including constriction of the efferent arterioles, as well as the oncotic plasma pressure drop or increase in the effective renal plasma flow; knowing these physiological factors, it is unknown why there are descriptions of specific acute renal lesions [11, 12]

It is not surprising then that the effect of a venomous snakebite on a pregnant would differ by species of snake.

General Complications

The most frequent complications described in patients envenomed by Viperidae species like *B. asper* are:

(a) Soft-tissue infection (11–30% of the cases), characterized by impetigo/cellulitis/abscesses/fasciitis, predominantly cellulitis and abscesses caused by gram-negative rods (*Morganella morganii*, *Proteus rettgeri*, *Klebsiella* spp., *Enterobacter* spp., *Aeromonas hydrophila*) or *Staphylococcus aureus* [7].
(b) Acute renal failure (ARF), which develops in 11–17% of patients, sometimes without oliguric phase (<400 ml/ day/1.73 m^2), hypertension, hyperkalemia, and metabolic acidosis. Clinically and pathophysiologically, ARF can be pre-renal or can be associated with acute glomerulonephritis, acute tubular necrosis, or acute cortical necrosis, the latter being unresponsive to dialysis during 3–4 weeks [7].

(c) Compartmental syndrome (CPS), occurring in 3% of patients. In severe local envenoming, extensive swelling can lead to CPS, mainly when the bite is on a finger, hand, and foot or in the anterior tibial compartment [7].

It is possible that some constituents of snake venom may cross the placenta, and there are case reports which suggest that venom may affect the fetus in the absence of, or before, manifestation of serious maternal envenoming [13].

Venomous snakebite in the pregnant female may lead to a poor outcome in both the mother and the fetus. Previous literature reviews found overall fetal deaths ranging from 38% to 43% [8, 9], with maternal deaths of approximately 10% after a venomous snakebite.

There are several possible mechanisms for abortion following snakebite during pregnancy: they include direct effects of the venom on the fetus, fetal hypoxia due to maternal shock, placental bleeding due to coagulopathy leading to abruptio placentae with evidence of fibrin deposition, and microthrombus formation in the spongy layer which led to placental cleavage and separation following a snakebite (*Bothrops* species); venom has been shown to cause uterine contractions in animals and, in isolated uterine tissue uterine contractions, may act directly on uterine muscle or may act indirectly by causing the release of or potentiating the effect of bradykinins on uterine muscle and pyrexia and cytokine release which occur following tissue damage. Maternal hemorrage with acute fetal anemia cause fetal death in utero, supine hypotension syndrome. And may also the antivenom cause potential maternal anaphylaxis [14, 15].

There were 213 cases of snakebite in pregnant females identified in the literature review, been the largest one. But with limited information on the type of envenomating snake, only was provided this information in 125 cases. Of the envenomation, there were 9 maternal deaths (9 of 213) reported. The maternal case fatality rate was aproximately 4.2%. There were 41 deaths of the fetus or neonate reported. The vast majority were in utero fetal deaths. The deaths in the neonates ocurred from 30 minutes to 8 days after birth. With neonatal case fatality rate aproximately 19.2% [16].

There were no maternal deaths reported from envenomation by US native species; it may reflect more rapid access to health care and availability of antivenom in the United States or possibly less venomous species. However, how soon the patient is seen and treated after the snakebite may have a more significant impact on maternal and/or fetal outcome than the species of snake involved in the envenomation [16].

Though the cause-effect relationship between envenomation and malformations in cases is unknown, it is possible that snake venom can cause embryotoxic and teratogenic effects. The venom of *Vipera aspis* has been shown to cause congenital anomalies in the form of cleft palate and facial deformities in pregnant mice [17]. *Naja nigricollis* venom injected into pregnant mice caused hepatic and myocardial damage as well as pulmonary vascular congestion and extravasated blood in the intestinal lumen of the fetuses [18].

From the largest research study done by Langley et al. (2020), of the taxa of snake involved in an envenomation during pregnancy; the number of reported cases, those who used antivenom, and findings of maternal and fetal outcomes were described. The overall rate of fetal loss is now around 20%, especially when there is systemic envenoming in the first trimester; and maternal case fatality rate is about 4% to 5% [16].

Treatment and Surveillance

First aid measures must be limited to immobilization of the extremity and rapid transfer of patient to the hospital. Tourniquets, suction devices, multiple punctures around the wound, or incisions increase the risk of ischemia and necrosis, the former two, and of hemorrhage and infection. Therefore, these interventions are strongly contraindicated.

Antivenom

The effect of antivenom on the fetus remains unclear. Seneviratne et al. reported 10 abortions and 1 malformation in 11 of 17 (64.7%) patients treated with antivenom. However, they did not find the administration of antivenom to be an independent risk factor for adverse fetal outcome [19]. The use of antivenom in pregnancy should balance its risks and benefits; no other treatment can reverse the venom's effect.

There are no reported epidemiological studies in toxicology or toxicological case series at the use of Crotalidae antivenom less of 24 hours during pregnancy for antidotes for which the risk is unknown [12].

Three kinds of antivenoms, based on the type of active substance, are currently produced in the world: (a) equine-derived, whole IgG antivenoms obtained by ammonium sulfate or caprylic acid fractionation of plasma, consisting of 2.1 g protein, 120 mg albumin, and 18% total antibody IgG (Polyvalent Snakes Venom Antiserum Liquid-Lyophilized); (b) equine-derived F(ab0)2 fragments, obtained by pepsin digestion of IgG and ammonium sulfate precipitation; and (c) Fab fragments obtained by papain digestion of ovine-derived IgG, only produced in North America and Europe.

And it is administered to patients with moderate or severe envenomation and unstable patients (i.e., those with hypotension, severe coagulopathy, respiratory distress) and when there is a progression in the wound or hematological parameters during observation.

A specific treatment for B. Asper bites is described, according to the envenoming grade to reduce from 100 to 300 milligrams of venom [20].

(a) Mild envenoming requires 2 or 4 vials of antivenom.
(b) Moderate envenoming requires 4 to 8 vials of antivenom.
(c) Severe envenoming requires 6 to 12 vials of antivenom.

Antivenom must be diluted in 0.9% NaCl solution (250 ml for adults), and the intravenous infusion should be completed within 30–60 min. Patients should be carefully observed for 24 h for the development of early adverse reactions. These appear within the first 24 h of antivenom therapy, predominantly during the infusion and within the first 2 h of treatment. And it is recommended briefly the antivenom infusion has to be stopped and adrenaline (0.01 mg/kg in children and 0.3–0.5 mg in adults) should be administered subcutaneously for mild/moderate and intravenously for severe early adverse reactions. Although some authors recommend intramuscular (i.m.) rather than subcutaneous (s.c.) adrenaline in terms of bioavailability, it must be kept in mind the risk of deep hematomas associated with i.m. injections in patients having coagulopathy [20]. Additionally, patients must receive hydrocortisone i.v. 100–200 mg every 6 h during 24 h any equivalent corticosteroid and one i.v. dose of antihistamine [20].

Those with mild or moderate envenoming can be treated in the emergency room during the first 24 hours, the latter with monitoring of vital signs, repeating blood coagulation tests by the first 6 hours; if there are no changes by this time, then the treatment is followed and finished in a hospitalization ward.

In the United States, a new antivenin is reported to have reduced potential for adverse reactions [21], and further study on the delayed treatment of antivenin has also been performed [22]. However, diagnosis of unknown snakebites is still a challenge for clinical physicians.

Ancillary Treatment

Patients with snakebite must be admitted and viewed as a true emergency, and the mainstay of hospital treatment for venomous snakebite is antivenom.

The emergency management of snakebites comprises cleaning of the wounds and administration of tetanus toxoid or tetanus immunoglobulin for under or nonimmunized patients, marking the leading edge of the swelling and recording the time of observation and measuring the circumference of extremity every 30 min.

If there is no proximal progression of local injury on the extremity and no coagulopathy after 12 hours of clinical observation and serial laboratory examination, the patient can be discharged with follow-up instructions.

The details of such ancillary treatment are the following:

(a) For the adequate correction of hypovolemia, two peripheral venous lines should be canalized, one for antivenom administration and the other to infuse crystalloids (normal saline solution or Ringer lactate solution), as needed (15–30 ml/kg or more in 30–60 min) to restore circulating volume.

    The measurement of the arterial oxygen saturation is recommended, in order to assess the need to provide oxygen therapy.

    In all cases, urinary output should be measured hourly, in severe cases, by means of a bladder catheter. Normally, adolescents and adults eliminate more than 0.5 ml/kg/h (30–40 ml/h). In severe envenoming, especially when there is anuria, the management of i.v. liquids are more difficult.

(b) The early use of antibiotics in moderate/severe bothropic envenoming (not prophylaxis, a term that implies the use of antibiotics before the trauma) is controversial for several reasons: (1) there have been few controlled clinical trials addressing this issue; (2) the venoms of different snake species differ in their proteolytic and necrotizing effects and, consequently, in their potential to promote infection; (3) the snake responsible for the accident is often not identified; (4) the time interval to seek medical attention at the hospital is often prolonged (>6 to 12 h), thus being too late for beginning antibiotic administration, considering that bacteria of high pathogenicity might have been injected with the venom in the affected tissues; (5) the groups of patients with mild, moderate, and severe envenoming described in several studies are not comparable; (6) antibiotics used were inadequate for the bacteria that cause infections in viperid bites; and (7) the indiscriminate use of broad-spectrum antibiotics promotes the development of bacterial resistance [20].
(c) Intramuscular injections should be avoided during the first 24–48 h of treatment or while coagulopathy persists. For an analgesic effect, tramadol or meperidine (1–2 mg/kg i.v. every 6–12 h) or acetaminophen per oral route is recommended.
(d) The affected extremity must rest at the level of bed, i.e., neither elevated nor pendant. Wound cleaning may be performed with saline solution and a soft antiseptic every day; then, it can be covered with sterile gauzes moistened with saline solution without bandage. Blister contents must be aspirated with sterile syringe at 12–24 h intervals because they contain high venom-antigen concentrations that can be reabsorbed. The search for infection is recommended, ordering cultures when necessary. Careful debridement of necrotic soft tissue, as well as amputations, must be performed under anesthesia and in a sequence indicated by clinical evolution, usually after the third day [7, 20].

Management decisions are difficult to make in these cases as care must be given to two "patients" with a complex interrelationship. The objective should be to ensure maternal survival and increase the chance of a successful pregnancy. The best chance for fetal survival is to guarantee maternal survival, although envenoming caused significant maternal morbidity. In series, treatment with it resulted in a good maternal outcome. After discharge from the hospital, patients should be asked to return for re-evaluation within the next 4 weeks and need to be instructed about the possible development of serum sickness within 5–24 days after antivenom infusion [2, 7, 20].

Scorpion Stings

The syndrome of scorpion envenoming is less heterogeneous than snake envenoming with all the major manifestations being autonomic neuroexcitatory (stimulation of both sympathetic and parasympathetic systems). The main target of venom is voltage-gated sodium channels.

Once the scorpion venom peptides (scorpion α toxins) bind to these channels, their inactivation is inhibited leading to prolonged depolarization with neuroexcitation. Envenoming is characterized by autonomic disturbances such as tachy-/

bradycardia, hyper-/hypotension, excessive salivation and lacrimation, urinary and fecal incontinence, and pulmonary edema. Deaths from scorpion stings are usually due to cardiogenic shock and pulmonary edema. Biochemical changes in the blood – such as hyperglycemia and increase on the level of sodium and on the creatinine concentration – are observed after scorpion sting in humans and experimental animals. Some studies in the literature demonstrate that the scorpion venom affects the maternal reproductive development in humans and in experimental animals, increasing the frequency and amplitude of uterine contraction and the number of resorptions.

Epidemiology

Scorpion envenomation is a public health issue in many places around the world, especially in tropical and subtropical countries, not only due to the high incidence of accidents but also because the venom can induce morbidity in stung patients [23].

There are approximately 1500 species of scorpions described worldwide and only about 30 of them belong to the Buthidae family, which is considered dangerous for humans and responsible for serious cases of envenomation and even death [24]. Obstetric patients are often young and healthy compared with other groups. These patients experience physical, psychological, and physiological changes with the progression of pregnancy. There is very limited information regarding the effects of therapies delivered for scorpion stings in pregnant women or the fetus [25].

Effects of Envenomation During Pregnancy on Prenatal Development

Scorpion envenomation is classified based on signs and symptoms shown by the victim:

- Mild – patients show local signs, such as edema, erythema, and sweating.
- Moderate – nausea, abdominal pain, tachypnea, tachycardia or bradycardia, mild hypertension, agitation, hypersalivation, fever, priapism, and hyperglycemia are present.
- Severe – characterized by cardiovascular complications (congestive heart failure, arrhythmia, or severe hypertension); pulmonary complications (edema and respiratory distress syndrome); gastrointestinal complications (acute pancreatitis); metabolic complications (hyperglycemia, hypocalcemia, hyperkalemia, or acid-base imbalance); and neurological symptoms (hypertensive encephalopathy, coma, or convulsion) [26].

However, scorpions do not release all of their venom in one bite. Scorpion stings therefore produce a mild clinical reaction.

This body system response, biochemical and hematological changes, as previously stated, such as hyperglycemia, hyperamylasemia, increase in serum activities of creatine kinase and aspartate aminotransferase, and increase in hematocrits, red blood cells count, and hemoglobin concentration, have been observed after the scorpion stings in humans and experimental animals [27, 28].

The experimental injection of *Buthus occitanus tunetanus* venom in pregnant rats caused similar effects on maternal blood parameters, including increase in sodium level and reduction in glucose level, increase in the concentration of creatinine, urea, and white blood cells. These observations suggest that the envenomation may cause disturbances in the gestational process and in the development and well-being of the fetus [29].

Alterations in the Maternal Reproductive System During Pregnancy

It was shown that the *Leiurus quinquestriatus* venom, from the Buthidae family, increases the frequency and amplitude of uterine contractions mediated by the release of kinins. Cytokines are important mediators in the gestational process, which lead to a successful pregnancy since they are involved in the implantation of the blastocyst, embryo formation and development, and especially development of the central nervous system [30].

Some studies demonstrated that scorpion venoms affect cytokines, which may be involved in the observed pregnancy losses [31, 32].

Those complications described in the literature like abortions, defects in ossification, skeletal malformations are based on animal models both goats and rats and extrapolations to humans are limited due to differences in the study designs, interspecies differences and responses to the envenomation; because few reports are documented in details regarding the effects of the scorpion venom in the perinatal phase, the available data are somewhat controversial.

Some authors state that a scorpion sting during pregnancy does not affect the mother or the fetus. In this sense Langley [9], in an extensive review of studies published between 1966 and 2002, showed that no adverse consequence was found in human mothers or their fetuses when they were stung by a scorpion during the pregnancy. Similarly, Kaplanoglu and Helvaci [33] described the clinical findings of scorpion stings in 11 pregnant women; all patients developed mild envenomation, and pregnancy complications were not observed. Although a retrospective study carried out in Tunisia from 1990 to 2004 with 20 pregnant women demonstrated neither maternal or fetal death nor preterm fetal delivery, it reported two patients who manifested intense pelvic pain, and one of them had vaginal bleeding [34].

Management

It is essential to be clear about the usefulness of current treatment strategies for scorpion envenoming. The main modes of therapy for scorpion stings historically were supportive treatment and immunotherapy in form of antivenom. However, whether antivenom added any advantage to standard supportive therapy has been debated.

The trials have been carried out in only a few countries, and recommendations are hence valid within the context of these locations, scorpion species, and age group of participants. Therefore, there are some parameters in addition to the level of evidence [35] within brackets of each recommendation [36].

For old world scorpions,

- *Steroids* have no benefit in management of scorpion stings (level of evidence, 2b; location, Tunisia; common species, *A. australis*, *B. occitanus*; applicable age group, children and adults over 10 years). The futility of steroids in scorpion envenoming is probably explained from the fact that toxins do not induce an extensive immune reaction in the immediate aftermath 4 hours when a majority manifest systemic envenoming). The envenoming is a result of functional disturbance of voltage-gated sodium ion channels that lead to autonomic hyperexcitability.
- *Pain Relief*. The pain perception and hence response to analgesia in severe envenoming can vary significantly from mild envenoming.

  *Local anesthesia by topical lidocaine patches may be superior to intravenous paracetamol or local ice application for pain relief in mild envenoming (level of evidence, 1b; location, Turkey; common species, *Androctonus crassicauda*, *Leiurus quinquestriatus*, *Mesobuthus gibbosus*, and *Mesobuthus eupeus*; applicable age group, adults over 18 years).
- *Prazosin* may be better than supportive therapy alone for stings by *M. tamulus* (level of evidence, 3b; location, India; applicable age group, in children).
- *Polyvalent antivenom* against *A. australis* and *B. occitanus* was ineffective when compared to placebo (level of evidence, 2a; location, Tunisia; applicable age group, children and adults over 10 years).
- Antivenom against *M. tamulus* may be better than prazosin alone (level of evidence, 2b; location, India; applicable age group, over 12 years of age).
- Antivenom (against *M. tumulus)* and prazosin combination is better than prazosin alone (level of evidence, 1b; location, India; applicable age group, both adults and children over 6 months of age).

For new world scorpions,

- Antivenom against *Centruroides* sp. are effective in reversing the clinical syndrome faster than no antivenom (level of evidence, 2a; location, Mexico and United States; applicable age group, children and young adults aged less than 18 years) [36].

Before the use of anti-venom therapy, the risks and benefits must be examined, considering the potential for Type 1 and Type 3 allergic reactions and complement activation [37]. The administration of anti-venom therapy is often recommended in the presence of systemic findings such as neurotoxicity, coagulopathy, kidney insufficiency, and hypotension.

Pregnancy is an exclusive period of life, during which physical, psychological, and physiological changes occur. Toxicity related to scorpion stings and anti-venom therapy during pregnancy have unknown effects both on the mother and the fetus. Prospective and multicenter studies are required to achieve generalizable results, along with monitoring of fetal outcomes during pregnancy.

References

1. Langley RL, Morrow WE. Deaths resulting from animal attacks in the United States. Wilderness Environ Med. 1997;8:8–16.
2. Otero Patiño R. Epidemiological, clinical and therapeutic aspects of Bothrops asper bites. Toxicon. 2009;54:998–1011.
3. White J. Bites and stings from venomous animals: a global overview. Ther Drug Monit. 2000;22:65–8.
4. Chippaux JP. Snake-bites: appraisal of the global situation. Bull World Health Org. 1998;176:515–24.
5. Chippaux JP. Snake Venoms and Envenomations. Malabar (FLA): Krieger Publishing Company; 2006. 287p
6. Kasturiratne A, Wickremasinghe AR, de Silva N, Gunawardena NK, Pathmeswaran A, Premaratna R, SAvioli L, Lalloo DG, da Silva HJ. The global burden of snakebite: a literature analysis and modelling based on regional estimates of envenoming and deaths. PLoS Med. 2008;5:e218. https://doi.org/10.1371/journal.pmed.0050218.
7. Otero-Patiño R. El accidente ofídico: realidades y perspectivas. In: Memorias VIII Congreso de APANAC, Panamá; 2008.
8. Dunnihoo DR, Rush BM, Wise RB, Brooks GG, Otterson WN. Snake bite poisoning in pregnancy. A review of the literature. J Reprod Med. 1992;37:653–8.
9. Langley R. A review of venomous animal bites and stings in pregnant patients. Wilderness Environ Med. 2004;15:207–15.
10. Pierini SV, Warrell DA, de Paulo A, Theakston RD. High incidence of bites and stings by snakes and other animals among rubber tappers and Amazonian Indians of the Jurua Valley, Acre State, Brazil. Toxicon. 1996;34:225–36.
11. Cunningham F, Leveno K, Bloom S, Spong CY, Dashe J. Williams obstetrics 24th Edition. McGraw Hill Professional. Chapter 5. Maternal changes; 2015.
12. Bailey B. Are there teratogenic risks associated with antidotes used in the acute management of poisoned pregnant women? Birth Defects Res A Clin Mol Teratol. 2003;67(2):133–40.
13. James RF. Snakebite in pregnancy. Lancet. 1985;ii:731.
14. Komori Y, Nikai T, Sugihara H. Biochemical and physiological studies on a kallikrein-like enzyme from the venom of Crotalus viridis viridis (prairie rattlesnake). Biochim Biophys Acta. 1988;967:92–102.
15. Nawar NN, Mohamed AH, Adieb N, Emad M. The effect of maternal Naja nigricollis envenomation on the placenta. An experimental study. Biol Struct Morphog. 1989;2:13–7.
16. Langley R. Snakebite during pregnancy: a literature review. Wilderness Environ Med. 2010;21:54–60.
17. Gabriel-Robez O, Clavert J. Teratogenic and lethal properties of the various fractions of venom of the viper, Vipera aspis. Acta Anat (Basel). 1980;108:226–9.
18. Mohamed AH, Nawar NNY, Hanna MM. Some effects of Naja nigricollis envenomation on developing fetal tissue. Toxicon. 1974;12:477–80.
19. Seneviratne SL, de Silva CE, Fonseka MMD, Pathmeswaran A, Gunatilake SB, de Silva HJ. Envenoming due to snake bite during pregnancy. Trans R Soc Trop Med Hyg. 2002;96:272–4.
20. Otero- Patiño R. Epidemiological, clinical and therapeutic aspects of Bothrops asper bites. Toxicon. 2010;54(2009):998–1011.
21. Spiller HA, Bosse GM, Ryan ML. Use of antivenom for snakebites reported to United States poison centers. Am J Emerg Med. 2010;28(7):780–5.
22. Larréché S, Mion G, Mayet A, Verret C, Puidupin M, Benois A, et al. Antivenin remains effective against African Viperidae bites despite a delayed treatment. Am J Emerg Med. https://doi.org/10.1016/j.ajem.2009.08.022.
23. Sbister GK. Scorpion envenomation. N Engl J Med. 2014;371:457–63.

24. Chippaux JP, Goyffon M. Epidemiology of scorpionism: a global appraisal. Acta Trop. 2008;107(2):71–9.
25. Langley RL. A review of venomous animal bites and stings in pregnant patients. Wilderness Environ Med. 2004;15:207e15.
26. Dorce ALC, et al. Perinatal effects of scorpion venoms: maternal and offspring development: review. J Venom Anim Toxins Incl Trop Dis. 2017;23:31. https://doi.org/10.1186/s40409-017-0121-z.
27. D'Suze G, Moncada S, González C, Sevcick C, Aguilar V, Alagón A. Relationship between plasmatic levels of various cytokines, tumor necrosis factor, enzymes, glucose and venom concentration following Tityus scorpion sting. Toxicon. 2003;41(3):367–75.
28. Cusinato DA, Souza AM, Vasconcelos F, Guimarães LF, Leite FP, Gregório ZM, et al. Assessment of biochemical and hematological parameters in rats injected with Tityus serrulatus scorpion venom. Toxicon. 2010;56(8):1477–86.
29. Ben Nasr H, Hammami S, Mion G, Sahnoun Z, Chouaiekh F, Rebai T, et al. Effects of Buthus occitanus tunetanus envenomation on an experimental murine model of gestation. C R Biol. 2007;330:890–6.
30. Meki AR, Nassar AY, Rochat H. A bradykinin-potentiating peptide (peptide K12) isolated from the venom of Egyptian scorpion Buthus occitanus. Peptides. 1995;16(8):1359–65.
31. Petricevich VL. Scorpion venom and the inflammatory response. Mediat Inflamm. 2010;2010:903295. https://doi.org/10.1155/2010/903295.
32. Magalhães MM, Pereira MES, Amaral CFS, Rezende NA, Campolina D, Bucaretchi F, et al. Serum levels of cytokines in patients envenomed by Tityus serrulatus scorpion sting. Toxicon. 1999;37(8):1155–64.
33. Kaplanoglu M, Helvaci MR. Scorpion stings in pregnant women: an analysis of 11 cases and review of literature. Clin Exp Obstet Gynecol. 2015;42(2):228–30.
34. Ben Nasr H, Hammami TS, Sahnoun Z, Rebai T, Bouaziz M, Kassis M, et al. Scorpion envenomation symptoms in pregnant women. J Venom Anim Toxins Incl Trop Dis. 2007;13(1):94–102. http://www.scielo.br/scielo.phpscript=sci_arttext&pid=S1678-91992007000100007
35. Levels of evidence. http://www.cebm.net/oxford-centre-evidence-basedmedicine-levels-evidence-march-2009/. Accessed 29 Mar 2017.
36. Chaturaka R, Gnanathasan A. Management of scorpion envenoming: a systematic review and meta-analysis of controlled clinical trials. Syst Rev. 2017;6(74)
37. Abroug F, Nouira S, Saguiga H. Envenomations scorpionniques: avences chimiques, physiopathologiques et therapeutiquis. MedTrop 2008:68:359–66.

Part VI
Respiratory

Chapter 24
Pregnant Patient with Acute Respiratory Failure Due to Thromboembolic Disease

Graciela Raquel Zakalik and Angela María Magali Sanchez

Introduction

In presence of patients with respiratory failure, it is necessary to consider the normal physiological alterations of pregnancy in order to quickly detect the evidence of pathology and to carry out an early and effective treatment.

Respiratory failure affects up to 0.2% of pregnancies, most commonly in the postpartum period [1]. It may be due to specific conditions of pregnancy (such as preeclampsia, embolism of amniotic fluid, or peripartum cardiomyopathy) as well as other diseases that may be exacerbated because of pregnancy such as pneumonia, pulmonary thromboembolic disease, asthma, etc. [2].

Dyspnea, cough, and edema of lower limbs are common clinical manifestations during pregnancy and puerperium and are attributed to physiological changes inherent to pregnancy. They can also be associated with potentially fatal disorders. Early recognition and the beginning of adequate therapy affect the prognosis, both maternal and fetal.

The incidence of venous thromboembolism (VTE) associated with pregnancy has been reported as 0.5–2.0 per 1000 pregnancies [3]. VTE is one of the leading causes of maternal mortality in the United States and accounts for 9.3% of all maternal deaths [1–4].

Deep vein thrombosis (DVT) and pulmonary embolism (PE) are collectively referred to as VTE. 75% to 80% of cases of VTE associated with pregnancy are caused by DVT, and 20–25% are caused by PE [4].

G. R. Zakalik (✉)
Department of Intensive Care, Hospital Lagomaggiore, Mendoza, Argentina

Argentine Society of Intensive Therapy (SATI), Buenos Aires, Argentina

A. M. M. Sanchez
Department of Intensive Care, Hospital Lagomaggiore, Mendoza, Argentina

C. Montufar et al. (eds.), *Obstetric Catastrophes*,
https://doi.org/10.1007/978-3-030-70034-8_24

Risk Factors

Pregnancy is associated with anatomical and physiological changes, which increas the risk of VTE. During gestation hypercoagulable state, increase in venous stasis, decreased venous return, compression of the inferior vena cava and pelvic veins for uterine enlargement, and decreased mobility can be observed. This thrombophilic state is transitory and disappears 6–8 weeks after birth, triggered by an imbalance between procoagulant and anticoagulant factors. The VTE risk in pregnant woman is higher in the third trimester, but is present from the first, even before anatomical changes of pregnancy occurs. It increases much more in the puerperium, especially during the first week of postpartum [5, 6].

The most important individual risk factor for VTE during pregnancy is the previous history of thrombosis, followed by the presence of hereditary or acquired thrombophilia. Approximately 50% of pregnant women with VTE have a history of thrombophilia, compared with 10% of the general population. Other additional risk factors are immobility, age over 35 years, multiparity, preeclampsia, pre- and postpartum hemorrhage, medical conditions (obesity, diabetes mellitus, smoking, lupus, nephrotic syndrome, hemoglobinopathies), assisted fertilization, cesarean, and recent surgery [7–8].

Diagnosis

Clinical suspicion is key to the diagnosis of VTE [4, 9]. The clinical presentation of PE in pregnancy is variable, with signs and symptoms similar to the general population. These include dyspnea (most frequent symptom), tachycardia, pain or edema in lower limbs, pelvic pain, and chest pain [8]. These clinical signs and symptoms lack specificity and may be present in other pathologies, making differential diagnosis difficult.

The existing clinical decision rule (CDR), Wells score, Geneva score, and PERC score, and the measurement of biomarkers such as D-dimer have a poor diagnostic accuracy for VTE in pregnant and postpartum women [5].

Due to the fact that the causes of respiratory distress in pregnancy are generally similar to those of the non-pregnant population, a portion of the non-obstetric population literature applies to pregnant women.

Recent publications have highlighted diagnostic by point-of-care ultrasound in the approach to acute respiratory failure during pregnancy [10]. Arbeid et al. described that despite physiological respiratory changes, lung ultrasound remains normal during the last weeks of pregnancy [11].

The USG widely disseminated in obstetric practice for fetal monitoring has also potential for maternal diagnosis and can be considered as an extension of clinic evaluation [12].

Ultrasound is a safe and fast diagnostic tool, and it's integration to clinical evaluation with point-of-care ultrasound is increasingly used in the evaluation of acute patients, surpassing conventional radiography in many cases.

Currently the use of ultrasound does not depend on external consultations to vascular specialists or radiologists [13], but any professional member of the multidisciplinary team with training and practice can achieve excellent results and improve their clinical practice. The lung ultrasound evaluation is a possible and useful diagnostic tool during pregnancy [11–12].

The BLUE protocol (bedside lung ultrasonography in emergency) enabled a reduction in time to diagnose most of the causes of dyspnea in patients admitted in the emergency department. It has the advantage of bedside speed in a noninvasive and non-ionizing way and in real time. It is not more specific than the CT, but in some cases it can be more than chest radiography [13].

In normal lung, the pleural line is identified as a horizontal hyperechoic sliding line. Beyond this pleural line, horizontal artifacts called lines A are usually seen.

In cases with interstitial disease (usually pulmonary edema), the greater density of the lung tissue creates reverberation artifacts called B lines. The B lines are defined as vertical hyperechoic lines of the comet-tail artifact type that begin in the pleural line, extend up to the lower part of the screen, and move synchronously with the sliding of the lung [11, 14–15].

Lichtenstein et al. have proposed a simplified lung ultrasonography algorithm that correctly classifies the majority of adult patients with dyspnea who go to the emergency department. The algorithm creates three profiles of pulmonary ultrasound. Acute pulmonary edema is strongly associated with anterior symmetric bilateral B lines (comet-tail artifact, interstitial syndrome). An asymmetrical profile (unilateral interstitial disease or pulmonary consolidation) suggests pneumonia. Acute dyspnea with a normal pulmonary ultrasound suggests a diagnosis of pulmonary embolism or bronchial disorder [13].

Figure 24.1 presents a diagnostic algorithm of the obstetric patient with dyspnea.

The asymmetry and pain in a lower limb are suggestive signs of DVT. Given this case, the recommended initial diagnostic test is compression ultrasound (CUS). In contrast to non-pregnant population, in which DVT is usually distal, a systematic review found high frequency of ileofemoral thrombosis (64%) and iliac (17%) in pregnant women with confirmed DVT [4]. In cases with abdominal pain and lumbar or generalized limb edema, additional images should be made with Doppler ultrasound of the iliac vein, venography, or MRI. See Fig. 24.2.

In presence of a pregnant patient with suspected PE without symptoms in the lower limbs or negative CUS for VTE, chest radiography (CXR) is the first image with ionizing radiation that must be performed in the diagnostic algorithm [16–17]. This is essential to accurately interpret an abnormal ventilation/perfusion scan (V/Q scan).

Current guidelines recommend the use of V/Q scan for pregnant women with suspected PE when CXR is normal and suggest the use of computed tomography pulmonary angiography (CTPA) when the CXR is abnormal [16–19].

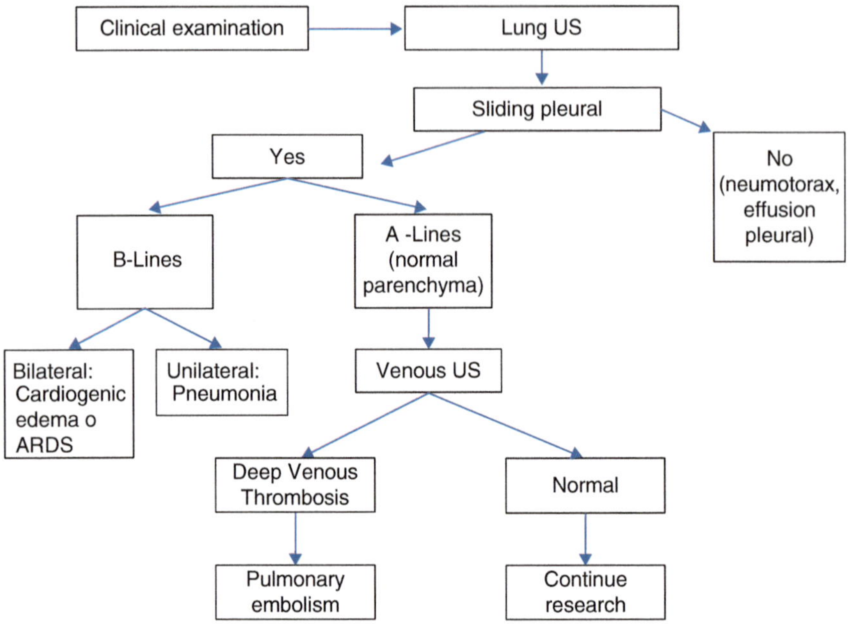

Fig. 24.1 Algorithm of the obstetric patient with dyspnea. Lung ultrasound (Lung US), venous ultrasound (Venous US), acute respiratory distress (ARDS)

Both diagnostic modalities have advantages and disadvantages with low radiation exposure risk [16]. In a recent review, Cochrane concludes that both the V/Q scan and the CTPA are reasonable test in order to dismiss PE in pregnancy [20]. The lack of prospective studies impedes a recommendation of choice, depending then on the availability and experience of each center [21].

The echocardiogram is not enough to establish a PE diagnosis; instead it is useful to confirm the diagnosis and guide the therapeutic decisions in front of a patient with massive PE [7].

The following figure shows the diagnostic algorithm in case of suspected PE (Fig. 24.3).

Treatment

In patients who are hemodynamically stable the first line of treatment consists in anticoagulant therapy. Both low molecular weight heparin (LMWH) and unfractionated heparin (UFH) do not go through the placenta, being safe for the fetus. LMWH has a longer average life, a more predictable anticoagulant effect, a lower incidence of heparin thrombocytopenia, and lower osteoporosis. These data make LMWH the elective treatment for VTE in pregnancy [4, 7]. The dose is adjusted

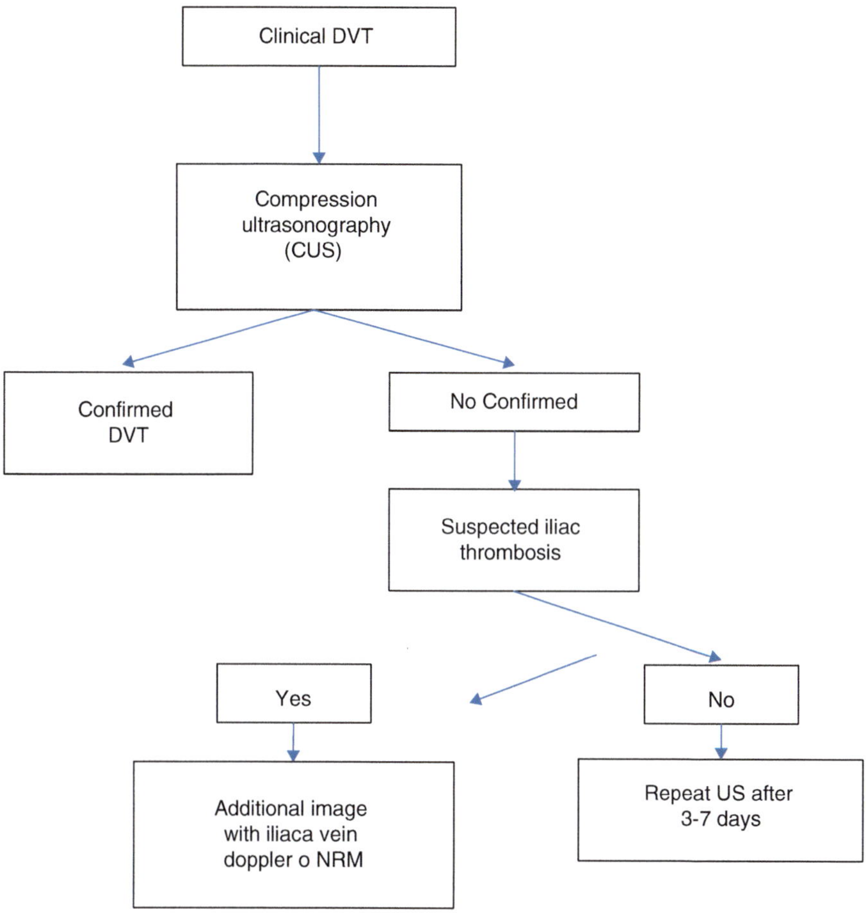

Fig. 24.2 Flowchart on the diagnostic approach in the suspicion of DVT in pregnancy. Deep vein thrombosis (DVT), ultrasound (US), nuclear magnetic resonance (NMR)

to weight, enoxaparin 1 mg/kg every 12 hours, dalteparin 200 units/kg once a day, or dalteparin 100 units/kg every 12 hours, to maintain a therapeutic level of anti-Xa. Current guidelines do not recommend routine monitoring of LMWH with anti-Xa levels, except in those patients with renal failure or extreme body weight [19].

Table 24.1 shows the anticoagulation regime [4, 19].

Heparin UFH is used in patients in whom thrombolysis can be considered (e.g., high risk or massive PE) and with renal failure or when a rapid reversal of anticoagulation is required (advanced pregnancy, risk of hemorrhage, or imminent surgery) [7, 10].

Patients with hemodynamic instability or severe hypoxemia should be treated with thrombolysis if there are no contraindications [7, 19].

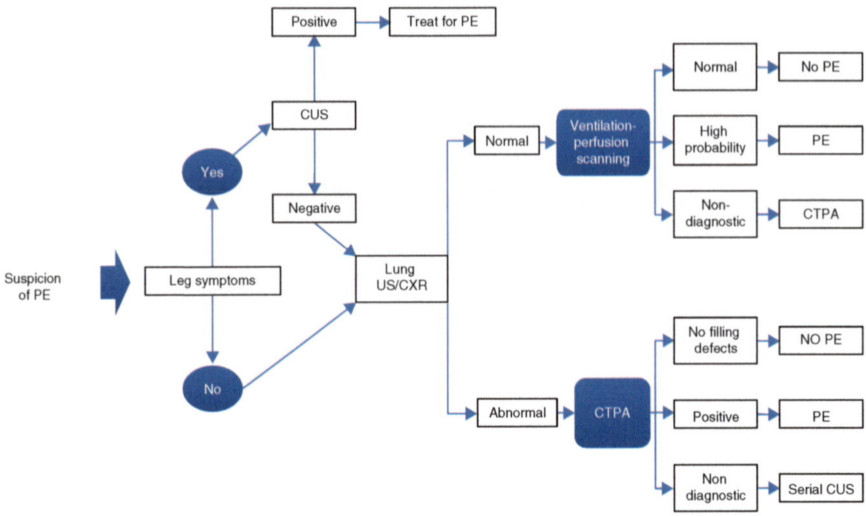

Fig. 24.3 Flowchart on the diagnostic approach in the suspicion of PE in pregnancy. Pulmonary embolism (PE), compression ultrasonography (CUS), lung ultrasound (Lung US), chest radiography (CXR), tomography pulmonary angiography (CTPA), compression ultrasonography (CUS)

Table 24.1 Anticoagulation regimen

Anticoagulation regimen	Anticoagulation dosage
Enoxaparin	1 mg/kg every 12 hours
Tinzaparin	175 U/kg once daily
Dalteparin	200 units/kg once daily 100 units/kg 12 hours
UFH	10,000 units or more SC every 12 hours or IV in doses adjusted to target aPTT in the therapeutic range 6 hours after injection IV

UFH unfractionated heparin, *SC* subcutaneously, *IV* intravenous, *aPTT* activated partial thromboplastin time

The temporal filter of the inferior vena cava is recommended in pregnant patients with VTE in whom anticoagulation is contraindicated, in those with recurrent VTE (despite anticoagulation), or in those with VTE close to delivery date with high thromboembolic risk (2 previous weeks) [4, 7, 19].

In anticoagulation management near delivery date, the switch to HNF is recommended [7, 19]. In case of no hemorrhagic complications LMWH can be restarted 12 hours after delivery. If an epidural catheter was left, the restart should be at least 4 hours after removing it. The initial dose is usually prophylactic, and then the anticoagulant dose is reinstated (at 24 hours) or sooner if you are sure of adequate hemostasis. Anticoagulation with LMWH or oral anticoagulants (OAC) is recommended for at least 6 weeks postpartum and until at least 3 months of treatment have been completed. From this period different risk factors are re-evaluated and determined whether to continue or suspend treatment. The use of elastic stockings is recommended in order to prevent post-thrombotic syndrome.

References

1. Lapinsky SE. Management of acute respiratory failure in pregnancy. Semin Respir Crit Care Med. 2017;38(2):201–7.
2. Mighty HE. Acute respiratory failure in pregnancy. Clin Obstet Gynecol. 2010;53(2):360–8.
3. Say L, Chou D, Gemmill A, Tuncalp O, Mollee AB, Daniels J, et al. Global causes of maternal death: a WHO systematic analysis. Lancet Glob Health. 2014;2(6):e323–33.
4. ACOG Practice Bulletin no.196: Thromboembolis in pregnancy. Obstet Gynecol. 2018;132(1):e1–e17.
5. Goodacre S, Horspool K, Shephard N, Pollard D, Hunt BJ, Fuller G, et al. Selecting pregnant or postpartum women with suspected pulmonary embolism for diagnostic imaging: the DiPEP diagnostic imaging: the DiPEP diagnostic study with decision-analysis modeling. Health Technol Assess. 2018;22(47):1–230.
6. Zakalik G, Sanchez M. Enfermedades tromboembólicas durante el embarazo. In: Editorial Medica Panamericana SA. Terapia Intensiva. Buenos Aires; 2015. p. 1365–7.
7. Dado CD, Levinson AT, Bourjeily G. Pregnancy and pulmonary embolism. Clin Chest Med. 2018;39(3):525–37.
8. Conti E, Zezza L, Ralli E, Comito C, Sada L, Passerini J, Caserta D, et al. Pulmonary embolism in pregnancy. J Thrombolysis. 2014;37(3):251–70.
9. Chan WS, Spencer FA, Ginsberg JS. Anatomic distribution of deep vein thrombosis in pregnancy. CMAJ. 2010;182(7):657–60.
10. Zieleskiewicz L, Bouvet L, Einav S, Duclos G, Leone M. Diagnostic point of care ultrasound: applications in obstetric anaesthetic management. Anaesthesia. 2018;73(10):1265–79.
11. Arbeid E, Demi A, Brogi E, Gori E, Giusto T, Soldati G, et al. Lung ultrasound pattern is Normal during the last gestational weeks: an observational pilot study. Gynecol Obstet Investig. 2017;82:398–403.
12. Zieleskiewicz L, Contargyris C, Brun C, Touret M, Vellin A, Antonini F, et al. Lung ultrasound predicts interstitial syndrome and hemodynamic profile in parturients with severe preeclampsia. Anesthesiology. 2014;120:906–14.
13. Volpicelli G, Elbarbary M, Blaivas M, Lichtenstein DA, Mathis G, Kirkpatrick AW, et al. International evidence-based recommendations for point-of-care lung ultrasound. Intensive Care Med. 2012;38:577–91.
14. Lichenstein DA, Meziere GA. Relevance of lung ultrasound in the diagnosis of acute respiratory failure: the BLUE protocol. Chest. 2008;134:117–25.
15. Lichtenstein DA, Goldstein I, Mourgeon E, Cluzel P, Grenier P, Rouby JJ. Comparative diagnostic performances of auscultation, chest radiography, and lung ultrasonography in acute respiratory distress syndrome. Anesthesiology. 2004;9(15):100.
16. Royal College of Obstetricians & Gynaecologists. Thromboembolic disease in pregnancy and the puerperium: acute management. In Royal College of Obstetricians & Gynaecologists, Green-top Guideline, No. 37b.2015. https://www.rcog.org.uk/globalassets/…/guidelines/gtg-37b.pdf. Accessed 15 Jun 2019.
17. ATS/STR Committee on Pulmonary Embolism in Pregnancy, American Thoracic Society documents: an official American Thoracic Society/Society of Thoracic Radiology Clinical Practice Guideline: evaluation of suspect pulmonary embolism in pregnancy. Radiology. 2012;262:635–46.
18. Linnemann B, Scholz U, Rott H, Halimeh S, Zotz R, Gerhardt A, et al. Treatment of pregnancy-associated venous thromboembolism-position paper from the working group in Women's Health of the Society of Thrombosis and Haemostasis (GTH). Vasa. 2016;45:103–18.
19. Bates SM, Middeldorp S, Rodger M, James AH, Greer I. Guidance for the treatment and prevention of obstetric-associated venous thromboembolism. J Tromb Thrombolysis. 2016;41:92–128.

20. van Mens TE, Schere LI, de Jong PG, Leeflang MM, Nijkeuter M, Middeldorp S, van Mens TE. Imaging for the exclusion of pulmonary embolism in pregnancy. Cochrane Database Syst Rev. 2017; https://www.ncbi.nlm.nih.gov/pubmed/28124411. Accessed 10 Jun 2019
21. Wan T, Skeith L, Karovitch A, Rodger M, Le Gal G. Guidance for the diagnsosis of pulmonary embolism during pregnancy: consensus and controversies. Thromb Res. 2017;157:23–8.

Chapter 25
Severe Acute Asthma

Amparo Aguilera, and Ariatna Aguilera

Introduction

Asthma is the most common respiratory disorder to complicate pregnancy. It remains a high-risk condition despite advances in therapy. In the USA, 5–8% of pregnant women have asthma, and asthma prevalence is increasing worldwide, affecting 2–13% of pregnancies with increasing healthcare utilization and costs [1]. The relationship between asthma status and pregnancy outcomes is complex, in part due to higher rates of smoking, obesity, and other comorbidities in patients with asthma that are independently associated with higher maternal and fetal obstetric risk. It is widely known that one-third of pregnant asthmatics improve, one-third remain stable, but the remaining third demonstrate a clinical worsening of their asthma during pregnancy [2].

Physiological Respiratory Changes in Pregnancy

Respiratory and cardiovascular changes that occur during pregnancy have been well documented. Minute ventilation is increased by 50% in late pregnancy secondary to progesterone effect. This hyperventilation usually results from the increased tidal volume with minimal changes in respiratory rate. Arterial blood gases often reveal a compensated respiratory alkalosis (pH, 7.40–7.45; PCO_2, 28–32 mm Hg) and a mild increase in PO_2 (106–110 mm Hg). The increase in pH secondary to respiratory alkalosis usually is blunted by an increase in renal excretion of bicarbonate [3]. Pregnancy also affects chest wall compliance with a fall in functional residual capacity (FRC) as pregnancy progresses (due to elevation of the diaphragm from the

A. Aguilera (✉) · A. Aguilera
Pulmonologist, Pulmonology Department, Irma de Lourdes Tzanetatos Hospital, Panama City, Panama

C. Montufar et al. (eds.), *Obstetric Catastrophes*,
https://doi.org/10.1007/978-3-030-70034-8_25

enlarging gravid uterus). Increasing dyspnea in late pregnancy is associated with a reduction in expiratory reserve volume, although an increase in inspiratory capacity results in total lung capacity remaining in the normal range. Healthy pregnant women show no change in forced expiratory volume in 1 second (FEV1), a very modest increase in forced vital capacity (FVC), of less than one-tenth of a liter, after 14–16 weeks gestational age, and no significant change in FEV1/FVC ratio throughout pregnancy. Therefore, in pregnant women with asthma, any decline in these spirometry parameters should be concerning.

Oxygen delivery to the fetus depends on uterine artery blood flow and maternal oxygen content. Since uterine artery blood flow is near maximal at baseline, the fetus is critically dependent on adequate maternal cardiac output for optimal oxygen delivery. Maternal fetal oxygen transfer occurs by an elegant concurrent exchange mechanism, with the difference in oxygen tension between the maternal and fetal circulations in the placenta determining oxygen transfer. Thus, maximization of maternal oxygen saturation and maintenance of maternal cardiac output best ensures appropriate fetal oxygen delivery when maternal respiratory compromise occurs [4].

Effects of Asthma on Pregnancy and Fetus

Over the past few years, a large systematic review and a series of meta-analyses have been published that summarize the literature on adverse perinatal outcomes among females with asthma. Asthma is strongly associated with preeclampsia, placental abruption and previa, and obstetric hemorrhage. The most common pediatric complications associated with poorly controlled maternal asthma include intrauterine growth retardation, preterm delivery, and low birth weight [5]. A large cohort of 36,587 women with asthma has also demonstrated increased prevalence of congenital malformations in women with severe asthma exacerbations during the first trimester [6]. A meta-analysis of studies from 1975 to 2012 also reported significant associations between maternal asthma and neonatal death, neonatal hospitalization, cleft lip/palate and minor malformations, but not major malformations or stillbirth [7].

Asthma Medications During Pregnancy

An Australian survey study of 102 pregnant females with asthma found that self-reported symptoms, both during the day and night, were worse during pregnancy than prior to pregnancy. Despite this, treatment of asthma by a medical professional was less likely during pregnancy than prior to pregnancy (79%), and the number using treatment for asthma was lower during pregnancy (76%) than prior to pregnancy (92%). Similarly, data from 2072 pregnant females using asthma medication in the Netherlands between 2004 and 2009 indicated that there was a significant decrease in prescriptions filled for asthma medication during the first 3 months of pregnancy compared to the 3 months prior to pregnancy [8]. In particular, a significant decrease in prescriptions filled for long-acting bronchodilators and combination medications was noted in the first trimester of pregnancy, which significantly increased in the postpartum period. 38.2% of pregnancies with three prescriptions of asthma medication in the year prior to pregnancy did not have any prescriptions for asthma medication during the first trimester [8]. While these differences might be explained by fluctuations in asthma course with pregnancy, they support other publications showing similar patterns of decreased asthma medication use in early pregnancy. This behavior puts pregnant females with asthma at risk of poor control and exacerbations during pregnancy.

Acute Asthma Exacerbation

Asthma exacerbation rates are higher during pregnancy, particularly for patients with a history of severe asthma. Acute asthma exacerbations have been identified as the most significant event to affect fetal morbidity and mortality in pregnancies complicated by asthma. Exacerbations can occur at any time during gestation but are most likely to occur in the second and third trimesters between weeks 17 and 34, with peak incidence at around 25 weeks of gestation [9]. Triggers for exacerbations include inhaled treatment non-adherence and viral infections.

Treating an acute exacerbation of asthma is similar for pregnant and non-pregnant patients. The first step in management is to identify the severity of the exacerbation and risk factors for respiratory failure. If close clinical follow-up is arranged, patients with mild exacerbations can be managed as an outpatient or discharged from the emergency department. For moderate and severe cases, inpatient monitoring is warranted. Beta-agonist bronchodilators and systemic corticosteroids are mainstays of treatment of acute exacerbations [10]. Bronchodilators in unstable patients can be delivered initially up to every 20 minutes; in severe cases, continuous delivery can be provided in an ICU setting. Systemic corticosteroids should be provided at the usual doses and early in the course of an exacerbation. Failure to adequately treat an acute exacerbation poses a much higher risk for the pregnant patient and fetus than does utilization of their standard medications daily [11].

An assessment of oxygenation, potential respiratory fatigue, and circulating volume is critical. Oxygen saturation should be maintained above 95%. As pregnant patients normally have a physiologic compensated respiratory alkalosis with partial pressure of carbon dioxide (PCO_2) range of 28–32 mm Hg, a seemingly normal PCO_2 on blood gas testing represents an acute respiratory acidosis and typically signals impending respiratory failure. Frank acidemia is a sign of imminent danger to the mother and fetus. Both cases warrant ICU-level care and should include close monitoring of the mother and fetus by obstetrics [12].

Acute Exacerbations and Indications for Admission to the ICU

Emergency department (ED) evaluation of dyspnea in an asthmatic patient must include acute exacerbation of asthma and whether a critical asthma syndrome is present, e.g., status asthmaticus (SA) or near-fatal asthma (NFA). Other causes of acute dyspnea must be excluded including pulmonary embolism, cardiogenic pulmonary edema, acute lung injury (ALI)/acute respiratory distress syndrome (ARDS), pneumonia, and pneumothorax among other possibilities [13].

Critical asthma syndrome, once diagnosed, can be defined as an acute and severe asthma exacerbation that does not respond promptly to intensive bronchodilator therapy. It can progress to NFA, where respiratory failure has ensued. Timely diagnosis and management is therefore of paramount importance because both the mother and fetus are at risk for morbidity and mortality from hypoxemia. A multidisciplinary team approach as previously described should be adopted. Overall, Cydulka et al. found that 12.6% of pregnant asthmatic women presented to the ED, and hospitalization occurred in 1.6% [14]. ICU admission should be considered for patients whose asthma continues to worsen despite maximal bronchodilator therapy.

Ventilatory Management

Non-invasive ventilation may be an alternative under the right clinical circumstance and may support ventilation while corticosteroids and maximal bronchodilator therapy take effect. Progressive or unremitting hypoxemia, respiratory acidosis, maternal fatigue, alteration in mental status, and other causes for increased work of breathing, despite maximal bronchodilator therapies and NIV, are indications for intubation and invasive mechanical ventilation [15].

Intubation, if indicated, in the pregnant asthmatic may be up to eight times more difficult when compared to non-pregnant women secondary to soft tissue edema and increased probability of aspiration of gastric contents of the gravid patient due to slow gastric emptying. Intratracheal intubation via the oral route should be favored over the nasal route because of hyperemia from capillary engorgement of the upper respiratory tract resulting in a narrower airway and relatively small endotracheal tubes may be required (6–7 mm) [12].

Since the basic pathophysiology of asthma involves air trapping, asthmatics should be ventilated with caution to avoid barotrauma and volutrauma that may occur in the presence of elevated airway pressures. Low minute ventilation with prolonged expiratory time avoids hyperinflation and is achieved with these recommended initial ventilator settings: low tidal volumes VT (6–8 cc/kg), low respiratory rate (8–12 breaths per minute), high inspiratory flow rates (up to 100 L/min in some cases), initial FIO_2 0.9–1 tritrated by PaO_2 values, and inspiratory times as short as 0.8 seconds may be required to achieve I:E ratios near 1:4. Frequently, sedation and even the use of muscle relaxants will be needed [16].

Treatment

Prior to discussing therapy recommendations, it may be useful to review the potential impact of asthma medications on pregnancy. In general, it is recommended that patients remain on the same drugs and dosages that are used outside of pregnancy. Inhaled agents are preferred over oral agents to reduce systemic effects and minimize any possible fetal effects.

Medications for asthma are divided into two types: (1) rescue (those used to treat acute bronchospasm and give symptomatic relief without treating the underlying cause of the bronchospasm) and (2) maintenance (those that help control airway hyperreactivity and treat the underlying inflammation) [17].

Rescue Medications

Short-Acting β_2-Agonists

These drugs are key to asthma management. Short-acting β_2-agonists include metaproterenol, terbutaline, and salbutamol (FDA Category C). These inhaled agents are good for acute and mild intermittent asthma, as they have a rapid onset resulting in maximum bronchodilation with minimal side effects. Side effects of these drugs include tremulousness, palpitations, and/or anxiety. However, such side effects can be minimized by the use of a spacer and mouth rinsing after inhalation. Studies have shown no association between short-acting β_2-agonist use and increased risk of congenital malformations or adverse pregnancy outcome. In acute setting salbutamol could be used nebulized or inhaled with spacer; there is no difference between them [18].

Anticholinergics

The main anticholinergic drug used in asthma therapy is ipratropium (FDA Category B) which has shown synergistic bronchodilator effect when added to inhaled β_2-agonists. It can be used nebulized as inhaled therapy.

Systemic Corticosteroids

In contrast to the low incidence of risk with inhaled corticosteroids, continuous use of systemic corticosteroid some studies have consistently shown increased risk of low birth weight, preterm delivery, pregnancy-induced hypertension, preeclampsia, and gestational diabetes, after the continuous use of systemic corticosteroids. Prednisone (FDA Category C) the recommended doses is 40 mg/day by 5-7days during exacerbation of Asthma [19].

Maintenance Medications

Inhaled Corticosteroids

Inhaled corticosteroids are considered the mainstay of treatment for persistent asthma. Studies have shown that the use of these inhaled steroids in standard doses is not associated with malformations, fetal growth restriction, stillbirth, or fetal mortality. Budesonide (FDA Category B) and beclomethasone (FDA Category C) are the two agents with the most data available regarding use during pregnancy [20].

Long-Acting β_2-Agonists

Currently, consensus recommendations support the use of long-acting β_2-agonists in patients with moderate to severe asthma who already are using inhaled steroids and who need additional therapy. Formoterol and salmeterol are the most common medications in this group (FDA Category C).

Leukotriene Modifiers

Leukotrienes are potent chemical mediators of the allergic response in asthma. They stimulate bronchoconstriction and mucus hypersecretion and promote microvascular leakage, edema formation, and eosinophil chemoattraction. Medications which modify and diminish the effects of leukotrienes have been to allow better asthma control. The most common drugs is montelukast (FDA Category B). While few data are available regarding their use in pregnancy, the Human Merck Registry has not shown any increased risk of malformation [21].

Summary

Asthma is common in pregnant women. While most women who have asthma during pregnancy have controlled disease, some may experience exacerbation of their disease necessitating immediate intervention. It is very important for the treating physicians to overcome the myth that pregnant women should not take any medications during pregnancy and work hard to keep asthma under control to minimize the risk of maternal and fetal hypoxia. Contrary to the common belief, almost all medications used in non-pregnant women are safe during pregnancy and should be continued. Patients with severe acute exacerbation should be managed in a monitored unit. Initial management should include the administration of repeated doses of inhaled β_2-agonist, systemic corticosteroid, and oxygen. Mechanical ventilation of patient with severe acute asthma should be performed in a controlled monitored setting to avoid complications of barotrauma or volutrauma. In very rare circumstances, termination of pregnancy maybe considered.

References

1. Murphy VE, Gibson PG. Asthma in pregnancy. Clin Chest Med. 2011;32:93–110.
2. McCallister JW. Asthma in pregnancy: management strategies. Curr Opin Pulm Med. 2013;19:13–7.
3. Grindheim G, Toska K, et al. Changes in pulmonary function during pregnancy: a longitudinal cohort study. BJOG. 2012;119(1):94–101.
4. Longo LD. Respiratory gas exchange in the placenta. Compr Physiol. 2011;13:351–401.
5. Kim S, Kim J, et al. Effect of pregnancy in asthma on health care use and perinatal outcomes. J Allergy Clin Immunol. 2015;136(5):1215–23.
6. Blais L, Kettani FZ, et al. Asthma exacerbations during the first trimester of pregnancy and congenital malformations: revisiting the association in a large representative cohort. Thorax. 2015;70(7):647–52.
7. Namazy JA, Murphy VE, et al. Effects of asthma severity, exacerbations and oral corticosteroids on perinatal outcomes. Eur Respir J. 2013;41(5):1082–90.
8. Sawicki E, Stewart K, et al. Management of asthma by pregnant women attending an Australian maternity hospital. Aust N Z J Obstet Gynaecol. 2012;52:183–8.
9. Powell H, Murphy VE, et al. Management of asthma in pregnancy guided by measurement of fraction of exhaled nitric oxide: a double-blind, randomized controlled trial. Lancet. 2011;378:983–90.
10. Chan AL, Juarez MM, Gidwani N, Albertson TE. Management of critical asthma syndrome during pregnancy. Clin Rev Allergy Immunol. 2015;48(1):45–53.
11. Breton MC, Beauchesne MF, Lemière C, Rey E, Forget A, Blais L. Risk of perinatal mortality associated with asthma during pregnancy. Thorax. 2009;64:101–6.
12. Peters JI, Stupka JE, Singh H, et al. Status asthmaticus in the medical intensive care unit: a 30-year experience. Respir Med. 2012;106(3):344–8.
13. Chan AL, Juarez MM, et al. Management of critical asthma syndrome during pregnancy. Clinic Rev Allergy Immunol. 2015;48:45–53.
14. Cydulka RK, Emerman CL, Schreiber D, et al. Acute asthma among pregnant women presenting to the emergency department. Am J Respir Crit Care Med. 1999;160:887–92.
15. Lapinsky SE, Rojas-Suarez JA, Crozier TM, et al. Mechanical ventilation in critically-ill pregnant women: a case series. Int J Obstet Anesth. 2015;24(4):323–8.
16. Leatherman JW, McArthur C, et al. Effect of prolongation of expiratory time on dynamic hyperinflation in mechanically ventilated patients with severe asthma. Crit Care Med. 2004;32(7):1542–5.
17. Liccardi G, Cazzola M, et al. General strategy for the management of bronchial asthma in pregnancy. Respir Med. 2003;97:778–89.
18. Cossette B, Forget A, Beauchesne MF, et al. Impact of maternal use of asthma-controller therapy on perinatal outcomes. Thorax. 2013;68(8):724–30.
19. Maselli DJ, Adams SG, et al. Management of asthma during pregnancy. Ther Adv Respir Dis. 2013;7:87–100.
20. Virchow JC. Asthma and pregnancy. Semin Respir Crit Care Med. 2012;33:630–44.
21. Sarkar M, Koren G, et al. Montelukast use during pregnancy: a multicentre, prospective, comparative study of infant outcomes. Eur J Clin Pharmacol. 2009;65(12):1259–64.

Chapter 26
Anaphylaxis During Pregnancy

Freddy Morales, José Mora, Miguel Chung Sang, and Ezio Villegas

Introduction

Anaphylaxis is the most serious and sudden clinical setting of an allergic reaction, which can result in hypersensitivity to an exogenous agent and characterized by developing cardiocirculatory instability (vasodilation and hypotension), in addition to hives, palpebral and labial swelling, laryngeal edema, and bronchial spasm, which in turn can result in suffocation, due to the massive release of histamine.

It is necessary to identify symptoms and alarm signs early, since a fatal outcome can easily occur and the patient may die within a few minutes, if treatment or adequate vital support is not given at the precise time.

The pregnant woman is not exempt from this noxa due to multiple etiologies; however, certain parameters must be taken into account when facing her presentation, usually sudden, such as the danger of loss of fetal well-being which can indicate the need to terminate pregnancy in the context of the therapeutic protocol, also taking into account gestational age and the consequences of prematurity [1].

F. Morales (✉) · J. Mora
Hospital de SOLCA – Manabí, Portoviejo, Ecuador
e-mail: freddy@moralesmd.com

M. Chung Sang
Hospital Gineco Obstétrico y Pediátrico Universitario de Guayaquil, Guayaquil, Ecuador

Universidad Católica de Santiago de Guayaquil, Guayaquil, Ecuador

E. Villegas
Hospital Gineco Obstétrico y Pediátrico Universitario de Guayaquil, Guayaquil, Ecuador

C. Montufar et al. (eds.), *Obstetric Catastrophes*,
https://doi.org/10.1007/978-3-030-70034-8_26

Epidemiology

It is complex to have an exact calculation of the population that presents or has presented an anaphylactic reaction, since the existing data have a variation that depends on the authors, study methods, and countries and other items.

However, worldwide the prevalence of anaphylactic reactions affects between 3 and 30 individuals per 100,000 people annually; and its mortality is between 0.05% and 2%. In such a way it is not a very frequent disease and few cases become fatal. Therefore, the notability of these figures indicates that this complication is avoidable with an early diagnosis, as well as timely and adequate treatment [2–4].

There is no literature that reliably indicates the incidence of anaphylaxis during pregnancy; however, allergen factors are analogous, except during labor, where allergic reaction to latex and antibiotics prevails (especially beta-lactams) [5].

There are also publications describing hypersensitivity or severe anaphylaxis (1/7000–1/13,000 anesthesia) during the perioperative stage, being a diagnostic challenge especially for the anesthesiologist and much more as it is a pregnant patient. All anesthetic inputs used in this perioperative period carry a potential danger of histamine release and therefore allergy, which mostly has no clinically important effect, but which in certain cases can induce serious cardiovascular and/or respiratory complications that can be deadly (between 3% and 6%) [6, 7].

Postpartum anaphylaxis, the period of onset of breastfeeding is rare, much less in Latin America; its etiology has been related to a lower production of the hormone progesterone and an increase in prolactin, which would develop a degranulation of mast cells in postpartum which is presumed to provide an exaggerated production of histamine.

There are few reports of such cases in the universal literature, the first report of a case on postpartum anaphylaxis being published in *Lancet* (1991); It was a 29-year-old woman who presented with generalized urticaria and angioedema of the upper respiratory tract, agreeing with breastfeeding 3 days after the birth of her son; being that, in the world literature until 2015, 5 cases were reported [8, 9].

Pathogeny

Anaphylaxis develops during the process of a massive release of substances inside the cells, such as mast cells and basophils, which will be the cause of the symptoms and signs characteristic of an allergic reaction.

These cells are impelled in a different way, the most frequent being an immediate allergic reaction given at the moment when an allergen adheres to the immunoglobulin E (IgE) antibodies, which are found on the surface of the cell membrane of the mast cells, and basophils; this coalition allows these substances to be released, triggering allergic symptoms.

Histamine stands out among the substances (tryptase, leukotrienes, prostaglandins, chemokines, and cytosines) that cause mast cell and basophil release, being able to cause blood vasodilation, with the consequent increase in capillary permeability and neuritic stimulation. This determines the appearance of edema, erythema and pruritus evidenced in the form of hives or hives of the skin, being also responsible for the development of bronchospasm.

The importance of anaphylactic reaction in pregnant women is given by the potential harmful effect that may have an impact on the product or fetus; otherwise its consequences are no different than those of non-pregnant women.

During anaphylactic shock the large amount of histamine released into placental and umbilical circulation has a more powerful vasoconstrictor effect than adrenaline, affecting fetal oxygenation directly as a consequence of maternal hypoxemia and indirectly peripheral vasoconstriction and resulting in arterial hypotension [2, 10].

Initially, the fetus can supply the decreased uterine flow by redistributing blood circulation to the target organs, increasing affinity for oxygen, releasing it to the tissues simply by reducing fetal movements. However, at the time the demand exceeds the compensatory mechanisms of the fetus, there is an increased danger for the appearance of hypoxic ischemic encephalopathy during childbirth with the consequent irreversible brain damage [2, 11, 12].

Most Frequent Etiology

Latex Exposure

Any woman who has had a history or allergic reactions to latex, such as itching when wearing gloves or inflating balloons, and pruritus from contact with condoms should notify her obstetrician, since this is one of the usual causes of anaphylaxis that have been reported in vaginal and cesarean deliveries. Allergic reactions to foods with cross-reactivity with latex have also been described, such as kiwi, avocado, banana, mango, papaya, chestnut, tomato, pineapple, melon, and potato.

Insect Bites in Sensitized People

Bee sting is a cause of fetal death due to systemic poisoning as it can beat the placental barrier. This situation usually occurs only in allergic women; otherwise, only a minor local inflammation would occur. But, once it triggers anaphylaxis, it can cause collateral fetal damage and placental insufficiency once the mother develops hypotension and therefore does not get enough irrigation to the placental circulation.

Medicine Administration

Among the drugs used during pregnancy, antibiotics are the most common causes of anaphylactic reactions; however, this type of complications has also been described with local anesthetics, medications for induction of general anesthesia, and even the same immunotherapy with the purpose of desensitizing some type of allergen.

Diagnosis

The initial clinical setting of anaphylaxis usually manifests in the places where there is a greater amount of mast cells, such as the skin and mucous membranes, heart, lungs, and digestive tract, being able to give signs and symptoms not as severe as tachycardia and hypotension not so marked, and the skin signs being easily generalized after their initial appearance in the chest commonly. However, when it progresses to anaphylactic shock, the most severe manifestation of anaphylaxis can end in a cardiac arrest, which can occur in any period of pregnancy, although more frequent in the third trimester, as well as in the perioperative period or during the delivery. The presentation of this complication is described in 50–80% during anesthetic induction and up to 30% in the post-anesthetic resuscitation room [13].

Postpartum anaphylaxis, despite being a rare presentation, however, still has lethal connotations, which require early recognition in order to avoid its life-threatening complications, since the clinical setting can manifest itself with a simple rash and evolve toward anaphylactic shock. Its presentation is given during the first 3 days of postpartum according to most reports (which are already mentioned to be few), but it is not well defined. It may be good advise to have in mind that this period could show itself as late presentations, based on its immunological etiology in postpartum [14–16].

In any case, it is established that the diagnosis of anaphylaxis is essentially clinical; however, pulmonary thromboembolism must be immediately ruled out, as well as amniotic fluid embolism, especially in front of a pregnant woman in the third trimester who has sudden respiratory distress with altered records of fetal heart rate. Another illness to consider is the gravidarum laryngitis attached to pregnant women with preeclampsia that may also give a similar respiratory symptomatology, but to a lesser extent than allergenic laryngospasm [16].

Treatment

The management and treatment of anaphylaxis in pregnant women does not differ from non pregnant ones and should be established as soon as possible and intense, to avoid fatal outcomes, based on the knowledge of its pathophysiology and the expertise of the professional who attends the patient during the anaphylactic episode; as it is an emergency, it will depend on available resources and accessibility to a hospital in order tu ensure such assistance.

In this context, the management of symptoms, specifically respiratory and cardiocirculatory, should be set as primary objectives, in addition to controlling the proliferation of histochemical mediators, as well as their involvement in target organs [2].

So the sequence of management and treatment of both anaphylaxis and anaphylactic shock includcs an ABCDE approach:

- The pregnant woman should be placed in the left lateral recumbency to avoid compression of the vena cava by the pregnant uterus.
- Verify the permeability of the airway, and ensure it definitively if it is necessary with tracheal intubation and ventilation with 100% FiO_2 in case it had not been performed.
- Determine the presence of signs of acute respiratory failure (frequency and respiratory pattern), oxyhemoglobin saturation, and if it is feasible to request an arterial gas study.
- Evaluate the circulatory state, taking into account that due to its physiological changes, hypotension is a late sign of shock; also observing semiological signs of poor tissue perfusion (sensory, capillary filling, diuresis).
- Establish the state of consciousness: disorientation, confusion, and agitation.
- Immediately discontinue any drug suspected of causing the reaction and change the venoclysis equipment if it had one [17].
- The first-line drug for the treatment of anaphylaxis is epinephrine (or adrenaline). Initial dose 0.2–0.5 mg/kg and repeat at a dose of 0.1–0.2 mg/kg until the desired effect is obtained. The total dose can reach 5–10 mg. It has been found that the intramuscular route (in the anteromedial of the thigh) is better than the subcutaneous one used previously, leaving intravenous route to be administered in medical centers with closer monitoring and specialized surveillance support. It relieves airway obstruction caused by beta-2 adrenergic effects given by mucosal edema, as well as smooth muscle constriction [18].
- Antihistamines are used to reverse the cutaneous symptoms, to which corticosteroids can be added, especially when trying to avoid the recurrence of symptoms several hours later, which is called biphasic anaphylaxis.
- In cases where bronchospasm does not yield with the administration of adrenaline, bronchodilators such as salbutamol aerosol and aminophylline intravenously and corticosteroids (1 g of methylprednisolone, 500 mg hydrocortisone) can be used.
- The use of sodium bicarbonate is indicated if severe metabolic acidosis coexists, previously assessing the acid/base state by arterial gasometry, which allows defining the necessary dose; however, its use in obstetrics is controversial.

- It is necessary to initiate vasopressor support (norepinephrine, dobutamine) in order to maintain acceptable haemodynamics, when hypotension is refractory to crystalloid therapy.
- Stop anesthesia if the reaction occurs at induction and end the intervention as quickly as possible; in patients at risk of developing histamine release, it is preferable to resort to inhalation anesthetics. However, there are more risks than benefits in the case of pregnant patients, because they can increase uterine contraction and possible fetal death, which adds to a potential vasodilation bleeding [19].
- In postpartum anaphylaxis, given by factors associated with breastfeeding (not specified due to their peculiarity), there is no clear evidence on the interruption of breastfeeding, since, in certain cases, after receiving an adequate treatment, the symptoms give way completely, but in other cases they show itching as a sequel [14, 20].

Patients who have presented anaphylaxis can keep hypotension, bronchial spasm, and laryngospasm present for several hours or days despite having received a correct and timely treatment. 20% of patients may have a recurrence of anaphylactic shock within the first 24 hours, so their in-hospital management must be done in an Intensive Care Unit [6].

Key Concepts

- Early recognition of anaphylactic shock alarm signs.
- Continuous monitoring of the mother and fetus.
- Place the patient in left lateral recumbency.
- Early and adequate resuscitation for pregnant women improves the prognosis of the fetus.
- The mother's life must be prioritized over the fetus.
- Interrupting the pregnancy can give the mother more opportunity, in case of a critical condition.
- The management and treatment should be early and urgent but does not differ from that of the non-pregnant woman.

Bibliography

1. Grabenhenrich L, et al. Implementation of anaphylaxis management guidelines: a register-based study. PLoS One. 2012;7:e35778.
2. Ferreres-García K, et al. Choque anafiláctico en una gestante en el tercer trimestre de embarazo. Ginecol Obstet Mex. 2014;82:188–93.
3. Beyer K, et al. Anaphylaxis in an emergency setting-elicitors, therapy and incidence of severe allergic reactions. Allergy. 2012;67:1451–6.

4. Adkinson NF, Middleton E. Middleton's allergy: principles & practice, vol. 46. 7th ed. Philadelphia: Mosby/Elsevier; 2009. p. 1765.
5. Berardi A, et al. Maternal anaphylaxis and fetal brain damage after intrapartum chemoprophylaxis. J Perinat Med. 2004;32:375–7.
6. Llanos Palmira LE, Fonseca León A, Carballo Alfaro JB, Benavides Vergara JE. Anafilaxia y anestesia en la paciente Obstétrica. A propósito de un caso. Revista Cubana Anestesiología y Reanimación. 2011;10(1):52–9.
7. Verill PJ. Adverse reactions to local anesthetics and vasoconstrictor drugs. Practitioner. 2005;214:380–7.
8. Mullins RJ, Russell A, McGrath GJ, Smith R, Sutherland DC. Breastfeeding anaphylaxis. Lancet. 1991;338(8777):1279–80.
9. Durgakeri P, Jones B. A rare case of lactation anaphylaxis. Australas Med J. 2015;8(3):103–5.
10. Reviriego J, Fernandez-Alfonso MS, Marin J. Actions of vasoactive drugs on human placental vascular smooth muscle. Gen Pharmacol. 1990;21:719–27.
11. Bytautiene E, et al. The effect of a mast cell degranulating agent on vascular resistance in the human placental vascular bed and on the tone of isolated placental vessels. Reprod Sci. 2008;15:26–32.
12. Sleth JC, et al. Anaphylaxis in terminal pregnancy: two case studies and review of the literature. Ann Fr Anesth Reanim. 2009;28:790–4.
13. Fulcher DA, Kateraris CH. Anaphylactic reactions to local anesthetics despite IgE deficiency. A case report. Asian Pac J Allergy Immunol. 2007;8(2):133–6.
14. Espín VL, Espín RG, Tigre-Guncay M, Quispe-Alcocer J, Silva PR. Anafilaxia post parto por lactancia materna: Reporte de caso. J Health Med Sci. 2018;4(2):77–9.
15. McCall SJ, Bunch KJ, Brocklehurst P, D'Arcy R, Hinshaw K, Kurinczuk JJ, Lucas DN, Stenson B, Tuffnell DJ, Knight M. The incidence, characteristics, management and outcomes of anaphylaxis in pregnancy: a population-based descriptive study. BJOG. 2018;25:965–71.
16. Simons FE, Schatz M. Anaphylaxis during pregnancy. J Allergy Clin Immunol. 2012;130(3):597–606.
17. Chaudhuri K, et al. Anaphylactic shock in pregnancy: a case study and review of the literature. Int J Obstet Anesth. 2008;17:350–7.
18. Pawankar R, Canonica GW, Holgate S, Lockey R, Blaiss M, editors. WAO white book on allergy update 2013. Milwaukee: World Allergy Organization; 2014.
19. Johnson WT, DeStigter T. Hypersensitivity to procaine, tetracaine, mepivacaine, and methylparaben: report of a case. J Am Dent Assoc. 2006;106:53–6.
20. Kang SH, Lee T, Lim H, Koo BS, Lee S, Park YH, Na S, Park SJ, Na HK, Cho YS. A case of breastfeeding anaphylaxis. Korean J Asthma Allergy Clin Immunol. 2011;31(1):55–8.

Part VII
Infectious Diseases

Chapter 27
Sepsis and Septic Shock in Pregnant Patient

Carlos E. Orellana-Jimenez, Jorge Hidalgo, Zulmi Aranda, and Adel Alsisi

General

The Third International Consensus Definitions for Sepsis and Septic Shock (Sepsis-3) defines sepsis as "a life-threatening organic disorder caused by a dysregulated host response to infection" and septic shock as "a subset of sepsis that includes circulatory and cellular/metabolic disorders associated with an increased risk of mortality" [1]. Despite advances in critical medicine, the global incidence of sepsis is high, according to estimates of around 50,000,000 cases per year, and the estimated global mortality secondary to septic shock is 11,000,000 per year [1]. This makes it a real emergency, making its early diagnosis and timely treatment imperative.

Terminology

Systemic inflammatory response syndrome (SIRS): a systemic inflammatory response manifested by two or more of the following conditions: (1) temperature >38 °C or <36 °C; (2) heart rate >90/min; (3) respiratory rate >20/min or CO_2

C. E. Orellana-Jimenez (✉)
Division of Critical Care, Salvadoran Social Security Institute, San Salvador, El Salvador

J. Hidalgo
Division of Critical Care, Karl Heusner Memorial Hospital, Belize City, Belize

Z. Aranda
Critical Care Unit, Instituto de Prevision Social, Asunción, Paraguay

A. Alsisi
Prime Healthcare Group LLC, Dubai, UAE
e-mail: dradel@primehospital.ae

C. Montufar et al. (eds.), *Obstetric Catastrophes*,
https://doi.org/10.1007/978-3-030-70034-8_27

arterial pressure ($paCO_2$) <32 mm Hg; and (4) white blood cell count >12,000 or <4000/mm^3 or >10% immature neutrophils.

Sepsis: a life-threatening organic disorder caused by a dysregulated host response to infection

Septic shock: a subset of sepsis that includes circulatory and cellular/metabolic disorders associated with an increased risk of mortality, in which there is hypotension that requires vasopressors to maintain mean arterial pressure (MAP) >65 mm Hg and a level of arterial lactate >2 mmol/L (18 mg/dL)

Maternal sepsis: organic dysfunction resulting from infection during pregnancy, birth, post-abortion, or postpartum

Organic dysfunction: is one that can be identified as an acute change in the total SOFA score >2 points, consistent with infection

Epidemiology

Globally, sepsis directly causes more than 260,000 maternal deaths a year. The incidence of sepsis varies from a developed country to a developing one and even within each country or city. Globally, 5% of maternal deaths occur in developed countries and 11% in developing countries [2]. This incidence is 0.47:1000 births in the UK; 0.2:1000 in the USA; and 0.1:1000 in Scotland [3]. Meanwhile, the prevalence of maternal mortality from sepsis is 0.8:100,000 births [4]. The prevalence of sepsis in pregnancy is 1:1000 pregnancies [5–8], of which half progress to multiple organ dysfunction and 3–4% to septic shock [8], with global mortality. Of approximately 1:100,000 pregnancies [9], urinary infections, community-acquired pneumonia, and acute appendicitis are the most frequent causes of non-obstetric sepsis [3]. In developing countries, endometriosis, chorioamnionitis, and septic abortion are the predominant infections [10], and with acute respiratory distress syndrome, they are the most frequent causes of maternal mortality [11]. The prevalence among deaths from sepsis in obstetric patients is mainly due to lung infection [12].

During pregnancy, infections caused by different microorganisms may occur; this as a consequence of the decreased immune response. There is an increased frequency of suffering sepsis from Gram-negative microorganisms, and morbidity and mortality are increased compared to that observed in women without pregnancy [13]. Likewise, among some patients, there is a genetic predisposition to suffer sepsis and increase the risk of mortality when the infection develops [14].

It should be borne in mind that the cesarean section increases the risk of infection by around five times among obstetric patients and that the prevalence increases by 50% if performed urgently [15]. It should also be borne in mind that the cesarean section involves the use of bladder catheterization that predisposes to urinary infections in those patients who use epidural anesthesia. Moreover, in those that undergo spinal anesthesia, it conditions respiratory infections because it can suppress the cough reflex for up to 4 hours after birth [16].

Among the main risk factors for maternal sepsis, the following are reported: cesarean delivery, obesity, home delivery, low socioeconomic status, malnutrition, anemia, immunosuppression, prolonged premature rupture of membranes, diabetes, history of cervical-vaginal infections, the performance of more than five vaginal touches during labor, cerclage, multiple pregnancies, bruising, assisted reproduction techniques, and instrumented labor [9, 17].

Sepsis and the Pregnant Patient

In the case of pregnant patients, there are physiological changes typical of their pregnancy, such as changes in heart rate, respiratory rate, and white blood cell count with respect to their non-pregnant controls (see Table 27.1).

T lymphocytes (thymus derivatives) represent cellular immunity, and B lymphocytes represent humoral immunity, which interacts collaboratively. The action of T lymphocytes is shown through two subgroups of cells: helper T lymphocytes (LThelper), which are subdivided into LTh1 and LTh2. LTH1s produce interferon-gamma, interleukin 2, and tumor necrosis factor, which are involved in macrophage activation and immune reactions against intracellular pathogens, as well as in

Table 27.1 Physiologic changes during pregnancy

System	Baseline changes	Physiologic impact
Cardiovascular	Decreased arterial pressure Increased heart rate and cardiac output	Increased risk of hypoperfusion in sepsis Abnormal baseline may mask signs of sepsis
Gastrointestinal	Decreased esophageal tone and delayed gastric emptying	Aspiration pneumonia risk Increased aspiration risk with airway interventions
Genitourinary	Decreased vaginal pH	Increased risk of chorioamnionitis
Hematology	Increased plasma volume without proportional increase in red cell mas, hemoglobin Increased production of factors VII, VIII, IX, X, XII and von Willebrand factor	Physiologic anemia, decreased O_2 supply to tissues Increased risk of disseminated intravascular coagulation and venous thromboembolic disease
Respiratory	Increased tidal volume and minute ventilation with typically unchanged respiratory rate Decreased residual volume due to elevate diaphragm	Decreased partial $paCO_2$ levels (a "normal" blood gas may therefore reflect impeding respiratory failure) Decreased oxygenation with faster rate of desaturation
Renal	Ureteral dilation and increased vesicoureteral reflux Increased renal plasma flow and glomerular filtration rate	Increase risk of pyelonephritis Abnormal baseline may mask renal injury in sepsis

$PaCO_2$ partial pressure of carbon dioxide
Reproduced from: Bridwell et al. [40]

late-type and cytotoxic hypersensitivity reactions, while both LTh2 release interleukins 4, 5, 6, 9, and 10 that facilitate the production of antibodies, necessary for immunity against extracellular microorganisms. Both groups complement and inhibit each other, depending on the circumstances. Furthermore, in pregnancy, there is a decrease in the number and action of T lymphocytes and natural killer cells (natural killer, NK), which is estimated to correlate with the reduction of cellular immunity [18].

Thus, the readjustment of the immune system during pregnancy is not antagonistic, but it becomes less aggressive but competent.

These physiological adaptations of pregnancy start from conception and can persist until 6 weeks after delivery [19]. Therefore, a significant proportion of sepsis-related morbidity and mortality occurs in the first trimester and the puerperium [20] (Table 27.2). There is evidence to suggest that childbirth and the puerperium may increase the risk 2–3 times when compared to the prenatal period, which in countries with low or lower middle income can increase the fatality rate by as much as 50% [21].

Diagnostic Tools

The World Health Organization defines maternal sepsis as "the organic dysfunction resulting from infection during pregnancy, birth, post-abortion or postpartum" [8].

Infection is defined as any process caused by the invasion of normally sterile tissues, liquids, or cavities, by pathogenic or potentially pathogenic microorganisms that initiate a systemic inflammatory response in the host [1].

When this response is dysregulated, it causes sepsis, which in the recent past was categorized as systemic inflammatory response syndrome (SIRS) that accompanied the infection, which was deprecated because it was nonspecific and because it could reflect a normal adaptive response of the host to localized infection [12].

In this sense, the early detection of sepsis in a pregnant patient is a more significant challenge that requires clinical suspicion and the help of simple diagnostic tools that can be used in different settings outside the intensive care unit (ICU). Thus, the Quick SOFA (qSOFA) arises, which is defined by the presence of at least two of the following clinical criteria [1, 5]:

- Respiratory rate is higher than 22 breaths per minute.
- Systolic blood pressure less than 100 mm Hg.
- Alteration of the mental state (Glasgow Coma Score less than 15 points).

Table 27.2 Common sources of infection in sepsis

Variables	Antepartum	Postpartum
Obstetric	Septic abortion Chorioamnionitis	Endometritis Wound infection
Nonobstetric	Urinary tract infection Pneumonia Appendicitis	Urinary tract infection Pneumonia Gastrointestinal

Reproduced from: Society for Maternal-Fetal Medicine (SMFM), Plante et al. [41]

Table 27.3 Obstetrically modified qSOFA score

	Score	
Parameter	0	1
Systolic blood pressure	≥90 mm Hg	<90 mm Hg
Respiratory rate	Less than 25 breaths/min	≥ 25 breaths/min or greater
Altered mentation	Alert (GCS 15 puntos)	No alert (GCS < 15 puntos)

Min minute, *mm Hg* millimeters of mercury, *qSOFA* quick Sequential (sepsis-related) Organ Failure Assessment score, *GCS* Glasgow Coma Score
Reproduced from: Bowyer et al. [4]

Table 27.4 Obstetrically modified Sequential Organ Failure Assessment (SOFA) score

		PUNTAJE		
System	Item	0	1	2
Respiration	PaO_2/FIO_2, mm Hg (kPa)	≥400 (53.3)	300 to <400	<300
Coagulation	Platelets, $\times 10^3/\mu L$	≥150	100–150	<100
Cardiovascular	Mean arterial pressure, mm Hg	≥70	<70	Vasopressors
Liver	Bilirubin, mg/dL (μmol/L)	≤1.2 (20)	1.2–1.9 (20–32)	>1.9 (>1.32)
Central nervous system	Glasgow Coma Scale	Alert	Rousable by voice	Rousable by pain
Renal	Creatinine, mg/dL (μmol/dL),	≤1.02 (< 90)	1.02–1.36 (90–120)	>1.36 (>120)

Adapted from: Bowyer et al. [4]

It must be taken into account that the qSOFA was performed from a population of which half were male with an average age of 61 years [4], a situation whereby the qSOFA variables were adapted to the obstetric population (Table 27.3). It should also be emphasized that this score should be used in scenarios outside the ICU since the SOFA (Sequential Organ Failure Assessment) score is recommended within it [1]. However, the SOFA score has not had adequate prospective validation in populations of pregnant and postpartum patients. The studies that exist to date have been small and retrospective and in environments with limited resources, so some modifications were made to the original SOFA score to adapt it to said population (Table 27.4).

There are other diagnostic tools that have been used to evaluate the early detection of sepsis in pregnant patients; among them, we have the Modified Early Warning Score (MEWS), which proved not to be useful in identifying the risk of sepsis, ICU admission, or death [6, 8]. Another score used is in the National Early Warning Score (NEWS), which has shown reasonable specificity among patients with sepsis, but has not been studied in pregnant patients. Because of the above, the Modified Early Obstetric Warning Score (MEOWS) was created to study the population of pregnant women [6]. However, it was not created to evaluate pregnant patients with sepsis.

Table 27.5 Sepsis obstetric score (SOS)

	Item	4	3	2	1	0	1	2	3	4
T°	°C	>40.9	39–40.9		38.5–38.9	36–38.4	34–35.9	32–33.9	30–31.9	<30
TAS	mm Hg					>90		70–90		<70
FC	beats/min	>179	150–179	130–149	120–129	<119				
FR	breaths/min	>49	35–49		25–34	12–24	10–11	6–9		<5
$SatO_2$	%					>92	90–91		85–89	<85
GB	$\times 10^3/\mu L$	>39.9		25–39.9	17–24.9	5.7–16.9	3.5–6	1–2.9		<1
Arterial lactate	mmol/L			>4		<4				

$SatO_2$ oxygen saturation, *mm Hg* millimeters of mercury, *°C* Celsius degrees
Adapted of: Knowles et al. [21]

Table 27.6 Sepsis signs continuum

Initial signs	Early hours	More than 24 hours
Impaired consciousness Shivering Hyperthermia Arterial hypotension Tachycardia Tachypnea	Cutaneous vasodilation Oliguria Dyspnea Rales Prolonged expiration Leukocytosis or leukopenia	Increase of the uremia Edema Hyponatremia Hepatic injury Adynamic ileus Thrombocytopenia

There are initial signs of sepsis, which, if not treated, progress to more severe signs of systemic compromise
Reproduced from: Malvino [42].

In 2014, the SOS (Sepsis in Obstetric Score) was described (Table 27.5), which is proposed to be used in obstetric or postpartum patients within the first 2 weeks with sepsis; those patients who achieve a score of at least 6 require ICU care [22].

Another parameter that can be used to detect sepsis is the Shock Index (HF), which is the ratio of heart rate to systolic blood pressure (HR/SAT); a recent study showed that the "worst" HF recorded has an excellent negative predictive value for maternal death in the context of sepsis [23].

A sequence of cellular responses to the presence of sepsis has been described [24] (Table 27.6).

Early diagnosis of sepsis through these signs allows:

- Establish if the clinical picture is of infectious origin.
- Determine if you meet the criteria for sepsis or septic shock.
- Predict the probable source focus.
- Consider the existence of underlying diseases and risk factors.

Septic Shock

Relative hypovolemia, myocardial dysfunction, peripheral vasodilation, and hyposensitivity to catecholamines by alpha-adrenergic receptors are causes that can lead to hypotension. The absence of hypotension does not rule out the existence of shock.

Septic shock refers mainly to a distributive shock, characterized by peripheral vasodilation with ineffective availability and oxygen extraction despite presenting low, normal, or increased cardiac output. There is an interaction between abnormal peripheral vasodilation, relative or absolute hypovolemia, abnormal ventricular function, and changes in the distribution of blood flow in the microcirculation [25]. Despite effectively replenishing intravascular volume and improving cardiac output, alterations in microcirculation can persist, severe conditioning alterations in tissue metabolism with tissue dysfunction (Table 27.7).

Another parameter that can be useful in determining the presence of systemic hypoperfusion is the value of the central venous oxygen saturation, which can be obtained with a conventional central venous catheter. This saturation will depend on cardiac output, arterial oxygen saturation, and hemoglobin concentration, as well as peripheral oxygen consumption. The importance of this parameter lies in highlighting the presence of inadequate resuscitation when it is decreased [26].

Septic shock during pregnancy is relatively rare, and mortality is lower when compared to non-pregnant patients. It has a frequency of 0.002–0.01% of all deliveries and 0.3–0.6% of pregnant women with sepsis. There are different causes that can cause septic shock, which is listed in Table 27.8.

In conclusion, septic shock is the most extreme and intense expression of microcirculatory compromise in sepsis, mainly due to less tissue oxygen extraction [27].

Management of Maternal Sepsis

The current management of sepsis is based on the extrapolation of sepsis scoring systems (except for the SOS score), investigation, and treatment in non-pregnant populations.

Table 27.7 Organ damage by sepsis

Organ system	Clinical features
Central nervous system	Altered mental status
Cardiovascular system	Hypotension from vasodilation and third spacing; myocardial dysfunction
Pulmonary system	ARDS
Gastrointestinal system	Paralytic ileus Hepatic failure or abnormal transaminases
Urinary system	Oliguria or acute kidney injury
Hematologic system	Thrombocytopenia or disseminated intravascular coagulopathy
Endocrine system	Adrenal dysfunction and increased insulin resistance

Adapted of: Society for Maternal-Fetal Medicine (SMFM), Plante et al. [41]

Table 27.8 Etiology of septic shock in pregnant patients

Puerperal endometritis	70–85%
Acute pyelonephritis	1–4%
Postpartum vaginal endometritis	1–4%
Septic abortion	1–2%
Surgical wound infections	1–2%
Pneumonia	2%
Chorioamnionitis	0.5–1%
Toxic shock syndrome	<1%
Other causes:	<1%
Appendicitis	
Cholecystitis	
Pelvic septic thrombophlebitis	
Infection secondary to invasive procedures	
Infected cerclage	
Necrotizing fasciitis	
Post-amniocentesis chorioamnionitis	

Adapted of: Albright et al. [22]

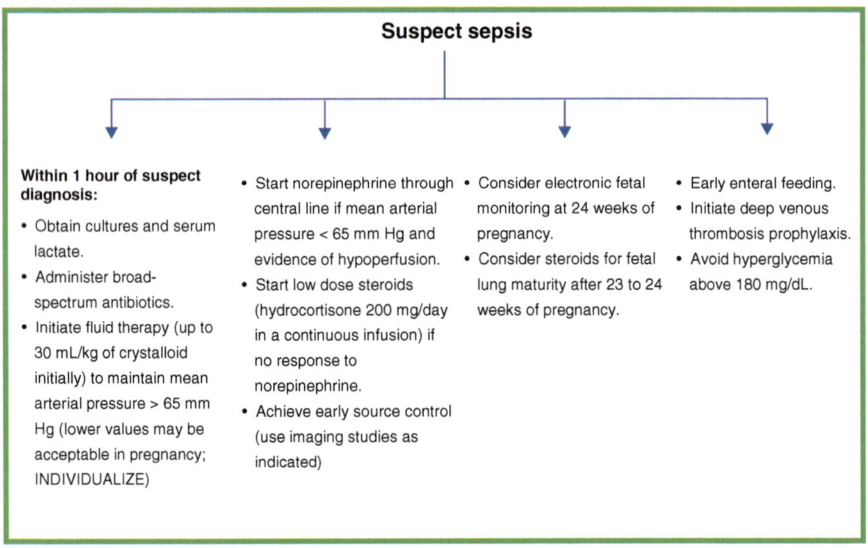

Fig. 27.1 Initial treatment of sepsis during pregnancy. (Adapted of Society for Maternal-Fetal Medicine (SMFM), Plante et al. [41])

Initial management should include simultaneous actions such as taking samples for cultures (if it does not imply a delay in the administration of antibiotics), judicious resuscitation with liquids, early initiation of antibiotics, and determination of infectious focus, among others (see Fig. 27.1; Table 27.9).

Table 27.9 Summary of recommendations in pregnant patients with sepsis

Number	Recommendation	Grade
1	We recommend that sepsis and septic shock be considered medical emergencies and that treatment and resuscitation for sepsis begin immediately	1B Strong recommendation, moderate-quality evidence
2	We recommend that providers consider the diagnosis of sepsis in pregnant patients with otherwise unexplained end-organ damage in the presence of an infectious process, regardless of the presence of fever	1B Strong recommendation, moderate-quality evidence
3	We recommend that empiric broad-spectrum antibiotics be administered as soon as possible, ideally within 1 hour, in any pregnant woman in whom sepsis is suspected	1B Strong recommendation, moderate-quality evidence
4	We recommend obtaining cultures (blood, urine, respiratory, and others as indicated) and serum lactate levels in pregnant or postpartum women in whom sepsis is suspected or identified. Early source control should be completed as soon as possible	1C Strong recommendation, low-quality evidence
5	We recommend early administration of 1–2 L of crystalloid solutions in sepsis complicated by hypotension or organ hypoperfusion	1C Strong recommendation, low-quality evidence
6	We recommend the use of norepinephrine as the first-line vasopressor during pregnancy and the postpartum period in sepsis with persistent hypotension and/or hypoperfusion despite fluid resuscitation	1C Strong recommendation, low-quality evidence
7	We recommend against immediate delivery for the sole indication of sepsis and that delivery should be dictated by obstetric indications	1B Strong recommendation, moderate-quality evidence

Reproduced from: Society for Maternal-Fetal Medicine (SMFM), Plante et al. [41]

Antibiotics

The most frequently isolated microorganisms in maternal sepsis are group A and group B *Escherichia coli* and *Streptococcus* [28, 29], although staphylococci, Gram-harmful, and anaerobic bacteria have been reported. Mixed infections are also possible and have been identified in 15% of maternal deaths from sepsis [30] (Table 27.10).

The use of broad-spectrum antibiotics is recommended to be administered as quickly as possible, ideally within 1 hour and hour, in any pregnant or postpartum patient in whom sepsis is suspected (Grade 1B) [5]. Antibiotics will be modified to a narrower spectrum and focused according to the results of the cultures. Molecular

Table 27.10 Proposed broad-spectrum empiric antibiotic coverage in sepsis complicating pregnancy

Source infection	Recommend antibiotics
Community-acquired pneumonia	Cefotaxime, ceftriaxone, ertapenem, or ampicillin plus azithromycin, clarithromycin, or erythromycin
Hospital-acquired pneumonia	Low-risk patients may be treated with piperacillin-tazobactam, meropenem, imipenem, or cefepime Patients at high risk may be need double coverage for *Pseudomonas* (beta-lactam plus an aminoglycoside or a quinolone) and MSRA coverage with vancomycin or linezolid
Chorioamnionitis	Ampicillin plus gentamicin. Add anaerobic coverage with clindamycin or metronidazole is cesarean delivery required
Endomyometritis	Ampicillin, gentamicin, and metronidazole (o clindamycin) Alternatively may use cefotaxime or ceftriaxone plus metronidazole
Urinary tract infections	Gentamicin with ampicillin Alternatively, may use monotherapy with a carbapenem or piperacillin-tazobactam
Abdominal infections	Ceftriaxone, cefotaxime, ceftazidime, or cefepime plus metronidazole Complicate cases may require monotherapy with a carbapenem or piperacillin-tazobactam
Skin and soft tissues (necrotizing)	Vancomycin plus piperacillin-tazobactam If *Streptococcus* group A or *Clostridium perfringens* are present, use penicillin G plus clindamycin.

MRSA methicillin-resistant *Staphylococcus aureus*
Reproduced from: Society for Maternal-Fetal Medicine (SMFM), Plante et al. [41]

techniques can improve the ability to identify undetected organisms based on culture methods.

As for monitoring the response to antibiotics in pregnant patients with sepsis, procalcitonin has a role in determining since the values have not been defined in this population, and these values must be considered individually, taking into account the clinical condition of the patient. A recent review [31] showed that the available evidence is of moderate quality with insufficient sample power per outcome, concluding that procalcitonin-guided antimicrobial therapy is not supported for patients with sepsis. More data is needed to support the use of procalcitonin in obstetric patients.

Resuscitation with Fluids

Fluid resuscitation should be part of the initial intervention if there is hypotension or hypoperfusion. Fever, venodilation, and capillary leak lead to inadequate preload in patients with sepsis. The Surviving Sepsis Campaign recommends an initial bolus of 30 mL/kg of crystalloid solution [32], but this recommendation may be too aggressive in pregnant patients, in whom the colloid-oncotic pressure is lower, and the risk of pulmonary edema is higher [5]. Only about 50% of hypotensive patients are fluid responders, and in those who are not, aggressive fluid administration can produce left ventricular dysfunction secondary to ventricular wall edema; pulmonary edema; cerebral edema; intestinal edema with increased pressure, intra-abdominal; and higher mortality [33].

In most pregnant patients, the initial administration of 1–2 L of crystalloids is reasonable. Patients who are responders to liquids must be identified after the initial bolus in order to continue with fluid resuscitation. It is recommended to use dynamic variables to monitor the preload, among which the variation of the pulse pressure, passive leg elevation, and point of care ultrasound (POCUS) can be mentioned.

Placement in Left Side Decube

Usually, pregnant patients with hypotension are placed in left lateral decubitus, mainly in the third trimester. One study showed that this intervention increased the diameter of the inferior vena cava (measured by ultrasound) by a maximum of 76% (average of 29%) among the study patients; however, 25% of patients achieved their largest inferior vena cava diameter by being in the supine position [34]. Another study found, via nuclear magnetic resonance imaging, that cardiac output in pregnant patients in the third trimester decreased by 16.4% when moving from the left lateral to the supine position, with a decrease in the diameter of the inferior vena cava at its origin in 85.3% and 44.4% at the level of the renal veins, with an increase in diameter of 220% in the azygos vein [35].

In conclusion, placing hypotensive pregnant women in left lateral decubitus improves venous return and, therefore, cardiac output.

Vasopressors and Inotropes

In pregnant patients with sepsis who are not responsive or who are not candidates for fluid resuscitation (e.g., patient with acute pulmonary edema), vasopressors should be used to increase blood pressure. The purpose of vasopressors is to constrict the pathologically dilated systemic circulation and to maintain adequate perfusion. The Surviving Sepsis Campaign recommends norepinephrine as the first-line drug, with the goal of mean arterial pressure (MAP) of at least 65 mm Hg, although this goal has not been studied in pregnant women with sepsis. Therefore, determining the goal of MAP in this type of patient should be individualized, considering the perfusion of all the organs. Health professionals should not hesitate to administer norepinephrine when indicated in a pregnant patient with sepsis.

Norepinephrine has been studied in pregnancy and is often used to maintain blood pressure in regional anesthesia in the case of cesarean section [36].

Dobutamine is an inotrope (increases cardiac output) and is recommended in the setting of myocardial dysfunction or continuous hypoperfusion despite therapy with fluids and vasopressors [32].

Steroids

Steroids are recommended in non-pregnant patients in whom hemodynamic instability does not respond with the use of vasopressors due to the possibility of sepsis-induced adrenal failure [32]. There is no evidence at the moment in pregnant patients. There is a recommendation in a guideline to use steroids in pregnant women with sepsis [5].

Indication of Labor in Patients with Sepsis

The only indication for delivery due to the mere presence of sepsis is in cases of chorioamnionitis.

The decision to carry the pregnancy to term must be individualized and will depend on the gestational age as well as the maternal and fetal conditions. In most cases, resuscitation improves maternal hemodynamics, which results in the improvement of uteroplacental perfusion and, consequently, in the improvement of the fetal condition. Delivery should be reserved for usual obstetric indications after the stabilization of the mother. There is no evidence that childbirth improves maternal outcomes [5].

The primary objective should be hemodynamic support therapy for the maternal benefit and antibiotic treatment with adequate control of the focus of infection.

Corticosteroids for fetal lung maturation are not contraindicated and may be used in sepsis if their use is indicated [5]. They are recommended in pregnant women with sepsis who are between weeks 24 and 33 with 6 days, with a risk of preterm delivery within the next 7 days [37].

Glycemic Control and Prophylaxis for Venous Thromboembolism

Maternal hyperglycemia can directly cause fetal hyperglycemia, and this can lead to acidosis, decreasing uterine blood flow, and fetal oxygenation [5]. Maternal serum glucose levels should be kept below 180 mg/dL.

Pregnancy itself increases the risk of deep vein thrombosis fivefold compared to non-pregnant patients [38]. In patients with septic shock who had prophylaxis for venous thrombosis, there was a 37% incidence of this pathology despite prophylaxis interventions. As pregnant patients are at high risk of venous thromboembolism, therefore, in patients without contraindications, they should use intermittent lower limb compression devices and either a daily dose of low molecular weight heparin or the administration of heparin 2–3 times a day. Unfractionated [5, 38].

Considerations on Studies in Progress

The Global Maternal Sepsis Study (GLOSS) [39] and the awareness campaign were implemented in 53 low-, middle-, and high-income countries in late 2017. The main objectives of the Global Maternal Sepsis Study (GLOSS) are:

1. Develop and validate a set of criteria for the identification of possible severe maternal infection (suspected maternal sepsis) and maternal sepsis (confirmed sepsis).
2. Evaluate the frequency and results of maternal sepsis in low- and middle-income countries compared to high-income countries.
3. Evaluate the frequency of use of a basic set of recommended practices for prevention, early identification, and management of maternal sepsis. Through the evaluation of the campaign we seek.
4. Explore the level of awareness of maternity and neonatal sepsis among healthcare providers, policymakers, and the general public, including pregnant women, mothers, and their families.

The results will provide global information on maternal sepsis. The final expected impact of the study is to improve early detection and management of women with sepsis.

Bibliography

1. Singer M, Deutschman CS, Seymour CW, et al. The third international consensus definitions for sepsis and septic shock (sepsis-3). JAMA. 2016;315(8):801–10. https://doi.org/10.1001/jama.2016.0287. PMID: 26903338.
2. Say L, Chou D, Gemmill A, et al. Global causes of maternal death: a WHO systematic analysis. Lancet Glob Health. 2014;2:e323–33. https://doi.org/10.1016/S2214-109X(14)70227-X.
3. Kramer H, Schutte J, Zwart J, Schuitemaker N, Steegers E, Roosmalen J. Maternal mortality and severe morbidity from sepsis in the Netherlands. Acta Obstet Gynecol. 2009;88:647–53. https://doi.org/10.1080/00016340902926734. PMID: 19412806.
4. Bowyer L, Robinson H, Barrett H, Crozier T, et al. SOMANZ guidelines for the investigation and management sepsis in pregnancy. Aust NZ J Obstet Gynaecol. 2017:1–12. https://doi.org/10.1111/ajo.12646. PMID: 28670748.
5. Plante L. Management of sepsis and septic shock for the obstetrician-gynecologistst. Obstet Gynecol Clin N Am. 2016;43:659–78. https://doi.org/10.1016/j.ogc.2016.07.010. PMID: 27816153.

6. Chebbo A, Tan S, Kassis C, Tamura L, et al. Maternal sepsis, and septic shock. Crit Care Clin. 2016;32:119–35. https://doi.org/10.1016/j.ccc.2015.08.010. PMID: 26600449.
7. Oud L. Pregnancy-associated severe sepsis. Curr Opin Obstet Gynecol. 2016;28(2):73–8. https://doi.org/10.1097/GCO.0000000000000250. PMID: 26825182.
8. Burlison C, Sirounis D, Walley K, Chau A. Sepsis in pregnancy and the puerperium. Int J Obstet Anesth. 2018;36:96–107. https://doi.org/10.1016/j.ijoa.2018.04.010. PMID: 29921485.
9. Cordioli R, Cordioli E, Negrini R, Silva E. Sepsis, and pregnancy: do we know to treat this situation? Rev Bras Ter Intensiva. 2013;25(4):334–44. https://doi.org/10.5935/0103-507X.20130056. PMID: 24553516.
10. Langford KS. Infectious disease and pregnancy. Curr Obstet Gynaecol. 2002;12:125–30. https://doi.org/10.1054/cuog.2001.0247.
11. Nelson PC. Infections in pregnancy. Curr Obstet Gynaecol. 2000;10:177.
12. Puertas Prieto A, Gallo J, Ruiz S. Identificación precoz de la sepsis obstétrica. Rev Latin Perinat. 2017;20(2):70–7.
13. Gonzalez J, Ofori E, Burd I, Chai J, Scholler N, Elovitz M. Maternal mortality from systemic illness: unraveling the contribution of the immune response. Am J Obstet Gynecol. 2009;200:430e1–8. https://doi.org/10.1016/j.ajog.2009.01.049.
14. Balk R. Optimum treatment of severe sepsis and septic shock. Disease-a-Month. 2004;50:163–213. https://doi.org/10.1016/j.disamonth.2003.12.003. PMID: 15133467.
15. Leth R, Moller J, Thomsen R, Uldbjerg N, et al. Risk of selected postpartum infections after cesarean section compared with vaginal birth. Acta Obstet Gynecol. 2009;88:976–83. https://doi.org/10.1080/00016340903147405. PMID: 19642043.
16. Belfort M, Clark S, Saade G, Kleja K, et al. Hospital readmission after delivery: evidence for an increased incidence of nonurogenital infection in the immediate postpartum period. Am J Obstet Gynecol. 2010;202:35.e1–7. https://doi.org/10.1016/j.ajog.2009.08.029. PMID: 19889389.
17. Spera AM, Bianco V, Simeone D, Vicente G, et al. Sepsis in pregnant and puerperal women living in high-income countries: an update for clinicians. J Gynecol Obstet. 2017;1:023.
18. Tejerizo López L, et al. Revisión de la respuesta inmunitaria materna a la infección. Clin Invest Ginecol Obstet. 2001;28(2):74–7.
19. Greer O, Shah NM, Sriskandan S, Johnson MR. Sepsis: precision-based medicine for pregnancy and the puerperium. Int J Mol Sci. 2019;20:5388. https://doi.org/10.3390/ijms20215388. PMID: 31671794.
20. Bonet M, Nogueira PV, Rijken MJ, Coomarasamy A, et al. Towards a consensus definition of maternal sepsis: results of a systematic review and expert consultation. Reprod Health. 2017;14:67. https://doi.org/10.1186/s12978-018-0451-5. PMID: 29310684.
21. Knowles SJ, O'Sullivan NP, Meenan AM, Hanni R, Robson M. Maternal sepsis incidence, etiology, and outcome for mother and fetus: A prospective study. BJOG. 2015;122:663–71. https://doi.org/10.1111/14710528.12892. PMID: 24862293.
22. Albright C, Ali T, Lopes V, Rouse D, et al. The sepsis in the obstetrics score: a model to identify the risk of morbidity from sepsis in pregnancy. Am J Obstet Gynecol 2014;211(1):39:e1–8. https://doi.org/10.1016/j.ajog.2014.03.010. PMID: 24613756.
23. Nathan HL, Seed PT, Hezelgrave NL, De Gree A, et al. Shock index thresholds to predict adverse outcomes in maternal hemorrhage and sepsis: A prospective cohort study. Acta Obstet Gynecol Scand. 2019;98:1178–86.
24. Malvino E. Obstetricia Crítica. (libro en Internet). 2ª Edición. Buenos Aires, Argentina. Eduardo Malvino, Publisher. 2019. Tomo IV. Infecciones Graves del Embarazo y Puerperio. Capítulo 1. Sepsis y Shock Séptico en Obstetricia (revisado 02/22/2020). Páginas 1–64. Disponible en: http://www.obstetriciacritica.com/doc/Infecciones_Graves.pdf.
25. Hollenberg S, Ahrens T, Annane D, Astiz M, et al. Practice parameters for hemodynamic support of sepsis in adult patients. Crit Care Med. 2004;32:1928–48. https://doi.org/10.1097/01.ccm.0000139761.05492.d6. PMID: 15343024.
26. Hernandez Poblete G. Consideraciones sobre el uso de drogas vasoactivas en el shock séptico. Programa de actualización en terapia intensiva. Ed Panamericana, Buenos Aires; 2001.

27. Mejía Monroy A, Moreno A, Tellez G, Turcios F. Sepsis y embarazo. FLASOG guía 1, 2013. (Revisado 02/22 2020). Disponible en: http://unimedudoanz.weebly.com/uploads/4/8/2/8/48281567/flasog.pdf.
28. Kramer HM, Schutte JM, Zwart JJ, Schuitemaker NW, et al. Maternal mortality and severe morbidity from sepsis in the Netherlands. Acta Obstet Gynecol Scand. 2009;88:647–53. https://doi.org/10.1080/00016340902926734. PMID: 19412806.
29. Acosta CD, Kurinczuk JJ, Lucas DN, Tuffnell DJ, Sellers S, Knight M. Severe maternal sepsis in the UK, 2011–2012: a national case-control study. PLoS Med. 2014;11:e1001672. https://doi.org/10.1371/journal.pmed.1001672. PMID: 25003759.
30. Bauer ME, Lorenz RP, Bauer ST, Rao K, Anderson FW. Maternal deaths due to sepsis in the state of Michigan, 1999–2006. Obstet Gynecol. 2015;126:747–52. https://doi.org/10.1097/AOG.0000000000001028. PMID: 26348189.
31. Andriolo BN, Andriolo RB, Salomão R, Atallah AN. Effectiveness and safety of procalcitonin evaluation for reducing mortality in adults with sepsis, severe sepsis, or septic shock. Cochrane Database Syst Rev. 2017;1:CD010959. https://doi.org/10.1002/14651858.CD010959.pub2. PMID: 28099689.
32. Rhodes A, Evans LE, Alhazzani W, et al. Surviving sepsis campaign: international guidelines for the management of sepsis and septic shock: 2016. Intensive Care Med. 2017;43:304–77. https://doi.org/10.1007/s00134-017-4683-6. PMID: 28101605.
33. Marik P, Bellomo R. A rational approach to fluid therapy in sepsis. Br J Anaesth. 2016;116:339–49. https://doi.org/10.1093/bja/aev349. PMID: 26507493.
34. Fields JM, Catallo K, Au AK, Rotte M, Leventhal D, Weiner S, Ku BS. Resuscitation of the pregnant patient: what is the effect of patient positioning on inferior vena cava diameter? Resuscitation. 2013;84:304–8. https://doi.org/10.1016/j.resuscitation.2012.11.011. PMID: 23178869.
35. Humphries A, Mirjalili SA, Tarr GP, Thompson JMD, Stone P. The effect of supine positioning on maternal hemodynamics during late pregnancy. J Matern Fetal Neonatal Med. 2019;32:3923–30. https://doi.org/10.1080/14767058.2018.1478958. PMID: 29772936.
36. Ngan Kee WD, Lee SW, Ng FF, Tan PE, Khaw KS. Randomized double-blinded comparison of norepinephrine and phenylephrine for maintenance of blood pressure during spinal anesthesia for cesarean delivery. Anesthesiology. 2015;122:736–45. https://doi.org/10.1097/ALN.0000000000000601. PMID: 25635593.
37. Roberts D, Brown J, Medley N, Dalziel SR. Antenatal corticosteroids for accelerating fetal lung maturation for women at risk of preterm birth. Cochrane Database Syst Rev. 2017;(3):CD004454. https://doi.org/10.1002/14651858.CD004454.pub3. PMID: 28321847.
38. Kaplan D, Casper TC, Elliott CG, et al. VTE incidence and risk factors in patients with severe sepsis and septic shock. Chest. 2015;148:1224–30. https://doi.org/10.1378/chest.15-0287. PMID: 26111103.
39. Bonet M, Souza JP, Abalos E, et al. The global maternal sepsis study and awareness campaign (GLOSS): study protocol. Reprod Health. 2018;15:16. https://doi.org/10.1186/s12978-017-0437-8. PMID: 29382352.
40. Bridwell RE, Carius BM, Long B, Oliver JJ, Schmitz G. Sepsis in pregnancy: recognition and resuscitation. West J Emerg Med. 2019;20:822–32. https://doi.org/10.5811/westjem.2019.6.43369.
41. Society for Maternal-Fetal Medicine (SMFM), Plante L, Pacheco LJM. SMFM Consult Series #47: Sepsis during pregnancy and the puerperium. Am J Obstet Gynecol. 2019;220:B2–B10. https://doi.org/10.1016/j.ajog.2019.01.216. PMID: 30684460.
42. Malvino E. Chapter 1: Sepsis and septic shock in pregnancy. In: Tome 4, Severe infections in pregnancy and puerperium. 2nd edition (Spanish). Buenos Aires: Eduardo Malvino Publisher; 2019, p. 13–44.

Chapter 28
Chorioamnionitis

Laura Pilar Vélez Batista

Chorioamnionitis (intra-amniotic infection) is an acute inflammation of the membranes, amniotic fluid, and chorion of the placenta, typically due to ascending polymicrobial bacterial infection in the setting of rupture of membranes. According to *Higgins* et al., it represents Intrauterine Infection and/or Inflammation (Triple-I) [1, 2].

Chorioamnionitis can occur with intact membranes, and this seems especially common with genital mycoplasmas, such as *Ureaplasma* species and *Mycoplasma hominis*, found in the lower genital tract of more than 70% of women [1].

Intraamniotic infection is present in 10–15% of patients with an episode of preterm birth and nearly 50% of very early preterm births [3]. Clinical infection also complicates 1% of term pregnancies.

The route of infection is usually migration (ascending bacterial invasion) from the cervicovaginal area, with progression to the amnion, decidua, and amniotic fluid [4].

The infection is typically polymicrobial; some common organisms associated with chorioamnionitis include *Ureaplasma* (47%), *Mycoplasma* (30%), *Gardnerella vaginalis* (25%), *Bacteroides* (30%), gram-negative rods including *Escherichia coli* (8%), and group B streptococcus (15%) [1]. GBS specifically has wide variability in prevalence among global populations [5]. Fungi can also be found; women who become pregnant while using intrauterine contraceptive devices are at high risk for intraamniotic infection with *Candida albicans* [6]. Bacteremia occurs in up to 10% of cases, especially with *E. coli* and group B streptococcal infection [4].

Intraamniotic infection also can occur, after invasive procedures (e.g., amniocentesis or chorionic villus sampling) [7] or by hematogenous pathway secondary to maternal systemic infection. Microorganisms such as *Listeria monocytogenes, Treponema pallidum, Yersinia pestis, Cytomegalovirus, Plasmodium*

L. P. Vélez Batista (✉)
Hospital Dr. Manuel Amador Guerrero (CSS), Colon City, Panama

C. Montufar et al. (eds.), *Obstetric Catastrophes*,
https://doi.org/10.1007/978-3-030-70034-8_28

species, and others can gain access through the maternal circulation to the intervillous space, from where they invade the villi and the fetal circulation. Bacteria involved in periodontal disease may use this pathway to reach the amniotic cavity [6].

Chorioamnionitis is a serious obstetric infection and is associated with increased risk of premature delivery and neonatal sepsis [4].

Table 28.1 Risk factors [1, 4]

Prolonged labor
Longer duration of rupture of membrane
Nulliparity
Multiple digital vaginal examinations
Presence of genital trace pathogens
Young age
Alcohol or drug abuse
Immunocompromised states

Clinical Signs and Symptoms

The patient presents sepsis, maternal tachycardia (>100 beats/min), fetal tachycardia (persistent elevation of fetal heart rate >160 beats/min), uterine tenderness, and purulent or foul vaginal discharge. *Fever* is present in almost all instances and is essential for diagnosis [4, 8].

Temperature greater than 100.4 °F (38 °C) is considered abnormal in pregnancy and warrants evaluation and appropriate intervention [1].

ACOG, in an expert workshop executive summary, defined *isolated maternal fever* as either a single oral temperature of 39 °C or greater, or an oral temperature of 38–38.9 °C that persists when the temperature is repeated after 30 minutes. Suspected intraamniotic infection is based on clinical criteria, which include maternal intrapartum fever and one or more of the following: maternal leukocytosis, purulent cervical drainage, or fetal tachycardia. The exact mechanism of such an effect remains unclear, although fetal hyperthermia (and associated changes in metabolic rate) is hypothesized to potentiate the negative effects of tissue hypoxia. Currently, given the potential benefits for the woman and newborn, antibiotics should be considered in the setting of isolated maternal fever unless a source other than intraamniotic infection is identified and documented [7].

Noninfectious causes of fever include use of epidural analgesia during labor, hyperthyroidism, dehydration, elevated ambient temperature, and the use of pyrogens such as prostaglandin E2 for the induction of labor [2].

Maternal tachycardia may be present in the absence of chorioamnionitis and requires careful assessment for alternative origins. Medications, such as ephedrine, antihistamines, and b-agonists, may raise maternal or fetal heart rate.

The combination of maternal fever and maternal or fetal tachycardia is strongly suggestive, however, of intrauterine infection and should be treated accordingly [1].

Diagnosis

It can be confirmed with Gram stain, culture of amniotic fluid, or both and biochemical analysis, but for most women at term who are in labor, the diagnosis is primarily made using *clinical criteria.*

Blood Tests

- Complete blood cell count: Maternal leukocytosis (white blood cell >15,000 cells/mm^3) or the presence of a left shift or bandemia (>9%) often supports the diagnosis of chorioamnionitis. Leukocytosis is reported in approximately 70–90% of cases of clinical chorioamnionitis. Isolated leukocytosis in the absence of other signs or symptoms, however, is of limited value because it may be induced by several other conditions, including labor and steroid use.
- High levels of C-reactive protein (CRP), lipopolysaccharide-binding protein, soluble intercellular adhesion molecule 1, and interleukin (IL)-6 are associated with a higher risk of chorioamnionitis in the setting of preterm premature rupture of membranes (PPROM) or preterm delivery. Their usefulness for the diagnosis or prediction of chorioamnionitis, however, as part of routine clinical practice is not established.

Amniotic Fluid Testing

Tests on amniotic fluid, usually obtained by amniocentesis, have been used for the diagnosis of chorioamnionitis. Culture of amniotic fluid is the most reliable test but is of limited use because culture results may not be available for up to 3 days. In addition, because of the invasive nature of the procedure, amniocentesis is not performed in the majority of cases of chorioamnionitis, which occur during labor. Some clinicians use amniocentesis to confirm clinically suspected chorioamnionitis to determine whether or not preterm delivery is warranted (thus avoiding iatrogenic prematurity) [1, 4].

Confirmed intraamniotic infection among women in labor at term will most commonly be made after delivery, based on histopathologic study of the placenta.

Histologically, it is staged on the basis of specific criteria, with increasing neutrophil infiltration and the development of necrosis, amnion basement membrane thickening, and chorionic microabscesses being seen with increasing disease severity. In addition, the fetal inflammatory response may progress from chorionic/umbilical vasculitis (neutrophil infiltration in the chorionic or umbilical vessels) to necrotizing funisitis (inflammation of the connective tissue of the umbilical cord) [8].

Treatment [7]

Empiric antibiotic coverage against aerobes and anaerobes should be initiated:

Table 28.2 Primary regimen includes

Ampicillin 2 g IV every 6 hours with Gentamicin 2 mg/kg IV load followed by 1.5 mg/kg every 8 hours *or* 5 mg/kg IV every 24 hours
Mild penicillin allergy
Cefazolin 2 g IV every 8 hours with Gentamicin 2 mg/kg IV load followed by 1.5 mg/kg every 8 hours *or* 5 mg/kg IV every 24 hours
Severe penicillin allergy
Clindamycin 900 mg IV every 8 hours or
Vancomycin 1 g IV every 12 hours with Gentamicin 2 mg/kg IV load followed by 1.5 mg/kg every 8 hours or 5 mg/kg IV every 24 hours

Alternative Regimens

Ampicillin–sulbactam 3 g IV every 6 hours

Piperacillin–tazobactam 3.375 g IV every 6 hours or 4.5 g IV every 8 hours

Cefotetan 2 g IV every 12 hours

Cefoxitin 2 g IV every 8 hours

Ertapenem 1 g IV every 24 hours

Clindamycin or metronidazole should be added to this regimen to enhance coverage of anaerobic organisms if the patient requires cesarean delivery. Failure to add anaerobic coverage in patients who undergo a cesarean delivery will result in treatment failure in up to 25% of patients [9].

Therefore, while antibiotic therapy cannot eradicate the infection, it is an important pillar of management to prevent exacerbation of disease prior to delivery [2].

Intrapartum antibiotics also have been shown to decrease maternal febrile morbidity and length of hospital stay. There is no benefit to continued oral antibiotics after parenteral therapy.

Intrapartum antimicrobial agents administered for suspected or confirmed intraamniotic infection should not be continued automatically postpartum; some cases need extension of antimicrobial therapy and should be based on risk factors or postpartum endometritis. Data suggest that women who have vaginal deliveries are less likely to have endometritis and may not require postpartum antibiotics. For women undergoing cesarean deliveries, at least one additional dose of antimicrobial agents after delivery is recommended. However, the presence of other maternal risk factors such as bacteremia or persistent fever in the postpartum period may be used to guide continuation of antimicrobial therapy [7].

Delivery will provide source control and prevent neonatal complications, but time to delivery does not appear to impact outcome. Cesarean delivery is not indicated and should be reserved for the usual obstetric indications [4].

Sepsis can lead to hypotension and decreased renal perfusion, with resultant prerenal ischemia, and potentially to acute tubular necrosis [10]. Persistent sepsis after delivery and antibiotic therapy should prompt a search for necrotizing myometritis or pelvic abscess [11].

Intraamniotic infection can be associated with long-term complications for the infant, such as bronchopulmonary dysplasia and cerebral palsy, potentially due to the effect of inflammation alone [8, 12]. More recently, severe maternal infections that include clinical chorioamnionitis have been linked to autism spectrum disorder in children [13].

When treating septic abortion or chorioamnionitis, evacuation of the uterine contents is necessary, because antibiotic penetration of the uterine cavity is suboptimal [14].

Prognosis

The prognosis for women diagnosed with chorioamnionitis is generally good; however, intra-amniotic infection does increase the likelihood of labor abnormalities and leads to a twofold to threefold increased risk of cesarean section. It also increases the risk for wound infection, pelvic abscess, and postpartum uterine atony with hemorrhage, endometritis, peritonitis, sepsis, adult respiratory distress syndrome, intensive care unit admission, and rare instances, maternal mortality [2, 15, 16].

References

1. Tita ATN, Andrews WW. Diagnosis and management of clinical chorioamnionitis. Clin Perinatol. 2010;37(2):339–54.
2. Higgins RD, Saade G, Polin RA, Grobman WA, Buhimschi IA, Watterberg K, et al. Chorioamnionitis Workshop Participants. Evaluation and management of women and newborns with a maternal diagnosis of chorioamnionitis: summary of a workshop. Obstet Gynecol. 2016;127:426–36.
3. Gravett MG. Successful treatment of intraamniotic infection/inflammation: a paradigm shift. Am J Obstet Gynecol. 2019;221(2):83–5.
4. Chebbo A, Tan S, Kassis C, et al. Maternal sepsis and septic shock. Crit Care Clin. 2015. https://doi.org/10.1016/j.ccc.2015.08.010.

5. Le Doare K, Heath PT. An overview of global GBS epidemiology. Vaccine. 2013;31(Suppl. 4):D7–D12.
6. Kim CJ, Romero R, Chaemsaithong P, Chaiyasit N, Yoon BH, Kim YM. Acute chorioamnionitis and funisitis: definition, pathologic features, and clinical significance. Am J Obstet Gynecol. 2015;213(4):S29–52.
7. The American College of Obstetricians and Gynecologists. Committee opinion: intrapartum management of intraamniotic infection, number 712; 2017.
8. Czikk MJ, McCarthy FP, Murphy KE. Chorioamnionitis: from pathogenesis to treatment. Clin Microbiol Infect. 2011;17:1304–11.
9. Black LP, Hinson L, Duff P. Limited course of antibiotic treatment for chorioamnionitis. Obstet Gynecol. 2012;119(6):1102–5.
10. Balofsky A, Fedarau M. Renal failure in pregnancy. Crit Care Clin. 2016;32(1):73–83. https://doi.org/10.1016/j.ccc.2015.08.003.
11. Lapinsky S. Obstetric infections. Crit Care Clin. 2013. https://doi.org/10.1016/j.ccc.2013.03.006.
12. Jobe AH. Mechanisms of lung injury and bronchopulmonary dysplasia. Am J Perinatol. 2016;33:1076–8.
13. Lee BK, Magnusson C, Gardner RM, et al. Maternal hospitalization with infection during pregnancy and risk of autism spectrum disorders. Brain Behav Immun. 2015;44:100–5.
14. Gammill HS, Jeyabalan A. Acute renal failure in pregnancy. Crit Care Med. 2005;33(Suppl):S372–84.
15. Morgan J, Roberts S. Maternal Sepsis. Obstet Gynecol Clin N Am. 2013;40(1):69–87. https://doi.org/10.1016/j.ogc.2012.11.007.
16. Rouse DJ, Landon M, Leveno KJ, Leindecker S, Varner MW, Caritis SN, et al. The Maternal-Fetal Medicine Units Cesarean registry: chorioamnionitis at term and its duration-relationship to outcomes. Am J Obstet Gynecol. 2004;191(1):211–6.

Chapter 29
Pneumonia During Pregnancy

Alex Dagoberto Loarca Chávez

Introduction

The community-acquired pneumonia is a potentially serious condition that can complicate particularly pregnant women; being the most common cause of fatal infection related causes nonobstetric pregnancy [1]. Pneumonia increases the risk of complications in the fetus also, as described by Madinger et al. [2]. Preterm labor occurs in 44% of patients with pneumonia, with a percentage of 36% of preterm births. The pregnant patient suffers anatomical, physiological, and immunological changes; related to the enlargement of the uterus and in response to physiological needs of pregnancy, these changes are occurred as the pregnancy progresses, which are reviewed in this chapter according to variants that can cause the pneumonia. The diagnosis is made in the same manner as in the general population, taking into account the limitations on radiation exposure. As ultrasound lung as a tool increasingly present in the clinical approach, it is presented. The treatment is focused on the most frequent etiologic microorganisms, which are similar to nonpregnant yet taken in drugs that can cause harm to the fetus. There are risk factors inherent in pregnancy both to acquire pneumonia, as complications thereof, which are discussed in this chapter which are similar to nonpregnant; however it takes into drugs that can cause harm to the fetus.

A. D. Loarca Chávez (✉)
Head of the Adult Intensive Care, Quetzaltenango Regional Hospital, Quetzaltenango, Guatemala

President of the Quetzaltenango Chapter, Guatemalan Society of Intensive Care, Guatemala City, Guatemala

C. Montufar et al. (eds.), *Obstetric Catastrophes*,
https://doi.org/10.1007/978-3-030-70034-8_29

Epidemiology

Different incidences have been reported associated with pneumonia in pregnancy, with variations in the course of recent decades. In the 1980s increased incidence was attributed to new immunodeficiencies HIV, drug abuse, and onset of chronic diseases in pregnant women, as the average age of pregnant patients was increasingly reported. Benedetti et al. [3] in 1982 reported 0.4 per 1000 deliveries; Mandiger et al. [4] reported in 1989 0.78 per 1000 deliveries; Berkowitz and LaSlasa [5] in 1990 reported 2.72 per 1000; Munn et al. [6] in 1999 reported 0.78 to 2.7 per 1000; Jin et al. [7] reported 1.47 per 1000 in Alberta, Canada; Plasencia W. et al. [8] in Gran Canaria, Spain, reported incidence of 0.79 per 1000.

Physiological and Anatomical Changes in Pregnancy

First of all cardiac physiology evolves in pregnant according to demand during pregnancy. Cardiac output is defined as the product of heart rate and stroke volume. Reaching even a 50% increase relative to the pregestational state, 16–20 weeks of gestation, thereafter, does not suffer significant changes [9]. This involves both increased moderate elevation in heart rate and more pronounced increase in stroke volume, the latter related to increased intravascular volume observed in normal pregnancy [10]. These changes are from a physiological point of view, driven by the need to increase the oxygen supply in both the fetal-placental unit as maternal tissue during pregnancy.

Changes in respiratory physiology during pregnancy are mainly in the volume of minute ventilation, not by increasing the respiratory rate if not tidal volume, increasing about 30–50% such volumes [11]. Non increases respiratory rate significantly during pregnancy. A pregnant woman breathes deeper but not faster. It is believed that this is due to increased production of progesterone by the placenta [10, 11]. There are changes in blood gases physiological response during pregnancy, to be taken into account for the assessment of the pregnant patient with pneumonia, not But should not skew the analysis of arterial blood gas analysis of critical patient, because changes that are abnormal in nonpregnant patients. They should also be considered abnormal in pregnant criticism. The blood gases values of a pregnant patient level sea are: PaO_2 of 101–106 mm Hg (nonpregnant 93), $PaCO_2$ 28–30, pH 7.42–7.46, bicarbonate 17–18 mEq/L by increasing renal excretion of the same in response to physiological decrease in $PaCO_2$ with slight changes from the first to the third trimester [12]. Regard to physiological changes of the airway, relevant in this topic are: hyperemia, edema plasma leakage stroma mucosal, glandular hypersecretion; since such changes cause a partial obstruction of the airway, during tracheal intubation should be considered [12, 13]. In Fig. 29.1 plotted are changes in lung volumes and capacities in pregnant compared to nonpregnant.

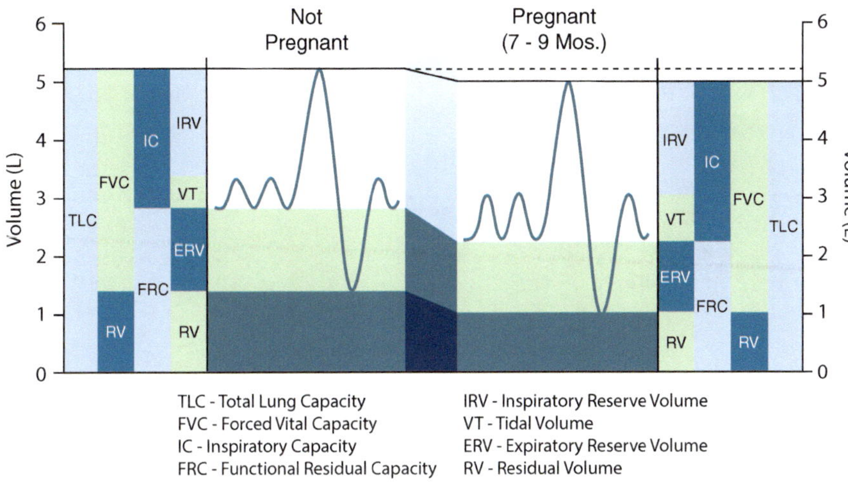

Fig. 29.1 Changes in lung volumes in pregnancy. The most significant changes are reductions in FRC and ERV and RV ITS subcomponents and increases in IC and VT [12]. (With permission of Matthew J. Hegewald)

The chest also suffers anatomical changes in response to physiological and mechanical changes by the increase in size of the uterus during the course of pregnancy. Mainly elevation up to 4 centimeters diaphragm, elevation of the subcostal angle and increase chest circumference. These changes cause restriction in the ribcage; however, apparently it does not change the pulmonary restriction [12]. Figure 29.2 exemplifies anatomical change during pregnancy.

Risk Factors

According to the discussion in relation to physiological changes, anatomical and immunological pregnant; these changes more risk factors for developing pneumonia during pregnancy are determining factors of clinical manifestations and course of the disease, different from the pregnant patient. However, we must note that there are factors in pregnancy that increase the risk of severe pneumonia. IDSA guidelines classifies Pneumonia according to criteria [15], severe pneumonia criteria are divided into major, invasive mechanical ventilation need and septic shock with the need for vasopressor, and minor criteria, respiratory rate greater than or equal to 30 minutes, PaO_2/FiO_2 ratio less than 250, infiltrates multilobe, confusion, increased nitrogen urea 20 mg/dL, leukopenia (WBC count <4000 cells/mm^3), thrombocytopenia (platelet count <100,000), hypothermia (core temperature, <36 °C), and hypotension requiring aggressive fluid resuscitation. Classifying severe pneumonia patients if they have at the least one major criterion or >3 minor criteria. The importance of classification and possible prediction of patients who develop severe

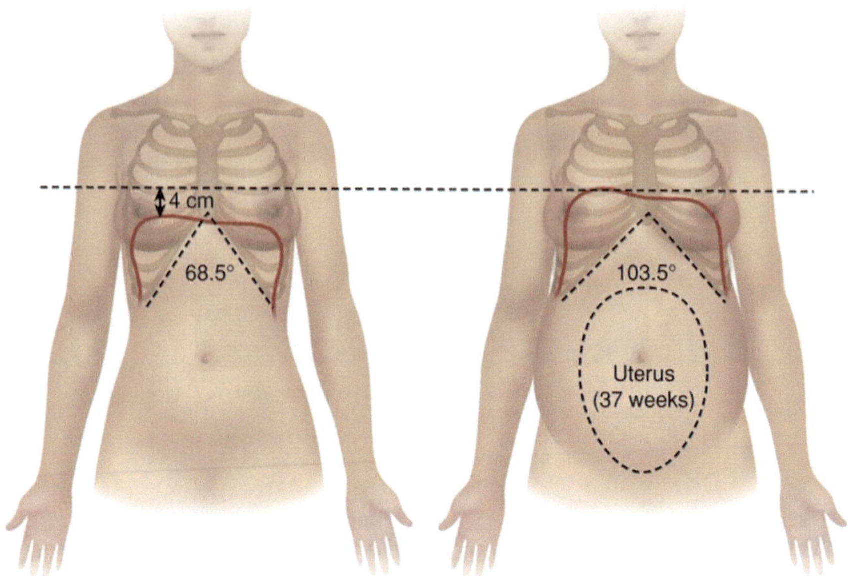

Fig. 29.2 Chest wall changes that occur during pregnancy. The subcostal angle increases, as does the anterior-posterior and transverse diameters of the chest wall and the chest wall circumference. These changes compensate for the 4 cm elevation of the diaphragm so that total lung capacity is not significantly reduced [12]. (With permission of Matthew J. Hegewald)

pneumonia during pregnancy not only lies in the increased mortality to the patient but also in the increasing bad outcomes in the product of gestation; as evidenced by Yanjun He et al. [14], the proportion of abortions and stillbirths was 42.9% in patients with severe pneumonia vs. 2.1% in patients with non-severe pneumonia during pregnancy. Also, the preterm births were in 31.4% of patients with severe pneumonia, while only 5% in patients with no severe pneumonia.

In the study published in 2019 by Yanjun He et al. [14], it was found that anemia, hypoalbuminemia, and BMI were the main predictors of severe pneumonia in pregnant patients because these factors showed statistically significant differences between patients with or without severity pneumonia. Low hemoglobin increases the risk of severe pneumonia as multivariate analysis OR: 0.87 (95% CI: 0.77–0.97) *p*: 0011; for body mass index (BMI) in multivariate analysis OR: 0.42 (95% CI: 0.22–0.81) *p*: 0.010; and for the OR albumin in multivariate analysis: 0.37 (95% CI: 0.19–0.69) [14].

Diagnosis

The diagnosis of acquired pneumonia in the community is basically clinical, supported by certain findings on chest x-ray or other techniques of radiological image, as mentioned guides the 2007 [15] and is not changed in El 2019 [1]. There are two

Table 29.1 Signs, symptoms, and radiological findings of pneumonia common in typical and atypical

	Typical pneumonia	Atypical pneumonia
Signs and symptoms	Sudden Fever (80%)[a] Shaking chills Purulent productive cough (38.6%)[a] Pleuritic pain (25.7%)[a] Murmur tubal	Insidious Fever No chills Nonproductive cough Headache Myalgia Arthralgia Dissociation clinical radiological Multilobar
Radiological images	Alveolar consolidation, usually single, homogeneous	Multiple infiltrates Interstitial

[a]Percentage reported in pregnant patients with typical and atypical pneumonia, the study of Yanjun He et al. [14]

major syndromes clinical and radiologic (Table 29.1), the typical and atypical, the first commonly caused by *Streptococcus pneumoniae* and the second by *Mycoplasma pneumoniae*, *Chlamydia psittaci*, *Coxiella burnetii*, *Chlamydia pneumoniae*, and respiratory virus. Microbiological studies support the diagnosis of pneumonia because it is caused by an infectious agent; however frequently studies give false negatives, so it is recommended not to studies as gram or cultures routinely in clinical practice, especially for know the epidemiology of every area [15, 16].

Procalcitonin (PCT) has been used to differentiate bacterial pneumonias of viral pneumonia. Some research levels have suggested <0.1 mg/L to indicate likelihood of viral infection and levels >0.25 mg/L to indicate bacterial pneumonia [17]. However the sensitivity thereof to detect bacterial infections ranges from 38% to 91%, making it risky based only on PCT to decide bacterial or viral etiology of pneumonia. However according to the systematic review of Cochrane, the use thereof to guide therapy reduces mortality (adjusted OR 0.83, 95% CI 0.70–0.99, $P = 0.037$) and the time of exposure to antibiotics (5.7 versus 8.1 days, 95% CI -2.15–2.71 A, $P < 0.001$) [18].

We note that the diagnosis of pneumonia during pregnancy may have a greater complexity because it can be difficult to distinguish between the symptoms of pneumonia with the physiological changes of pregnancy, which is already discussed in this chapter. However, it should be noted that physiological changes do not limit the daily activity of the child, and gradually appear, are changing during pregnancy. So, all abrupt onset of respiratory symptoms, not falling in the concept of "physiological change" should be investigated, taking into account differential diagnoses such as pneumonia, thromboembolism, aspiration, pneumonitis, and pulmonary edema cardiogenic or non-cardiogenic, which are entities that can occur relatively frequently during pregnancy [8].

The diagnosis of pneumonia in nonpregnant and pregnant patients, accurate radiological confirmation, as previously exposed. Although confirmation of the same is achieved in 39% of the request cases [19]. A chest radiograph in the pregnant patient, it is always considered radiation the patient, but especially the uterus and the fetus will get. So, it is important to clarify the concepts. Considering radiation represents a factor of teratogenic risk, the embryo or fetus should receive more than 50–10 mGy. However, it has been reported that the dose to the fetus of a chest radiograph is less than 0.1 mGy. And conceptual dose chest radiography is affected by the selected kVp, filtration of the X-ray tube, and film screen combinations. It has been shown that the chest apron has a limited value in chest radiography to reduce the radiation dose, since most of the dose results from internal dispersion in the maternal y fetal tissues [20].

He currently has the pulmonary ultrasound for clinical use, so it can also be done by the same radiological confirmation, according to several published protocols. The sensitivity and specificity even are superior to chest radiography for diagnosis of pneumonia. According to a study published in the EMJ in 2010, the sensitivity of chest X-ray was 67% (95% CI 56.4–76.9%) and specificity 85% (95% CI 73.3–95.9%), while sensitivity of ultrasound was 98% (95% CI 93.3–99.9%) and specificity 95% (95% CI 82.7–99.4%) [21]. Therefore, it is a diagnostic tool that can be used in radiological confirmation of pneumonia during pregnancy.

Etiology

The microorganisms that cause pneumonia in patients without pregnancy are the same that cause pneumonia during pregnancy. The etiological diagnosis is not always possible for several reasons, principally because in the 58.7–68.7% of patients with pneumonia or hospital outpatient treatment respectively, the microorganism is not identified by the present methods of isolation [22].

Studies have been published concerning the epidemiology of the etiology of pneumonia during pregnancy; they have several methodological limitations; however, the results are similar with those published in pneumonia without pregnancy. However, there have also been published case series, demonstrating a role of other microorganisms associated with factors of pregnancy, including mumps, infectious mononucleosis, swine flu, influenza, *Legionella*, varicella, *Chlamydophila pneumoniae*, coccidioidomycosis, and other fungal pneumonias [23]. It is not known whether infection with any of these agents is more common in pregnancy than in the nonpregnant, but certain pathogens, such as influenza and chickenpox, can pose a greater risk to the pregnant woman because of their physiological defect's cellular immunity [1].

Pneumonias methicillin-resistant *Staphylococcus aureus* (CA-MRSA) are not commonly reported but can cause severe forms of pneumonia after infection influenza [25]. The organism can lead to severe bilateral necrotizing infection due to production of a variety of toxins, including Panton-Valentine leukocidin, microorganism responsible for infections of skin and soft tissue, but can be associated with boxes septic pelvic thrombophlebitis.

Treatment

Treatment for bacterial pneumonia in pregnant, this based on empirical antimicrobial therapy directed to common microorganisms, as previously discussed, *Streptococcus pneumoniae*, *H. influenzae*, and atypical microorganisms are most frequents [16]. The treatment should include antibiotics covering the spectrum of pathogens, with particular care that are safe in pregnancy for both mother and fetus.

Penicillins, cephalosporins, and erythromycin are safe and effective. Current guidelines suggest the option of fluoroquinolones to treat pneumonia in nonpregnant; however during pregnancy these should not be used because of the risk of arthropathy and malformations in the fetus, which have been sporadically reported, unless they are very necessary, in the absence of another alternative [16, 26].

For the treatment of community-acquired pneumonia, requiring outpatient treatment, is recommended the use of a beta-lactam as amoxicillin oral (incidence *Streptococcus* resistant less than 25%) plus a macrolide, ideally azithromycin orally, which is better tolerated to erythromycin, clarithromycin as not indicated in pregnancy, through its association with fetal malformations [16].

Patients admitted, who need intensive care unit, without risk of comorbidities or resistant *Streptococcus* (known resistance less than 25%) should receive amoxicillin IV azithromycin or erythromycin plus intravenous; if they risk resistant *Streptococcus*, comorbidities, recent use of antibiotics, should receive intravenous beta-lactam as ceftriaxone, cefotaxime or ceftaroline, more azithromycin, or erythromycin [15, 16].

For patients requires admission to ICU, you must differentiate whether or not pseudomonad risk based on what previously exposed, if there is no risk of pseudomonas can be used as intravenous beta-lactam ceftriaxone, cefotaxime, plus intravenous macrolide. If there is risk for pseudomona, can be used anti-psuedomona: cefepime, meropenem, piperacillin tazobactam or imipenem, although the latter is rated C, while the others are B; amikacin plus an aminoglycoside such as gentamycin or which should be used with caution and strict indication, the risk of nephrotoxicity and ototoxicity for mother and fetus; In addition to adding the macrolide for atypical pathogens [15, 16].

Patients at high risk of methicillin-resistant *Staphylococcus aureus* must be associated with vancomycin, although there is much experience of use during pregnancy. Linezolid does not have much experience, yet it is an inhibitor of protein synthesis, which means that the risk adverse effects on pregnant is minimal, so it may be an option.

Most pneumonias are etiology viral [27]. In the case of viral pneumonia Influenza A, current guidelines recommend the use of antivirals such as oseltamivir, in either the outpatient or inpatient, as it has shown to reduce mortality and results adverse. However, in such pneumonias is also indicated to antibiotics, since most of cases, patients with viral pneumonias were superinfecting with bacteria, mainly *Streptococcus*, *H. influenzae*, and methicillin-resistant *Staphylococcus aureus*, so

Table 29.2 Antimicrobial treatment, classification, suggested dose, and duration of pneumonia during pregnancy

Regime	Antibiotic	Classification	Dose	Duration
Regime primary	Ceftriaxone Cefazolin + Azithromycin	B B B	02.01 gm IV q24 h 600 mg IV q12 h 500 mg IV q24 h	Until stabilization. No more than 5 days or guided by PCT
Alternatives	Ampicillin-sulbactam Azithromycin	B B	3 gm IV q6h	Until stabilization. No more than 5 days or guided by PCT
For methicillin-resistant *Staph. aureus*	Vancomycin Linezolid	C C	15–20 mg/kg q8–12 h 600 mg IV q12 h	7 days 7 days
Pseudomonas aeruginosa for	Piperacillin-tazobactam Meropenem Cefepime Ceftazidime	B B B B	4.5 gm IV q 6 h 1 gm IV q8 h 2 gm IV q8 h 2 gm IV q8 h	Until stabilization. No more than 5 days or guided by PCT
Influenza A	Oseltamivir	C	75 mg q12 h	7 days 10 or more if pneumonia complicated

References: Lionel A. Mandell [15], Joshua P. Metlay [16], S. Jain [27], Stern A. Skalsky [28], and Richrd G. Wunderink [29]

must add antibiotics covering said germens [16]. Table 29.2 summarizes the different regimens, classification, dose, and duration of the recommended antibiotics during pregnancy.

Corticosteroids

A number of studies that have published results for the use of corticosteroids for adjuvant treatment of pneumonia; however there is evidence that they can reduce mortality in patients with severe pneumonia, as well as improvement in the results of radiographic progression and stability clinic 5–8 days in patients with non-severe and severe pneumonia [27, 28]. These results have not been replicated in other meta-analyses. So, for the risks posed by the routine use of corticosteroids, they are not currently recommended in guidelines [15, 16, 27].

Bibliography

1. Brito V, Niederman MS. Pneumonia complicating pregnancy. Clin Chest Med. 2011;32:121–32. https://doi.org/10.1016/j.ccm.2010.10.004.
2. Madinger NE, Greenspoon JS, Ellrodt AG. Pneumonia during pregnancy: Has modem technology improved maternal and fetal outcome? Am J Obstet Gynecol. 1989;161(3):657–62.

3. Benedetti TJ, Valle R, Ledger WJ. Antepartum pneumonia in pregnancy. Am J Obstet Gynecol. 1982;144:413e7.
4. Madinger NE, Greenspoon JS, Elrodt AG. Pneumonia during pregnancy: has modern technology improved maternal and fetal outcome? Am J Obstet Gynecol. 1989;161:657e62.
5. Berkowitz K, LaSala A. Risk factors associated with increasing prevalence of pneumonia during pregnancy. Am J Obstet Gynecol. 1990;163:981e5.
6. Munn MB, Groome LJ, Atterbury JL, et al. Pneu- monia as a complication of pregnancy. J Matern Fetal Med. 1999;8:151e4.
7. Jin Y, Carriere KC, Marrie TJ, et al. The effects of community acquired pneumonia during pregnancy ending in a live birth. Am J Obstet Gynecol. 2003;18:800e6.
8. Plasencia W, Eguiluz I, Barber MA, Martín A, Medina N, Goya M, García-Hernández JA. Neumonía y Gestación. Clin Invest Ginecol Obst. 2006;33(1):15–21.
9. Halla ME, Georgeb EM, Grangerb JP. El corazón durante el embarazo. Rev Esp Cardiol. 2011;64(11):1045–50.
10. Frye D, Clark SL, Piacenza D, Shay-Zapien G. Pulmonary complications in pregnancy considerations for care. J Perinat Neonat Nurs. 2011;25(3):235–44.
11. Gustavo C, Mónica G, Teresa B, et al. Ventilatory drive and respiratory muscle function in pregnancy. Am Rev Respir Dis. 1991;144(4):837–41.
12. Hegewald MJ, Crapo RO. Respiratory physiology in pregnancy. Clin Chest Med. 2011;32:1–13.
13. Bende M, Gredmark T. Nasal stuffiness during pregnancy. Laryngoscope. 1999;109(7 Pt 1):1108–10.
14. He Y, Li M, Mai C, et al. Anemia and low albumin levels are associated with severe community-acquired pneumonia in pregnancy: a case-control study. Tohoku J Exp Med. 2019;248:297S–305.
15. Mandell LA, Wunderink RG, Anzueto A, et al. Infectious Diseases Society of America/ American Thoracic Society consensus guidelines on the management of community-acquired pneumonia in adults. Clin Infect Dis. 2007;44:S27–72.
16. Metlay JP, Waterer GW, Long AC, et al. Diagnosis and treatment of adults with community-acquired pneumonia. American Thoracic Society Documents. Am J Respir Crit Care Med. 2019;200(7):e45–67.
17. Christ-Crain M, Stolz D, Bingisser R, et al. Procalcitonin guidance of antibiotic therapy in community acquired pneumonia: a randomized trial. Am J Respir Crit Care Med. 2006;174:84–93.
18. Schuetz P, Wirz Y, Sager R, et al. Procalcitonin to initiate or discontinue antibiotics in acute respiratory tract infections (review). Cochrane Database Syst Rev 2017;(10):Art. No.: CD007498.
19. Diethelm L, Xu H. Diagnostic imaging of the lung during pregnancy. Clin Obstet Gynecol. 1996;39:36–55.
20. Damilakis J, Perisinakis K, Prassopoulos P, et al. Conceptus radiation dose and risk from chest screen-film radiography. Eur Radiol. 2003;13:406–12.
21. Cortellaro F, Colombo S, Coen D, et al. Lung ultrasound is an accurate diagnostic tool for the diagnosis of pneumonia in the emergency department. Emerg Med J. 2012;29:19–23.
22. Cilloniz C, Martin-Loeches I, Garcia-Vidal C, et al. Microbial etiology of pneumonia: epidemiology, diagnosis and resistance patterns. Int J Mol Sci. 2016;17:2120.
23. Goodnight WH, Soper DE. Pneumonia in pregnancy. Crit Care Med. 2005;33:S390–7.
24. Rotas M, McCalla S, Liu C, Minkoff H. Methicillin-resistant Staphylococcus aureus necrotizing pneumonia arising from an infected episiotomy site. Obstet Gynecol. 2007;109:533–6.
25. Micek ST, Dunne M, Kollef MH. Pleuropulmonary complications of Panton-Valentine leukocidin-positive community-acquired methicillin-resistant Staphylococcus aureus. Chest. 2005;128(4):2732–8. https://doi.org/10.1378/chest.128.4.2732.
26. Loebstein R, Addis A, HoE, et al. Pregnancy outcome following gestational exposure to fluoroquinolones: a multicenter prospective controlled study. Antimicrob Agents Chemother. 1998;42:1336–9.

27. Jain S, Self WH, Wunderink RG, et al. Community-acquired pneumonia requiring hospitalization among U.S. adults. N Engl J Med. 2015;373(5):415–27.
28. Stern A, Skalsky K, Avni T, Carrara E, Leibovici L, Paul M. Corticosteroids for pneumonia (review). Cochrane Database of Syst Rev. 2017; (12):Art. No.: CD007720.
29. Wunderink RG, Waterer GW. Community-acquired pneumonia. N Engl J Med. 2014;370:543–51.

Chapter 30
Tetanus in the Pregnant Woman

Sabrina Da Re Gutiérrez, Jorge Sinclair Ávila, Jorge E. Sinclair De Frías, and Jose Miguel Jauregui

Introduction

The evidence indicates that "...inadequate maternal vaccination and (...) poor perinatal hygiene" propitiate the appearance of maternal and neonatal tetanus [11].

Therefore, in the second half of the twentieth century, medicine recommended and practiced the generalized immunization – routine – of pregnant women [9] until the 1980s when, for reasons of "caution, efficacy and preparation of vaccine components," reserved in industrialized countries for "… certain high-risk groups" [3].

Following this criterion, the initiative of the World Health Organization (WHO) for the elimination of maternal and neonatal tetanus (MNT), founded on the "... immunization of women and the improvement of childbirth hygiene..." [9], vaccinated and protected "…between 1999 and 2016 (…) 148 million women…" from 59 countries [9], 94% of women of childbearing age, achieving the elimination of MNT [6].

S. Da Re Gutiérrez (✉)
Critical and Intensive Care Medicine, Maternal and Child Hospital, Caja Nacional de Salud (CNS), La Paz, Bolivia

J. Sinclair Ávila
Critical Medicine, UCI Hospital Pacífica Salud/Johns Hopkins Medicine, Faculty of Medicine University of Panamá, Panamá City, Panama

J. E. Sinclair De Frías
Santo Tomas Hospital, Faculty of Medicine University of Panamá, Panamá City, Panamá

J. M. Jauregui
Gynecological Obstetric and Pediatric University Hospital, Espíritu Santo Specialties University Hospital, Guayaquil, Ecuador

C. Montufar et al. (eds.), *Obstetric Catastrophes*,
https://doi.org/10.1007/978-3-030-70034-8_30

Epidemiology

It is possible to find *Clostridium tetani* spores in "...human and animal feces, soil and manure, (...) worldwide" [11], which is why natural environmental phenomena can "...increase the risk of tetanus infection..." [11].

Mortality from tetanus – depending on its severity – ranges from 10% to 80%. Trudy et al. describe a lethality of 16% to more than 50% [4] and Roper et al. one of 8–50% that "...increases with age" [8].

Neonatal disease is fatal in most cases [9]. According to Roper et al., in the 1980s, neonatal tetanus mortality approached 100% [8].

Currently, neonatal tetanus mortality ranges from 10% to 60% with hospital care [8]. WHO stated that in 1988, 787,000 died with tetanus, reducing the figure to 34,000 by 2015 [6]. However, "the estimated deaths from tetanus at all stages of life totaled around 73,000" [6].

Fortunately, Bolivia was not contemplated by WHO within the 16 countries of concern: Afghanistan, Angola, Central African Republic, Chad, DR Congo, Guinea, Kenya, Mali, Nigeria, Pakistan, Papua New Guinea, Philippines, Somalia, Sudan, South, Sudan, and Yemen [6].

The Elimination of Maternal and Neonatal Tetanus from the Americas

Since tetanus is not transmitted from person to person but rather that the human being becomes infected in the environment with "...spores on the ground or in medical instruments" [6], it is impossible to eradicate "...since the environmental reservoir will never disappear" [6] since it is widespread throughout the world [11].

Therefore, precisely, WHO coined a new meaning – less ambitious – for the term "elimination", stating that "...tetanus is eliminated when the annual rate of neonatal tetanus is less than one case per 1000 live births in a district" [6].

Etymology

The word "tetanus" comes from the Latin *tetănus* and this, in turn, from the Greek ζέζανος ([7], p. 2168) which means "contract" [9]. It is described as a pathological entity since 1600 A.C. [9].

Definition

Citing the Centers for Disease Control and Prevention (CDC) Thwaites et al. define tetanus as "The acute onset of hypertonia or (...) painful muscle contractions (almost always of the jaw and neck muscles) and generalized muscle spasms with no other obvious medical cause" ([10], p. 1197).

Etiology

The *Clostridium tetani* is a gram-positive and spore-forming anaerobic bacillus ([10], p. 1197) that contaminate the soil and gastrointestinal tract of animals [5]. These spores are so resistant that their destruction "...requires autoclave or prolonged exposure to iodine, hydrogen peroxide, formalin or glutaraldehyde" [8].

This bacillus produces two exotoxins, tetanolysin and tetanospasmin. The latter is the neurotoxin that causes tetanus. The evidence indicates that the genes that encode tetanospasmine and its regulator exist in an intracellular plasmid [5] called PE88 [11].

Chemically, tetanospasmine (or tetanus toxin) "...is a 150 kDa protein that divides to give rise to the heavy (100 kDa) and light (50 kDa) chains" ([10], p. 1197).

The evidence proves that the minimum lethal human dose is 2.5 ng/kg [10].

Pathogeny

Clostridium spores enter the body due to existing skin or mucous lesions and germinate and proliferate in the "...sites poor in oxygen (for example, necrotic tissue or wounds),..." [4] causing disease in subjects without circulating antibodies [11]. The existence of blood, foreign bodies, and chemicals (e.g., lactic acid, calcium salts, quinine) favors such proliferation [8].

In about 20% of cases, "...there is no obvious entry site..." [9] of the bacillus in the human body.

Incubation

The evidence indicates various incubation periods ranging from 0 to 112 days after the injury [4].

Toxin Release

When the bacillus crosses its stationary phase of growth [11] or dies, the toxin is released and is transformed into its active form by a bacterial protease [5].

Tetanospasmin binds through the carboxyl group of its heavy chain to the "polysialogangliosides and membrane proteins" ([10], p. 1197) in the "presynaptic nerve endings α" ([10], p. 1197) until it is introduced into the neuron.

Then, it is transported at the speed of 3–13 mm/hour [8] to the neuronal body by the "…same pathways as the brain-derived neurotrophic factor, p75 neurotrophin receptor and kinase related to tropo-myosin B" [11] and then transferred "… through the synapse to the terminations of the GABA-ergic presynaptic inhibitory interneurons" ([10], p. 1197) where the light chain "…unfolds to the vesicle-related protein VAMP2, (vesicle associated membrane protein 2).

This molecule is necessary for presynaptic binding and neurotransmitter release; consequently, the tetanus toxin prevents the release of neurotransmitter and blocks the discharge of the inhibitory interneuron. The result is the uncontrolled activity of the motor nervous system" ([10], p. 1197). The same phenomenon disrupts the autonomous system.

Toxic properties depend on the light chain [5].

Acute immune changes during pregnancy, some of them modulated by estrogen and progesterone [3], increasing the susceptibility of pregnant women to infection. There is "…a change from a T helper (Th) -1 response to a response more favored by Th2, which allows tolerance to fetal antigen but potentially increases vulnerability to infectious diseases" [6].

The same change in behavior of maternal T lymphocytes increases the vulnerability of decidua to infections [3].

During pregnancy, there is also a decrease in immunoglobulin G (IgG) in plasma.

Fortunately, the evidence states that "...pregnant women can generate antibody responses and develop immune memory similar to non-pregnant women after vaccination or infection" [3].

Regarding the infant, immune immaturity probably generates "…tolerogenic immune responses" [6] that increase their vulnerability to tetanus. Therefore, precisely, before 6 months of age, active immunization of the infant is less efficient, a fact that makes multiple doses of a certain vaccine necessary to protect [3].

Likewise, due to immune immaturity, the protection of the infant against viruses depends predominantly on their innate immune system, non-specific cytotoxicity, and the "...placental transfer of maternal immunoglobulin's during the third trimester of pregnancy" [3]. The test of this transfer allowed passive immunization of the infant by active immunization of the mother, although "…the antigens in the infant can fall substantially…" [3].

Particularities in the Natural History of the Disease

Trudy et al. [4] and Thwaites et al. ([10], p. 985) describe that there is a higher mortality when the incubation period of the disease is short.

Also, the literature states that there is a direct relationship between the increase in circulating catecholamines and cardiovascular complications ([10], p. 985).

Maternal or Obstetric Tetanus

Maternal tetanus is one that occurs during pregnancy "...or in the six weeks following its final term (either by childbirth or spontaneous or induced abortion)" ([10], p. 984).

Historical evidence shows the close relationship between high lethality rates and post-abortion tetanus [4], because it usually occurs "...after abortion, spontaneous abortions or non-hygienic delivery practices" [11].

Epidemiologically, Roper et al. state that maternal tetanus shares risk factors and means of prevention with neonatal tetanus [8].

Neonatal Tetanus

Citing WHO Thwaites et al. define neonatal tetanus as the disease "…that occurs in an infant who has normal ability to suck and cry in the first two days of age, but who loses this ability between days 3 and 28 of age, and becomes stiff at the time experiencing spasms" ([10], p. 984). Trudy et al. affirm that "...it is associated with contamination of the umbilical stump" [4].

Incubation is "5 to 7 days (range 3 to 24) after birth" [11]; 90% of cases appear "…in the first 3-14 days of life" [5]; ergo, in most cases it occurs during the first month of life, more precisely between 3 and 14 days after birth. Signs and symptoms are irritability, difficulty feeding, spasm, and "...ascending muscle stiffness..." [5].

Depending on the severity of the respiratory disorder suffered during the disease, surviving infants may suffer cerebral palsy and psychomotor retardation. On the point, Roper et al. "…neurological abnormalities or cognitive impairment were described in 4 to 50% of patients; severe disabilities are identified in 10-20%" [8]. Sepsis can be associated with tetanus making the disease worse [8]. Evidence indicates that low birth weight increases the risk of death [8].

Signs and Symptoms

The clinical manifestations of tetanus are classified as generalized and local ([10], p. 1198). In both classes "...conscience is conserved,..." [8].

In the generalized manifestations that occur in 80% of cases [4], frequently associated with severe tetanus, muscle spasm first affects the muscles of the face and jaw, resulting in muscle trism, pain, and stiffness, low back pain, and dysphagia. Abdominal muscle pain is an early symptom [5]. The literature states that there are "...reports of spasms strong enough to produce tendon tears and crush fractures..." ([10], p. 1198). At first, muscle spasms begin "...in response to sensory stimuli" [5]. The involvement of the laryngeal muscles can cause "...complete airway obstruction..." ([10], p. 1198). In addition, respiratory muscle spasm causes respiratory failure [4], and episodes of apnea and cyanosis are described [8].

Tetanus also involves the autonomic nervous system generating unstable blood pressure (hyper and hypotension), "...tachycardia. (...) Bradycardia (...) heart block, (...), sweating, increased tracheal secretions and kidney failure (often high expense)" ([10], p. 1198). In this regard, "…the electrocardiograms of 33 patients in Dakar (Senegal) showed more than one abnormality in 93% of patients, despite normal echocardiography" [11].

In local manifestations – which usually denote mild tetanus – only "...small regions of local muscle spasm are observed" ([10], p. 1198), although if the spasm compromises the pharyngeal or laryngeal muscles, the result may be ominous.

At first, muscle spasms begin "...in response to sensory stimuli" [5].

Evolution

Nosocomial infections (e.g., pneumonia, etc.) and other diseases (e.g., pulmonary embolism, bedsores, etc.) usually complicate the patient's evolution with tetanus.

The literature asserts that recovery can last several weeks. Since "Relatively little is known about the processes of recovery of tetanus" ([10], p. 1198), it is speculated that in tetanus the recovery is given by "...degradation of the toxin" ([10], p. 1198) and would probably involve "...germination of peripheral nerves ..." ([10], p. 1198) as in botulism.

Diagnosis

It is eminently clinical [5] with support in the cultivation of *Clostridium tetani* ([10], p. 1198) in agar with blood with low oxygen content or meat broth [11] or in PCR detection of tetanus toxin in plasma or wound exudate [11], since *Clostridium tetani* is not frequently detected in the cultures (e.g., of wounds) of patients with tetanus

[8] and, worse still, *Clostridium tetani* "...occasionally grows in cultures of patients without tetanus" [5].

Differential Diagnosis

Thwaites et al. and Roper et al. state that when the manifestations of tetanus are local oropharyngeal infection (e.g., tonsillitis, dental infections, etc.), mumps, rabies [1], diphtheria [1], and temporomandibular joint disease should be taken into account as differential diagnostic possibilities ([8], ([10], p. 1198)). On the other hand, when they are generalized in the adult patient, strychnine poisoning, dystonic reactions to dopamine drugs ([10], p. 1198), phenothiazine poisoning, rigid man syndrome, psychogenic tetanus, epilepsy, retroperitoneal abscess, and postpartum eclampsia [1] constitute the differential diagnostic possibilities.

Generalized manifestations in infants suggest hypocalcemia, hypoglycemic, and meningoencephalitis as diagnostic possibilities ([8], ([10], p. 1198)).

Treatment

Preventively, any contaminated wound should be treated "…with vaccination with or without antitoxin" [9].

With tetanus diagnosed, whenever possible, it is necessary to identify the entrance wound, clean it, debride it, and remove the necrotic material "...to remove anaerobic foci of infection" ([10], p. 1199) because "The impossibility eliminating reservoirs with active infection could lead to recurrent or prolonged tetanus" (([10], p. 1199), [11]).

In addition, using metronidazole rectally (400 mg) or intravenously (500 mg) every 6 hours for 7 days, "...is the preferable antibiotic" ([10], p. 1199). Penicillin (100,000–200,000 IU/Kg per day) is an alternative; however, the evidence indicates that "...can exacerbate spasms" ([10], p. 1199). The evidence shows that "of 45 isolates of C. tetani in Vietnam (...) all isolates are sensitive to metronidazole and penicillin, but resistant to cotrimoxazole" [11].

Also, antitoxin (human or equine) should be administered early to neutralize the circulating toxin and "...prevent its uptake into the nervous system" ([10], p. 1199). The doses remain controversial [11]. Because of its lower probability of causing anaphylactic reactions [9], the best option is human tetanus immunoglobulin (TIG) from 3000 to 6000 IU in a single intramuscular dose ([10], p. 1199). If there is no TIG, the equine antitoxin is administered from 10,000 to 20,000 IU in a single intramuscular dose. However, Thwaites et al., citing Blake, affirm that "…there were no differences in the result in those who received less than 500 IU of tetanus immunoglobulin compared to higher doses" [11]. In addition, Thwaites et al. state that "the difficulties caused by the restricted availability of tetanus immunoglobulin supplies have led to a new guideline that indicates that normal human immunoglobulin can be used instead. This decision is based on theoretical considerations…" [11].

Regarding intrathecal infusion of antitoxin, based on some meta-analysis, Thwaites et al. affirm that "Although the mortality rates were not different (…), hospital stay and disease progression were reduced in the intrathecal group and treatment with intrathecal antitoxin significantly reduced the costs of both the intensive care unit and the hospitalization. A reported side effect during intrathecal administration was mild headache and reversible paraparesis was reported only once" [11].

Deep sedation controls spasms. To induce it, benzodiazepines are used. Propofol has also been used to sedate and relax the muscles.

Intravenous magnesium sulfate is useful for producing muscle relaxation, vasodilation, and negative chronotropic effect [11]. Thwaites et al. cite a randomized trial that concluded that magnesium sulfate would only be useful "...in milder cases of tetanus, although magnesium reduces the need for other muscle relaxants and improves cardiovascular stability" [11].

The literature also suggests as chlorpromazine and phenobarbital sedatives nasogastrically or intravenously, because of their affordability [11].

Cardiovascular instability caused by tetanus "...is very difficult to control" ([10], p. 1199). To treat it, it is useful to intensify sedation with intravenous magnesium sulfate (2–4 mmol/L in plasma), morphine, or other sedatives ([10], p. 1199).

If drugs with cardiovascular effect are used "Short-acting ones that allow rapid dose adjustment are preferable; special care should be taken with long-acting β antagonists, since their use is related to cardiac arrest related to hypotension" ([10], p. 1199).

Also, the airway must always be controlled in severe tetanus ([10], p. 1199), especially knowing that the drugs used to achieve muscle sedation cause respiratory depression, making it necessary to use mechanical respirators ([10], p. 1199) and the consequent admission to an intensive care unit [8]. Thwaites et al. suggest control of muscle spasm with intramuscular paraldehyde when mechanical ventilation is not available [11].

Prevention

Reliable immunization is performed with the tetanus toxoid antigenic vaccine that is safely applicable during pregnancy [6], including immunocompromised subjects, since – combined (Tdap) – "…no risks are known for administration during first quarter" [2]. However, its application is recommended "…preferably at the end of the second or third quarter" [2].

The duration of protection conferred depends on the number of doses, age of vaccination, potency of the vaccine, and immune competence of the recipient [8]; after 5 or 6 doses, it seems to be "20–25 years in populations that receive primary doses in childhood and reinforcements in childhood and adolescence" [8].

Protection arises from the second dose for "90% of people" [8].

Serious adverse reactions are rare.

Roper et al., citing WHO, recommended that at least five doses of the vaccine be administered from childhood for 12–15 years, plus a sixth dose in early adulthood [8].

Infants "...born to mothers with tetanus antibodies are protected against tetanus..." [8].

The aforementioned maternal immunoglobulin G antibodies are transferred placentally – over-all – during the third trimester of pregnancy into the fetal circulation. Protection is achieved with two doses in women "...previously unimmunized and their (...) newborns" [8].

It is recommended the course of 6 weeks between the first and second dose.

Since the peak of antibody transfer is reached at "…60 days or more after the second dose, (…)" [8], it should be vaccinated several weeks before delivery to ensure the "…Protective concentrations of antibodies in the newborn" [8].

Therefore, recommendations for vaccination of pregnant women indicate:

(a) For pregnant women with an unknown or incomplete tetanus vaccine:

- Pregnant women who have never been vaccinated against tetanus should receive the series of three vaccines during pregnancy, with the following scheme: initial vaccine, 4 weeks after the second dose, and then 6–12 months later the third dose. The Tdap vaccine should preferably be used at the end of the second trimester or during the third trimester of pregnancy.

(b) For pregnant women who should receive a tetanus booster:

- Indicated for women who have not previously received Tdap or who received the Td vaccine 10 years before. They should be given Tdap during pregnancy, preferably at the end of the trimester or during the third trimester [2].

There is evidence that malaria "...decreases the response of antibodies to tetanus toxoid in children, although prophylaxis against malaria seems to preserve the response" [8].

Evidence indicates that the tetanus toxoid stimulates protective response in children and adult women not pregnant with HIV, but with a smaller amount of antibodies to control subjects, even lower, when the CD4 T cell count is less than 300 cells/μL.

During a study conducted in Brazilian women infected with HIV, a minor placental transfer of IgG was found, which was not found during a similar study carried out in Malawi; however, infants born, in both studies, had a protective amount of IgG against tetanus [8].

It is clear that antibodies decrease with the progression of the disease [8]. Therefore, the literature suggests frequent reinforcements for those infected with HIV.

Science also suggests that prematurity, severe maternal hypergammaglobulinemia, and malaria "...affect the transplacental transfer of antibodies against tetanus" [8].

Roper et al. conclude that the vaccine is "...sufficiently immunogenic (...) even in the presence of disorders that affect maternal and neonatal antibodies (...)" [8], conventionally being understood that the concentration of "... 0.01 IU/mL by neutralization test in vivo or 0.10–16.1 IU/mL by ELISA" protect against tetanus [8].

Additionally, Roper et al. emphasize that "Hygienic deliveries and umbilical cord care clearly reduce neonatal tetanus and have the additional benefit of reducing maternal and neonatal sepsis caused by other bacterial pathogens" [8], used for care of the umbilical cord stump chlorhexidine and topical antibiotics.

References

1. Fauveau V, Mamdani M, Steinglass R, Koblinsky M. Maternal tetanus: magnitude, epidemiology and potential control measures. (R. Adanu, Ed.). Int J Gynaecol Obstet. 1993;XL:3–12.
2. Fortner K, Kuller J, Rhee E, Edwards K. Influenza and tetanus, diphtheria, and acellular pertussis vaccinations during pregnancy. Obstet Gynecol Surv. 2012;67:251–7.
3. Kachikis A, Englund J. Optimizing protection for the mother and infant. (T. B. Association, Ed.). J Infect. 2016;72:S83–90.
4. Murphy T, Slade B, Broder K, Kretsinger K, Tiwari T, Joyce P, et al. Prevention of pertussis, tetanus, and diphtheria among pregnant and postpartum women and their infants. (C. f. Prevention, Ed.). Morb Mortal Wkly Rep Recomm Rep. 2008;57(04):1–47,51.
5. Otoikhian C, Osakwe A, Akporhuarho J, Ogwezi R. Clostridium tetani in maternal and neonatal infections (TETANUS). Int J Pharma Med Biol Sci. 2014;III(3):51.
6. Perrett K, Nolan T. Immunization during pregnancy: impact on the infant. (R. McNab, Ed.). Pediatr Drugs. 2017;19:313–24.
7. Real Academia Española. Diccionario de la Lengua Española (Vigésima segunda ed., vol I). Madrid: Editorial Espasa Calpe S. A; 2001.
8. Roper M, Vandelaer J, Gasse F. Maternal and neonatal tetanus. Lancet. 2007;370(9603):1947–59.
9. Thwaites L, Loan H. Eradication of tetanus. (O. U. Press, Ed.). Br Med Bull. 2015;116:69–77.
10. Thwaites L, Mihn L. In: Longo D, Kasper D, Jameson L, Fauci A, Hauser S, Loscalzo J, editors. Tétanos, en Harrison Principios de Medicina Interna (Decimoctava ed., vol I). México D. F.: McGraw-Hill Interamericana Editores, S. A. de C. V; 2012.
11. Thwaites L, Beeching N, Newton C. Maternal and neonatal tetanus. Lancet. 2015;385(9965):362–70.

Chapter 31
Malaria in the Pregnant Women

Juan Ignacio Silesky-Jiménez and Jorge Hidalgo

Introduction

Malaria is a parasitic infectious disease, caused by the *Plasmodium* parasite. It is transmitted through the *Anopheles* mosquito. This disease causes a life-threatening condition, in which at least 2 million people are at risk of presenting it in 90 endemic countries and it also infects 125 million travelers [1].

It is important to consider that with the phenomenon of global warming, as well as climate changes, endemic areas of malaria will be increased, which is estimated to increase the incidence of malaria in 50–80 million people [2].

Plasmodium produces an infection with its own particularities: with its multi-stage life cycle, which produces cyclic fevers, with adequate treatment, sick individuals have a rapid resolution of symptoms; however, they can also present serious complications such as cerebral malaria, severe malarial anemia, coma, and death. The treatment and chemoprophylaxis varies according to the species of the parasite, geography, sensitivity, and demography of the patient. Latent or reactive infections have been reported even years after exposure.

J. I. Silesky-Jiménez (✉)
Critical Care Medicine, Clinical Nutrition, Health Services Administration, Hospital San Juan de Dios and Hospital CIMA, San José, Costa Rica

Costa Rica University, San José, Costa Rica

AMICOR and COCECATI, San José, Costa Rica

J. Hidalgo
Division of Critical Care, Karl Heusner Memorial Hospital, Belize City, Belize

C. Montufar et al. (eds.), *Obstetric Catastrophes*,
https://doi.org/10.1007/978-3-030-70034-8_31

Epidemiology and Transmission

The risk of becoming infected by this parasite is high for humans, since 40% of the world's population is at risk annually because they inhabit or visit malaria-endemic regions [3].

There are five species that are capable of infecting humans, with characteristics of virulence and different worldwide distribution [4]:

1. *Plasmodium falciparum*, which is the one with the highest morbidity and mortality, is found in Africa, specifically in the West and in sub-Sahara areas.
2. *Plasmodium vivax*, which is found in South Asia, the West Pacific and Central America.
3. *Plasmodium ovale*, which is in the sub-Saharan African region.
4. *Plasmodium malariae*, with the same distribution as *P. ovale*.
5. *Plasmodium knowlesi*, which is present in Southeast Asia.

About 500 million people annually present this infection, with a mortality between 1.5 and 2.7 million, that is 0.3–0.54% [4]; however, the highest mortality, about 90%, occurs in Africa [1], especially in children, pregnant women, travelers, etc. [1, 4, 5]. It is important to note that of the 125 million people who visit endemic areas per year, 10–30 thousand individuals become infected with this parasite, with a mortality of 1% [4, 5].

This infection occurs after the female of the *Anopheles* mosquito becomes infected after ingesting the parasite gametes from the bloodstream of an infected patient, and then the sporozoites replicate in the gut of the mosquito. Subsequently, the mosquito infected with the parasite, in the following "bloodmeals," release these sporozoites into the bloodstream of the new host. At 60 minutes, these sporozoites invade the livers (hepatocytes) and divide rapidly forming the merozoites [6].

These merozoites reenter the bloodstream, invading erythrocytes and that is where *Plasmodia* consumes hemoglobin and develops its immature trophozoite form, which evolve into mature trophozoites or gametocytes. These immature trophozoites replicate forming schizonts, which break the erythrocyte membrane and produce endothelial adhesion in the capillaries and cell lysis.

An untreated malaria can last from 2 to 24 months, where infected individuals can have a resolution of the symptoms; however, they can present severe complications such as cerebral malaria, severe anemia, and death.

It is known that *P. ovale* and *P. vivax* can enter a kind of wintering, or "dormant schozogony," where inactive intrahepatic parasites can remain months or years, before reactivating, reporting latent or reactivated infections years after exposure [6] (Fig. 31.1).

The incubation period is different between species [1]:

1. 8–11 days for *P. falciparum*
2. 8–17 days for *P. vivax*
3. 10–17 days for *P. ovale*
4. 18–40 days for *P. malariae* (including for several years)
5. 9–12 days by *P. knowlesi*

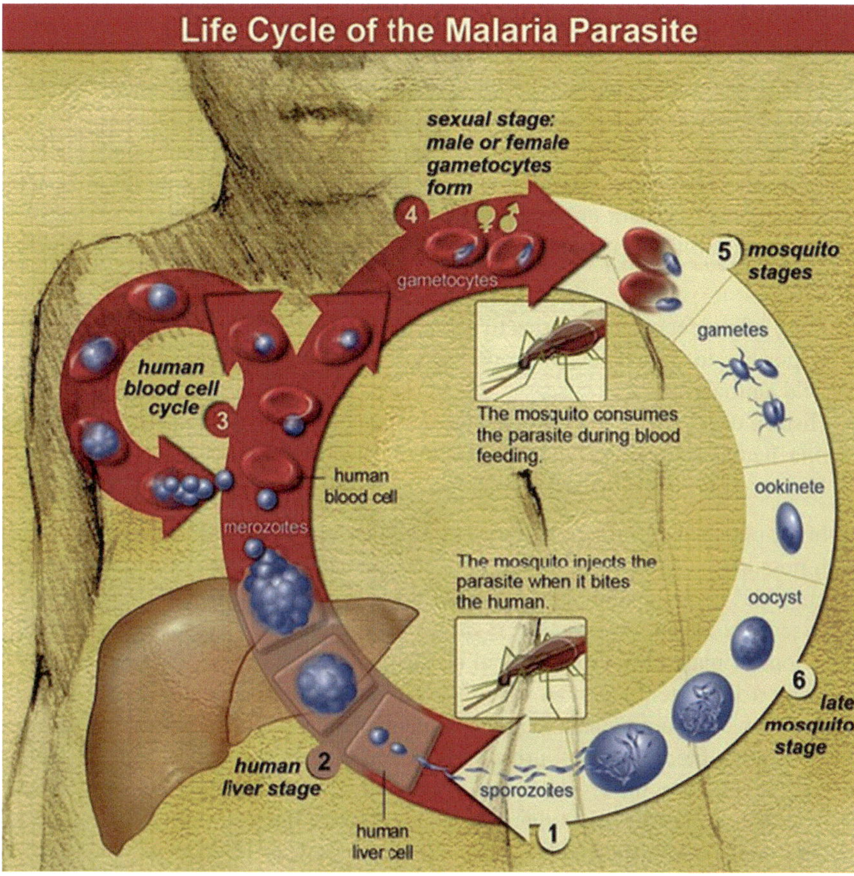

Fig. 31.1 Life cycle of the malaria parasite. (Contributed by Wikimedia Commons, National Institute of Health (NIH) (Public Domain))

The life cycle of this parasite dictates the periodicity of the clinical manifestation of "malarial paroxysm" of rigors, followed by several hours of fever, and then presents diaphoresis and return to a body temperature. Classically, in *P. vivax*, it has been described that it occurs every 48 hours; however, it is rare to persist this behavior by diagnosis and early treatment [1].

The symptoms and their severity depend on the parasitemia and the type of host: it has been described that the symptoms in native individuals develop with 0.002% and in previously exposed individuals with 0.2%. Severe infections occur with parasitemia greater than 5% [1, 7].

These manifestations occur due to the secretion of IFN-gamma and TNF-alpha, released by the action of parasite toxins. These responses are mediated by innate immunity given by phagocytosis of monocytes and macrophages in the splenic red pulp; and in addition, the adaptive immune response is developed by IFN-gamma and TNF-alpha, which induce a class change of CD4 lymphocytes [7].

Clinical Evaluation

Malaria is suspected when an individual who inhabits or has visited endemic regions presents fever, especially if it lasts for 7 or more days [5].

Other symptoms present are fever, malaise, weakness, gastrointestinal distress, upper respiratory symptoms, and myalgias; in severe cases jaundice, seizures, confusion, and coluria (dark urine) may occur [1, 4].

At this point it is very important to collect the following data from the clinical history:

1. Place of residence, recent trips to endemic areas, and use of chemoprophylaxis
2. Exposure to insect or arthropod bites, freshwater, caverns, domestic, or wild animals
3. History of HIV infection, pregnancy, G6PD deficiency, sickle cell anemia, anemia, hematological malignancies, or other cancers
4. History of previous malaria infections, including their treatment and evolution

In the physical examination, a patient who is acutely ill with fever can be found, with possible hepatosplenomegaly, jaundice, paleness, or signs of dehydration. In severe cases hemodynamic instability, drowsiness, and coma can be observed. The most severe cases may be due to *P. falciparum* infection or concomitant bacterial infections or malaria-induced adrenal insufficiency [4].

From a laboratory point of view, the patient should be treated as any febrile patient with exposure to malaria as a complete blood count, metabolic panel, coagulation studies, blood cultures, urine analysis, chest radiography, and thick and thin smears. In addition, the level of lactate, arterial gases, and lumbar puncture should be assessed, especially when there is an alteration of the state of consciousness or cerebral malaria is suspected [4].

Regarding the results of patients with malaria, you can find:

1. Thrombocytopenia in 60–70%.
2. Anemia in 29% of adults, being more severe in *P. falciparum* infections, by invasion of all erythrocytes, capillaries, and splenic sequestration of erythrocytes due to the decrease in their flexibility and cytoadherence [1]. In the cases of *P. vivax* and *P. malariae*; a moderate anemia occurs due to preferential invasion of reticulocytes and older erythrocytes.
3. The metabolic panel can show hepatocellular lesion secondary to the invasion of parasites to the liver: indirect hyperbilirubinemia by hemolysis. Hydroelectrolytic abnormalities are observed due to release of intracellular content, dehydration, and renal injury secondary to glomerular damage [4].
4. Coagulation abnormalities can be documented due to liver dysfunction and severe thrombocytopenia.
5. The urinalysis shows proteinuria as an indicator of glomerular lesion or can even cause a nephrotic syndrome [1].

The gold standard diagnostic test for malaria is the evaluation of Giemsa-stained thick and thin smears of a free-flowing venipuncture blood specimen [1, 4], which is done with immersion oil that must be completed 100-times and 1000-times magnification to avoid the loss of low levels of parasitemia or "delicate ring forms" [1].

Parasitemia is estimated by the number of organisms per high power field, after counting between 500 and 2000 red blood cells [8]. The appearance of infected erythrocytes varies according to the stage and type of *Plasmodium* [9]:

- The ring stage in *P. falciparum* appears as a "purple spot with a thin ring"; in *P. vivax* as a "purple spot with a deformed body"; in *P. ovale* as a "ring with a large purple spot"; in *P. malariae* as a "purple spot with a thick body"; and in *P. knowlesi* as a "purple spot (or spots) with an amorphous thick ring."
- The trophozoite stage in *P. falciparum* appears as "a bigger spot [growing] around a smaller spot"; in *P. vivax* as "a misshapen circle which contains an extended spot"; in *P. ovale* as "an oval circle (sometimes with small corners) which contains a purple spot with undefined shapes"; in *P. malariae* as "basket or band-shaped [without a] spot"; and in *P. knowlesi* as a "purple branched spot."
- The schizont stage in *P. falciparum* is not established; in *P. vivax* it appears as "not defined purple spots inside a circle"; in *P. ovale* as "more than one spot inside an oval circle (sometimes with small corners)"; in *P. malariae* as "diffuse purple spots around a darker spot"; and in *P. knowlesi* as "defined purple spots [that are] easy to count."

The gametocyte stage in *P. falciparum* appears as "banana [or] sausage-shaped"; in *P. vivax* as an "extended, big spot"; in *P. ovale* as a "row of accumulated spots"; in *P. malariae* as a "big stained spot which almost fill[s] the circle"; and in *P. knowlesi* as a "big spot which contains small spots."

A negative test does not rule out malaria, because infected erythrocytes may be sequestered in the intravascular compartment. If suspicion is maintained, the test should be repeated in 12–24 hours [4, 8]. In addition, it can be seen in monocytes and neutrophils, a malarial pigment manifested in blood smear, especially in patients with cerebral malaria [1].

There are also other specific diagnostic tests, such as:

1. Rapid diagnostic testing (RDT): This study is based on the determination of the antigens of the parasite histidine-rich-protein-2, lactate dehydrogenase, and aldolase, which are used for the diagnosis of *P. falciparum* infection [4, 10]. It has a 100% sensitivity, although it is always important, to follow the recommendation to perform the microscopic examination at the time of presentation and at 12 and 24 hours. Limitations are as follows: it is only useful for *P. falciparum* infection, there may be false positives weeks after infection due to persistent blood of the antigens, and it is not able to quantify the parasitic load [4].
2. Microhematocrit centrifugation: This technique separates the infected erythrocytes, which binds to acridine in the test tube, producing fluorescence of the parasites [1].
3. Polymerase chain reaction (PCR): this method is particularly useful, when there is a low level of parasitemia and speciation [1].

Malaria in Pregnancy

Malaria infection in pregnant women causes an increase in maternal morbidity and mortality. Although the mechanisms are not well-known, the pregnant woman presents a decrease in the immune response and is also less effective for malaria infection; in addition, *Plasmodium* is sequestered and replicates in the placenta.

Pregnant women have three times the risk of developing severe malaria, than non-pregnant women in the same region. For the product, this infection produces abortions, premature births, low birth weight, congenital infection, and/or perinatal death.

The risk of fetal death is greater when an infection with *P. falciparum* or *P. vivax* occurs [11].

The disease presentation is different in regions where transmission is low and unstable versus in areas where the infection is high and stable, due to the immunity developed by the mother. In places where transmission is low, women would seldom become infected, but since they have low immunity, the disease evolves rapidly to severe conditions, with a high risk of presenting severe malaria (cerebral malaria and ARDS) and death [12, 13]. In areas with stable transmission by *P. falciparum*, approximately 50 million pregnancies occur per year, where women are semi-immune and can carry the disease with few or no symptoms.

Women who have a semi-immunity may present an insidious process for the mother and the product, which impact on the prognosis of the mother and the product, such as severe maternal anemia and low birth weight. For first time pregnant women, there is a high risk of complications of this infection, which is reduced in future pregnancies by the development of a natural resistance acquired to *P. falciparum*, thanks to the development of antibodies against parasitized erythrocytes that bind to chondroitin sulfate A (CSA) of the placenta Fig. 31.2 [14, 15]. It has been observed that in areas where malaria control and incidence has decreased, a decrease in specific antibodies against malaria has been observed, with an increase in parasite burden and sequelae of the disease [16].

In areas of stable transmission, benefits have been observed in chemoprophylaxis, such as decreased parasitemia and improvement in hematocrit [17–19], with the subsequent beneficial effect of improving LBW, preterm delivery (PTD), perinatal mortality, and neonatal mortality, because maternal anemia increases the risk of the above. In addition, severe anemia is the greatest risk factor for mortality when women have postpartum hemorrhage in low-income countries [20]. In addition, chemoprophylaxis has a positive impact on the fetal prognosis during pregnancy and after birth, reducing perinatal mortality [18, 21].

Diagnosis of Malaria During Pregnancy

Diagnosis of malaria during pregnancy can be difficult. In *P. falciparum* infection, especially in semi-immune women who are asymptomatic, the parasites accumulate in the placenta and may have a low blood density, making it difficult to detect by microscopy (BS microscopy).

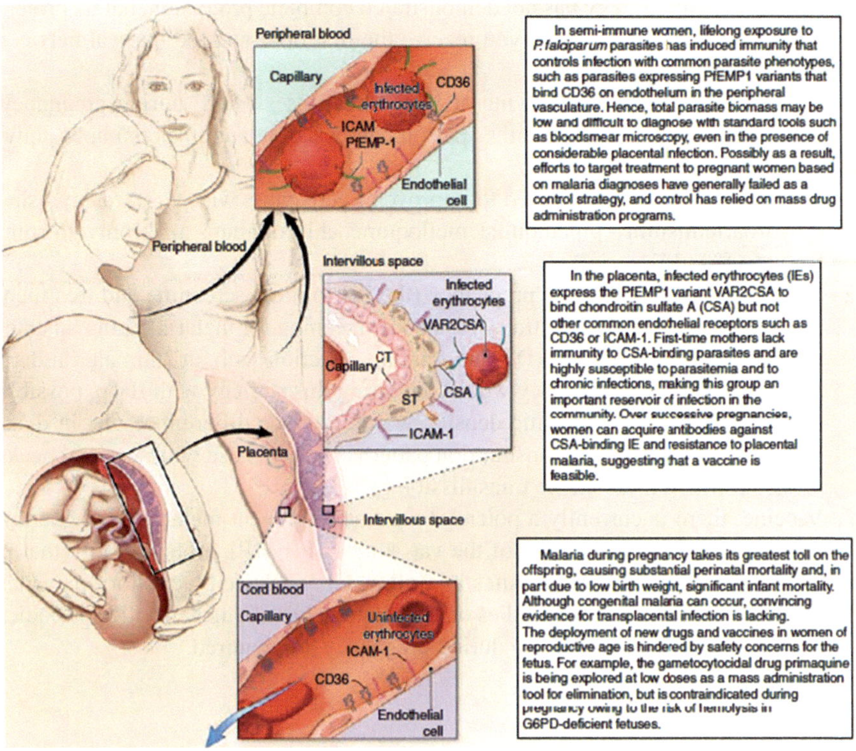

Fig. 31.2 Malaria during pregnancy features several unique host-parasite interactions that require special attention for elimination strategies. Although malaria is more common in pregnant women than other adults, it is difficult to diagnose and therefore to control. The few drugs known to be safe during pregnancy are losing efficacy to drug-resistant *Plasmodium falciparum* parasites, and the use of new drugs or other interventions is hindered by concerns for fetal safety. Based on the knowledge of malaria immunity during pregnancy, vaccine approaches appear promising for the control of PM, but first-generation candidates are only now entering clinical trials, and it is unclear whether these products will interrupt malaria transmission in pregnant women

The rapid diagnostic test (RDT) is a test that has gained acceptance in the general population, with adequate levels of sensitivity and specificity in pregnant women. Different studies have determined a sensitivity between 15% and 97% and a specificity between 91% and 98% [22–24].

However, because malaria antigens remain for a long period in the bloodstream, it is limited for the management and monitoring of the effectiveness of treatment during pregnancy [25–28].

Thus, strategies for the prevention of this pathology have been designed in pregnant women who live in areas with high risk of transmission:

1. Intermittent presumptive treatment (IPTp): This strategy currently reduces the incidence of malaria in pregnancy and/or the parasite load in some areas of West Africa, however, in areas with low or moderate SP (sulfadoxine-pyrimethamine)

resistance, this strategy has not demonstrated complete protection, but its protective effect depends on when you receive the first dose and the interval between treatments [29].

WHO recommends receiving at least three doses of SP during pregnancy, with each dose at least 1 months apart; it can be safely administered until delivery [30].

Other drugs have been used to improve effectiveness with this strategy using dihydroartemisinin – piperaquine, mefloquine, chloroquine – azithromycin combination [31–35].

2. Screening and treatment in pregnancy (the intermittent screening and treatment in pregnancy (ISTp)): this strategy is about screening for malaria during an antenatal clinic visit using an RDT and treating infection with an antimalarial drug studies with different efficacy when comparing this strategy with IPTp, possibly due to differences in parasitic density, which produce different results in diagnostic tests and different transmission patterns such as those with seasonal peaks vs. those with a more stable transmission [36–38].
3. Vaccine: there is currently a potential vaccine to prevent malaria in pregnancy, called VAR2CSA, a member of the var gene or PfEMP1 protein family that is upregulated in placental parasites as well as CSA-selected laboratory parasites [39, 40]. However, further studies on the relationship of other specific antibodies and protection against malaria during pregnancy are required.

Treatment/Management

The pillars of malaria treatment are:

1. Hospitalization for high-risk patients:

   Children and naive adults require 24 hours of hospitalization to assess evolution with clinical antimalarial treatment and evaluation of parasitemia. When there is a presence of a high initial parasitemia and a slow decrease in it, an increase in the risk of fluid imbalances, renal injury, and acute respiratory distress syndrome have been associated.
2. Support measures, especially in unstable patients, with respiratory distress and cerebral malaria. These patients must be admitted to intensive care [4].

   Patients with any of the following clinical criteria for severe disease should receive aggressive intravenous treatment [8]:

   (a) Alteration of the state of consciousness
   (b) Severe normocytic anemia (less than 7 Hb)
   (c) Renal injury
   (d) ARDS (Acute Respiratory Distress Syndrome)
   (e) Hypotension
   (f) DIC (Disseminated Intravascular Coagulation)
   (g) Spontaneous bleeding
   (h) Metabolic Acidosis

(i) Hemoglobinuria
(j) Jaundice
(k) Repetitive generalized seizures
(l) Parasitemia >5%.

3. Antiparasitic treatment:
   This treatment is necessary to fight parasites in all its forms, both in the liver and in erythrocytes.
   There are several antimalarial medications:

   (a) Chloroquine and hydroxychloroquine: both synthetic drugs derived from quinine interfere with parasitic hemoglobin metabolism and produce an increase in intracellular pH, causing a disruption of the erythrocyte stage [41, 42]. Usually 2 days of treatment are required, ensuring better tolerance and short hospitalizations. However, chloroquine can contribute to resistance, as it helps gametogenesis. This is a concern in South Asia.
   (b) Primaquine: is a hypnozointocidal, which is added for the eradication of liver parasites and the prevention of dormancy and relapse. In *P. vivax* or *P. ovale* infections [4, 43]. Contraindicated in pregnancy due to fetal teratogenicity and in difficulty of G6PD due to hemolytic reaction (bite cells an Heinz bodies on blood smear is observed) [5].
   (c) Artemisinin-base combination therapy (ACT): it is active against parasites in all life cycle states [4]
   (d) Atovaquone-proguanil: its objective is to inhibit the production of ATP, by inhibiting the electronic cellular transporter. Proguanil improves the response of the atovaquones, by means of sensitizing parasitic mitochondria [44]. It is active against erythrocytic and extra erythrocytic forms [44, 45].

The choice of antimalarial treatment depends on the *Plasmodium* species, clinical condition, age, and regional sensitivity of the parasite. The 2019 CDC Guidelines [8] provide the following recommendations:

Stable uncomplicated patients:

1. Infections with *P. falciparum*, *P. malariae*, or *P. knowlesi*; in chloroquine-sensitive areas, chloroquine phosphate 600 mg loading dose and then 300 mg at 6.24.48 hours or hydroxychloroquine 620 mg of loading dose, followed by 310 mg at 6.24.48 hours
2. *P. falciparum* infections in areas resistant to chloroquine or with unknown resistance can be treated with:

   (a) Atovaquone-proguanil 250 mg/100 mg, 4 tablets daily for 4 days
   (b) Artemetherlumefantrine 20 mg/120 mg, 4 tablets initial dose, then 8 hours later and then twice a day for 2 days
   (c) Quinine sulfate 542 mg three times a day for 3 days (in Southeast Asia it should take 7 days) + doxycycline 100 mg a day for 7 days
   (d) Tetracycline 250 mg daily for 7 days
   (e) Clindamycin 20 mg/kg/day, divided into three times a da
   (f) Mefloquine 684 mg loading dose, followed by 456 mg every 6–12 hours for a total of 1250 mg

3. *P. vivax* or *P. ovale* infections in chloroquine-sensitive regions should be treated with chloroquine phosphate or hydroxychloroquine as indicated + primaquine phosphate 30 mg daily for 14 days or tafenoquine 300 mg one dose.
4. *P. vivax* infections in chloroquine-resistant regions (Indonesia, Papua New Guinea) are treated with the following combinations:

   (a) Quinine sulfate (as previously described) + doxycycline, primaquine, or tafenoquine
   (b) Atovaquone-proguanil + primaquine or tafenoquine
   (c) Mefloquine + primaquine or tafenoquine

5. Infections of any species in pregnant women in areas sensitive to chloroquine are treated with chloroquine or hydroxychloroquine.
6. Infections of any species in pregnant women in areas resistant to chloroquine are treated with:

   (a) In any trimester of pregnancy: quinine sulfate + clindamycin or mefloquine. Quinine treatment should be continued for 7 days in infections acquired in Southeast Asia and for 3 days in other places, and treatment with clindamycin should be continued for 7 days regardless of where the infection was acquired.
   (b) Only in the 2 and 3 quarter with artemether-lumefantrine.
   (c) The use of doxycycline or tetracycline in combination with quinine sulfate is not recommended, but sometimes where there is no other option, it can be used if the benefits outweigh the risks.
   (d) Infections caused by *P. falciparum* resistant to chloroquine; atovaquone-proguanil does not have adequate safety studies; however, it could be used if there are no other treatment options and when the benefits are considered to outweigh the risks.
   (e) In pregnant women with *P. vivax* or *P. ovale*, they should continue during their pregnancy with the administration of prophylaxis with chloroquine of 300 mg base (= 500 mg salt) PO per week. Radical treatment should not be given for hypnozoites with primaquine phosphate and tafenoquine.
   (f) After delivery and if the patient does not have G6PD deficiency, the treatment decision for hypnozoites should be taken depending on whether the mother is going to breastfeed: in case of breastfeeding with children with normal G6PD activity, she should receive primaquine phosphate; the use of tafenoquine is not recommended. In case of not breastfeeding, treatment with primaquine phosphate and tafenoquine is started.

Patients with Severe Malaria

In unstable and nonpregnant patients, in any region: artesunate IV 2.4 mg/kg at 0.12.24 and 48 hours and then continue with any of the following: artemether-lumefantrine, atovaquone-proguanil, doxycycline, or mefloquine. If there is no oral tolerance, you can continue with artesunate, a daily dose up to 7 days.

The use of clindamycin or intravenous doxycycline is not recommended due to its slow antimalarial action, which is observed 24 hours after its onset.

Although the data are limited in terms of the use of artesunate in the first trimester of pregnancy, no adverse effects have been observed, and also, taking into account that severe malaria is a fatal condition for the pregnant woman and the fetus, it is estimated that the benefit outweighs the risks, with the understanding that there are no other treatment options [8].

The only contraindication for artesunate IV is the known allergy to artemisinins.

Forecast

The duration of the untreated infection and the time of recurrence varies by location and species [1]:

1. *P. falciparum* and *P. ovale*, the infection lasts 2–3 weeks and relapse can occur 6–18 months after the primary infection.
2. *P. vivax*, the infection can last between 3 and 8 weeks and can relapse in months up to 5 years later.
3. *P. malariae*, the infection can last at least 3–24 weeks and relapse about 20 years later.

Relapse is when recurrence of symptoms occurs, months to years after the resolution of erythrocytic organisms by reinfection or activation of hypnozoites [1, 4]. The resurgence is defined as recurrent symptoms in the days or weeks of an acute infection due to the permanence of parasitemia after ineffective or incomplete treatment or due to failure of the immune response, which is more common in *P. falciparum* infection.

A complete and appropriate treatment causes a complete resolution of the symptoms.

Complications

The severe complications of this infectious disease are three:

1. Cerebral malaria
2. Severe malarial anemia
3. Nephrotic syndrome

Cerebral Malaria

This complication occurs in 80% of fatal cases, especially with *P. falciparum* infection. It is presented as an alteration of the state of consciousness of slow appearance, violent shaking, headache, and very high fever (about 42 C), followed by coma, metabolic acidosis, and hypoglycemia, and in addition, seizures and death can be observed [1, 7].

Its pathogenesis is due to the formation of malarial rosettes, which is the formation resulting from an infected erythrocyte surrounded by three uninfected erythrocytes, which produce kidnapping and vasodilation at the cerebral level, causing an extreme inflammatory response by the action of IFN-gamma, TNF-alpha, and oxygen-free radicals. The above causes congestion, decreased cerebral perfusion, endothelial activation, impaired blood-brain barrier, and cerebral edema, producing an increase in brain volume and intracranial pressure, which is the cause of death in this complication [46].

Severe Malarial Anemia

This complication is due to an increase in destruction and a decrease in erythrocyte production due to several mechanisms mediated by THF-alpha. These are cell lysis by the replication and exit of the erythrocyte parasites, removal and splenic lysis mediated by erythrocytes marked by immune mechanisms, poor incorporation of iron into the forming HEME molecules, and a suppression of the bone marrow.

Blackwater fever is a clinical presentation caused by severe anemia with hemoglobinuria and renal injury in the context of patients with massive intravascular hemolysis who have had repeated *P. falciparum* infections and who have been treated with quinine in a chronic manner, a rare condition and which has been thought to be associated with G6PD deficiency [1, 3, 47].

Nephrotic Syndrome

This complication occurs due to the accumulation of immune antigen-antibody complexes in the glomerulus and produces a syndrome similar to membranoproliferative glomerulonephritis with proteinuria and decreased renal function.

It is commonly observed in *P. malariae* and *P. knowlesi*; it is less frequent with *P. vivax* and very rare with *P. falciparum* and *P. ovale* [48].

Other complications described, typical of this infection are:

(a) Bilious remittent fever: presents with abdominal pain and persistent vomiting, which can cause dehydration, jaundice, and dark urine.
(b) Algid malaria, it is an adrenal insufficiency due to congestion of the gland by the parasite and subsequent necrosis of the adrenal glands.
(c) Acute respiratory distress syndrome, circulatory collapse, DIC, pulmonary edema, coma, and death.

Prevention

Regarding the prevention of this disease, the two most important points:

1. Vector control: there are several measures in this regard such as the use of bed nets impregnated with insecticides, clothes treated with permethrin, and application of DEET on the skin, as well as not traveling to endemic areas.
2. Chemoprophylaxis: the three drugs used for this purpose:

   - Atovaquone-proguanil (Malarone): it is taken once a day during and 1 week after the trip to an endemic area; this drug suppresses the liver stage and is not approved in pregnancy [2].
   - Doxycycline: It is taken once a day during and 1 month after the trip, it works by suppressing the blood phase. It has the benefit of having a prophylactic effect against rickettsias, Q fever, leptospirosis, and traveler's diarrhea. However, it causes gastrointestinal upset and photosensitivity and increases the risk of candidiasis.
   - Mefloquine: it is taken once a week during and 1 month after the trip; it suppresses the blood stage. It can be used safe in the second and third trimesters of pregnancy; however, it has a much higher risk of neuropsychiatric adverse effects.

The US military uses doxycycline if they are found in areas with known drug sensitivity.

For women pregnant in the first trimester or who are breastfeeding, prophylaxis with chloroquine or mefloquine is preferable; the safety of atovaquone-proguanil in pregnancy is limited [49].

References

1. Garcia LS. Malaria. Clin Lab Med. 2010;30(1):93–129. [PubMed].
2. Ikemoto T. Tropical malaria does not mean hot environments. J Med Entomol. 2008;45:963–9.
3. Lou J, Lucas R, Grau GE. Pathogenesis of cerebral malaria: recent experimental data and possible applications for humans. Clin Microbiol Rev. 2001;14:810–20.
4. Fletcher TE, Beeching NJ. Malaria. J R Army Med Corps. 2013;159(3):158–66. [PubMed].
5. López Del Prado GR, Hernán García C, Moreno Cea L, Fernández Espinilla V, Muñoz Moreno MF, Delgado Márquez A, Polo Polo MJ, Andrés García I. Malaria in developing countries. J Infect Dev Ctries. 2014;8(1):1–4. [PubMed].
6. Krotoski WA, Garnham PCC, Bray RS, et al. Observations on early and late post sporozoite tissue stages in primate malaria. 1. Discovery of a new latent form of Plasmodium cynomolgi (the hypnozoite), and failure to detect hepatic forms within the first 24 hours after infection. Am J Trop Med Hyg. 1982;31:24–35.
7. Carlton JM. Malaria parasite evolution in a test tube. Science. 2018;359(6372):159–60.[PMC free article] [PubMed].
8. https://www.cdc.gov/malaria/resources/pdf/clinicalguidance.pdf.

9. Ortiz-Ruiz A, Postigo M, Gil-Casanova S, Cuadrado D, Bautista JM, Rubio JM, Luengo-Oroz M, Linares M. Plasmodium species differentiation by non-expert on-line volunteers for remote malaria field diagnosis. Malar J. 2018;17(1):54. [PMC free article] [PubMed].
10. Mathison BA, Pritt BS. Update on malaria diagnostics and test utilization. J Clin Microbiol. 2017;55(7):2009–17. [PMC free article] [PubMed].
11. Moore K, Simpson J, Scoullar M, McGready R, Fowkes F. Quantification of the association between malaria in pregnancy and stillbirth: a systematic review and meta-analysis. Lancet Glob Health. 2017;5:e1101–12.
12. Duffy PE, Desowitz RS. Pregnancy malaria throughout history: dangerous labors. In: Duffy PE, Fried M, editors. Malaria in pregnancy: deadly parasite, susceptible host. New York: Taylor & Francis; 2001. p. 1–25.
13. Nosten F, ter Kuile F, Maelankirri L, Decludt B, White NJ. Malaria during pregnancy in an area of unstable endemicity. Trans R Soc Trop Med Hyg. 1991;85:424–9.
14. Fried M, Nosten F, Brockman A, Brabin BJ, Duffy PE. Maternal antibodies block malaria. Nature. 1998;395:851–2.
15. Fried M, Duffy P. Malaria during pregnancy. Cold Spring Harb Perspect Med. 2017;7:a025551.
16. Mayor A, Bardaji A, Macete E, Nhampossa T, Fonseca AM, Gonzalez R, Maculuve S, Cistero P, Ruperez M, Campo J, et al. Changing trends in P. falciparum burden, immunity, and disease in pregnancy. N Engl J Med. 2015;373:1607–17.
17. Greenwood BM, Greenwood AM, Snow RW, Byass P, Bennett S, Hatib-N'Jie AB. The effects of malaria chemoprophylaxis given by traditional birth attendants on the course and outcome of pregnancy. Trans R Soc Trop Med Hyg. 1989;83:589–94.
18. Greenwood AM, Armstrong JR, Byass P, Snow RW, Greenwood BM. Malaria chemoprophylaxis, birthweight and child survival. Trans R Soc Trop Med Hyg. 1992;86:483–5.
19. Menendez C, Todd J, Alonso PL, Lulat S, Francis N, Greenwood BM. Malaria chemoprophylaxis, infection of the placenta and birth weight in Gambian primigravidae. J Trop Med Hyg. 1994;97:244–8.
20. Tort J, Rozenberg P, TraoreM FP, Dumont A. Factors associated with postpartum hemorrhage maternal death in referral hospitals in Senegal and Mali: A cross-sectional epidemiological survey. BMC Pregnancy Childbirth. 2015;15:235.
21. Garner P, Gulmezoglu AM. Drugs for preventing malaria in pregnant women. Cochrane Database Syst Rev. 2006. https://doi.org/10.1002/14651858.CD000169.pub2.
22. Mankhambo L, Kanjala M, Rudman S, Lema VM, Rogerson SJ. Evaluation of the OptiMAL rapid antigen test and species-specific PCR to detect placental Plasmodiumfalciparum infection at delivery. J Clin Microbiol. 2002;40:155–8.
23. VanderJagt TA, Ikeh EI, Ujah IO, Belmonte J, Glew RH, VanderJagt DJ. Comparison of the OptiMAL rapid test and microscopy for detection of malaria in pregnant women in Nigeria. Tropical Med Int Health. 2005;10:39–41.
24. Tagbor H, Bruce J, Browne E, Greenwood B, Chandramohan D. Performance of the OptiMAL dipstick in the diagnosis of malaria infection in pregnancy. Ther Clin Risk Manag. 2008;4:631–6.
25. Wongsrichanalai C, Chuanak N, Tulyayon S, Thanoosingha N, Laoboonchai A, Thimasarn K, Brewer TG, Heppner DG. Comparison of a rapid field immunochromatographic test to expert microscopy for the detection of Plasmodium falciparum asexual parasitemia in Thailand. Acta Trop. 1999;73:263–73.
26. Mayxay M, Pukrittayakamee S, Chotivanich K, Looareesuwan S, White NJ. Persistence of Plasmodium falciparum HRP-2 in successfully treated acute falciparum malaria. Trans R Soc Trop Med Hyg. 2001;95:179–82.
27. Tjitra E, Suprianto S, McBroom J, Currie BJ, Anstey NM. Persistent ICT malaria P.f/P.v panmalarial and HRP-2 antigen reactivity after treatment of Plasmodium falciparum malaria is associated with gametocytemia and results in false-positive diagnoses of Plasmodium vivax in convalescence. J Clin Microbiol. 2001;39:1025–31.
28. Kattenberg JH, Tahita CM, Versteeg IA, Tinto H, Traore-Coulibaly M, Schallig HD, Mens PF. Antigen persistence of rapid diagnostic tests in pregnant women in Nanoro, Burkina

Faso, and the implications for the diagnosis of malaria in pregnancy. Tropical Med Int Health. 2012;17:550–7.

29. Nosten F, McGready R. Intermittent presumptive treatment in pregnancy with sulfadoxine-pyrimethamine: A counter perspective. Malar J. 2015;14:248.
30. https://www.who.int/malaria/areas/preventive_therapies/pregnancy/en/.
31. Kakuru A, Jagannathan P, Muhindo MK, Natureeba P, Awori P, Nakalembe M, Opira B, Olwoch P, Ategeka J, Nayebare P, et al. Dihydroartemisinin–piperaquine for the prevention of malaria in pregnancy. N Engl J Med. 2016;374:928–39.
32. Briand V, Bottero J, Noel H, Masse V, Cordel H, Guerra J, Kossou H, Fayomi B, Ayemonna P, Fievet N, et al. Intermittent treatment for the prevention of malaria during pregnancy in Benin: A randomized, open-label equivalence trial comparing sulfadoxine-pyrimethamine with mefloquine. J Infect Dis. 2009;200:991–1001.
33. Gonzalez R, Desai M, Macete E, Ouma P, Kakolwa MA, Abdulla S, Aponte JJ, Bulo H, Kabanywanyi AM, Katana A, et al. Intermittent preventive treatment of malaria in pregnancy with mefloquine in HIV-infected women receiving cotrimoxazole prophylaxis: A multicenter randomized placebo-controlled trial. PLoS Med. 2014b;11:e1001735.
34. Denoeud-Ndam L, Zannou DM, Fourcade C, Taron-Brocard C, Porcher R, Atadokpede F, Komongui DG, Dossou- Gbete L, Afangnihoun A, Ndam NT, et al. Cotrimoxazole prophylaxis versus mefloquine intermittent preventive treatment to prevent malaria in HIV-infected pregnant women: two randomized controlled trials. J Acquir Immune Defic Syndr. 2014;65:198–206.
35. Evaluate azithromycin plus chloroquine and sulfadoxine plus pyrimethamine combinations for intermittent preventive treatment of falciparum malaria infection in pregnant women in Africa. ClinicalTrials.gov Identifier: NCT01103063.
36. Desai M, Gutman J, L'Lanziva A, Otieno K, Juma E, Kariuki S, Ouma P, Were V, Laserson K, Katana A, et al. Intermittent screening and treatment or intermittent preventive treatment with dihydroartemisinin–piperaquine versus intermittent preventive treatment with sulfadoxine-pyrimethamine for the control of malaria during pregnancy in western Kenya: an open-label, three-group, randomised controlled superiority trial. Lancet. 2015;386:2507–19.
37. Tagbor H, Cairns M, Bojang K, Coulibaly SO, Kayentao K, Williams J, Abubakar I, Akor F, Mohammed K, Bationo R, et al. A non-inferiority, individually randomized trial of intermittent screening and treatment versus intermittent preventive treatment in the control of malaria in pregnancy. PLoS One. 2015;10:e0132247.
38. Fried M, Muehlenbachs A, Duffy PE. Diagnosing malaria in pregnancy: an update. Expert Rev Anti-Infect Ther. 2012;10:1177–87.
39. Salanti A, Dahlback M, Turner L, Nielsen MA, Barfod L, Magistrado P, Jensen AT, Lavstsen T, Ofori MF, Marsh K, et al. Evidence for the involvement of VAR2CSA in pregnancy-associated malaria. J Exp Med. 2004;200:1197–203.
40. Ndam NT, Denoeud-Ndam L, Doritchamou J, Viwami F, Salanti A, Nielsen MA, Fievet N, Massougbodji A, Luty AJ, Deloron P. Protective antibodies against placental malaria and poor outcomes during pregnancy, Benin. Emerg Infect Dis. 2015;21:813–23.
41. Ben-Zvi I, Kivity S, Langevitz P, Shoenfeld Y. Hydroxychloroquine: from malaria to autoimmunity. Clin Rev Allergy Immunol. 2012;42(2):145–53. [PubMed].
42. Slater AF. Chloroquine: mechanism of drug action and resistance in Plasmodium falciparum. Pharmacol Ther. 1993;57(2–3):203–35. [PubMed].
43. Commons RJ, Simpson JA, Thriemer K, Humphreys GS, Abreha T, Alemu SG, Añez A, Anstey NM, Awab GR, Baird JK, Barber BE, Borghini-Fuhrer I, Chu CS, D'Alessandro U, Dahal P, Daher A, de Vries PJ, Erhart A, Gomes MSM, Gonzalez-Ceron L, Grigg MJ, Heidari A, Hwang J, Kager PA, Ketema T, Khan WA, Lacerda MVG, Leslie T, Ley B, Lidia K, Monteiro WM, Nosten F, Pereira DB, Phan GT, Phyo AP, Rowland M, Saravu K, Sibley CH, Siqueira AM, Stepniewska K, Sutanto I, Taylor WRJ, Thwaites G, Tran BQ, Tran HT, Valecha N, Vieira JLF, Wangchuk S, William T, Woodrow CJ, Zuluaga-Idarraga L, Guerin PJ, White NJ, Price RN. The effect of chloroquine dose and primaquine on Plasmodium vivax recurrence: a WorldWide Antimalarial Resistance Network systematic review and individual patient pooled meta-analysis. Lancet Infect Dis. 2018;18(9):1025–34. [PMC free article] [PubMed].

44. Staines HM, Burrow R, Teo BH, Chis Ster I, Kremsner PG, Krishna S. Clinical implications of Plasmodium resistance to atovaquone/proguanil: a systematic review and meta-analysis. J Antimicrob Chemother. 2018;73(3):581–95. [PMC free article] [PubMed].
45. Delves M, Plouffe D, Scheurer C, Meister S, Wittlin S, Winzeler EA, Sinden RE, Leroy D. The activities of current antimalarial drugs on the life cycle stages of Plasmodium: a comparative study with human and rodent parasites. PLoS Med. 2012.9(2):e1001169. [PMC free article] [PubMed].
46. Seydel KB, Kampondeni SD, Valim C, Potchen MJ, Milner DA, Muwalo FW, Birbeck GL, Bradley WG, Fox LL, Glover SJ, Hammond CA, Heyderman RS, Chilingulo CA, Molyneux ME, Taylor TE. Brain swelling and death in children with cerebral malaria. N Engl J Med. 2015;372(12):1126–37. [PMC free article] [PubMed].
47. Shanks GD. The multifactorial epidemiology of blackwater fever. Am J Trop Med Hyg 2017;97(6):1804–7. [PMC free article] [PubMed].
48. van Velthuysen MLF, Florquin S. Glomerulopathy associated with parasitic infections. Clin Microbiol Rev. 2000;13:55–66.
49. Mayer RC, Tan KR, Gutman JR. Safety of atovaquone-proguanil during pregnancy. J Travel Med. 2019;26(4):tay138. [PMC free article] [PubMed].

Chapter 32
Dengue in Pregnant Women

Juan Ignacio Silesky-Jiménez and Jorge Hidalgo

Introduction

Dengue is a self-limited viral infection due to an arbovirus that affects humans and is transmitted by mosquitoes, mainly by *Aedes aegypti*, which also carries other arboviruses such as Zika, Yellow Fever, and Chikungunya, thus, as another vector to a lesser extent such as *Aedes albopictus*.

This viral infection can cause subclinical conditions producing asymptomatic seroconversion, even severe clinical conditions that are life-threatening, such as severe dengue which can lead the individual to a condition of deep shock, with thrombocytopenia, hypoxia, and acidosis, with multiorgan dysfunction and death [1].

In addition, in special conditions such as pregnant women, this infection presents a diagnostic challenge making the differential diagnosis with some conditions of pregnancy, such as HELLP syndrome, vertical product infection, peripartum problems especially with the increased risk of bleeding, and, finally, the clinical management of severe dengue presentations in this group of patients [2].

The dengue virus belongs to the Flaviviridae family and has four different serotypes such as DEN-1, DEN-2, DEN-3, and DEN-4, which are the cause of different clinical manifestations of the virus.

This disease presents in tropical and subtropical areas, especially in urban and suburban areas, due to many causes such as rain fall, the increase in temperature due

J. I. Silesky-Jiménez (✉)
Critical Care Medicine, Clinical Nutrition, Health Services Administration, Hospital San Juan de Dios and Hospital CIMA, San José, Costa Rica

Costa Rica University, San José, Costa Rica

AMICOR and COCECATI, San José, Costa Rica

J. Hidalgo
Division of Critical Care, Karl Heusner Memorial Hospital, Belize City, Belize

C. Montufar et al. (eds.), *Obstetric Catastrophes*,
https://doi.org/10.1007/978-3-030-70034-8_32

to the global warming phenomenon, globalization (with the transport of the virus by infected subjects or vectors), rapid urban development without planning, and the characteristics of the vectors that make them resistant to many environmental conditions [3].

It's most serious presentation, the severe dengue, has been known since the 1950s of the last century, in an epidemic in the Philippines and Thailand; it is currently a cause of hospitalization and mortality in many regions of Latin America and Asia.

Another important point of this disease is its capacity for hyperendemicity, which produces an important impact not only on human health but also on local, national, regional, and global economies. In addition, infected travelers spread this virus.

Epidemiology and Transmission

WHO has determined a significant increase in the incidence of this infectious disease in recent decades. It is important to emphasize that many of these cases are asymptomatic and that in other parts of the world, they are not diagnosed or reported.

It has been determined that there is an incidence of about 390 million cases per year (with a 95% confidence interval between 284 and 528 cases annually); of which 96 million are diagnosed (variation of 67–136). It is possible that 400,000 cases of severe dengue occur annually, with a mortality of 5%; however, with proper treatment, it can be reduced by 1% [4, 5].

It has been estimated that 3.9 billion people in 128 countries are at risk of infection with this virus, which represents at least half of the world's population.

Dengue is an endemic infection in regions of Africa, America, the Eastern Mediterranean, Southeast Asia, and Western Pacific [6].

This infection has had an important worldwide spread in recent decades; before the 1970s, it was known that only nine countries in the world had severe dengue epidemics. Currently more than 100 have had epidemic peaks, and it is estimated that at least 128 are the risk of infection [4, 6].

From 2008 to 2018, there were significant outbreaks in different parts of the world:

1. In 2008, more than 1.2 million cases were recorded in total in the Americas, Southeast Asia, and Western Pacific regions and, in 2015, more than 3.2 million (according to official data submitted by Member States to the WHO).
2. In 2012, an outbreak of dengue in the Madeira archipelago (Portugal) caused more than 2000 cases, and imported cases were registered in 10 other European countries, in addition to continental Portugal
3. In 2015, 2.35 million cases were reported in the Region of the Americas alone, of which more than 10,200 cases were diagnosed as severe dengue and caused 1181 deaths. On this same year in Delhi (India), the worst outbreak has been recorded since 2006, with more than 15,000 cases. The island of Hawaii, in the

homonymous state of the United States, was affected in 2015 by an outbreak with 181 cases, and transmission continued in 2016. Cases have continued to be recorded in Pacific island states: Fiji, Tonga, and French Polynesia.
4. 2016 had large outbreaks of dengue throughout the world. The Americas region reported more than 2,380,000 cases, and in Brazil alone there were just under 1,500,000 cases, that is, about three times more than in 2014. There were 1032 reported deaths from dengue in this region. The Western Pacific Region had 375,000 cases reported, 176,411 of them in the Philippines and 100,028 in Malaysia, figures that represent a similar number to that of previous years in both countries. The Solomon Islands declared an outbreak with more than 7000 suspected cases. In the African Region, Burkina Faso reported a localized outbreak with 1061 probable cases

During 2017, there was a significant reduction in the incidence, especially in the Americas, with a 73% reduction (from 2177,171 cases in 2016 to 584,263 in 2017), as well as a decrease in severe dengue by 53% [6].

The most important dengue vectors have important characteristics to consider that affect the spread of the disease:

1. *Aedes aegypti* is the main vector of this disease, which is infected with asymptomatic and symptomatic humans on day 4 or 5, until day 12. Infected females transmit the virus, after an incubation period of 4–10 days; it is important to emphasize that the mosquito can transmit the disease for life.

   This vector inhabits urban sites and reproduces in artificial containers. However, eggs can remain in dry places for more than a year and hatch when in contact with water. Female mosquitoes bite many people mainly in the early morning and evening.
2. *Aedes albopictus* is the secondary vector. It is important in Asia, Canada, and North America and in 25 countries in Europe. The above due to the commercial trade of used tires, which are artificial breeding grounds, and materials such as bamboo and for the ability of this mosquito to survive cold temperatures, since they survive temperatures below zero degrees Celsius and it's adaptability to microhabitats [6]

Pathogenesis

When the virus is introduced by the bite of the mosquito, it is directed through the lymphatic vessels to the lymph nodes where they replicate before producing viremia. Any serotype (DEN-1, DEN-2, DEN-3, and DEN-4) can initially cause any manifestation of the disease, from asymptomatic cases to severe conditions. An infection can produce permanent immunity.

However, in the recovery phase of an infection, a new infection by another serotype potentially produces a new production of antibodies that combine with the previous ones, producing a heterogeneous combination that activates dendritic, monocyte, and macrophage cells, which produces a release of vasoactive substances, which produce an increase in vascular permeability and hemorrhagic manifestations, making the presentation of hemorrhagic dengue (DHF) and dengue shock syndrome (DSS) more likely [7, 8].

This activation of complement and cytokines through the virus/antibody complex causes endothelial dysfunction, platelet destruction, and consumption of coagulation factors, which produces hemorrhagic manifestations and capillary leakage [7, 9]. In addition, there is a soluble viral protein, called DengueNS, which binds to the endothelial glycocalyx, contributing to capillary leakage. To all of the above, it has been demonstrated that in patients with severe dengue, an elevation of substances such as platelet activating factor, leukotrienes, vascular endothelial growth factor, and angiopoietin-2 [10].

An interesting fact is that the person recovering from dengue has a lifelong immunity for the particular serotype; but, because the immunity against other serotypes is temporary and partial, there is a risk that in future infections by other serotypes, the risk of having a severe dengue presentation is increased.

Classification

The World Health Organization (Fig. 32.1) has simplified the classification of dengue in:

1. Dengue fever (DF): in which there is the presence of fever and at least two of the typical clinical signs or any of the warning signs. It is required for the diagnosis of epidemiological and serological evidence.
2. Severe dengue: defined as dengue that has the following [12]:
   (i) Severe plasma leakage leading to shock or respiratory distress
   (ii) Severe hemorrhage
   (iii) Any organ failure

Hemorrhagic Dengue

Severe dengue presentations have been classically referred to as Hemorrhagic Dengue Fever (DHF) or Dengue Shock Syndrome (DSS); the risk factors for developing them are:

1. Life extremes in infants and the elderly [13].
2. Presence of chronic diseases such as diabetes mellitus, bronchial asthma, sickle cell anemia [14].
3. Serotypes DEN-1 and DEN-2 have a worse prognosis [15].
4. It has been observed that variations in the HLA-A locus in the host, increase susceptibility to DHF, and alleles of specific sensitivity and resistance in HLA-A have also been identified [16].

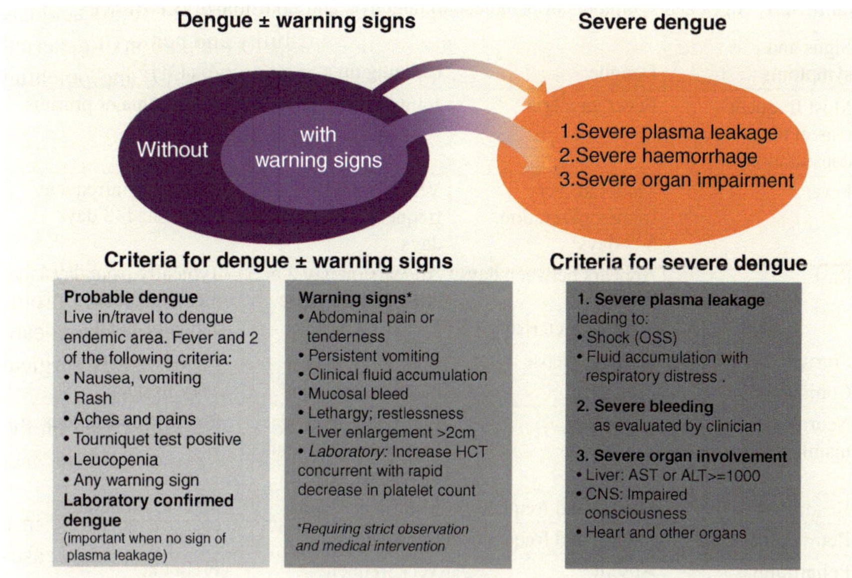

Fig. 32.1 Dengue case classification by severity [11]. ALT alanine aminotransferase, AST aspartate aminotransferase, CNS central nervous system, DSS dengue shock syndrome, HCT hematocrit

Clinical Manifestations

The dengue virus produces a range of clinical manifestations, from an asymptomatic seroconversion, through a feverish condition, to severe conditions that put the patient's life at risk (severe dengue).

It is important to know the dynamics of the disease, since an adequate knowledge of the different phases of the disease lead to a rational approach in the management of the patient.

After the mosquito inoculates the virus, an incubation period occurs between 4 and 10 days. The classic symptoms of the disease are fever, nausea, vomiting, rash, headache, retroocular pain, myalgias, arthralgia, petechiae, leukopenia, and positive tourniquet test [17].

Many of these symptoms are shared by other arboviruses such as Zika and chikungunya, as they can also coexist with dengue infection.

Some differences of these diseases, from a clinical point of view, can be listed in the following table, obtained from WHO/PAHO [18] (Table 32.1).

The disease begins with a sudden fever, which produces three clinical phases (Fig. 32.2):

Table 32.1 Signs and symptoms of dengue, chikungunya, and Zika arbovirus infections

Signs and symptoms	Dengue	Chikungunya	Zika
Most frequent reason for consultation	Fever, myalgia	Joint pain, fever	Exanthema or pruritus
Fever	Moderate Very frequent Duration: 5–7 days[a]	Very high very frequent duration: 3–5 days	Mild very infrequent duration: 1–3 days
Rash	Appears between days 5 and 7 Non-characteristic	Appears on day 2 or 3 Non-characteristic	Typically from day 1: maculopapular, cephalocaudal
Pruritus	Mild to intense	Mild to moderate	Moderate to intense
Conjunctivitis	Infrequent	Not very frequent[b]	Very frequent
Neurological manifestations	Infrequent	Infrequent (can be frequent and serious in neonates)	Possible and serious
Headache	Intense and frequent	Mild to moderate	Mild to moderate
Retro-ocular pain	Intense and frequent	Infrequent	Infrequent
Poliartralgias	Absent	Very frequent	Frequent
Polyarthritis	Absent	Frequent	Frequent
Edema in hands and feet	Infrequent	Frequent	Infrequent
Evolution to chronic form	No	Very frequent	Not described
Myalgia	Very frequent and intense	Frequent moderate to intense	Infrequent
Hepatomegaly	Warning sign	Very infrequent	Very infrequent
Frequent vomiting	Warming sign	Very infrequent	Very infrequent
Diarrhea	Frequent	Very infrequent	Very infrequent
Intense abdominal pain	Warming sign	Not present	
Skin bleeding	Frequent	Very infrequent	Very infrequent
Mucosal bleeding	Warning sign	Very infrequent (when present, it is serious)	Very infrequent
Shock	More frequent in the severe form[c]	Infrequent	Unknown
Leukopenia	Moderate to intense	Mild to moderate	Mild to moderate
C-Reactive protein	Normal	Elevated	Elevated
High hematocrit level	Warning sign	Infrequent	Infrequent
Platelet count	Normal to very low	Normal to low	Normal to low
Special considerations	Risk of death	Can evolve to chronic arthropathy	Risk of congenital infection and GBS

[a]With dengue, a drop in fever between days 3 and 5 of the disease can actually be associated with onset of severity

[b]Conjunctivitis is uncommon in CHIKV infection, but this symptom is more frequent in children

[c]The onset of shock is sudden, and it occurs most often between days 3 and 7 of the disease

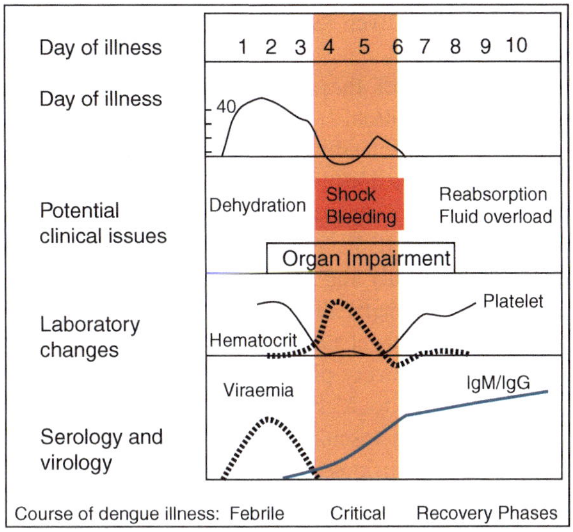

Fig. 32.2 The course of dengue illness. IgM immunoglobulin M, IgG immunoglobulin G. Temperature is given in degrees Celsius (°C). (Source: adapted from Yip, 1980 [2] by authors)

1. Febrile phase (febrile)
2. Critical phase (critical)
3. Recovery phase (recovery)

 1. In the febrile phase, the patient presents a sudden and high fever condition, which can last between 2 and 7 days, associated with the symptoms of cutaneous erythema, facial flushing, myalgia, arthralgia, retroorbital pain, headache, conjunctival injection, sore throat, nausea, and vomiting. Pain and hepatomegaly can be found upon liver palpation [19], as well as petechiae and small hemorrhages in mucous membranes. Major bleeding from venipuncture sites may occur.

    The tourniquet test may have a diagnostic value at this stage, but does not predict severity [20].

    Blood work can show: leukopenia, mild to moderate thrombocytopenia, and moderate elevation of liver enzymes.

    In addition, it can produce alterations in the ability to perform the daily tasks of the person, such as their work, attending school, interpersonal relationships [21].

 2. In the critical phase, it occurs at the time when the fever starts to diminish, typically between day 3 and 7, when the warning signs are manifested, namely, capillary leakage, bleeding, shock, and organic dysfunction can be observed, lasting at least 24–48 hours, being the most affected young patients and children. In this phase in addition to the fall of fever, hypoproteinemia and hemoconcentration with pleural effusions and ascites may also appear.

    In this phase, Dengue Shock Syndrome develops, characterized by a decrease in pulse pressure, hemodynamic collapse, and metabolic acidosis and disseminated intravascular coagulation and organic dysfunction such as hepatitis, liver failure, acute kidney injury, encephalitis, and myocarditis [22–29].

Many of these clinical conditions can improve with appropriate fluid administration.

Severe bleeding may occur in patients without DSS, who have received NSAIDs, aspirin, or corticosteroids. As well as in patients who have previous duodenal or gastric ulcers [30, 31].

APACHE II, SOFA Score, arterial lactate, and serum albumin can predict the mortality and prognosis of a high-risk patient [32, 33].

Fortunately, the majority of patients who develop dengue fever do not develop this phase, evolving to their recovery.

3. In the recovery phase, a gradual redistribution of extravascular fluid occurs within 48 to 72 hours after the end of the critical phase; however, despite improving vascular permeability, patients may persist with dyspnea due to pleural effusions and pulmonary edema due to fluid resuscitation. In addition, a maculopapular rash can be seen by a leukocytoclastic vasculitis; a rash that surrounds areas of normal skin called "isles of white in the sea of red" can be observed [34]. And electrocardiographic changes and bradyarrhythmia.

Laboratory Diagnosis

Dengue's laboratory diagnosis is not necessary for the clinical management of the patient; its usefulness is based on confirming the diagnosis in atypical cases that requires excluding this cause in a differential diagnosis and providing information for epidemiological surveillance.

Dengue's diagnostic laboratory tests are able to detect the virus or any of its components (virus antigen, virus, or virus genome) or by determining a serological response of the patient after infection, such as IgM and IgG levels (Table 32.2) [2].

To choose the best method to use of these diagnostic tools, it is important to consider three important factors:

1. Serological and virological markers in relation to the time of the evolution of dengue infection (Fig. 32.3) [2]
2. Type of diagnostic method in relation to the disease
3. Type of clinical sample (Table 32.3)

When the virus enters the host, the virus replicates, and the individual's immune response occurs; the latter may vary if it is a primary or secondary infection.

Viremia is detected at the same time that symptoms appear and are not detectable at the time of symptom reduction.

When an individual is infected for the first time, that is, he has a primary infection, viremia appears 1–2 days before the fever develops, up to 4–5 days later. IgM antibody develops with the disappearance of fever and viremia [35]; is detected 3–6 days after the onset of fever, detected on average in 50% of cases on days 3–5

Table 32.2 Dengue diagnostics and sample characteristics

	Clinical sample	Diagnostic method	Methodology	Time to results
Virus detection and its components	Acute serum (1–5 days of fever) and necropsy tissues	Viral isolation	Mosquito or mosquito cell culture inoculation	One week or more
		Nucleic acid detection	RT-PCR and real-time RT-PCR	1 or 2 days
		Antigen detection	NS1 Ag rapid tests	Minutes
			NS1 Ag ELISA	1 day
			Immunohistochemistry	2–5 days
Serological response	Paired sera (acute serum from 1–5 days and second serum 15–21 days after)	IgM or IgG seroconversion	ELISA HIA	1–2 days
			Neutralization test	Minimum 7 days
	Serum after day 5 of fever	IgM detection (recent infection)	ELISA	1 or 2 days
			Rapid tests	Minutes
	IgG detection	IgG ELISA HIA	1 or 2 days	

ELISA enzyme-linked immunosorbent assay, *HIA* hemagglutination inhibition assay, *IgG* immunoglobulin G, *IgM* immunoglobulin M, *NS1 Ag* nonstructural protein 1 antigen, *RT-PCR* reverse transcriptase polymerase chain reaction

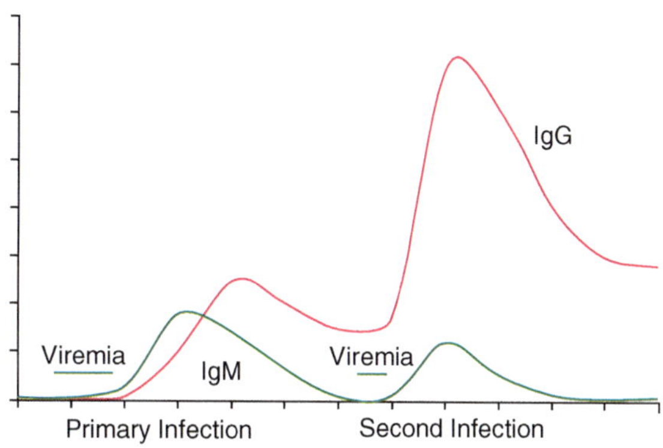

Fig. 32.3 Virological and serological markers of dengue infection according to time of illness. IgG immunoglobulin G, IgM immunoglobulin M

after the onset of the disease; and increases up to 95–98% on days 6–10, and low titers can be detected up to 1–3 months. In addition, in this infection they develop slowly and with low levels of specific anti-dengue IgG, from day 9–10; however, these remain present for decades and indicate a previous dengue infection [11, 36–40].

During a secondary infection, a rapid and high concentration in specific anti-dengue IgG antibodies occurs, with a slow increase and decreased in IgM. High levels of IgG remain high for 30–40 days. In addition, a shorter, but more intense viremia has been recognized in this type of infection [11, 36–40].

Table 32.3 Confirmed and probable dengue diagnosis, interpretation of results, and sample characteristics

	Method	Interpretation	Sample characteristics
Confirmed dengue infection	Viral isolation	Virus isolated	Serum (collected at 1–5 days of fever) necropsy tissues
	Genome detection	Positive RT-PCR or positive real-time RT-PCR	
	Antigen detection	Positive NS1 Ag	
		Positive immunohistochemical	Necropsy tissues
	IgM seroconversion	From negative IgM to positive IgM in paired sera	Acute serum (days 1–5) and convalescent serum (15–21 days after first serum)
	IgG seroconversion	From negative IgG to positive IgG in paired sera or 4-fold increase IgG levels among paired sera	
Probable dengue infection	Positive IgM	Positive IgM	Single serum collected after day 5
	High IgG levels	High IgG levels by ELISA or HI (≥1280)	

ELISA enzyme-linked immunosorbent assay, *IgG* immunoglobulin G, *IgM* immunoglobulin M, *NS1 Ag* nonstructural protein 1 antigen, *RT-PCR* reverse transcriptase-polymerase chain reaction

Confirmation of a dengue diagnosis is confirmed by (Table 32.3) [2]:

1. Virus detection
2. Detection of the viral genome or NS1 antigen
3. Seroconversion of IgM or IgG: from negative to positive IgM/IgG or increase of four times the specific antibody titer

The determination of NS1 antigen, using rapid kits or ELISA (enzyme-linked immunosorbent assay), is important for diagnosis in the first 1–5 days of the disease; its sensitivity in the febrile phase is about 90% and is detected even several days after the patient is afebrile [41].

Detection of viral nucleic acid, using reverse transcriptase-polymerase chain reaction (RT-PCR) is the most sensitive and specific test when used in the first 5 days of fever onset [42].

A positive serology by IgM and a hemagglutination inhibition assay (HIA) antibody titer of 1280 or higher are criteria of a probable infection by dengue.

A compilation of the above is included in Fig. 32.4 [43].

Clinical Management

All patients with dengue should be evaluated systematically and completely, following the following steps (Table 32.4), proposed by the WHO [2].

Step I: Overall assessment:

1. The medical history should include the date of onset of symptoms, the amount of oral fluids ingested, the presence of diarrhea, urinary output, assessment of alarm symptoms, changes in mental status, presence of seizures, or dizziness.

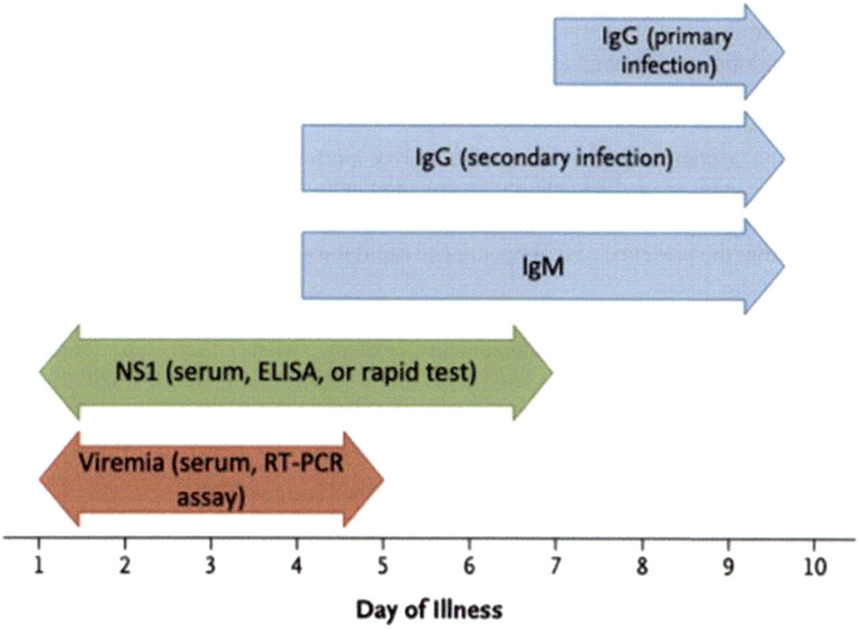

Fig. 32.4 Laboratory diagnostic options in a patient with suspected dengue infection. Detection of viral nucleic acid, nonstructural protein 1 (NS1), or IgM seroconversion is a confirmatory finding in patients in whom dengue is a possible diagnosis. Day 0 is the first day when the patient noted any symptom during this illness. ELISA denotes enzyme-linked immunosorbent assay and RT-PCR reverse transcriptase-polymerase chain reaction

Table 32.4 A stepwise approach to the management of dengue

Step I – Overall assessment	
1.1	History, including symptoms, past medical and family history
1.2	Physical examination, including full physical and mental assessment
1.3	Investigation, including routine laboratory tests and dengue-specific laboratory tests
Step II – Diagnosis, assessment of disease phase and severity	
Step III – Management	
III.1	Disease notification
III.2	Management decisions. Depending on the clinical manifestations and other circumstances, patients may [1]:
	be sent home (Group A)
	be referred for in-hospital management (Group B)
	require emergency treatment and urgent referral (Group C)

Epidemiological data on exposure to dengue of relatives or trips to endemic areas of dengue, comorbidities (pregnancy, chronic diseases, obesity, etc.), or risks to other diseases such as zoonosis, jungle trips, and water exposure (such as malaria, leptospira, etc.) and drug abuse or unprotected sexual exposure (consider acute HIV seroconversion).

2. In the physical examination it is important to evaluate the mental state, the level of hydration and hemodynamic condition; assess for tachypnea, pleural effusion, or acidotic respiration; assess for abdominal pain, hepatomegaly, or ascites; determine if there are rash or hemorrhagic manifestations. Perform the tourniquet test.
3. Ideally, a complete blood count should be performed in the first evaluation, which can be normal and should be repeated daily until the critical phase passes. The hematocrit should be assessed to assess whether there is a capillary leak. In addition, the presence of leukopenia and rapid thrombocytopenia are observed as part of the disease.
   Dengue-specific laboratories are indicated to confirm the diagnosis; they are not required for patient management, except when there are unusual manifestations.
   Other specific tests for the comorbidities that the patient may present in the laboratory and images should be considered.

Step II: Diagnosis, assessment of disease phase, and severity

- With the data obtained in Step I, the clinician is able to diagnose dengue, as well as assess the phase of the disease and its severity.

Step III: Management

1. Disease notification
   This disease must be notified in suspected, probable, or confirmed cases, even before laboratory confirmation, especially in countries in endemic areas.
   In non-endemic areas, it is recommended to report only confirmed cases.
2. Management decisions
   As proposed the management of patients in three groups A, B, and C, depending on their condition and clinical characteristics and with adequate management, mortality can be reduced to less than 1%:

Group A

They are the group of patients that can be managed on an outpatient basis.

These patients can drink fluids properly, have urination at least every 6 hours, and have no warning sign.

Ideally, after the third day of illness should be assessed daily, to determine disease progression.

In addition to oral fluids, paracetamol can be administered, without exceeding 3 grams per day in adults. Any NSAIDs or intramuscular injections should be avoided.

They should consult the hospital, if any of the following situations occur: clinical worsening, deterioration near the time of diminishing of the fever, severe abdominal pain, persistent vomiting, cold and clammy limbs, lethargy, irritability or restlessness, bleeding, dyspnea, and not passing urine for more than 4–6 hours. Admission during the febrile phase is indicated in patients who cannot manage hydration in their home and children and who have coexisting conditions.

Group B
This group includes patients who require hospital management, with close observation.

They are patients with warning signs, with coexisting conditions that make the disease or its management more complicated (pregnant, elderly, obese, diabetic, hypertensive, heart failure, immunosuppressed, etc.) or with patients with circumstances or social problems.

These patients benefit from an early and adequate fluid replacement to prevent progression to shock and modify the course and severity of the disease.

Resuscitation with isotonic saline solutions such as 0.9% saline, Ringer's lactate, or Hartmann solution is recommended.

Using the initial hematocrit as a reference, before replacement with liquids, a replacement from 5 to 7 cc/kg/hour can be used for 1–2 hours until the infusion rate is maintained at 2–3 cc/kg/hour or less depending on of the clinical response. It is of utmost importance the maintenance of perfusion, an adequate water balance, and a urinary output of 0.5 cc/kg/hour.

Fluids are usually not required for more than 24–48 hours, and adequate control of vital signs, perfusion, and urinary output, which should be maintained in patients with alarm signs.

Group C
This group includes patients with severe dengue who require emergency management because they present with:

1. Severe capillary leak leading to shock or accumulation of fluid with respiratory distress
2. Severe hemorrhages
3. Severe organic dysfunction such as kidney injury, liver injury, cardiomyopathy, encephalopathy, or encephalitis.

These patients must be admitted to hospitals with access to a blood bank. Fluid therapy should be adequately managed to maintain adequate central and tissue perfusion (decrease in heart rate, improving blood pressure and pulse pressure, improve capillary filling >2 seconds, with pink and warm limbs), as well as organic perfusion (improve the level of consciousness, decrease metabolic acidosis, urinary output greater than 0.5 cc/kg/hour).

Patients should be managed individually, administering rescue boluses of 10–20 cc/kg. The use of colloids in patients with decompensated shock should be assessed. This hydration can be guided with hematocrit.

Blood transfusion transfusion is performed only in case of severe confirmed or suspected bleeding, especially if there is unexplained arterial hypotension, such as:

1. Persistent or severe bleeding in the presence of hemodynamic instability, regardless of hematocrit level
2. Decreased hematocrit after resuscitation boluses associated with hemodynamic instability

3. Refractory shock that does not respond after the administration of liquids of 40–60 cc/kg
4. Shock with hypotension with an inappropriately low or normal hematocrit
5. Persistent or worsening metabolic acidosis, despite adequate systolic blood pressure, especially with severe abdominal pain and distention

The transfusion of red blood cells or fresh blood should be done early, without using the hemoglobin level criteria. The use of platelets, fresh frozen plasma, and cryoprecipitate; they will be used under the context of mass transfusion.

It is important to clarify that in special situations such as the pregnant patient or patients who require surgery, transfusion of platelets or frozen fresh plasma can be anticipated to the procedure, to avoid severe bleeding.

In cases of shock, WHO proposes the following management algorithms (Figs. 32.5 and 32.6) [2]:

Fluid therapy can result in overhydration as a complication; it must stop under the following proposed conditions:

1. Capillary leak detection
2. Stabilization of blood pressure, pulse, and perfusion
3. Decrease of the hematocrit in the presence of an adequate pulse pressure
4. Afebrile patient, without antipyretics for more than 24–48 hours

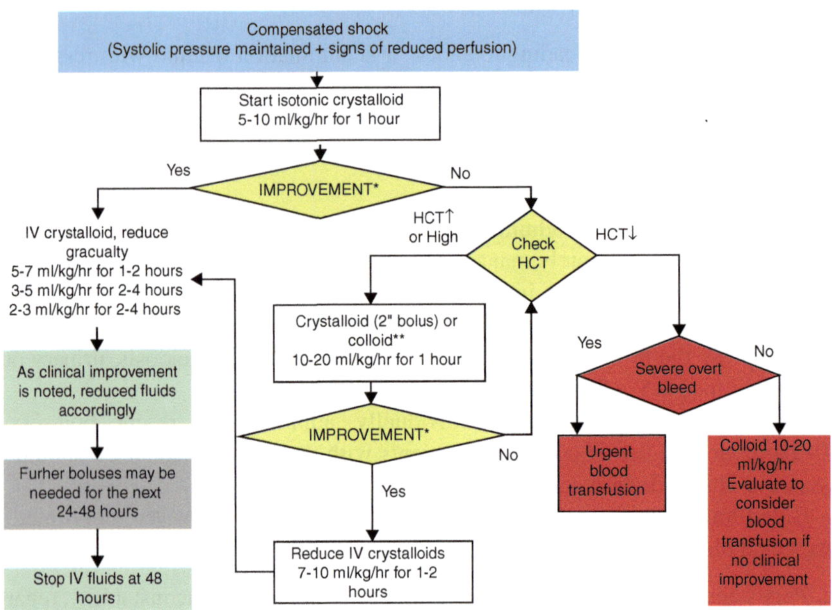

Fig. 32.5 Algorithm for fluid management of compensated shock: in adults. *Reassess the patient's clinical condition, vital signs, pulse volume, capillary refill time, and temperature of extremities. **Colloid is preferable if the patient has already received previous blouses of crystalloid. IV intravenous, HCT hematocrit, ↑ increased, ↓ decreased

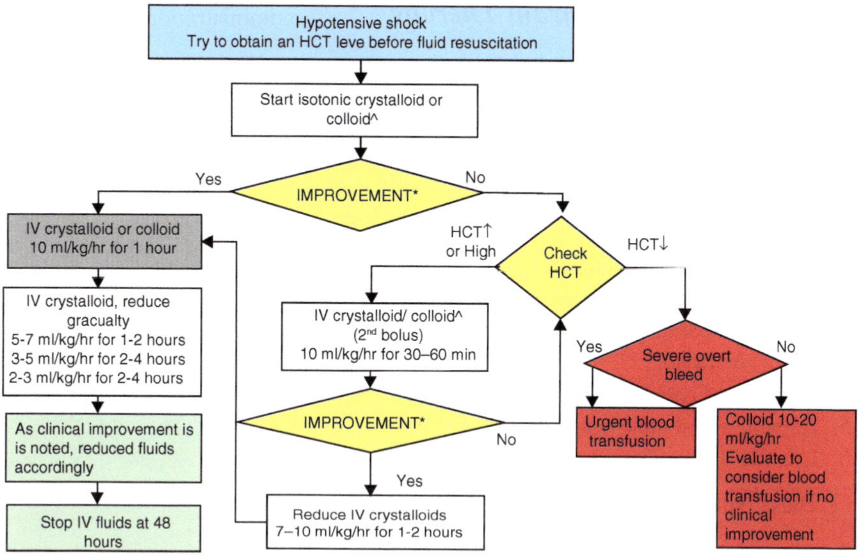

Fig. 32.6 Algorithm for fluid management in hypotensive shock – infants, children, and adults. ^Colloid is preferable if the patient has already received previous blouses of crystalloid. *Reassess the patient's clinical condition, vital signs, pulse volume, capillary refill time, and temperature of extremities. IV intravenous, HCT hematocrit, ↑ increased, ↓ decreased

5. Resolution of abdominal and intestinal symptoms
6. Adequate urinary output

It is also very important to consider the following points in the treatment of these patients:

1. Glucose: hyperglycemia and hypoglycemia may occur, which are corrected with isotonic fluids without glucose and with boluses of dextrose solution 0.1–0.5 g/kg.
2. Hydroelectrolyte and acid/base disbalances: hyponatremia (with a mechanism not fully known) can occur frequently, potassium disorders such as hyperkalemias due to metabolic acidosis or associated renal injury or hypokalemia due to gastrointestinal or stress losses (hypercortisolemia). Calcium should be monitored, especially in the context of massive transfusions or administration of sodium bicarbonate.
3. Metabolic acidosis: it is due to hypovolemia and shock caused by lactic acidosis. An adequate resuscitation of the patient corrects the disorder; however, if it persists, a red blood cell transfusion should be evaluated. The administration of sodium bicarbonate is not recommended if the pH is ≥7.10, since it is related to sodium and liquid overload, increase in lactate and pCO_2, decrease in ionized calcium, and deviation to the left of the dissociation curve of hemoglobin that increases tissue hypoxia.

Hyperchloremia due to resuscitation with saline solutions causes metabolic acidosis with normal lactate levels [44], which can be improved with the use of Ringer's lactate solutions or Hartmann's solution.

Critical Care and Adjuvant Therapy

Patients whom present organic dysfunction due to late diagnosis, inadequate monitoring or interpretation of vital signs, inadequate monitoring of water balance, late recognition of shock or severe bleeding, as well as inadequate resuscitation (little or much administration of liquids) or poor aseptic techniques, which produces complications that require critical care and adjuvant support therapies.

These conditions can be:

1. Prolonged and/or deep shock
2. Severe bleeding with DIC
3. Water overload
4. Failure and respiratory distress
5. Hepatic, renal, and neurological dysfunction
6. Irreversible shock and death

These patients may require:

1. Optimization of fluid therapy
2. Noninvasive or invasive ventilatory support
3. Use of vasopressors and inotropics, according to requirements and hemodynamic profile
4. Blood products
5. Renal support, ideally continuous renal support
6. Treatment of coexisting nosocomial infections
7. Drug toxicity, as in the case of the use of high doses of paracetamol

Medications

Some medications used in this infectious disease have not shown benefit, such is the case of factor VIIa [45], steroids [46–48], and immunoglobulins IV [49, 50].

Other medications that have been used require more research such as:

1. Carbazochrome reduces vascular capillary permeability, but has not shown benefit in dengue [51].
2. Chloroquine, which produces an interference with viral replication in a pH dependent step, does not reduce the duration of the disease and produces many adverse effects [52].
3. Lovastatin does not produce benefits, despite the theoretical benefit of statins in their endothelial anti-inflammatory effects and possible antiviral effects against dengue; it did not affect viremia nor clinical manifestations [53].
4. Some antivirals such as balapiravir and celgosivir showed no benefits [54, 55].

5. Other antivirals, with different mechanisms of action such as MTase inhibitors, nucleoside analogs, helicase inhibitors, protease inhibitors, and NS4B inhibitors, are currently being studied [56].

6. Serum human monoclonal antibodies and polyclonal antibodies (IgG), against all dengue serotypes, are promising treatments under investigation [56].

Dengue in Pregnancy

The clinical manifestations, the treatment and prognosis of pregnant women with Dengue are similar to women who are not; however they have different conditions to consider [57, 58]. There should be a high index of suspicion of this infection in pregnant patients who have traveled or live in endemic areas of dengue, being the most frequent cause of fever in these areas [59].

The diagnosis can be difficult, since it has some findings of diseases that occur in pregnancy such as preeclampsia, eclampsia, HELLP syndrome (hemolysis, elevated liver enzymes, and low platelet count), pneumonia, pulmonary embolism, other infectious diseases, as well as other causes of transvaginal bleeding.

It is still uncertain, the effect of dengue, in the prognosis of pregnancy in terms of preterm births, low birth weight, and caesarean sections [58, 60–63]; in some reports, it has been associated with high maternal and fetal mortality [64], above all, in patients with severe dengue presentations such as DSS/DHS [65]. If the vertical transmission of the virus from the mother to the child is recognized, in the perinatal period in up to 90% of the cases [58, 66–69] and the risk of bleeding in the critical phase [62, 70].

Management of dengue during pregnancy:

- In general terms, these patients should be managed early in the hospital, especially if they are in labor or if they have completed the pregnancy.
- Conservative medical and obstetric management is preferred during dengue infection during pregnancy [66].

There are some changes of the pregnancy to consider and that may affect the recognition of dengue conditions:

1. Hyperemesis gravidarum of the first trimester can be confused with a dengue alarm symptom, which can delay the recognition of a severe dengue.
2. After the second trimester, pregnancy changes such as the increase in circulating volume and heart rate, as well as the decrease in blood pressure and hematocrit; it may delay the diagnosis of decompensated shock. Hence the importance of serial hematocrit control.

3. Signs of capillary leakage of pleural effusion and ascites can be difficult to detect with a gravid uterus.

Regarding the management of these patients, the following should be taken into account:

1. Monitoring and close care are of the utmost importance, with adequate targeted therapy during all phases of care: prepartum, intrapartum, and postpartum.
2. The late recognition of shock in these patients can lead to prolonged shock, massive bleeding, and multiorgan dysfunction.
3. There is no difference in the resuscitation of these patients; however, the gravid uterus can reduce the tolerance of accumulation of fluid in pleurae and peritoneum of the capillary leak, so excess fluid should be avoided.
4. The normal changes at the end of pregnancy of increase in heart rate and decrease in blood pressure can lead to overhydration when trying to normalize these hemodynamic parameters, producing an fluid overload with respiratory worsening.
5. There is an increased risk of bleeding during the critical phase of dengue (thrombocytopenia, coagulopathy, and vasculopathy), in the presence of wounds or trauma [71].
6. Prophylactic platelet transfusion is not indicated, except for some obstetric indication.
7. In case of severe bleeding, transfusion of red blood cells or fresh whole blood should be initiated.
8. The delivery must be done in a hospital with access to the blood bank, with an adequate team of obstetricians and neonatologists.
9. The use of tocolytics and other measures to postpone delivery should be evaluated, especially in the critical phase of dengue.

If labor is inevitable during the critical phase:

1. Bleeding should be anticipated and monitored.
2. Blood products should be reserved for childbirth.
3. The trauma should be reduced during the procedure.
4. Platelet transfusion should be initiated during or at the start of labor, since platelet count is maintained for a few hours with transfusion in the critical phase [72, 73].
5. If significant bleeding occurs, a transfusion of fresh red blood cells or fresh whole blood should be initiated early. Do not wait hematocrit results or blood losses exceeding 500 cc before transfusion.
6. Infusions of ergotamine and oxytocin should be indicated, to produce a uterine contraction that prevents postpartum hemorrhage.

In postpartum, it is recommended:

1. The mother and the newborn should be monitored in the hospital, given the risk of vertical transmission [66, 74].

2. A severe neonatal or fetal dengue may occur and death, at or near birth, due to insufficient time for the formation of protective maternal antibodies.
3. It must be aware that the presentation of dengue in the mother or the newborn can be atypical
4. The congenital infection can be suspected clinically and then confirmed by laboratory tests.

Prevention (Dengue)

Regarding the prevention and control of this infectious disease, there are some strategies such as avoiding contact with the disease vector, vector control, and the development of vaccines.

It is important to bear in mind that at the moment, none of these strategies alone are highly effective, and furthermore, other tools are under development and research.

We can summarize the above as follows:

1. Avoid contact with the vector:

   The World Health Organization [75] establishes measures to avoid or reduce the contact of the vector that transmits dengue among humans. Some of these recommendations are:

   - Avoid visiting endemic areas.
   - Wear clothing that reduces the amount of exposed skin, especially during the day, when mosquitoes are most active, particularly during dengue outbreaks.
   - Use of insect repellants, adhering to the recommended use of the product.
   - Place mosquito nets, ideally treated with insecticides, especially with people who sleep during the day such as infants, bedridden people, and people who work at night.
   - Use of household insecticides or environmental repellants.
   - Placement of metal fabric screens on doors and windows, as well as air conditioning.

2. Vector control:

   These activities focus on the control of the *Ae. aegypti* and *Ae. albopictus*, from their immature stages to adulthood, in the environments in which humans find themselves.

   These controls are based on:

   - Environmental management: attempts to diminish the habitats of the vectors, through the manipulation of containers (destruction, alteration, removal or recycling), the physical or infrastructure transformation, and the placement of barriers that reduce the contact between vectors and people (mosquito nets, racks of metallic screens, etc.). The improvement of the water supply and storage systems, the protection of the water storage containers against mosquitoes, and the management of solid waste are also contemplated, the cleaning of streets and the construction of structures without habitats for these vectors.

- Chemical control: chemicals with effect on larvae and adult mosquitoes action have been used extensively; however, they are complementary measures to environmental control. These measures range from the use of chemicals to control the storage and distribution of water, as well as for fumigation and chemicals with residual effect on surfaces, which control the density and longevity of the mosquitoes, as well as the transmission parameters.
- Biological control: it is based on the introduction of organisms that predate or parasitize mosquitoes, in order to reduce their population. They have developed from autochthonous larvivorous fish such as guppies (*Poecilia reticulata*) or predatory copepods (small crustaceans). As well as the use of a biological larvicide, with *Bacillus thuringiensis israelensis* (Bti), with efficacy in the entomological indices; however, its impact on the transmission of the disease is not clear [76–79].

Other new tools for mosquito control, in which a biological, genetic, and behavioral strategy is mixed, are:

- *Wolbachia* bacteria adapted to infect *A. aegypti* mosquitoes, in adult stage or in eggs, which are subsequently released and which have an impact on decreasing the mosquito's fertility, its life expectancy, and blocking the replication of the dengue virus [80], thereby suppressing the *Aedes* population over a long period of time and reducing the transmission of other infections transmitted by this vector.
- Genetic modifications have been made to the mosquito, with the introduction in male *Aedes* of a gene known as RIDL (Release of Insects Carrying to Dominant Lethal), through which it is transmitted to embryos that experience death in larval stages before being adults. Tests were carried out in Brazil in 2011, in which it has also been considered for the control of Zika [81].

Finally, there is another approach that includes tools based on the behavior of the mosquito, in terms of its appearance, chemical signals, and its swarm, which can synergize different methods, producing a more effective control [82]. For all of the above, it is important to continue with research based on the behavior, ecology, and epidemiology of the vector [83]; in order to obtain programs for the integral management of the vector, which are cost-effective [77, 84].

It is important to clarify that in systematic reviews, there is no clear association between vector indices and dengue transmission [77].

3. Vaccines:

There is been attempts to produce several vaccines for the prevention of dengue, through live attenuated viruses, inactivated viruses, recombinant proteins, and DNA vaccines.

A vaccine against dengue, CYD-TDV or Dengvaxia®, which is a recombinant tetravalent vaccine with live attenuated viruses has been evaluated [85, 86].

The post-use analysis is that the vaccine works dependent on the sero-status of the individual. To those who have had previous dengue infection, that is, they are seropositive, the vaccine is safe and effective. However, for seronegatives, after 3 years of vaccination, the risk of developing severe dengue is increased when the individual develops a natural dengue infection. Therefore, the World Health Organization recommends its application in HIV-positive individuals.

Other vaccines are under investigation [87].

Bibliography

1. Amin P, Acicbe Ö, Hidalgo J, Jiménez JIS, Baker T, Richards GA. Dengue fever: report from the task force on tropical diseases by the World Federation of Societies of Intensive and Critical Care Medicine. J Crit Care. 2018;43:346–51. https://doi.org/10.1016/j.jcrc.2017.11.003.
2. WHO/TDR. Handbook for clinical management of dengue. 2012. http://www.who.int/tdr/publications/handbook_dengue/en/.
3. Gubler DJ. The global emergence/resurgence of arboviral diseases as public health problems. Arch Med Res. 2002;33(4):330–42.
4. Brady OJ, Gething PW, Bhatt S, Messina JP, Brownstein JS, Hoen AG, et al. Refining the global spatial limits of dengue virus transmission by evidence-based consensus. PLoS Negl Trop Dis. 2012;6(8):e1760.
5. Senior K. Dengue fever: what hope for control? Lancet Infect Dis. 2007;7(10):636.
6. WHO. Dengue y Dengue Severo. 2019. https://www.who.int/es/news-room/fact-sheets/detail/dengue-and-severe-dengue.
7. Guzman MG, Kouri G. Dengue: an update. Lancet Infect Dis. 2002;2(1):33–42.
8. Leong AS, Wong KT, Leong TY, Tan PH, Wannakrairot P. The pathology of dengue hemorrhagic fever. Semin Diagn Pathol. 2007;24(4):227–36.
9. Pang T, Cardosa MJ, Guzman MG. Of cascades and perfect storms: the immunopathogenesis of dengue haemorrhagic fever-dengue shock syndrome (DHF/DSS). Immunol Cell Biol. 2007;85(1):43–5.
10. Malavige GN, Ogg GS. Pathogenesis of vascular leak in dengue virus infection. Immunology. 2017;151(3):261–9.
11. Dengue. Guidelines for diagnosis, treatment prevention and control. Geneva: World Health Organization; 2009, WHO/HTM/NTD/DEN/2009.
12. Srikiatkhachorn A, Rothman AL, Gibbons RV, Sittisombut N, Malasit P, Ennis FA, et al. Dengue--how best to classify it. Clin Infect Dis. 2011;53(6):563–7.
13. Guzman MG, Kouri G, Bravo J, Valdes L, Vazquez S, Halstead SB. Effect of age on outcome of secondary dengue 2 infections. Int J Infect Dis. 2002;6(2):118–24.
14. Bravo JR, Guzman MG, Kouri GP. Why dengue haemorrhagic fever in Cuba? Individual risk factors for dengue haemorrhagic fever/dengue shock syndrome (DHF/DSS). Trans R Soc Trop Med Hyg. 1987;81(5):816–20.
15. Guzman MG, Kouri GP, Bravo J, Soler M, Vazquez S, Morier L. Dengue hemorrhagic fever in Cuba, 1981: a retrospective seroepidemiologic study. Am J Trop Med Hyg. 1990;42(2):179–84.
16. Loke H, Bethell DB, Phuong CX, Dung M, Schneider J, White NJ, et al. Strong HLA classI--restricted T cell responses in dengue hemorrhagic fever: a double-edged sword? J Infect Dis. 2001;184(11):1369–73.
17. Gubler DJ. Dengue and dengue hemorrhagic fever. Clin Microbiol Rev. 1998;11(3):480–96.
18. Pan American Health Organization/WHO. Tool for the diagnosis and care of patients with suspected arboviral diseases. 2017. http://iris.paho.org/xmlui/bitstream/handle/123456789/33895/9789275119365_eng.pdf?sequence=1&isAllowed=y.

19. Kalayanarooj S, Vaughn DW, Nimmannitya S, Green S, Suntayakorn S, Kunentrasai N, et al. Early clinical and laboratory indicators of acute dengue illness. J Infect Dis. 1997;176(2):313–21.
20. Cao XT, Ngo TN, Wills B, Kneen R, Nguyen TT, Ta TT, et al. Evaluation of the World Health Organization standard tourniquet test and a modified tourniquet test in the diagnosis of dengue infection in Viet Nam. Tropical Med Int Health. 2002;7(2):125–32.
21. Lum LCS, et al. Quality of life of dengue patients. Am J Trop Med Hyg. 2008;78(6):862–7.
22. Wills BA, Oragui EE, Stephens AC, Daramola OA, Dung NM, Loan HT, et al. Coagulation abnormalities in dengue hemorrhagic fever: serial investigations in 167 Vietnamese children with dengue shock syndrome. Clin Infect Dis. 2002;35(3):277–85.
23. Mairuhu AT, Mac Gillavry MR, Setiati TE, Soemantri A, ten Cate H, Brandjes DP, et al. Is clinical outcome of dengue-virus infections influenced by coagulation and fibrinolysis? A critical review of the evidence. Lancet Infect Dis. 2003;3(1):33–41.
24. Lum LC, et al. Fulminant hepatitis in dengue infection. Southeast Asian J Trop Med Public Health. 1993;24(3):467–71.
25. Nguyen TL, Nguyen TH, Tieu NT. The impact of dengue haemorrhagic fever on liver function. Res Virol. 1997;148(4):273–7.
26. Poovorawan Y, et al. Dengue virus infection: a major cause of acute hepatic failure in Thai children. Ann Trop Paediatr. 2006;26(1):17–23.
27. Ooi ET, et al. Gastrointestinal manifestations of dengue infection in adults. Med J Malays. 2008;63(5):401–5.
28. Kumar R, et al. Prevalence of dengue infection in north Indian children with acute hepatic failure. Ann Hepatol. 2008;7(1):59–62.
29. Trung DT, et al. Liver involvement associated with dengue infection in adults in Vietnam. Am J Trop Med Hyg. 2010;83(4):774–80.
30. Tsai CJ, et al. Upper gastrointestinal bleeding in dengue fever. Am J Gastroenterol. 1991;86(1):33–5.
31. Chiu YC, et al. Endoscopic findings and management of dengue patients with upper gastrointestinalbleeding. Am J Trop Med Hyg. 2005;73(2):441–4.
32. Juneja D, Nasa P, Singh O, Javeri Y, Uniyal B, Dang R. Clinical profile, intensive care unit course, and outcome of patients admitted in intensive care unit with dengue. J Crit Care. 2011;26(5):449–52.
33. Jog S, Prayag S, Rajhans P, Zirpe K, Dixit S, Pillai L, et al. Dengue infection with multiorgan dysfunction: SOFA score, arterial lactate and serum albumin levels are predictors of outcome. Intensive Care Med. 2015;41(11):2029–30.
34. Nimmannitya S. Clinical spectrum and management of dengue haemorrhagic fever. Southeast Asian J Trop Med Public Health. 1987;18(3):392–7.
35. Vaughn DW, et al. Dengue viremia titer, antibody response pattern, and virus serotype correlate with disease severity. J Infect Dis. 2000;181:2–9.
36. Guzman MG, Rosario D, Kouri G. Diagnosis of dengue virus infection. In: Kalitzky M, Borowski P, editors. Molecular biology of the flaviviruses. Wymondham: Horizon Bioscience; 2009.
37. Buchy F, et al. Laboratory tests for the diagnosis of dengue virus infection. Geneva, TDR/Scientific Working Group, 2006. TDR/SWG/08.
38. Guzman MG, Kouri G. Dengue diagnosis, advances and challenges. Int J Infect Dis. 2004;8:69–80.
39. Pan American Health Organization. Dengue and dengue hemorrhagic fever in the Americas: guidelines for prevention and control. Washington, DC: Pan American Health Organization; 1994: 548.
40. Vazquez S, et al. Kinetics of antibodies in sera, saliva, and urine samples from adult patients with primary or secondary dengue 3 virus infections. Int J Infect Dis. 2007;11:256–62.

41. Chaterji S, Allen JC Jr, Chow A, Leo YS, Ooi EE. Evaluation of the NS1 rapid test and the WHO dengue classification schemes for use as bedside diagnosis of acute dengue fever in adults. Am J Trop Med Hyg. 2011;84(2):224–8.
42. Dussart P, Petit L, Labeau B, Bremand L, Leduc A, Moua D, et al. Evaluation of two new commercial tests for the diagnosis of acute dengue virus infection using NS1 antigen detection in human serum. PLoS Negl Trop Dis. 2008;2(8):e280.
43. Simmons C, Farrar J, Vinh Chau N, Wills B. Dengue. N Engl J Med. 2012;366:1423–32.
44. Burdett E, Roche AM, Mythen MG. Hyperchloremic acidosis: pathophysiology and clinical impact. Transfus Altern Transfus Med. 2003;5(4):424–30.
45. Chuansumrit A, Wangruangsatid S, Lektrakul Y, Chua MN, Zeta Capeding MR, Bech OM, et al. Control of bleeding in children with dengue hemorrhagic fever using recombinant activated factor VII: a randomized, double-blind, placebo-controlled study. Blood Coagul Fibrinolysis. 2005;16(8):549–55.
46. Sumarmo D, Talogo W, Asrin A, Isnuhandojo B, Sahudi A. Failure of hydrocortisone to affect outcome in dengue shock syndrome. Pediatrics. 1982;69(1):45–9.
47. Panpanich R, Sornchai P, Kanjanaratanakorn K. Corticosteroids for treating dengue shock syndrome. Cochrane Database Syst Rev. 2006;(3):CD003488.
48. Tam DT, Ngoc TV, Tien NT, Kieu NT, Thuy TT, Thanh LT, et al. Effects of short-course oral corticosteroid therapy in early dengue infection in Vietnamese patients: a randomized, placebo-controlled trial. Clin Infect Dis. 2012;55(9):1216–24.
49. Ostronoff M, Ostronoff F, Florencio R, Florencio M, Domingues MC, Calixto R, et al. Serious thrombocytopenia due to dengue hemorrhagic fever treated with high dosages of immunoglobulin. Clin Infect Dis. 2003;36(12):1623–4.
50. Dimaano EM, Saito M, Honda S, Miranda EA, Alonzo MT, Valerio MD, et al. Lack of efficacy of high-dose intravenous immunoglobulin treatment of severe thrombocytopenia in patients with secondary dengue virus infection. Am J Trop Med Hyg. 2007;77(6):1135–8.
51. Tassniyom S, Vasanawathana S, Dhiensiri T, Nisalak A, Chirawatkul A. Failure of carbazochrome sodium sulfonate (AC-17) to prevent dengue vascular permeability or shock: a randomized, controlled trial. J Pediatr. 1997;131(4):525–8.
52. Tricou V, Minh NN, Van TP, Lee SJ, Farrar J, Wills B, et al. A randomized controlled trial of chloroquine for the treatment of dengue in Vietnamese adults. PLoS Negl Trop Dis. 2010;4(8):e785.
53. Whitehorn J, Nguyen CVV, Khanh LP, Kien DTH, Quyen NTH, Tran NTT, et al. Lovastatin for the treatment of adult patients with dengue: a randomized, double-blind, placebo-controlled trial. Clin Infect Dis. 2016;62(4):468–76.
54. Nguyen NM, Tran CN, Phung LK, Duong KT, Huynh Hle A, Farrar J, et al. A randomized, double-blind placebo controlled trial of balapiravir, a polymerase inhibitor, in adult dengue patients. J Infect Dis. 2013;207(9):1442–50.
55. Kaptein SJ, Neyts J. Towards antiviral therapies for treating dengue virus infections. Curr Opin Pharmacol. 2016;30:1–7.
56. Chan CY, Ooi EE. Dengue: an update on treatment options. Future Microbiol. 2015;10(12):2017–31.
57. Waduge R, et al. Dengue infections during pregnancy: a case series from Sri Lanka and review of literature. J Clin Virol. 2006;37(1):27–33.
58. Tan PC, et al. Dengue infection in pregnancy: prevalence, vertical transmission, and pregnancy outcome. Obstet Gynecol. 2008;111(5):1111–7.
59. Chansamouth V, et al. The aetiologies and impact of fever in pregnant inpatients in Vientiane, Laos. PLoS Negl Trop Dis. 2016. https://doi.org/10.1371/journal.pntd.0004577.
60. Carles G, et al. Dengue fever in pregnancy. A study of 38 cases in French Guiana. Eur J Obstet Gynecol Reprod Biol (Paris). 2000;29(8):758–62.

61. Seneviratne SL, Perera J, Wijeyaratne C. Dengue infections and pregnancy: caution in interpreting high rates of premature deliveries and maternal mortality. Southeast Asian J Trop Med Public Health. 2007;38(1):195–6.
62. Basurko C, et al. Maternal and fetal consequences of dengue fever during pregnancy. Eur J Obstet Gynecol Reprod Biol. 2009;147(1):29–32.
63. Pouliot SH, et al. Maternal dengue and pregnancy outcomes: a systematic review. Obstet Gynecol Surv. 2010;65(2):107–18.
64. Sharma S, Jain S, Rajaram S. Spectrum of maternofetal outcomes during dengue infection in pregnancy: an insight. Infect Dis Obstet Gynecol. 2016;2016:Article ID 5046091.
65. Agarwal K, Malik S, Mittal P. A retrospective analysis of the symptoms and course of dengue infection during pregnancy. Int J Gynaecol Obstet. 2017;139(1):4–8.
66. Sirinavin S, et al. Vertical dengue infection: case reports and review. Paediatr Infect Dis J. 2004;23(11):1042–7.
67. Kerdpanich A, et al. Perinatal dengue infection. Southeast Asian J Trop Med Public Health. 2001;32(3):488–93.
68. Fernandez R, et al. Study of the relationship dengue-pregnancy in a group of Cuban-mothers. Rev Cubana Med Trop. 1994;46:76–8.
69. Arragain L, et al. Vertical transmission of dengue virus in the peripartum period and viral kinetics in newborns and breast milk: new data. J Pediatr Infect Dis Soc. 2017;6(4):324–31.
70. Thaithumyanon P, et al. Dengue infection complicated by severe hemorrhage and vertical transmission in a parturient woman. Clin Infect Dis. 1994;18(2):248–9.
71. Carroll ID, Toovey S, Van Gompel A. Dengue fever and pregnancy – a review and comment. Travel Med Infect Dis. 2007;5:183–8.
72. Hashmi M, Zainab G, Khan F. Anticipated and unanticipated complications of severe dengue in a primigravida. Indian J Crit Care Med. 2015;19:678–80.
73. Dat T, et al. Dengue fever during pregnancy. Nagoya J Med Sci. 2018 May;80(2):241–7.
74. Perret C, et al. Dengue infection during pregnancy and transplacental antibody transfer in Thai mothers. J Infect. 2005;51(4):287–93.
75. https://www.who.int/denguecontrol/control_strategies/es/.
76. Bowman LR, Runge-Ranzinger S, McCall PJ. Assessing the relationship between vector indices and dengue transmission: a systematic review of the evidence. PLoS Negl Trop Dis. 2014;8:e2848.
77. Horstick O, Runge-Ranzinger S, Nathan MB, Kroeger A. Dengue vector-control services: how do they work? A systematic literature review and country case studies. Trans R Soc Trop Med Hyg. 2010;104:379–86.
78. Tan AW, Loke SR, Benjamin S, Lee HL, Chooi KH, Sofian-Azirun M. Spray application of Bacillus thuringiensis israelensis (Bti strain AM65-52) against Aedes aegypti (L) and Ae albopictus Skuse populations and impact on dengue transmission in a dengue endemic residential site in Malaysia. Southeast Asian J Trop Med Public Health. 2012;43:296–310.
79. Boyce R, Lenhart A, Kroeger A, Velayudhan R, Roberts B, Horstick O. Bacillus thuringiensis israelensis (Bti) for the control of dengue vectors: systematic literature review. Tropical Med Int Health. 2013;18:564–77.
80. Hoffmann AA, Montgomery BL, Popovici J, et al. Successful establishment of wolbachia in Aedes populations to suppress dengue transmission. Nature. 2011;476:454–7.
81. Carvalho DO, McKemey AR, Garziera L, et al. Suppression of a field population of Aedes aegypti in Brazil by sustained release of transgenic male mosquitoes. PLoS Negl Trop Dis. 2015;9:e0003864.
82. Benelli G, Mehlhorn H. Declining malaria, rising of dengue and Zika virus: insights for mosquito vector control. Parasitol Res. 2016;115:1747–54.
83. Paul R, Sousa C, Sakuntabhai A, Devine G. Mosquito control might not bolster imperfect dengue vaccines. Lancet. 2014;384:1747–8.

84. WHO. Dengue: guidelines for diagnosis, treatment, prevention, and control. France: World Health Organization; 2009.
85. L'Azou M, Moureau A, Sarti E, Nealon J, Zambrano B, Wartel TA, et al. Symptomatic dengue in children in 10 Asian and Latin American countries. N Engl J Med. 2016;374(12):1155–66.
86. Capeding MR, Tran NH, Hadinegoro SR, Ismail HI, Chotpitayasunondh T, Chua MN, et al. Clinical efficacy and safety of a novel tetravalent dengue vaccine in healthy children in Asia: a phase 3, randomised, observer-masked, placebo-controlled trial. Lancet. 2014;384(9951):1358–65.
87. Wilder-Smith A. Dengue vaccine development: status and future. Bundesgesundheitsblatt Gesundheitsforschung Gesundheitsschutz. 2020;63(1):40–4.

Chapter 33
Rickettsiosis in Pregnant Women

Juan Ignacio Silesky-Jiménez and Jorge Hidalgo

Introduction

Rickettsia is an infectious disease caused by small gram-negative microorganisms, obligated intracellular bacilli, transmitted to humans by hematophagous arthropod vectors such as ticks, lice, mites, and fleas [1, 2].

Due to their high prevalence in nature and that they have a large worldwide distribution, both in tropical and subtropical areas, they are a potential cause of emerging and re-emerging febrile illness, which unfortunately produces a febrile condition that is not differentiated with other diseases and that in many occasions is overlooked. This feverish picture can sometimes be accompanied with rash and eschar [3, 4].

The difficulty for the recognition of this infectious disease is very large, because a confirmatory test is not available during the acute phase of the disease and its diagnosis is usually confirmed, retrospectively by serological means.

The recognition of this infectious disease is important and at the beginning of the specific treatment is associated with a rapid clinical improvement and also with a decrease in mortality in severe cases [5, 6].

J. I. Silesky-Jiménez (✉)
Critical Care Medicine, Clinical Nutrition, Health Services Administration, Hospital San Juan de Dios and Hospital CIMA, San José, Costa Rica

Costa Rica University, San José, Costa Rica

AMICOR and COCECATI, San José, Costa Rica

J. Hidalgo
Division of Critical Care, Karl Heusner Memorial Hospital, Belize City, Belize

C. Montufar et al. (eds.), *Obstetric Catastrophes*,
https://doi.org/10.1007/978-3-030-70034-8_33

Etiology

This infectious disease is caused by bacteria of the genus *Rickettsia*, which, as mentioned, are obligated intracellular gram-negative bacilli, which have been classified into four categories, according to their genetic characteristics:

1. Spotted fever group (SFG) rickettsiae: this group corresponds to the *Rickettsia rickettsii*, the cause of the Rocky Mountain spotted fever, which is responsible for one of the most severe and well-known presentations in North America, as well as others, such is the case of *Rickettsia africae* that produces the African tick bite fever in sub-Sahara Africa and *Rickettsia conorii*, which produces the Mediterranean spotted fever in Europe and North Africa. This group is currently responsible for at least 15 diseases.
2. Typhus group rickettsiae, this group includes *Rickettsia prowazekii* and *Rickettsia typhi*.
3. Ancestral group includes *Rickettsia bellii* and *Rickettsia canadensis*.
4. Transitional group, named because it consists of members with genetic characteristics between the SFG and typhus group. In this group are *Rickettsia akari*, *Rickettsia australis*, and *Rickettsia felis* [7–11].

The List of Prokaryotic Names with Standing in Nomenclature [12] contains 27 species of *Rickettsia*, and of which 17 more are capable of producing infections in humans (Table 33.1) [4]. However, some *Rickettsia*, such as *R. peacockii* and *R. buchneri*, are symbiotic bacteria from ticks and have little capacity to cause infections in humans; on the other hand, others such as *R. parkeri*, *R. slovaca*, and *R. massilliae* were considered nonpathogenic to humans in the past and are now known to cause human infections. There are other isolated *Rickettsia* such as *R. amblyommatis* and R. philipii, which are associated with human infections [13–20].

Epidemiology

Rickettsia is an infection transmitted by ticks, lice, and fleas; hence, in many cases, humans are accidental guests.

The clinical picture will depend on the region in which the patient is, the type of vector, and the mechanism in which the disease is transmitted. Hence, it is that rickettsial infection is more common during the warmer months and people are exposed or do outdoor activities; as is the case, for example, of the *Dermacentor variabilis* (American dog tick), *Dermacentor andersoni* (Rocky Mountain wood tick), and Amblyomma americanum (lone star tick) that have been associated in many cases of Rocky Mountain spotted fever in the United States; *Amblyomma cajennense*, associated with spotted fever in South America; and *Amblyomma hebraeum* or *Amblyomma variegatum* in South Africa. Other pictures are related to poor hygiene

Table 33.1 Named organisms of the genus *Rickettsia* and rickettsial diseases

Organism	Group	Disease
Rickettsia rickettsii	SFG	Rocky Mountain spotted fever
Rickettsia prowazekii	Typhus	Epidemic louse-borne typhus
Rickettsia conorii	SFG	Mediterranean spotted fever
Rickettsia typhi	Typhus	Murine typhus
Rickettsia sibirica	SFG	Siberian tick typhus
Rickettsia australis	Transitional	Queensland tick typhus
Rickettsia akari	Transitional	Rickettsialpox
Rickettsia slovaca	SFG	Tick-borne lymphadenopathy
Rickettsia parkeri	SFG	Maculatum disease
Rickettsia japonica	SFG	Japanese spotted fever
Rickettsia honei	SFG	Flinders Island spotted fever
Rickettsia africae	SFG	African tick bite fever
Rickettsia massiliae	SFG	Unnamed spotted fever
Rickettsia aeschlimannii	SFG	Unnamed
Rickettsia heilongjiangensis	SFG	Far Eastern spotted fever
Rickettsia monacensis	SFG	Unarmed
Rickettsia helvetica	SFG	Unnamed
Rickettsia felis	Transitional	Flea-borne spotted fever
Rickettsia raoultii	SFG	
Rickettsia asiatica	SFG	
Rickettsia bellii	Ancestral	
Rickettsia buchneri	SFG	
Rickettsia canadensis	Ancestral	
Rickettsia hoogstraalii	Transitional	
Rickettsia montanensis	SFG	
Rickettsia peacockii	SFG	
Rickettsia rhipicephali	SFG	
Rickettsia tamurae	SFG	
Rickettsia amblyommatis	SFG	Unnamed

Abbreviation: SFG spotted fever group

conditions such as epidemic typhus, *R. prowazekii* transmitted by body lice, and murine typhus caused by *R. typhi* caused by flea bites in tropical and subtropical areas [21–24].

In the following figure (Fig. 33.1), the distribution of the most frequent Rickettsia infections is summarized, as well as the syndrome that causes and the vector or vectors involved in its transmission [25].

Table 33.2 [4] shows the heterogeneity of this infectious disease, since there is a lot of diversity in terms of severity, known name of the disease, distribution, the causative vector, and the clinical presentation of it.

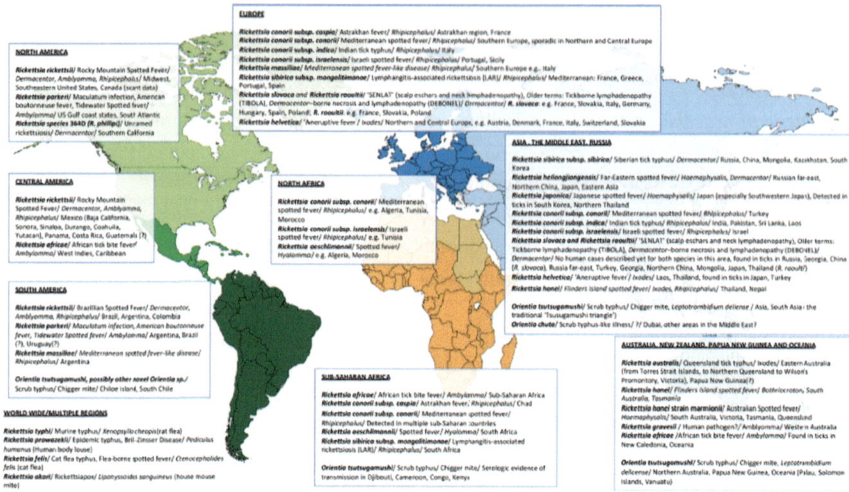

Fig. 33.1 Major rickettsioses described by causative agent, clinical syndrome, and vector by region. (From Refs. [2, 14–16, 29, 64], and the CDC Yellow Book (https://wwwnc.cdc.gov/travel/yellowbook/2018/infectious-diseases-related-to-travel/rickettsial-spotted-and-typhus-fevers-and-related-infections-including-anaplasmosis-and-ehrlichiosis). The map was created using mapchart.net

Transmission and Pathophysiology

The transmission of this disease to the host requires of a vector. The mechanism of transmission will depend on the type of vector and the species of *Rickettsia*.

Four mechanisms for the transmission of this disease have been described:

1. Transmission by saliva during the bite and feeding of ticks and mites, the cabbage is the most frequent mechanism in the rickettsias SFG.
2. Transmission by entry of fecal material into bite sites and cuts in the skin of the host. This mechanism is characteristic of the flea- and louse-borne rickettsiae [26].
3. TG rickettsiae can cause infection by inhalation via aerosolization or contamination of dust particles in the air [27].
4. Finally, a rare route of inoculation is through the conjunctiva, through exposure of contaminated tick hemolymph on fingers from crushed ticks [26].

Rickettsia after entering the host organism has a rapid entry of the organisms into the cell and the downregulation of immune pathways allowing for persistence of infection. At the site of inoculation, a localized rickettsial infection, manifested by an eschar ("tache noir"), where a greater inflammatory reaction to achieve local control of the infection, can be observed [28] (Fig. 33.2) [1].

Table 33.2 Clinical and epidemiologic features of rickettsial diseases

Severity	Disease	Organism	Distribution	Vector	Rash (%)	Eschar (%)
+++++	Rocky Mountain spotted fever	*R rickettsii*	Americas	Tick	90	<1
++++	Typhus	*R prowazekii*	South America, Africa, Eurasia	Body louse, ectoparasites of flying squirrels	80	None
+++	Mediterranean spotted fever	*R conorii*	Europe, Africa, Asia	Tick	97	50
+++	Murine typhus	*R typhi*	Worldwide	Flea	60	None
++	Siberian tick typhus	*R sibirica*	Eurasia, Africa	Tick	95	100
++	Japanese spotted fever	*R japonica*	Japan, eastern Asia	Tick	100	94
++	Flinders Island spotted fever	*R honei*	Australia, Asia	Tick	76	42
++	Far Eastern spotted fever	*R heilongjiangensis*	Eastern Asia	Tick	92	92
++	Queensland tick typhus	*R australis*	Eastern Australia	Tick	95	65
++	African tick bite fever	*R africae*	Sub-Saharan Africa	Tick	50	90
++	Maculatum disease	*R parkeri*	Americas	Tick	88	94
++	Rickettsialpox	*R akari*	North America, Eurasia	Mouse mite	100	90
+[a]	Flea-borne spotted fever	*R felis*	Worldwide	Flea	75	13
+	Tick-borne lymphadenopathy	*R slovaca*	Europe, Asia	Tick	5	100
+[b]	Unnamed spotted fever	*R massiliae*	South America, Europe	Tick	75	75
+[b]	Unnamed spotted fever	*Candidatus R* philipii	United States	Tick	14	100
+[b]	Unnamed spotted fever	*R aeschlimannii*	Africa	Tick	80	60
+[b]	Unnamed spotted fever	*R monacensis*	Europe	Tick	67	33
+[b,c]	Unnamed spotted fever	*R helvetica*	Europe	Tick	None	13
+/−[c]	Asymptomatic or mild illness with seroconversion	*R amblyommatis*	Americas	Tick	Probably few	None

[a]*R felis* has been identified from blood, eschar, and cerebrospinal fluid specimens by polymer as a chain reaction in patients with febrile illness, but the detection of *R felis* DNA from the blood and skin of asymptomatic humans causes some ambiguity with regard to its pathogenic nature
[b]Clinical data based on a limited number of patients reported in the literature
[c]Implicated as a cause of asymptomatic infection or self-limited illness with subsequent seroconversion

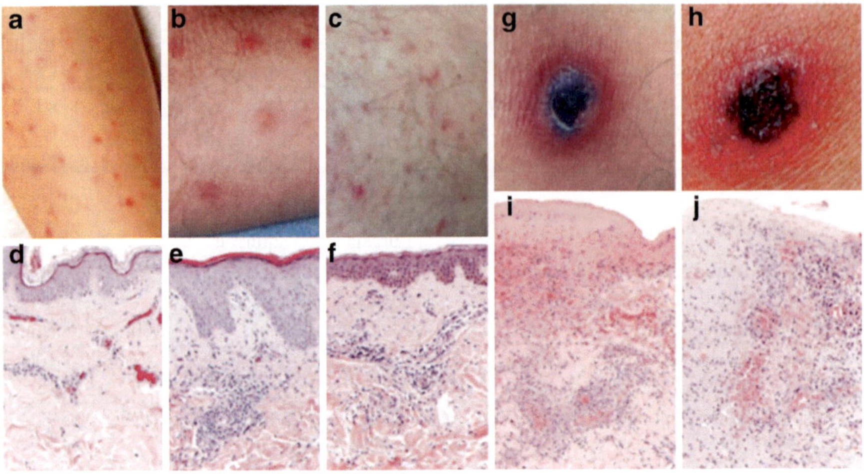

Fig. 33.2 Maculopapular rashes caused by spotted fever group rickettsias (SFGR) are clinically and histologically identical with prominent perivascular mononuclear infiltrates. Likewise, the eschars produced by SFGR are both clinically and histologically identical, featuring mononuclear perivascular infiltrates in the deep dermis and microvascular fibrin thrombi-induced ischemic necrosis of superficial dermis with loss of epidermis. *R. rickettsii* (**a** and **d**), *R. parkeri* (**b** and **e**, **h** and **j**), *R. akari* (**c** and **f**, **g** and **i**), Photomicrographs: hematoxylin and eosin, 25×. (Image adapted from Denison et al. [58])

This infection produces in the vascular endothelium of the small and medium vessels of the organism, a disseminated inflammation, with loss of the barrier function and alteration in vascular permeability. This increase in vascular permeability is related to bacterial load and tumor necrosis factor, which produce disruptions of endothelial cell junctions [29, 30]. Vasculitis, and the endothelial damage produced, produces the clinical manifestations of fever, myalgia, symptoms in the central nervous system such as headache and confusion, rash and cardiovascular instability, cutaneous necrosis, digital gangrene, pneumonitis, meningoencephalitis, and multiorgan failure, which can cause death. A case of antineutrophil cytoplasmic autoantibody (ANCA)-positive vasculitis associated with Rocky Mountain spotted fever (RMSF) has been described [31].

Clinical Evaluation

Classically, patients have a triad of fever, headache, and a petechial or macular rash within 4–10 days after exposure to vectors, usually by bites of fleas or ticks. However, it is important to remember that patients may have flu-like symptoms in the summer months, where the possibility of contact between the host and the vector increases, since exposure to the latter may be brief or unnoticed by the patient, so it is very important to maintain a high index of suspicion.

Symptoms may include lymphadenopathy, changes at the level of the central nervous system such as confusion or nuchal stiffness, hearing at the inoculation site, myalgias, arthralgias, hepatitis, vomiting, and cardiovascular instability.

Although the classical triad is consistent with rickettsial species, the specific etiology must be defined according to the specific symptoms and geography where the exposure occurred. A detailed history about travel and outdoor exposure is important.

It is of interest that depending on the category of *Rickettsia*, the manifestations and severity of the disease can vary:

1. Spotted Fever Group Rickettsioses (SFG rickettsiae):

   This category has a broad presentation spectrum, from a disease with mild manifestations such as the case of *R. slovaca* to fatal cases such as those caused by *R. rickettsii* [32, 33]. In this group it is known for the seroconversion of patients, with very mild symptoms and even without them, in such a way that this infection can simulate other infections especially in tropical areas where other infections are prevalent [34].

   Prominent symptoms include fever, headache, and myalgia. In addition, patients may experience nausea, vomiting, and abdominal pain, despite not being a gastrointestinal disease. The presence of rash is variable, being very frequent between 90 and 97% in RMSF and MSF, 46% in ATBF, and only 2% in TIBOLA [32, 35–38], which is usually macular or maculopapular; however it can vary, for example, in RMSF the rash can start on the wrists and ankles before the trunk or start on the trunk or be diffuse. The involvement of palms of the hands and feet is considered as characteristic of the RMSF. In ATBF the rash is papulovesicular and papulopustular.

   It is also characteristic in the skin, the formation of the inoculation eschar or tache noir, which is observed in 95% in ATBF and in 72% in the MSF [35, 38].

   Lymphadenopathy is observed in 27% of the RMSF; in other less severe diseases the nodal involvement can be observed in the drainage nodules of the eschar inoculation area.

   In the case of TIBOLA, the clinical picture is less severe, and they even have asymptomatic seroconversion, with local symptoms such as eschar, with 100% local lymphadenopathy, with alopecia around the eschar and asthenia, with few constitutional symptoms [15, 39].

   In severe cases such as RMSF, mortality has been reported between 4% and 30% in Mexico, and 40% have been reported in Brazil; the MSF is 2.5% [29, 33, 40].

   In these cases, multiorgan compromise may occur manifested by:

   (a) Lung compromise manifested by cough, dyspnea, and respiratory failure, which requires mechanical ventilation
   (b) Acute renal injury due to prerenal azotemia that can cause acute tubular necrosis, requiring renal support
   (c) Neurological commitment, which can occur with delirium, coma, stupor, and seizures
   (d) Gangrene in limbs or fingers

The risk factors for severe manifestations are glucose-6-phosphate dehydrogenase deficiency, alcoholism, older age, and use of sulfonamide antibiotics.

2. Typhus Group Rickettsioses:

   The typical clinical manifestations of this group are the appearance of sudden fever, accompanied by myalgia and headache. They present rash in variable incidence, and it has also been described to listen in this group, although the latter is not recognized as a manifestation of the typhus group rickettsioses [41–43]. About half of the patients develop nausea and vomiting [41, 42].

   Louse-borne typhus is the most severe manifestation, associated with neurological symptoms such as delirium, seizures, stupor, and coma, with a mortality between 13% and 50% [41]. Murine typhus has a mortality of 0.4–4%; the latter mortality is observed in severe cases that are not hospitalized; the less severe forms of this group are flying squirrel-associated typhus and recrudescent typhus (Brill-Zinsser disease), to which mortality is not associated [44, 45].

3. Transitional Group Rickettsioses:

   This group produces what has been called rickettsialpox; during the subsequent days of the mite bite, there is a papulovesicular lesion, which progresses to an eschar with induration and edema around. Then, between 1 and 2 weeks, the patient presents constitutional symptoms of fever, headache, and myalgia. Subsequently, days after the appearance of these symptoms, a skin rash occurs in the form of maculae, which evolves into papules that become papulovesicles and then crusted lesions [46].

   The clinical presentation of Queensland tick typhus is similar to SFG rickettsioses with maculopapular rash in 90% and with eschar over 65% associated with regional lymphadenopathy, which are usually mild; however, severe and fatal cases have been reported [47, 48].

   Flea-borne spotted fever is a disease that has mild manifestations compared to another rickettsioses SFG, in which rash has been reported in 75% and 13% eschar [49].

Clinical Evaluation and Diagnosis

The clinical diagnosis is based on a high suspicion of this disease in patients presenting with symptoms of fever, rash, and headache, with the history of possible exposure to infected arthropods or from trips to endemic areas.

Due to the limitations of laboratory data, empirical treatment should be initiated promptly, if there is a suspicion of this disease.

General laboratories may show thrombocytopenia, hyponatremia, and pleocytosis in the cerebrospinal fluid; in addition, leukograms can show high, normal, or low counts, unable to rule out a rickettsia infection.

Depending on the samples taken and the evolution of the symptoms, different diagnostic methods of this disease can be used, including immunohistochemical

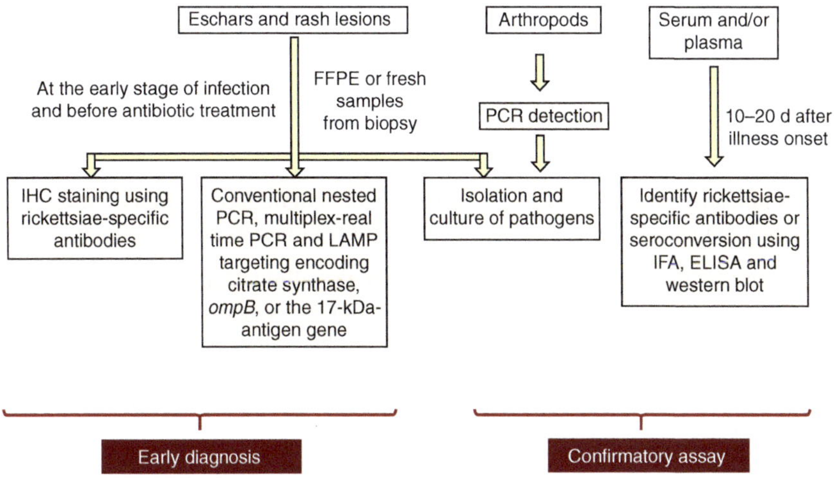

Fig. 33.3 A diagnostic algorithm for laboratory diagnosis of rickettsial diseases. ELISA enzyme-linked immunosorbent assay, FFPE formalin-fixed, paraffin-embedded, IFA immunofluorescence assay, IHC staining, immunohistochemical staining, LAMP loop-mediated isothermal amplification, OmpB outer membrane protein B, PCR polymerase chain reaction

analysis, molecular detection, isolation and culture of pathogens, and serology (Fig. 33.3) [4].

1. Detection of Rickettsial Antigen by Immunohistochemical Staining

   It is based on the determination of rickettsial antigen present in the rash or eschar, by means of a skin biopsy, particularly in the acute phase of the disease. After the biopsy in formalin and paraffin embedded is established, immunohistochemical staining can show rickettsias, by means of antibodies directed or cross-reactive against these rickettsial species. [13, 49–53]

   These techniques can be helpful in autopsy specimens, in tissues such as the skin, liver, spleen, lung, heart, kidney, and brain [54, 55].

   However, this technique is not sensitive after 48 hours or more of the administration of antibiotic treatment [56]
2. Molecular Genetic Approaches for Diagnosis

   It has been possible to detect nucleic acid molecules of rickettsia, using techniques such as blood and skin PCR. However, the sensitivity and specificity are higher in the skin samples, due to the tropism of these intracellular bacteria to the endothelium; blood samples have poor sensitivity [57–62] U-Z).

   The research and use of new molecular techniques have improved the sensitivity and specificity in the detection of this disease.
3. Isolation and Culture

   The culture and isolation of rickettsias can be performed by cell cultures of the skin, blood, and arthropod samples. However, this type of diagnostic technique requires expertise and special conditions.

   Because small amounts of aerosolized rickettsia can cause disease, a laboratory with level 3 biosecurity is required. In addition, appropriate host cells for cultivation is required, and many skin samples or arthropods are not sterile, requiring processes or treatments to be cultured [4].

4. Serology

   The detection of antibodies in serum or plasma is the gold standard assay to confirm infection by Rickettsiae.

   This detection can be performed by several methods such as enzyme-linked immunosorbent assay (ELISA), Western blot, and indirect immunofluorescence assay (IFA); the latter is the gold standard for the diagnosis of RMSF [56, 63, 64]

The antibody production response is after the clinical manifestations, usually after 7–10 days, but in some cases, it may be after 2–3 weeks. In the case of RMSF, the increase in IgM and IgG occurs almost simultaneously, in the second week of the disease [63]; IgM has a cross-reaction with nonrecreational antigens and therefore does not offer great sensitivity or specificity during the acute phase of the disease.

Seroconversion or a fourfold increase, from the acute phase to the convalescence phase, confirms the diagnosis of rickettsiosis [56].

Rickettsiosis in Pregnancy

In Southeast Asia, especially in rural areas, more than 1 million people a year suffer from scrub typhus and murine typhus, being one of the probable causes of treatable fever, with a mortality of 50–80,000 deaths per year.

97 cases of pregnant women with typhus have been described, of which 82 prognosis is known, with maternal death occurring in two cases. However, the neonatal prognosis was worse, occurring in more than 40% of pregnancies: stillbirth, prematurity, and low birth weight [65].

There are no large studies describing the infection during FMSR pregnancy, and it is unknown if it can cause infection in utero [66]. In addition, many laboratory abnormalities may be due to other diseases resulting from pregnancy such as preeclampsia and HELLP syndrome [66, 67].

In a report of four women with RMSF in Sonora, Mexico, between the years 2015 and 2016, it was found that the four pregnant women and one infant survived at 36 weeks' gestation; however, in the other pregnancies that were in the first trimester, they suffered spontaneous abortion [68].

Treatment/Management

The onset of treatment for this disease is based on suspicion and clinical recognition, with early empirical treatment with effective antibiotic treatment [6].

The class of antibiotics of choice for all rickettsiosis are tetracyclines, and although there are few prospective studies to evaluate antibiotic treatments for rickettsiosis and none specific for RMSF, many decades of experience support the efficacy of these antibiotics [69, 70].

Other antibiotics, such as penicillins, cephalosporins, and sulfonamides, are ineffective for *Rickettsia* spp., and in the case of sulfonamides, poor prognosis has been associated [71, 72].

Quinolones are effective, in less severe conditions; however, their use in pregnancy or in pediatric patients is not recommended [73].

Doxycycline is not related to staining of permanent teeth in children, such as tetracycline. Therefore, doxycycline is recommended in pediatric patients [56].

As for pregnant women, their management is transformed into a real challenge, due to the following facts:

1. Tetracyclines are deposited in the fetal skeleton and may cause temporary inhibition of bone growth [74].
2. Tetracyclines are associated with pancreatitis and maternal hepatotoxicity [75].
3. In advanced pregnancy, chloramphenicol has a high transplacental concentration, which can cause a gray baby syndrome (abdominal distention, pallor, cyanosis, and vasomotor collapse) [76].
4. In pregnant women, with less severe disease, azithromycin can be considered as a safe but unproven option.

The treatment for this infection is outline[4] in Table 33.3.

Prevention

There is no vaccine for the prevention of SFG and typhus rickettsioses.

Prevention is based on avoiding contact with possible vectors and controlling them. The use of repellents or protective clothing that protects exposed skin is recommended.

Different strategies have been used with positive impacts in the control of some epidemics:

1. The use of clothes treated with permethrin has been effective for the prevention of tick bites [77].
2. In the 1940s DDT was used in rat harborages, with a decrease in the incidence of murine typhus in the United States.
3. In some local outbreaks of louse-borne typhus, washing sheets and clothes with hot water kills lice and their eggs.
4. WHO recommends mass treatment by compressed air dusting of permethrin on clothing [78].
5. In Arizona, Brazil, and Sonora, Mexico, ticks have been reduced by treating animals and the environment with acaricides [79–81].

Table 33.3 Treatment of rickettsial diseases

	Medication	Adult dose	Pediatric dose	Duration
First choice for virtually all rickettsioses	Doxycycline oral or intravenous[a]	100 mg twice daily	2.2 mg/kg (maximum 100 mg) twice daily	≥3 d after defervescence (minimum course 5–7 d)[b]
Severe RMSF or other severe rickettsial illness[a]	Doxycycline intravenous	200 mg loading dose followed by 100 mg twice daily	2.2 mg/kg (maximum 100 mg) twice daily	≥3 d after defervescence (minimum course 5–7 d)[b]
Alternative for RMSF and other rickettsioses[c]	Chloramphenicol oral or intravenous	500 mg every 6 h	12.5 mg/kg every 6 h	≥3 d after defervescence (minimum course 5–7 d)[b]
Alternative for MSF and other less severe SFG rickettsioses	Oral fluoroquinolones:			
	Ciprofloxacin	500 mg twice daily	Not recommended	5–7 d
	Levofloxacin Oral macrolides:	500 mg daily	Not recommended	
	Clarithromycin	500 mg twice daily	7.5 mg/kg twice daily	7 d
	Azithromycin	500 mg daily	10 mg/kg daily	3 d
		500 mg × 1 then 250 mg daily	10 mg/kg × 1 then 5 mg/kg daily	5 d
Alternative for epidemic louse-borne typhus[d]	Short-course oral doxycycline	200 mg once		
Alternative for murine typhus	Oral fluoroquinolones			
	Ciprofloxacin	500 mg twice daily	Not recommended	
	Levofloxacin	500 mg daily	Not recommended	

[a]The bioavailability of doxycycline is excellent. The decision to choose the parenteral form should be made if gastrointestinal upset precludes its oral use or if absorption is thought to be compromised during critical illness

[b]The duration of treatment of RMSF is based on experience, because there are no controlled trials to guide the optimal duration

[c]Chloramphenicol is inferior to doxycycline for RMSF. Its oral form is not available in the United States, and the parenteral form is exceedingly hard for hospital pharmacies to stock. It is also associated with gray baby syndrome in neonates and aplastic anemia

[d]Relapses have been documented. Only recommended if needed for mass treatment to curtail an outbreak and if medications are in limited supply

Bibliography

1. Adem PV. Emerging and re-emerging rickettsial infections. Semin Diagn Pathol. 2019;36(3):146–51.
2. Tello-Martin R, Dzul-Rosado K, Zavala-Castro J, Lugo-Caballero C. Approaches for the successful isolation and cell culture of American *Rickettsia* species. J Vector Borne Dis. 2018;55(4):258–64.
3. Parola P, Paddock CD, Socolovschi C, et al. Update on tick-borne rickettsioses around the world: a geographic approach. Clin Microbiol Rev. 2013;26(4):657–702.
4. Fang R, Blanton LS, Walker DH. Rickettsiae as emerging infectious agents. Clin Lab Med. 2017;37(2):383–400.
5. Drexler NA, Yaglom H, Casal M, et al. Fatal Rocky Mountain spotted fever along the United States-Mexico Border, 2013–2016. Emerg Infect Dis. 2017;23(10):1621–6.
6. Regan JJ, Traeger MS, Humpherys D, et al. Risk factors for fatal outcome from Rocky Mountain spotted fever in a highly endemic area–Arizona, 2002–2011. Clin Infect Dis. 2015;60(11):1659–66.
7. Dehhaghi M, Kazemi Shariat Panahi H, Holmes EC, Hudson BJ, Schloeffel R, Guillemin GJ. Human tick-borne diseases in Australia. Front Cell Infect Microbiol. 2019;9:3.
8. Diop A, Raoult D, Fournier PE. Paradoxical evolution of rickettsial genomes. Ticks Tick Borne Dis. 2019;10(2):462–9.
9. Laroche M, Raoult D, Parola P. Insects and the transmission of bacterial agents. Microbiol Spectr. 2018;6(5): https://doi.org/10.1128/microbiolspec.MTBP-0017-2016.
10. Hardstone Yoshimizu M, Billeter SA. Suspected and confirmed vector-borne rickettsioses of North America associated with human diseases. Trop Med Infect Dis. 2018;3(1):e2.
11. Gillespie JJ, Williams K, Shukla M, et al. Rickettsia phylogenomics: unwinding the intricacies of obligate intracellular life. PLoS One. 2008;3(4):e2018.
12. Parte AC. LPSN – list of prokaryotic names with standing in nomenclature (bacterio.net), 20 years on. Int J Syst Evol Microbiol. 2018;68:1825–9.
13. Paddock CD, Sumner JW, Comer JA, et al. Rickettsia parkeri: a newly recognized cause of spotted fever rickettsiosis in the United States. Clin Infect Dis. 2004;38(6):805–11.
14. Shapiro MR, Fritz CL, Tait K, et al. Rickettsia 364D: a newly recognized cause of eschar-associated illness in California. Clin Infect Dis. 2010;50(4):541–8.
15. Raoult D, Lakos A, Fenollar F, et al. Spotless rickettsiosis caused by Rickettsia slovaca and associated with Dermacentor ticks. Clin Infect Dis. 2002;34(10):1331–6.
16. Niebylski ML, Schrumpf ME, Burgdorfer W, et al. Rickettsia peacockii sp. nov., a new species infecting wood ticks, Dermacentor andersoni, in western Montana. Int J Syst Bacteriol. 1997;47(2):446–52.
17. Kurtti TJ, Felsheim RF, Burkhardt NY, et al. Rickettsia buchneri sp. nov., a rickettsial endosymbiont of the blacklegged tick Ixodes scapularis. Int J Syst Evol Microbiol. 2015;65(Pt 3):965–70.
18. Vitale G, Mansuelo S, Rolain JM, et al. Rickettsia massiliae human isolation. Emerg Infect Dis. 2006;12(1):174–5.
19. Dahlgren FS, Paddock CD, Springer YP, et al. Expanding range of Amblyomma americanum and simultaneous changes in the epidemiology of spotted fever group rickettsiosis in the United States. Am J Trop Med Hyg. 2016;94(1):35–42.
20. Walker DH, Paddock CD, Dumler JS. Emerging and re-emerging tick-transmitted rickettsial and ehrlichial infections. Med Clin North Am. 2008;92(6):1345–61, x.
21. Khamesipour F, Dida GO, Anyona DN, Razavi SM, Rakhshandehroo E. Tick-borne zoonoses in the Order Rickettsiales and Legionellales in Iran: a systematic review. PLoS Negl Trop Dis. 2018;12(9):e0006722.
22. Weitzel T, Aylwin M, Martínez-Valdebenito C, Jiang J, Munita JM, Thompson L, Abarca K, Richards AL. Imported scrub typhus: first case in South America and review of the literature. Trop Dis Travel Med Vaccines. 2018;4:10.

23. Eldin C, Parola P. Update on tick-borne bacterial diseases in travelers. Curr Infect Dis Rep. 2018;20(7):17.
24. Moreira J, Bressan CS, Brasil P, Siqueira AM. Epidemiology of acute febrile illness in Latin America. Clin Microbiol Infect. 2018;24(8):827–35.
25. Abdad MY, Abou Abdallah R, Fournier P-E, Stenos J, Vasoo S. A concise review of the epidemiology and diagnostics of rickettsioses: Rickettsia and Orientia spp. J Clin Microbiol. 2018;56:e01728–17.
26. Walker DH, Ismail N, Olano JP, Valbuena GA, McBride J. Chapter 2: pathogenesis, immunity, pathology, and pathophysiology in rickettsial diseases. In: Raoult D, Parola P, editors. Rickettsial diseases. New York: Informa Healthcare; 2007.
27. Raoult D, Woodward T, Dumler JS. The history of epidemic typhus. Infect Dis Clin N Am. 2004;18:127–40.
28. Parola P, Paddock C, Socolovschi C, Labruna M, Mediannikov O, Kernif T, Abdad MY, Stenos J, Bitam I, Fournier PE, Raoult D. Update on tick-borne rickettsioses around the world: a geographic approach. Clin Microbiol Rev. 2013;26:657–702.
29. Valbuena G, Walker DH. Changes in the adherens junctions of human endothelial cells infected with spotted fever group rickettsiae. Virchows Arch. 2008;446:379–82.
30. Woods ME, Olano JP. Host defenses to Rickettsia rickettsii infection contribute to increased microvascular permeability in human cerebral endothelial cells. J Clin Immunol. 2008;28:174–85.
31. Nickerson A, Marik PE. Life-threatening ANCA-positive vasculitis associated with rickettsial infection. BMJ Case Rep. 2012;2012:bcr0320125993. https://doi.org/10.1136/bcr.03.2012.5993.
32. Silva-Pinto A, de Lurdes Santos M, Sarmento A. Tick-borne lymphadenopathy, an emerging disease. Ticks Tick Borne Dis. 2014;5(6):656–9.
33. Alvarez-Hernandez G, Roldan JFG, Milan NSH, et al. Rocky Mountain spotted fever in Mexico: past, present, and future. Lancet Infect Dis. 2017;17(6):e189–96.
34. Traeger MS, Regan JJ, Humpherys D, et al. Rocky Mountain spotted fever characterization and comparison to similar illnesses in a highly endemic area-Arizona, 2002–2011. Clin Infect Dis. 2015;60(11):1650–8.
35. Jensenius M, Fournier PE, Kelly P, et al. African tick bite fever. Lancet Infect Dis. 2003;3(9):557–64.
36. Helmick CG, Bernard KW, D'Angelo LJ. Rocky Mountain spotted fever: clinical, laboratory, and epidemiological features of 262 cases. J Infect Dis. 1984;150(4):480–8.
37. Kaplowitz LG, Fischer JJ, Sparling PF. Rocky Mountain spotted fever: a clinical dilemma. In: Remington JB, Swartz HN, editors. Current clinical topics in infectious diseases, vol. 2. New York: McGraw-Hill; 1981. p. 89–108.
38. Raoult D, Weiller PJ, Chagnon A, et al. Mediterranean spotted fever: clinical, laboratory and epidemiological features of 199 cases. Am J Trop Med Hyg. 1986;35(4):845–50.
39. Dubourg G, Socolovschi C, Del Giudice P, et al. Scalp eschar and neck lymphadenopathy after tick bite: an emerging syndrome with multiple causes. Eur J Clin Microbiol Infect Dis. 2014;33(8):1449–56.
40. Walker DH. Changing dynamics of human-rickettsial interactions. Am J Trop Med Hyg. 2016;94(1):3–4.
41. Bechah Y, Capo C, Mege JL, et al. Epidemic typhus. Lancet Infect Dis. 2008;8(7):417–26.
42. Tsioutis C, Zafeiri M, Avramopoulos A, et al. Clinical and laboratory characteristics, epidemiology, and outcomes of murine typhus: a systematic review. Acta Trop. 2017;166:16–24.
43. Blanton LS, Lea AS, Kelly BC, et al. An unusual cutaneous manifestation in a patient with murine typhus. Am J Trop Med Hyg. 2015;93(6):1164–7.
44. Pieracci EG, Evert N, Drexler NA, et al. Fatal flea-borne typhus in Texas: a retrospective case series, 1985–2015. Am J Trop Med Hyg. 2017;96(5):1088–93.
45. Dumler JS, Taylor JP, Walker DH. Clinical and laboratory features of murine typhus in South Texas, 1980 through 1987. JAMA. 1991;266(10):1365–70.

46. Kass EM, Szaniawski WK, Levy H, et al. Rickettsialpox in a New York City hospital,1980 to 1989. N Engl J Med. 1994;331(24):1612–7.
47. Stewart A, Armstrong M, Graves S, et al. Rickettsia Australis and Queensland tick typhus: a rickettsial spotted fever group infection in Australia. Am J Trop Med Hyg. 2017;97(1):24–9.
48. Graves SR, Stenos J. Tick-borne infectious diseases in Australia. Med J Aust. 2017;206(7):320–4.
49. Parola P. Rickettsia felis: from a rare disease in the USA to a common cause of fever in sub-Saharan Africa. Clin Microbiol Infect. 2011;17(7):996–1000.
50. Walker DH, Feng HM, Ladner S, et al. Immunohistochemical diagnosis of typhus rickettsioses using an anti-lipopolysaccharide monoclonal antibody. Mod Pathol. 1997;10:1038–42.
51. Walker DH, Parks FM, Betz TG, et al. Histopathology and immunohistologic demonstration of the distribution of Rickettsia typhi in fatal murine typhus. Am J Clin Pathol. 1989;91:720–4.
52. Paddock CD, Zaki SR, Koss T, et al. Rickettsialpox in New York City: a persistent urban zoonosis. Ann N Y Acad Sci. 2003;990:36–44.
53. Lepidi H, Fournier PE, Raoult D. Histologic features and immunodetection of African tick-bite fever eschar. Emerg Infect Dis. 2006;12(9):1332–7.
54. Rutherford JS, Macaluso KR, Smith N, et al. Fatal spotted fever rickettsiosis, Kenya. Emerg Infect Dis. 2004;10(5):910–3.
55. Paddock CD, Greer PW, Ferebee TL, et al. Hidden mortality attributable to Rocky Mountain spotted fever: immunohistochemical detection of fatal, serologically unconfirmed disease. J Infect Dis. 1999;179(6):1469–76.
56. Chapman AS, Bakken JS, Folk SM, et al, Tickborne Rickettsial Diseases Working Group, CDC. Diagnosis and management of tickborne rickettsial diseases: Rocky Mountain spotted fever, ehrlichioses, and anaplasmosis—United States: a practical guide for physicians and other health-care and public health professionals. MMWR Recomm Rep. 2006;55(RR-4):1–27.
57. La Scola B, Raoult D. Laboratory diagnosis of rickettsioses: current approaches to diagnosis of old and new rickettsial diseases. J Clin Microbiol. 1997;35:2715–27.
58. Denison AM, Amin BD, Nicholson WL, et al. Detection of Rickettsia rickettsii, Rickettsia parkeri, and Rickettsia akari in skin biopsy specimens using a multiplex real-time polymerase chain reaction assay. Clin Infect Dis. 2014;59(5):635–42.
59. Sexton DJ, Kanj SS, Wilson K, et al. The use of a polymerase chain reaction as a diagnostic test for Rocky Mountain spotted fever. Am J Trop Med Hyg. 1994;50:59–63.
60. Mouffok N, Socolovschi C, Benabdellah A, et al. Diagnosis of rickettsioses from Es char swab samples, Algeria. Emerg Infect Dis. 2011;17:1968–9.
61. Kondo M, Akachi S, Kawano M, et al. Improvement in early diagnosis of Japanese spotted fever by using a novel Rick PCR system. J Dermatol. 2015;42(11):1066–71.
62. Znazen A, Sellami H, Elleuch E, et al. Comparison of two quantitative real time PCR assays for Rickettsia detection in patients from Tunisia. PLoS Negl Trop Dis. 2015;9(2):e0003487.
63. Clements ML, Dumler JS, Fiset P, et al. Serodiagnosis of Rocky Mountain spotted fever: comparison of IgM and IgG enzyme-linked immunosorbent assays and indirect fluorescent antibody test. J Infect Dis. 1983;148:876–80.
64. Jensenius M, Fournier PE, Vene S, et al. Comparison of immunofluorescence, Western blotting, and cross-adsorption assays for diagnosis of African tick bite fever. Clin Diagn Lab Immunol. 2004;11(4):786–8.
65. McGready R, et al. Pregnancy outcome in relation to treatment of murine typhus and scrub typhus infection: a fever cohort and a case series analysis. PLoS Negl Trop Dis. 2014;8(11):e3327.
66. Dotters-Katz SK, Kuller J, Heine RP. Arthropod-borne bacterial dis-eases in pregnancy. Obstet Gynecol Surv. 2013;68:635–49.
67. Stallings SP. Rocky Mountain spotted fever and pregnancy: a case report and review of the literature. Obstet Gynecol Surv. 2001;56:37–42.
68. Licona-Enriquez JD, et al. Case report: Rocky Mountain spotted fever and pregnancy: four cases from Sonora, Mexico Mexico. Am J Trop Med Hyg. 2017;97(3):795–8.

69. Biggs HM, Behravesh CB, Bradley KK, et al. Diagnosis and management of tickborne rickettsial diseases: Rocky Mountain spotted fever and other spotted fever group rickettsioses, ehrlichioses, and anaplasmosis – United States. MMWR Recomm Rep. 2016;65(2):1–44.
70. Dumler JS. Clinical disease: current treatment and new challenges. In: Palmer GH, Azad AF, editors. Intracellular pathogens II: Rickettsiales. Washington, DC: ASM Press; 2012. p. 1–39.
71. Rolain JM, Maurin M, Vestris G, et al. In vitro susceptibilities of 27 rickettsiae to 13 antimicrobials. Antimicrob Agents Chemother. 1998;42(7):1537–41.
72. Ruiz Beltran R, Herrero Herrero JI. Deleterious effect of trimethoprimsulfamethoxazole in Mediterranean spotted fever. Antimicrob Agents Chemother. 1992;36(6):1342–3.
73. Ruiz Beltran R, Herrero Herrero JI. Evaluation of ciprofloxacin and doxycycline in the treatment of Mediterranean spotted fever. Eur J Clin Microbiol Infect Dis. 1992;11(5):427–31.
74. Cohlan SQ. Teratogenic agents and congenital malformations. J Pediatr. 1963;63:650–9.
75. Herbert WN, Seeds JW, Koontz WL, et al. Rocky Mountain spotted fever in pregnancy: differential diagnosis and treatment. South Med J. 1982;75(9):1063–6.
76. Ross S, Burke FG, Sites J, et al. Placental transmission of chloramphenicol (Chloromycetin). J Am Med Assoc. 1950;142(17):1361.
77. Vaughn MF, Funkhouser SW, Lin FC, et al. Long-lasting permethrin impregnated uniforms: a randomized-controlled trial for tick bite prevention. Am J Prev Med. 2014;46(5):473–80.
78. Epidemic typhus risk in Rwandan refugee camps. Wkly Epidemiol Rec. 1994;69:259.
79. Straily A, Drexler N, Cruz-Loustaunau D, et al. Notes from the field: communitybased prevention of Rocky Mountain spotted fever – Sonora, Mexico, 2016. MMWR Morb Mortal Wkly Rep. 2016;65(46):1302–3.
80. Brites-Neto J, Nieri-Bastos FA, Brasil J, et al. Environmental infestation and rickettsial infection in ticks in an area endemic for Brazilian spotted fever. Rev Bras Parasitol Vet. 2013;22(3):367–72.
81. Drexler N, Miller M, Gerding J, et al. Community-based control of the brown dog tick in a region with high rates of Rocky Mountain spotted fever, 2012-2013. PLoS One. 2014;9(12):e112368.

Part VIII
Cardiology

Chapter 34
Acute Coronary Syndromes in Pregnancy

Rania Magdi Ali, Bahaa El-Din Ewees Hassan, and Noura M. Youssri Mahmoud

Introduction

Acute coronary syndrome (ACS) is a seldom event in women of childbearing age. However, in pregnancy, the relative risk is three- to fourfold higher than that of non-pregnant age-matched women [1]. Profound physiological changes in the peripartum period can augment the strain on the heart, especially in the presence of risk factors for myocardial infarction. ACS complicating pregnancy is relatively uncommon and varies between countries. Yet, it accounts for >20% of all maternal cardiac deaths [2]. Historically, the maternal mortality has been reported to be about half the women in the peripartum period. Thereafter it dropped to 5–11% of affected patients most probably due to early detection and the invasive interventions executed, as well as the intensive care units, anaesthesia, and high-risk obstetric practice advancements [3].

Physiologic Changes on the Cardiovascular System

Pregnancy is a natural stress challenge because the cardiovascular system undergoes adaptations to sustain a high-volume load. These changes that occur during pregnancy increase myocardial oxygen demand [4].

There is augmentation in plasma volume and reduction in peripheral vascular resistance that starts as early as 6 weeks and continues until it reaches a plateau at around 32 weeks of gestation. These changes are attributed to activation of the renin-angiotensin system and a mild reduction of the plasma atrial natriuretic

R. M. Ali (✉) · B. E.-D. E. Hassan · N. M. Y. Mahmoud
Anesthesia, Intensive Care and Pain Management, Faculty of Medicine, Ain Shams University, Cairo, Egypt

C. Montufar et al. (eds.), *Obstetric Catastrophes*,
https://doi.org/10.1007/978-3-030-70034-8_34

peptide levels. Instantly, cardiac output rises steadily until 25 weeks of gestation, initially secondary to the increase in stroke volume and later because of an increase in maternal heart rate [5].

On the other hand, blood pressure exhibits fluctuations during pregnancy; it initially decreases then increases in the third trimester, in addition to postural hypotensive attacks that occur during the second and third trimesters due to aorto-caval compression that potentially reduce the venous return to the heart [6].

During labour and delivery, there are dramatic haemodynamic changes. The heart rate and blood pressure increase significantly as a result of pain, anxiety, and uterine contractions. The rise in heart rate during labour mimics the increase in heart rate that occur during moderate to heavy physical exercise. Besides, the cardiac output increases up to 50% with each contraction, and there is a marked fluid shift from the uterus into the maternal circulation with each uterine contraction and at delivery of the placenta [7].

Later, diuresis and natriuresis start 48 hours post-delivery, and maternal hemodynamic state generally returns to the pre-pregnancy state 3–6 months after delivery [8].

Haematological and Metabolic Changes

In pregnancy, erythropoiesis increases red blood cell mass 20–30%; however this increase is proportionally lower than the increase in plasma volume, resulting in physiologic anaemia from haemodilution [5].

Pregnancy is associated with amplified thrombogenic state and many changes that increase the risk of thromboembolism, including hypercoagulability, venous stasis, compression of the pelvic veins by the enlarging uterus, and decreased mobility. Simultaneously, pregnancy increases the levels of procoagulants and reduces the levels of natural anticoagulants. These changes in the coagulation system persist 8 weeks postpartum. Accordingly, the risk of thrombosis continues in the postpartum period [8].

From a metabolic standpoint, pregnancy is a catabolic state that leads to insulin resistance and an atherogenic lipid profile with elevated serum fatty acids. Dyslipidaemia may be worsened because high-density lipoprotein cholesterol (HDL) is significantly decreased during pregnancy. However, there is no significant change in low-density lipoprotein cholesterol (LDL) or triglyceride levels in pregnancy [9].

Impact of Physiological Changes on Risk of Myocardial Infarction

The increased stroke volume and heart rate during pregnancy lead to significantly increased myocardial oxygen demand. At the same time, the physiological anaemia of pregnancy, hypercoagulability, and decrease in diastolic blood pressure may reduce the myocardial oxygen supply and contribute to the aggravation of myocardial ischaemia where the coronary arterial blood supply is already compromised [8]. Further, the augmentation of the cardiac output in the immediate postpartum period, as a result of decompression of the inferior vena cava and shift of blood flow from the uterus back to the systemic circulation, results in further stress on the myocardium and makes the peripartum period of particularly high risk [9].

Aetiology

The Risk Factors in Pregnancy

The overall effect of the increased cardiac output, enhanced stroke volume, and hypercoagulability favour the development or unmasking of underlying coronary artery disease. Risk factors for acute coronary syndrome during pregnancy include traditional and pregnancy-specific features such as smoking, maternal age, hypertension, diabetes, obesity, and dyslipidaemia and cocaine use. Additional risk factors include pre-eclampsia, thrombophilia, transfusion, post-partum infection, multiparity, and post-partum haemorrhage [10].

As the birth rate in women older than 40 years increases, the frequency of ACS complicating pregnancy increases with 20% increase in MI risk for every year increase in maternal age [2].

Oral contraceptives especially in combination with smoking increase significantly the risk for developing myocardial infarction in young women, whereas assisted reproductive technology helps to achieve pregnancy in older women with multiple coronary risk factors or already having coronary artery disease [11].

Pathophysiology

ACS is classified based on electrocardiogram (ECG) findings as non-ST elevation ACS and ST elevation myocardial infarction (STEMI). Non-ST elevation ACS can be further subdivided as non-ST elevation myocardial infarction (NSTEMI) with elevated myocardial injury biomarkers or unstable angina. Partial occlusion of a vessel causes findings consistent with NSTEMI, while total occlusion of the vessel presents as STEMI [11].

The aetiology of coronary artery diseases in pregnancy differs from the general population. Most of the cases have non-atherosclerotic mechanisms, including coronary artery occlusion related to aortic dissection, embolism, spasm, arteritis, and in addition to takotsubo (stress) cardiomyopathy [1]. Coronary artery dissection is the most common cause of pregnancy-associated ACS. It can occur at any time during pregnancy, typically in the early postpartum period [12]. It predominantly involves the left-sided coronaries. Potential precipitating factors include fluctuating oestrogen and progesterone levels resulting in structural changes in coronary vasculature and increased coronary shear stresses associated with labour [13]. Pregnancy-related hypertension, along with physiologic increase in blood volume and cardiac output in pregnancy, augments the stress on blood vessels and increases the risk of coronary dissection.

Coronary thrombosis in the absence of atherosclerosis is most likely due to the hypercoagulability of pregnancy and can result from paradoxical embolization. Smoking during pregnancy may further increase the risk of thrombosis due to enhanced platelet aggregability and additional release of tissue plasminogen activator (t-PA) inhibitor [14].

The mechanisms of ACS with angiographically normal coronary arteries remain unclear and include transient coronary spasm due to increased vascular reactivity. Besides, drugs used in and around pregnancy such as terbutaline, ergotamine, and bromocriptine can induce continuous coronary vessel spasm [12, 15].

Furthermore, the progress in management of medium size autoimmune arteritis patients, Kawasaki disease, and the higher survival rate presents an additional risk. Relevant Kawasaki disease manifestations include aneurysms, coronary blood flow alteration, coronary stenoses, myocardial ischaemia/fibrosis, congestive cardiac failure, and valvular abnormalities [16].

Diagnosis

Clinical Features

Diagnosis of ACS in pregnancy may be a great challenge due to its low prevalence. Also, as the presenting symptoms and signs can be interpreted as normal manifestations of pregnancy or be concealed during labour, thus delaying proper diagnosis and consequently low index of suspicion is mandatory.

Clinical presentation is the same as in the non-pregnant population. Every pregnant or postpartum patient with chest pain or cardiac symptoms should have consideration of ACS. Patients who have an ACS can present with typical (chest pain or shortness of breath) or atypical symptoms (vomiting, reflux, or diaphoresis) that mimic physiological changes of pregnancy [17]. Simultaneously, typical features of pregnancy such as epigastric pain, vomiting, or dizziness, in the presence of known ACS risk factors, should be further investigated because it is usually hard to differentiate common symptoms of pregnancy, such as mild shortness of breath or oedema, from ischaemia or heart failure [8].

Also, some patients first present with haemodynamic compromise and complications. Potential complications of maternal ACS include heart failure, cardiogenic shock, ventricular arrhythmias, recurrent myocardial infarction, maternal mortality, and intrauterine foetal death [1].

Investigations

Electrocardiography

Electrocardiographic (ECG) changes in ACS reveal ST-segment elevations or depression. ECG interpretation can be challenging, as new ST depressions, T wave inversions, and left axis deviation can be normally seen in pregnancy. Importantly, ST elevations are never seen in normal pregnancy and should prompt further investigation. The differential diagnosis includes pericarditis, pulmonary embolism, and electrolyte abnormalities. Caution should be taken as NSTEMI is more common than STEMI in pregnancy-related ACS [18].

Blood Cardiac Markers

Elevated troponins have high sensitivity and specificity for myocardial damage, whereas a negative troponin test at presentation does not exclude cardiac damage, as it can take 12 hours to reach peak level. Besides, the troponin levels may be elevated in pre-eclampsia but never above the standard threshold set for MI. Thus, serum troponin rise should suggest myocardial ischaemia, even in pre-eclampsia [19]. In contrast, other cardiac markers such as creatinine kinase and creatinine kinase isoenzyme MB can be increased significantly in labour.

Echocardiogram

When the ECG is non-diagnostic, echocardiography is safe and can be helpful [20]. It can exclude differential diagnoses of ACS in pregnancy like pulmonary embolism and aortic dissection. During pregnancy, some changes in echo parameters are expected, such as mild dilatation of the chambers, a change in LV wall thickness, and an increase in valve gradient [21]. However, segmental wall motion abnormalities cannot occur in normal pregnancy and, if observed, indicate myocardial ischaemia or injury [3].

Coronary Angiography

Coronary angiography remains the standard for diagnosis in patients with ACS. The potential risks of ionizing radiation exposure to the foetus depend on the stage of pregnancy and the absorbed dose. Risks are highest during organogenesis in the first trimester. It is reassuring to note that the estimated foetal and maternal effective doses for diagnostic coronary angiography are 1.5 mGy and 7 mGy, respectively, whereas for percutaneous coronary intervention (PCI) are 3 mGy and 15 mGy, respectively. Hence, they will not cross the threshold that has been reported to be associated with foetal malformations with first trimester exposure, 50–100 mGy [22]. Nevertheless, if coronary angiography is planned, radial access is recommended with the abdomen shielded and fluoroscopic time minimized.

On the other hand, there is a high incidence of iatrogenic coronary artery dissection in pregnant women during performing coronary angiography. Hence, some protective measures should be performed if possible, such as avoiding deep catheter intubation, minimizing the number of low-pressure contrast injections, and limiting the use of fractional flow reserve pressure guidewires, suction devices, and balloons. Imaging techniques, such as intravascular ultrasound or optical coherence tomography, may be used during angiography to aid in clarifying the extent of coronary artery injury or the presence of coronary artery dissection and guiding intervention [3].

Another concern with coronary angiography is the use of iodinated contrast agents and the associated clinical risk of foetal congenital hypothyroidism. Although there are no reports to date suggest that contrast dye is teratogenic, evaluating foetal thyroid function at time of birth or within the first week of delivery is still recommended [23]. Despite these reassuring data, it is preferred to avoid coronary angiography in stable patients with preserved global left ventricular function because of the risk of complications [12, 16].

CT Coronary Angiography

CT coronary angiography provides an alternative diagnostic method; however, it requires radiation and potentially high-dose beta-blockade and may fail to demonstrate limited coronary artery dissection [24].

Management

ACS management in pregnancy is like that in the general population aims to re-establish normal coronary blood flow. However, in pregnancy there are added restrictions and considerations. ACS during pregnancy is best managed in a high-dependency or intensive care unit by multidisciplinary team, including emergency, obstetric, and cardiovascular teams. Any revascularization must be performed by the most experienced operator due to the risks associated with coronary intervention in this patient population [22].

Management of the maternal condition should receive priority. While maternal evaluation and initial therapy are proceeding, an unstable patient should be placed in a left lateral tilt ranging from 30° to 90° to increase uteroplacental perfusion. Initial medical management usually includes oxygen supplementation, nitrates, aspirin, intravenous unfractionated heparin, and beta-blocker therapy. If symptoms persist, coronary angiography is the preferred investigation and should be performed without delay [17].

Close monitoring of the foetus is required, and corticosteroids to enhance foetal lung maturation are recommended for appropriate gestational ages. Delivery strategy should be ready in case there is sudden maternal or foetal deterioration. The type of intervention should be individualized based on the aetiology of acute coronary syndrome, patient characteristics, and facilities available at the presenting medical centre [17].

ACS occurs at all stages of pregnancy with increasing in the incidence as the gestational age advances reaching a peak incidence during the postpartum period [25]. There are treatment challenges for ACS throughout the pregnancy and postpartum. Early in pregnancy is the peak of organogenesis, and the teratogenic risk of pharmacologic therapy and radiation exposure during cardiac catheterization are the leading concern. In the later stages of pregnancy, weighing the risk of bleeding during delivery against the risk of stent thrombosis if dual antiplatelet therapy (DAPT) is discontinued is the main concern [3].

ST Elevation Myocardial Infarction STEMI

Coronary angiography and primary PCI are the treatment of choice to restore coronary blood flow promptly and tissue reperfusion especially if the cause is atherosclerotic coronary disease [17]. The effects of ionizing radiation should not prevent primary PCI in pregnant patients with standard indications for revascularization. However, the radiation dose must be minimized.

Non-ST Elevation Myocardial Infarction (NSTEMI)

In stable, low-risk NSTEMI, a noninvasive approach should be considered [12]. Antiplatelet drug treatment aim is preventing further thrombus formation, facilitating clot dissolution and increasing blood flow to the myocardium.

PCI is considered if the symptoms of coronary ischaemia continue despite medical treatment or with newly developed haemodynamic instability. Patients whose symptoms settle on medical treatment but have high-risk features may also be considered for angiography following discussion of the risks and benefits by the multidisciplinary team [8].

In patients suffering from coronary artery dissection, vascular vulnerability should be considered when applying revascularization strategies. The results of PCI in women with coronary dissection are suboptimal and associated with high risk of propagation of the existing dissection. For this reason, a conservative approach is recommended in stable patients with coronary artery dissection [26]. Beta-blockade may be beneficial in reducing shear stress in such cases [22].

Ongoing chest pain or ischaemic changes on ECG, cardiogenic shock requiring inotropes or mechanical support, sustained ventricular tachycardia or ventricular fibrillation, and left main dissection are all clinical criteria in patients with coronary dissection necessitate percutaneous revascularization with a stent [3].

Medical Management

Antiplatelet Therapy During Pregnancy

There is little information regarding the foetal safety of antiplatelet drug therapy in ACS [27]. Low-dose aspirin appears to be safe, but there is little information regarding $P2Y_{12}$ inhibitors usage in pregnant patients. Hence, Clopidogrel should be used only when strictly necessary and for the shortest duration [1]. Whereas prasugrel, and ticagrelor, their routine use is not recommended.

In the absence of data regarding glycoprotein IIb/IIIa inhibitors, abciximab, eptifibatide, and tirofiban, their routine use is not recommended, and it is better to reserve their use during PCI for patients at high ischaemic risk, including those with prior myocardial infarction, high thrombus burden, and complex PCI [22].

Anticoagulation During Pregnancy

Unfractionated heparin (UFH) is commonly used in pregnancy owing to its relative safety in pregnancy, fast onset, short half-life, and ease of dose adjustment. In addition, UFH does not cross the placenta; therefore, it does not cause foetal bleeding and foetal malformations [3].

Pregnancy leads to alterations in heparin's pharmacokinetic parameters because of increased levels of heparin-binding proteins, factor VIII, and fibrinogen. However, its effect is subject to close monitoring by measurement of the activated clotting time or activated partial thromboplastin time (aPTT) that aid in adjusting the dose of heparin [28].

Low-molecular-weight heparin (LMWH) safety in pregnancy is less well studied than UFH. Besides, its pharmacokinetics is also affected by the physiological changes associated with pregnancy as the increase in maternal weight, renal clearance, and volume of distribution of LMWH. Dosing may be monitored and adjusted according to the anti-Xa activity target level. However, the optimal target level for anticoagulation in ACS is not well defined, and bedside testing assays are not readably available [29].

Direct thrombin inhibitors (DTI) are as effective as UFH but with less bleeding complications in patients with ACS undergoing PCI. Furthermore, DTI have a more predictable dose response than UFH. The lower rate of bleeding complications, fast onset of activity, and short half-life about 25–45 minutes, all these factors make it an attractive option in pregnancy. However, there are limited data on its safety during pregnancy (pregnancy category B) [30].

There are no published reports to date on bivalirudin utilization during pregnancy, whereas several case reports document the use of argatroban for the treatment of venous thromboembolism in pregnant patients with heparin-induced thrombocytopenia, and there were no adverse effects that have been described. Accordingly, argatroban is recommended to be used only in those with heparin-induced thrombocytopenia owing to the limited data on the foetal effects [31].

Switching between LMWH and UFH results in an increase in both catheter-related bleeding and adverse ischaemic outcomes [32]. On the other hand, switching to bivalirudin during PCI from either UFH or LMWH is associated with similar rates of ischaemic events and significantly lower rates of bleeding; however, there are no data refer to the safety of bivalirudin in pregnancy [33]. Therefore, anticoagulation with UFH is recommended from time of presentation until conclusion of PCI while avoiding switching to antithrombin therapy [3].

Thrombolytic Therapy

Thrombolytic therapy in pregnancy produces several complications including maternal haemorrhage, preterm delivery, foetal loss, spontaneous abortion, placenta abruption, uterine bleeding, and postpartum haemorrhage. As the coronary dissection is relatively common in pregnancy, thrombolytic therapy may be harmful, increasing the risk of bleeding and progression of the dissection. For these reasons, thrombolytic therapy is rarely utilized for acute myocardial infarction treatment in pregnancy [34].

Nonetheless, thrombolysis is a suitable alternative if a significant delay is expected in accessing PCI. The thrombolytic agent of choice is intravenous t-PA as it does not cross the placenta. However, one must bear in mind that there is an associated risk of maternal haemorrhage. Thus, when a patient with STEMI presents to a medical centre that does not have interventional cardiac catheterization facilities, options include emergent transfer to a centre that has these capabilities or emergent thrombolysis according to the situation [17].

Percutaneous Therapy

If an intervention is necessary, the best time is after the fourth month in the second trimester. By this time, organogenesis is complete, and the uterine volume is still small, so there is a greater distance between the foetus and the chest than in later months [22].

Procedures should use as low as reasonably achievable radiation by applying the following manoeuvres; use echo guidance when possible, place the source as distant as possible from the patient and the receiver as close as possible to the patient, use only low-dose fluoroscopy, favour anteroposterior projections, avoid direct radiation of the abdominal region, collimate as tightly as possible to the area of interest, minimize fluoroscopy time, and utilize an experienced cardiologist [35].

Notably, abdominal shielding lowers the radiation dose to the foetus to some degree; however, the presence of lead in the field of the primary beam may on the other hand increase scattered radiation. As the benefit of shielding is limited, it should not interfere with an optimal intervention [22].

The benefits of short-term heparinization during PCI probably outweigh the risk of bleeding complications. Unfractionated heparin (UFH) must be given at 40–70 U/kg intravenous targeting an activated clotting time of 200–300 seconds or an aPTT two times normal values [22].

Old balloon angioplasty is no longer recommended in pregnancy as it is associated with high restenosis rates and high frequency of recurrent myocardial infarction [3].

Bare-metal stents (BMS) are commonly employed in pregnancy. BMS require short duration of dual antiplatelet therapy (DAPT) for at least uninterrupted 4 weeks. Therefore, during the third trimester of pregnancy, a BMS is most appropriate. This allows for interruption of dual antiplatelet therapy at the time of delivery and reduces the potential bleeding complications in the peripartum period [3].

However, drug-eluting stents (DES) are associated with further reductions in revascularization compared with BMS and are recommended according to the 2017 AMI STEMI Guidelines [18]. The optimal duration of DAPT with a second-/third-generation DES is at least uninterrupted 3 months duration. There is less experience using the newer-generation DES in pregnancy; nevertheless, modern DES may be used in the first two trimesters with anticipated interruption of DAPT near time of delivery [36]. Bioabsorbable stent usage has been reported in spontaneous coronary artery dissection; however, there is currently no evidence to recommend them in pregnancy [3].

Cardiac Surgery with Cardiopulmonary Bypass

Cardiac surgery is recommended only when medical therapy or interventional procedures fail, and the mother's life is threatened. The best period for surgery is the second trimester. Maternal mortality during cardiopulmonary bypass is now like that in non-pregnant women. However, foetal mortality remains high up to 20% [37]. The risks to both the mother and the foetus can be minimized by full maternal and foetal monitoring, minimizing the time of cardiopulmonary bypass and using pulsatile perfusion [38].

Of note, the use of an intra-aortic balloon pump to improve left ventricular output and coronary perfusion is also considered safe, although the patient should be positioned in the left lateral decubitus position to reduce compression of the inferior vena cava [3].

Timing and Mode of Delivery

Data regarding timing and mode of delivery are limited. Timing of delivery must be individualized based on maternal cardiac status and gestational age. However, treatment of ACS should not be delayed for delivery. If possible, delivery should be postponed for at least 2 weeks post the acute attack to facilitate maternal management [9]. If preterm delivery is anticipated, maternal steroid injections must be administered as early as possible.

Gestational age has a large impact on neonatal outcome [39]. When gestational age is beyond 28 weeks, delivery before surgery should be considered, but when the gestational age is between 26 and 28 weeks, the advantages of delivery before cardiopulmonary bypass for the baby at this gestational age is query and depends on estimated weight, prior administration of corticosteroids before delivery, and the outcome statistics of the neonatal unit concerned [37].

In terms of the mode of delivery, vaginal delivery is generally preferred. Vaginal delivery is associated with less blood loss and lower risk of infection, venous thrombosis, and embolism. Elective caesarean section carries no maternal benefit, and it is better to be reserved for the usual obstetric indications or if the patient is haemodynamically unstable [40].

During labour, the patient should be kept in the left lateral position to attenuate the impact of the aorto-caval compression. Labour can negatively influence the myocardial workload with higher increases in the preload from uterine contractions. If induction of labour is considered, synthetic prostaglandin analogues including misoprostol (25 μg), prostaglandin E1, or dinoprostone (1–3 mg) or slow-release formulation of 10 mg prostaglandin PGE2 may be used after considering the theoretical risk of coronary vasospasm and arrhythmias [41]. Blind intramyometrial injection of dinoprostone can cause profound hypotension; thus it is preferable to avoid this route of administration [42]. Infusion of oxytocin also can be used although some haemodynamic adverse effects have been reported in association with continuous infusion and bolus dosing of oxytocin [22].

Ultimately, spontaneous onset of labour is favoured. Shortening the second stage with instrumental delivery is recommended to avoid the unwanted haemodynamic effect of the contractions [22].

All through delivery, supplementary oxygen should be provided as well as continuous maternal cardiovascular monitoring, including pulse oximetry, blood pressure, and ECG. Continuous foetal monitoring is also mandatory. If left ventricular function is significantly impaired or in women with a recent cardiac event, invasive monitoring with an arterial catheter may be appropriate [8].

For prevention or treatment of myocardial ischaemia during delivery, intravenous nitroglycerin, beta-blockers, and calcium antagonists can be used. However, nitroglycerin and calcium antagonists do have tocolytic properties and may prolong labour [8].

To reduce the risk of postpartum haemorrhage, intravenous infusion of oxytocin, less than 2 U/min, can be administered slowly after placental delivery to avoid systemic hypotension. Ergometrine is contraindicated because of the increased risk of coronary artery spasm. Prostaglandin F analogues should be avoided. PGE analogues, sulprostone, 100–500 μg/h, and misoprostol, 200–1000 μg, can be used but with caution [43].

After delivery, maternal monitoring should take place in a high- dependency or intensive care unit for at least 24–48 hours as significant haemodynamic changes and fluid shift occur in this period [40].

Antiplatelet Interruption During Delivery

Patients who suffer a STEMI during pregnancy typically require at least temporary cessation of DAPT before delivery. There is no consensus on the best approach to manage DAPT during delivery. A minimum of 12 months of DAPT for the treatment of STEMI after BMS or DES implantation remains a class I indication, whereas discontinuation after 6 months of treatment in those who are deemed at high risk of bleeding is a class IIb recommendation in the 2016 American College of Cardiology/American Heart Association guideline update on the duration of DAPT inpatients with CAD [36].

Hence, if the patient received DAPT for less than 6 months prior to delivery, clopidogrel should be resumed as soon as it is deemed safe after delivery to complete at least 12 months of DAPT. If the patient received at least 6 months of DAPT prior to delivery, it may be reasonable to withheld reinitiating clopidogrel after delivery if the risk of bleeding outweighs the benefits of continued DAPT [3].

If the patient is receiving DAPT near the time of delivery, it is recommended to discontinue clopidogrel 5 days prior to planned delivery and only bridging with GP IIb/IIIa inhibitors, tirofiban, or eptifibatide, in instances in which the risk of stent thrombosis is high, including those with prior MI, complex PCI, or high thrombosis risk. Tirofiban and eptifibatide should be continued up to 4–6 hours before delivery [28]. Reinitiating GP IIb/IIIa inhibitors after delivery is not recommended, expect in rare cases of complex PCI that are deemed of very high thrombotic burden.

Delivery in Anticoagulated Women

For women with a planned caesarean section, therapeutic LMWH dosing can be simply omitted for 24 hours prior to surgery. If delivery must be performed earlier, then anti-Xa activity can guide the timing of the procedure. If vaginal delivery is planned, moderate- and high-risk patients can be converted to an infusion of UFH with regular checkup of aPTT to optimize control, and the infusion stops at least 4–6 hours prior to anticipated delivery, while for women at low-risk, therapeutic LMWH can be omitted 24 hours prior to anticipated delivery. Anticoagulation can be restarted at 6 hours post-delivery in high-risk women using therapeutic

UFH. Whereas in women at moderate or low-risk, a single prophylactic dose of LMWH can be given 6 hours post-delivery, before restarting therapeutic LMWH 12 hours later [22].

Urgent delivery in a patient taking therapeutic anticoagulation carries a high-risk of maternal haemorrhage. For UFH, protamine sulphate should be given, the exact dose depending on the mode of administration and time since the last dose of UFH. In the case of LMWH, protamine sulphate could be given; however, repeated doses or an infusion of protamine sulphate may be required as the half-life of LMWH is longer and absorption after subcutaneous injection is longer [44].

Anaesthesia Considerations

ACS patients may require an elevated level of monitoring and anaesthetic care for delivery. Neuraxial analgesia for labour and neuraxial anaesthesia for caesarean delivery in the form of spinal, epidural, or combined spinal-epidural is generally preferred. However, it can cause systemic hypotension, which can be minimized by low-dose local anaesthetic techniques and careful titration of vasoconstrictors and intravenous fluids [3].

Another major concern is the risk of epidural hematoma formation and consequent neurological impairment in patients receiving DAPT and anticoagulation [3]. The American Society of Regional Anesthesia and Pain Medicine (ASRA) suggested a new recommendation concerning the higher-dose UFH therapeutic anticoagulation in the pregnant patient that neuraxial block occur 24 hours after SC heparin administration, in case of single dose greater than 10,000 USC or total daily dose greater than 20,000 U, subsequent heparin administration is allowed 1 hour after puncture, catheter manipulation, or removal. The safety of indwelling neuraxial catheters in patients receiving doses greater than 5000 U or greater than 15,000 U of UFH daily has not been established, and the risk and benefits should be assessed on an individual basis. Conversely, there is no change in the recommendation concerning intravenous heparin as to discontinue heparin infusion 4–6 hours prior to neuraxial blockade or removal of the indwelling neuraxial catheters and to delay heparin administration for 1 hour after needle placement or catheter removal [45].

LMWH, 1 mg/kg of enoxaparin BID or 1.5 mg/kg once daily, should be discontinued for at least 12 hours before placement or removal of a neuraxial catheter. A post procedure dose of enoxaparin should usually be given no sooner than 4 hours after catheter removal. Neuraxial anaesthesia can be performed safely in patients receiving aspirin therapy alone. The recommended time interval for discontinuation of clopidogrel is 5–7 days, and it may be reinstituted 24 hours postoperatively, and it may be resumed immediately after needle placement or catheter removal. In patients receiving DTI, ASRA recommends against the performance of neuraxial techniques [45].

Pre-pregnancy Counselling

Women with pre-established ACS are at risk of serious adverse cardiac events during pregnancy, the highest risk of which is seen in atherosclerotic coronary disease. Adverse obstetric outcomes and adverse foetal events are common in them [46].

Pregnancy may be considered in patients with known coronary disease in the absence of residual ischaemia and clinical signs of LV dysfunction. Although there are no high-quality data defining how long pregnancy should be delayed post-ACS, however, delaying pregnancy for 12 months post ACS is recommended. This allows optimization of comorbidities and cardiovascular status as well as adjustment of the medical therapy [22].

There is no definitive evidence that previous coronary artery dissection increases recurrence risk. However, avoidance of further pregnancy is advised, and, if the patient chooses to proceed, close monitoring is recommended [12].

Cardiac patient that wish to get pregnant should be carefully examined and investigated prior to any pregnancy. Investigations should include both ECG at rest and stress ECG, echocardiography, and even coronary CT angiography in certain cases. Women with significantly decreased ejection fraction, symptoms of heart failure, angina pectoris, and advanced coronary artery disease should be discouraged from getting pregnant for fear of aggravating the symptoms and developing serious complications. Antenatal plan for meticulous supervision by both cardiologist and obstetrician and checkup visits all through the pregnancy should be established, noting that all medicines used by women planning to become pregnant should be reviewed [46].

References

1. Elkayam U, Jalnapurkar S, Barakkat MN, Khatri N, Kealey AJ, Mehra A, Roth A. Pregnancy-associated acute myocardial infarction: a review of contemporary experience in 150 cases between 2006 and 2011. Circulation. 2014;129:1695–702.
2. Bush N, Nelson-Piercy C, Spark P, Kurinczuk JJ, Brocklehurst P, Knight M. Myocardial infarction in pregnancy and postpartum in the UK. Eur J Prev Cardiol. 2013;20:12–20.
3. Ismail S, Wong C, Rajan P, Vidovich MI. ST-elevation acute myocardial infarction in pregnancy: 2016 update. Clin Cardiol. 2017;40(6):399–406.
4. Nelson-Piercy C, Adamson D, Knight M. Acute coronary syndrome in pregnancy: time to act. Heart. 2012;98:760–1.
5. Poh CL, Lee CH. Acute myocardial infarction in pregnant women. Ann Acad Med Singap. 2010;39:247–53.
6. Savu O, Jurcut R, Giusca S, Van Mieghem T, Gussi I, Popescu BA, Ginghină C, Rademakers F, Deprest J, Voigt JU. Morphological and functional adaptation of the maternal heart during pregnancy. Circ Cardiovasc Imaging. 2012;5(3):289–97.
7. Söhnchen N, Melzer K, Martinez de Tejada B, Jastrow-Meyer N, Othenin-Girard V, Irion O, Boulvain M, Kayser B. Maternal heart rate changes during labour. Eur J Obst Gynecol Reprod Biol. 2011;158:173–8.

8. Wuntakal R, Shetty N, Ioannou E, Sharma S, Kurian J. Myocardial infarction and pregnancy. Obstet Gynaecol. 2013;15:247–55.
9. Roth A, Elkayam U. Acute myocardial infarction associated with pregnancy. J Am Coll Cardiol. 2008;52:171–80.
10. James AH, Jamison MG, Biswas MS, Brancazio LR, Swamy GK, Myers ER. Acute myocardial infarction in pregnancy: a United States population-based study. Circulation. 2006;113:1564–71.
11. Janion-Sadowska A, Sadowski M, Kurzawski J, Zandecki L, Janion M. Pregnancy after acute coronary syndrome: a proposal for patients' management and a literature review. BioMed Res Int. 2013;2013, Article ID 957027:7 pages.
12. Tweet MS, Hayes SN, Gulati R, Rose CH, Best PJ. Pregnancy after spontaneous coronary artery dissection: a case series. Ann Intern Med. 2015;162:598–600.
13. Vijayaraghavan R, Verma S, Gupta N, Saw J. Pregnancy-related spontaneous coronary artery dissection. Circulation. 2014;130:1915–20.
14. Goland S, Elkayam U. Anticoagulation in pregnancy. Cardiol Clin. 2012;30:395–405.
15. Agewall S, Beltrame JF, Reynolds HR, Niessner A, Rosano G, Caforio AL, De Caterina R, Zimarino M, Roffi M, Kjeldsen K, Atar D, Kaski JC, Sechtem U, Tornvall P. ESC working group position paper on myocardial infarction with non-obstructive coronary arteries. Eur Heart J. 2017;38:143–53.
16. Gordon CT, Jimenez-Fernandez S, Daniels LB, Kahn AM, Tarsa M, Matsubara T, Shimizu C, Burns JC, Gordon JB. Pregnancy in women with a history of Kawasaki disease: management and outcomes. BJOG. 2014;121:1431–8.
17. Practice Bulletin No ACOG. 212: pregnancy and heart disease. Obstet Gynecol. 2019;133(5):e320–56. https://doi.org/10.1097/AOG.0000000000003243.
18. Ibanez B, James S, Agewall S, Antunes MJ, Bucciarelli-Ducci C, Bueno H, Caforio ALP, Crea F, Goudevenos JA, Halvorsen S, Hindricks G, Kastrati A, Lenzen MJ, Prescott E, Roffi M, Valgimigli M, Varenhorst C, Vranckx P, Widimský P, ESC Scientific Document Group. 2017 ESC guidelines for the management of acute myocardial infarction in patients presenting with ST-segment elevation: the task force for the management of acute myocardial infarction in patients presenting with ST-segment elevation of the European Society of Cardiology (ESC). Eur Heart J. 2018;39:119–77.
19. Joyal D, Leya F, Koh M, Besinger R, Ramana R, Kahn S, Jeske W, Lewis B, Steen L, Mestril R, Arab D. Troponin I levels in patients with preeclampsia. Am J Med. 2007;120:819.e13–4.
20. Lancellotti P, Price S, Edvardsen T, Cosyns B, Neskovic AN, Dulgheru R, Flachskampf FA, Hassager C, Pasquet A, Gargani L, Galderisi M, Cardim N, Haugaa KH, Ancion A, Zamorano JL, Donal E, Bueno H, Habib G. The use of echocardiography in acute cardiovascular care: recommendations of the European Association of Cardiovascular Imaging and the Acute Cardiovascular Care Association. Eur Heart J Acute Cardiovasc Care. 2015;4(1):3–5.
21. Cornette J, Ruys TP, Rossi A, Rizopoulos D, Takkenberg JJ, Karamermer Y, Opic P, Van den Bosch AE, Geleijnse ML, Duvekot JJ, Steegers EA, Roos-Hesselink JW. Hemodynamic adaptation to pregnancy in women with structural heart disease. Int J Cardiol. 2013;168:825–31.
22. Regitz-Zagrosek V, Roos-Hesselink JW, Bauersachs J, Blomström-Lundqvist C, Cífková R, De Bonis M, Iung B, Johnson MR, Kintscher U, Kranke P, Lang IM, Morais J, Pieper PG, Presbitero P, Price S, Rosano GMC, Seeland U, Simoncini T, Swan L, Warnes CA, ESC Scientific Document Group. 2018 ESC guidelines for the management of cardiovascular diseases during pregnancy. Eur Heart J. 2018;39(34):3165–241.
23. Thomsen HS. European Society of Urogenital Radiology (ESUR) guidelines on the safe use of iodinated contrast media. Eur J Radiol. 2006;60:307–13.
24. Colletti PM, Lee KH, Elkayam U. Cardiovascular imaging of the pregnant patient. AJR Am J Roentgenol. 2013;200:515–21.
25. Yilmaz S, Sahinkus S, Kilic H, Gunduz H, Akdemir R. Acute coronary syndrome during pregnancy: a case report and literature review. Turk J Emerg Med. 2016;14(3):135–8.

26. Havakuk O, Goland S, Mehra A, Elkayam U. Pregnancy and the risk of spontaneous coronary artery dissection: an analysis of 120 contemporary cases. Circ Cardiovasc Interv. 2017;10:e004941.
27. Frishman WH, Elkayam U, Aronow WS. Cardiovascular drugs in pregnancy. Cardiol Clin. 2012;30:463–91.
28. Amsterdam EA, Wenger NK, Brindis RG, Casey DE, Ganiats TG, Holmes DR, Jaffe AS, Jneid H, Kelly RF, Kontos MC, Levine GN, Liebson PR, Mukherjee D, Peterson ED, Sabatine MS, Smalling RW, Zieman SJ. 2014 AHA/ACC guideline for the management of patients with non-ST-elevation acute coronary syndromes: a report of the American College of Cardiology/American Heart Association Task Force on Practice Guidelines. Circulation. 2014;130:e344–426.
29. Bates SM, Greer IA, Hirsh J, Ginsberg JS. Use of antithrombotic agents during pregnancy: the Seventh ACCP Conference on Antithrombotic and Thrombolytic Therapy. Chest. 2004;126(3):627S–44S.
30. Stone GW, White HD, Ohman EM, Bertrand ME, Lincoff AM, McLaurin BT, Cox DA, Pocock SJ, Ware JH, Feit F, Colombo A, Manoukian SV, Lansky AJ, Mehran R, Moses JW, Acute Catheterization and Urgent Intervention Triage strategy (ACUITY) trial investigators. Bivalirudin in patients with acute coronary syndromes undergoing percutaneous coronary intervention: a subgroup analysis from the Acute Catheterization and Urgent Intervention Triage strategy (ACUITY) trial. Lancet. 2007;369:907–19.
31. Ekbatani A, Asaro LR, Malinow AM. Anticoagulation with argatroban in a parturient with heparin-induced thrombocytopenia. Int J Obstet Anesth. 2010;19:82–7.
32. White HD, Kleiman NS, Mahaffey KW, Lokhnygina Y, Pieper KS, Chiswell K, Cohen M, Harrington RA, Chew DP, Petersen JL, Berdan LG, Aylward PE, Nessel CC, Ferguson JJ 3rd, Califf RM. Efficacy and safety of enoxaparin compared with unfractionated heparin in high-risk patients with non-ST-segment elevation acute coronary syndrome undergoing percutaneous coronary intervention in the Superior Yield of the New Strategy of Enoxaparin, Revascularization and Glycoprotein IIb/IIIa Inhibitors (SYNERGY) trial. Am Heart J. 2006;152:1042–50.
33. Gibson CM, Ten Y, Murphy SA, Ciaglo LN, Southard MC, Lincoff AM, Waksman R. Association of prerandomization anticoagulant switching with bleeding in the setting of percutaneous coronary intervention (A REPLACE-2 analysis). Am J Cardiol. 2007;99:1687–90.
34. Tawfik MM, Taman ME, Motawea AA, Abdel-Hady E. Thrombolysis for the management of massive pulmonary embolism in pregnancy. Int J Obstet Anesth. 2013;22:149–52.
35. Ntusi NA, Samuels P, Moosa S, Mocumbi AO. Diagnosing cardiac disease during pregnancy: Imaging modalities. Cardiovasc J Afr. 2016;27:95–103.
36. Levine GN, Bates ER, Bittl JA, Brindis RG, Fihn SD, Fleisher LA, Granger CB, Lange RA, Mack MJ, Mauri L, Mehran R, Mukherjee D, Newby LK, O'Gara PT, Sabatine MS, Smith PK, Smith SC Jr. 2016 ACC/AHA guideline focused update on duration of dual antiplatelet therapy in patients with coronary artery disease: a report of the American College of Cardiology/ American Heart Association Task Force on Clinical Practice Guidelines. J Am Coll Cardiol. 2016;68:1082–115.
37. Kapoor MC. Cardiopulmonary bypass in pregnancy. Ann Card Anaesth. 2014;17:33–9.
38. Hosseini S, Kashfi F, Samiei N, Khamoushi A, Ghavidel AA, Yazdanian F, Mirmesdagh Y, Mestres CA. Feto-maternal outcomes of urgent open-heart surgery during pregnancy. J Heart Valve Dis. 2015;24:253–9.
39. John AS, Gurley F, Schaff HV, Warnes CA, Phillips SD, Arendt KW, Abel MD, Rose CH, Connolly HM. Cardiopulmonary bypass during pregnancy. Ann Thorac Surg. 2011;91:1191–6.
40. Ruys TP, Roos-Hesselink JW, Pijuan-Domenech A, Vasario E, Gaisin IR, Iung B, Freeman LJ, Gordon EP, Pieper PG, Hall R, Boersma E, Johnson MR. Is a planned caesarean section in women with cardiac disease beneficial? Heart. 2015;101:530–6.
41. Ramsey PS, Hogg BB, Savage KG, Winkler DD, Owen J. Cardiovascular effects of intravaginal misoprostol in the mid trimester of pregnancy. Am J Obstet Gynecol. 2000;183:1100–2.

42. Kilpatrick AW, Thorburn J. Severe hypotension due to intramyometrial injection of prostaglandin E2. Anaesthesia. 1990;45:848–9.
43. Cauldwell M, Steer PJ, Swan L, Uebing A, Gatzoulis MA, Johnson MR. The management of the third stage of labour in women with heart disease. Heart. 2017;103:945–51.
44. Van Veen JJ, Maclean RM, Hampton KK, Laidlaw S, Kitchen S, Toth P, Makris M. Protamine reversal of low molecular weight heparin: clinically effective? Blood Coagul Fibrinolysis. 2011;22:565–70.
45. Horlocker TT, Vandermeuelen E, Kopp SL, Gogarten W, Leffert LR, Benzon HT. Regional anesthesia in the patient receiving antithrombotic or thrombolytic therapy American Society of Regional Anesthesia and Pain Medicine evidence-based guidelines (fourth edition). Reg Anesth Pain Med. 2018;43:263–309.
46. Burchill LJ, Lameijer H, Roos-Hesselink JW, Grewal J, Ruys TP, Kulikowski JD, Burchill LA, Oudijk MA, Wald RM, Colman JM, Siu SC, Pieper PG, Silversides CK. Pregnancy risks in women with pre-existing coronary artery disease, or following acute coronary syndrome. Heart. 2015;101:525–9.

Chapter 35
Aortic Dissection in Pregnancy

Juan Carlos Barrientos Rojas

Introduction

Acute aortic dissection is the most common life-threatening disorder affecting the aorta [1], the immediate mortality rate in aortic dissection is as high as 1% per hour over the first several hours [2], and an early diagnosis is important to improve survival. It is uncommon to complicate pregnancy but potentially fatal for the mother and fetus [3]. Although hormonal changes in the aortic wall have been theorized as potentially playing a role, cystic medial degeneration is the pathology underlying many thoracic aortic aneurysms and dissection, and abnormalities in the transforming growth factor-B pathway and abnormalities in smooth muscle cell contractile element function may underlie certain aortic dissections. Classification for aortic dissection is based on anatomic involvement of the aortic dissection. In the DeBakey classification, type I dissections originate in the ascending aorta and extend to at least the aortic arch, type II dissections involve the ascending aorta only, and type III dissections begin in the descending aorta, usually just distal to the left subclavian artery. In the Stanford classification, type A dissections involve the ascending aorta, and type B dissections are those that do not involve the ascending aorta. The patient must undergo emergency cesarean section and aortic dissection repair in most cases [4].

The incidence of aortic complications was 5.5 per million patients during pregnancy and the postpartum period versus 1.4 per million during the control period (incidence rate ratio, 4.0; 95% confidence interval, 2.0–8.2). Pregnant women face a several-fold higher risk of venous thromboembolism, myocardial infarction, and stroke than nonpregnant women of childbearing age. These risks extend for several months into the postpartum period [5–8].

J. C. B. Rojas (✉)
Head of the Critical Obstetrics Unit, Gynecology and Obstetrics Department, Hospital General San Juan de Dios, University of San Carlos de Guatemala, Guatemala City, Guatemala

C. Montufar et al. (eds.), *Obstetric Catastrophes*,
https://doi.org/10.1007/978-3-030-70034-8_35

Risk Factors

Case series suggest that pregnancy may trigger aortic dissection or rupture, but few population-based data exist to support an association between pregnancy and aortic complications. Pregnancy and the postpartum state cause hemodynamic changes, such as increases in heart rate, stroke volume, cardiac output, and left ventricular dimensions, which may affect the forces on the aortic wall. This may be exacerbated by increased outflow resistance in the distal aorta attributable to compression by the gravid uterus. Pregnancy also causes hormonal and biochemical changes that may modify the ability of the aorta to withstand the hemodynamic effects placed on it.

Estrogen receptors are present in aortic tissue and may mediate the effect of pregnancy-induced hormonal changes on the weakening of elastic fibers [9–12] organization and vascular integrity.

Is uncommon that acute aortic dissection complicates pregnancy and usually occurs during labor, delivery, or in the early postpartum period.

Other causes of hypertension like preeclampsia, pheochromocytoma, and heavy weight lifting are associated [13, 14]. Women with uncontrolled hypertension from preeclampsia, compounded by the stress and hemodynamic changes accompanying labor, are predisposed to dissection as the aorta experiences increased shearing forces [15].

Motor vehicle accident in the context of thoracic trauma may increase the risk of acute aortic dissection, and cocaine use is also a risk factor because acute hemodynamic stress and both are usually present at the same time.

Genetic disorders affecting the aorta with aneurysm and/or dissection, like Marfan syndrome, Loeys-Dietz aneurysm syndrome, vascular Ehlers-Danlos syndrome, and bicuspid aortic valve, are associated in about 10%. Turner syndrome and familial heterozygous mutation in *MYH11* are often underrecognized because they are less common, and a mutation analysis may detect and confirm familial thoracic aortic aneurysm/dissection (TAA/D) [13, 16].

Coarctation of the aorta and tetralogy of Fallot are congenital diseases potentially to aortic dissection, and prior cardiovascular surgery, aortic valve replacement, angiography or stenting, intra-aortic balloon pump, coronary artery bypass surgery, and atherosclerosis ulcer are under-considered risk factors.

In general patients with thoracic aneurisms from any cause are at risk for aortic dissection, with absolute size, especially more than 5 to 6 cm, age, body surface area, sex, rate of growth, and specific genetic disorder as modulating risks of dissection.

Infrequently inflammatory diseases like giant cell arteritis, Takayasu arteritis, aortitis, and Behcet disease are related, as well as infectious diseases like syphilis.

Aortic complications are particularly common in those with connective tissue disorders and in those with a family history but may also occur in the absence of these risk factors [17–19]. The lack of knowledge of underlying Marfan syndrome diagnosis in almost 50% of registry women with aortic dissection related to pregnancy is a common finding in the existing literature and underscores the need for early diagnosis, prepregnancy risk counseling, and multidisciplinary peripartum management [20, 21].

Clinical Presentation and Diagnosis

The clinical manifestations are sudden onset of severe chest, back, or abdominal pain, which may be migratory or radiate to the abdomen or inferior extremities, and shortness of breath, making early diagnosis and treatment critical for survival, so a high index of suspicion is important in the early identification and better outcomes, especially when risk factors are present or signs and symptoms suggest it [22, 23].

Hypertension is present in about 75% of cases, especially in patients with type B dissections, contrary to type A dissection which are normotensive or hypotensive [4], so preeclampsia is a risk factor to consider strongly. Acute aortic dissection with hypotension is related to cardiac tamponade, aortic rupture, or heart failure associated with severe aortic regurgitation.

Chest X-ray shows an abnormal aortic contour or widening of the aortic silhouette, present in more than 80%. However, 12–15% will be normal, the ECG changes are nonspecific.

D-dimer levels are elevated, but its accuracy in pregnancy is lowest because of physiology changes. However, within the first 24 h of symptom onset, a D-dimer level <500 ng/ml had a negative likelihood ratio of 0.07 and a negative predictive value of 95% [24].

Multidetector computed tomography, transesophageal echocardiogram, and magnetic resonance imaging are highly accurate in the diagnosis of aortic dissection [13, 25].

Pregnancy increases the risk of aortic complications in women with an aortic root diameter <40 mm or <45 mm, which are the thresholds currently recommended for deciding on the safety of pregnancy in women with Marfan syndrome or other connective tissue disorders [26, 27]. Pyeritz recommended against pregnancy in women with aortic diameters over 40 mm [28]. However, in more recently based data, the investigators suggested that pregnancy in the absence of preexisting aortic dissection is safe up to 45 mm [20].

Other manifestations are symptoms of heart failure from acute aortic regurgitation, neurological deficits like stroke, spinal cord ischemia, ischemic neuropathy, and hypoxic encephalopathy are more common in type A dissections, syncope, or vascular insufficiency may be caused by cardiac tamponade, aortic rupture with left pleural effusions or hemothorax signals, cerebral vessel obstruction, or activation of cerebral baroreceptors. Sudden chest or back pain with pulse deficits, aortic regurgitation, or neurological manifestations should alert the clinician to the diagnosis of acute aortic dissection.

Coronary artery dissection presents in the postpartum period. Myocardial infarction or coronary ischemia is a particularly dangerous complication, because of the dissection flap obstructing coronary flow. Renal ischemia or renovascular hypertension is a result of the dissection process.

Management

The multidisciplinary evaluation of the patient with acute aortic dissection should be carried out in conjunction with the cardilogist and cardiovascular surgeon.

Initially includes stabilization of the patient, using beta blockers as the first drugs of choice reducing ventricular force and stress on the aorta and for long-term medical management. Control of hypertension with multiple agents is required, and angiotensin receptor blockers, by antagonizing transforming growth factor-B, may be beneficial in certain genetically disorders. When refractory hypertension exists, renovascular hypertension related to the dissection flap must be considered [20, 21, 29, 30].

Ascending dissections type requires emergency surgical repair and is the most common in pregnancy, whereas medical therapy is usually for uncomplicated acute type B dissections [13]. The patient must undergo emergency cesarean section and aortic dissection repair, which includes excision of the intimal tear when possible, obliteration of entry into the false lumen, and interposition graft replacement in the ascending aorta. The aortic valve may need to be replaced [31].

Most type B dissections are managed medically during pregnancy, although indications for operative intervention include fetal distress, expanding dissection, and evidence of compromised end-organ perfusion. The thoracic endovascular aortic repair is safe in women diagnosed with type B aortic dissections late in the third trimester of pregnancy [32].

The mortality rate of patients undergoing surgery for type A dissection is 26% and for those treated medically is 58% related with malperfusion, shock, or cardiac tamponade. Uncomplicated type B dissection has a mortality rate of about 10%, but those whom require emergency surgery have a mortality rate of about 25–50%, which includes aortic rupture and visceral or branch vessel ischemia. Endovascular grafts are the first option [4].

Prognosis

Lifelong imaging with regular intervals is important to detect complications like aneurysmal enlargement. Limitations on physical activity and certain types of employment are important [33].

Short- and long-term survival in acute type A dissection has ranged between 52% and 94% at 1 year and 45% and 88% at 5 years [34]. The 10-year actual survival rate of patients with acute dissection who survive initial hospitalization is reported as 30–60% in various studies. Other study reported a 10-year survival of 55% and 20-year survival of 30% after type A dissection [35].

Screening first-degree relatives of the patient with acute aortic dissection for thoracic aortic disease must be considered, because about 20% will be affected [36]. Obtaining this information is important for assessing risks in pregnancy counseling, prenatal care, and peripartum care.

Women who are aware of their underlying diagnosis may receive prepregnancy counseling, choose to forego pregnancy, have careful monitoring and take beta-blockers during pregnancy, or undergo prophylactic aortic surgery in anticipation of pregnancy, if indicated [37].

References

1. Baverman AC. Acute aortic dissection, clinician update. Circulation. 2010;122:184–8.
2. Hagan PG, et al. International Registry of Acute Aortic Dissection (IRAD): new insights from an old disease. JAMA. 2000;283:897–903.
3. Curry RA, Gelson E, Swan L, Dob D, Babu-Narayan SV, Gatzoulis MA, Steer PJ, Johnson MR. Marfan syndrome and pregnancy maternal and neonatal outcomes. Br J Obstet Gynaecol. 2014;121:610–7.
4. Milewicz DM, Guo DC, Tran-Fadulu V, Lafont AL, Papke CL, Inamoto S, Kwartler CS, Pannu H. Genetic basis of thoracic aortic aneurysms and dissections: focus on smooth muscle cell contractile dysfunction. Annu Rev Genomics Hum Genet. 2008;9:283–302.
5. Heit JA, Kobbervig CE, James AH, Petterson TM, Bailey KR, Melton LJ 3rd. Trends in the incidence of venous thromboembolism during pregnancy or postpartum: a 30-year population-based study. Ann Intern Med. 2005;143:697–706.
6. James AH, Jamison MG, Biswas MS, Brancazio LR, Swamy GK, Myers ER. Acute myocardial infarction in pregnancy: a United States population-based study. Circulation. 2006;113:1564–71.
7. Kittner SJ, Stern BJ, Feeser BR, Hebel R, Nagey DA, Buchholz DW, Earley CJ, Johnson CJ, Macko RF, Sloan MA, Wityk RJ, Wozniak MA. Pregnancy and the risk of stroke. N Engl J Med. 1996;335:768–74.
8. Kamel H, Navi BB, Sriram N, Hovsepian DA, Devereux RB, Elkind MS. Risk of a thrombotic event after the 6-week postpartum period. N Engl J Med. 2014;370:1307–15.
9. Immer FF, Bansi AG, Immer-Bansi AS, McDougall J, Zehr KJ, Schaff HV, Carrel TP. Aortic dissection in pregnancy: analysis of risk factors and outcome. Ann Thorac Surg. 2003;76:309–14.
10. Ohlson L. Effects of the pregnant uterus on the abdominal aorta and its branches. Acta Radiol Diagn (Stockh). 1978;19:369–76.
11. Manalo-Estrella P, Barker AE. Histopathologic findings in human aortic media associated with pregnancy. Arch Pathol. 1967;83:336–41.
12. Loeys BL, et al. Aneurysm syndromes caused by mutations in the TGF-beta receptor. N Engl J Med. 2006;355:788–98.
13. Braverman AC, Thompson R, Sanchez L. Diseases of the aorta. In: Bonow RO, Mann DL, Zipes DP, Libby P, editors. Braunwald's heart disease. 9th ed. Philadelphia: Elsevier; 2011.
14. Sawlani N, Shroff A, Vidovich MI. Aortic dissection and mortality associated with pregnancy in the United States. J Am Coll Cardiol. 2015;65:1600–1. https://doi.org/10.1016/j.jacc.2014.12.066.
15. Huang J, Liu H, Ding YL. Two cases of acute aortic dissection following preeclampsia in non-Marfan patients. Chin Med J. 2012;125:2073–5.

16. Braverman AC, Beardslee MA. The bicuspid aortic valve. In: Otto C, Bonow R, editors. Valvular heart disease: a companion to Braunwald's heart disease. Philadelphia: Saunders/Elsevier; 2009. p. 169–86.
17. Gelpi G, Pettinari M, Lemma M, Mangini A, Vanelli P, Antona C. Should pregnancy be considered a risk factor for aortic dissection? Two cases of acute aortic dissection following cesarean section in non-Marfan nor bicuspid aortic valve patients. J Cardiovasc Surg. 2008;49:389–91.
18. Weissmann-Brenner A, Schoen R, Divon MY. Aortic dissection in pregnancy. Obstet Gynecol. 2004;103(5 pt 2):1110–3.
19. Snir E, Levinsky L, Salomon J, Findler M, Levy MJ, Vidne BA. Dissecting aortic aneurysm in pregnant women without Marfan disease. Surg Gynecol Obstet. 1988;167:463–5.
20. Meijboom LJ, Vos FE, Timmermans J, Boers GH, Zwinderman AH, Mulder BJM. Pregnancy and aortic root growth in the Marfan syndrome: a prospective study. Eur Heart J. 2005;26:914–20.
21. Donnelly RT, Pinto NM, Kocolas I, Yetman AT. The immediate and long-term impact of pregnancy on aortic growth rate and mortality in women with Marfan syndrome. J Am Coll Cardiol. 2012;60:224–9.
22. Husebye KO, Wolff HJ, Freidman LL. Aortic dissection in pregnancy: a case of Marfan's syndrome. Am Heart J. 1958;55:662–76.
23. Sutinen S, Piiroinen O. Marfan syndrome, pregnancy, and fatal dissection of aorta. Acta Obstet Gynecol Scand. 1971;50:295–300.
24. Suzuki T, et al. For the IRAD-Bio Investigators. Diagnosis of acute aortic dissection by D-dimer: the International Registry of Acute Aortic Dissection Substudy on Biomarkers (IRAD-bio) experience. Circulation. 2009;119:2702–7.
25. Hiratzka LF, et al. Guidelines for the diagnosis and management of patients with thoracic aortic disease: a report of the 2010 ACCF/AHA/AATS/ACR/ASA/SCA/SCAI/SIR/STS/SVM. Circulation. 2010;121(13):e266–369.
26. Regitz-Zagrosek V, et al. ESC guidelines on the management of cardiovascular diseases during pregnancy. Eur Heart J. 2011;32:3147–97.
27. Baumgartner H. ESC guidelines for the management of grownup congenital heart disease (new version 2010). Eur Heart J. 2010;31:2915–57.
28. Pyeritz RE. Maternal and fetal complications of pregnancy in the Marfan syndrome. Am J Med. 1981;71:784–90.
29. Rossiter JP, Repke JT, Morales AJ, Murphy EA, Pyeritz RE. A prospective longitudinal evaluation of pregnancy in the Marfan syndrome. Am J Obstet Gynecol. 1995;173:1599–606.
30. Oskoui R, Lindsay J Jr. Aortic dissection in women < 40 years of age and the unimportance of pregnancy. Am J Cardiol. 1994;73:821–3.
31. Pacini L, Digne F, Boumendil A, Muti C, Detaint D, Boileau C, Jondeau G. Maternal complication of pregnancy in Marfan syndrome. Int J Cardiol. 2009;136:156–61.
32. Shu C, Fang K, Dardik A, Li X, Li M. Pregnancy-associated type B aortic dissection treated with thoracic endovascular aneurysm repair. Ann Thorac Surg. 2014;97:582–7. https://doi.org/10.1016/j.athoracsur.2013.09.009.
33. Rosenblum NG, Grossman AR, Gabbe SG, Mennuti MT, Cohen AW. Failure of serial echocardiographic studies to predict aortic dissection in a pregnant patient with Marfan's syndrome. Am J Obstet Gynecol. 1983;146:470–1.
34. Tsai TT, et al. International registry of acute aortic dissection. Circulation. 2006;114:2226–31.
35. Stevens LM, Madsen JC, Isselbacher EM, Khairy P, MacGillivray TE, Hilgenberg AD, Agnihotri AK. Surgical management and long-term outcomes of acute ascending aortic dissection. J Thorac Cardiovasc Surg. 2009;138:1349–57.
36. Albornoz G, Coady MA, Roberts M, Davies RR, Tranquilli M, Rizzo JA, Elefteriades JA. Familial thoracic aortic aneurysms and dissections:incidence, modes of inheritance, and phenotypic patterns. Ann Thorac Surg. 2006;82:1400–5.
37. Roman MJ, et al. Aortic complications associated with pregnancy in Marfan syndrome: the NHLBI National Registry of Genetically Triggered Thoracic Aortic Aneurysms and Cardiovascular Conditions (GenTAC). J Am Heart Assoc. 2016;5:e004052.

Chapter 36
Cardiac Tamponade

Juan Carlos Barrientos Rojas

Introduction

Cardiac tamponade is characterized by hemodynamic instability due to heart compression by accumulation of fluid, blood, clots, or gas in the pericardial space, secondary to infectious diseases, autoimmune disorders, radiation-induced diseases, malignancies, chronic myxedema, renal failure, trauma, iatrogenic, anticoagulation, uremia, neoplasm, pneumopericardium and hemopericardium in aortic dissection, and rupture of the heart after acute myocardial infarction. The context of pregnancy is associated with preeclampsia [1–4]. The incidence of pericardial effusion during pregnancy is about 40%, usually in the third trimester, asymptomatic, incidental echo finding, and often resolves by 2 months postpartum [4]. It has been reported that hypertension of pregnancy is an etiological factor of pericardial effusion although the presence of such effusions is generally asymptomatic, and no treatment is required [5].

Pathophysiology

Normally, 30ml or less of pericardial fluid exists between the two layers. When intrapericardial pressure exceeds intracardiac pressures, cardiac tamponade develops. The stability depends on intrapericardial pressure not exceeding right heart filling pressures.

Pericardial effusion is found in 15%, 19.2%, and 40% of pregnant women in the first, second, and third trimesters, respectively, and disappears spontaneously within 50–60 days after labor. An increase in total body fluid volume during the pregnancy is likely to be one of the mechanisms for this phenomenon. The rate of pericardial

J. C. B. Rojas (✉)
Head of the Critical Obstetrics Unit, Gynecology and Obstetrics Department, Hospital General San Juan de Dios, University of San Carlos de Guatemala, Guatemala City, Guatemala

C. Montufar et al. (eds.), *Obstetric Catastrophes*,
https://doi.org/10.1007/978-3-030-70034-8_36

effusion was higher among pregnant women with preeclampsia than among unaffected pregnant women. However, pericardial effusion during pregnancy is generally asymptomatic, and the presence of such effusion is not attributed to maternal cardiac dysfunction [6–11].

In pregnancy the result of excessive salt and body fluid retention may increase the risk to develop cardiac tamponade. Haiat and Halphen pointed out that the mean weight gain is significantly higher in women showing signs of pericardial effusion than in others whose echocardiograms are free of any effusion at the same stage of gestation. Abduljabbar et al. showed that subjects who gained more than 12 kg during pregnancy have an increased risk of developing pericardial effusions [6–8]. Hypoalbuminemia and an increase in peripheral vascular permeability together with excessive volume of fluid transfusion may have augmented retention of pericardial effusions.

Reddy et al. described three phases of hemodynamic changes in tamponade. In phase I, the accumulation of pericardial fluid "stiffens" the ventricles and impairs their relaxation. Ventricular filling pressures are increased but remain higher than the intrapericardial pressure. In phase II, further fluid accumulation increases intrapericardial pressure above right ventricular filling pressure. Systemic venous pressure is unable to fill the right heart, resulting in a decrease in cardiac output. In phase III, a further decrease in cardiac output leading to circulatory collapse occurs when intrapericardial pressure equilibrates with left ventricle filling pressure. Low-pressure tamponade develops when intrapericardial pressure exceeds right heart filling pressure in a hypovolemic patient. Here, the low right ventricular filling pressure may be normalized by volume loading. The increase in systemic venous return restores right heart filling pressure, allowing forward flow of blood [12, 13].

Interventricular interdependence, an increase in right ventricle size during spontaneous inspiration, will induce a septal shift of the interventricular septum toward the left ventricle, resulting in decreased left ventricle dimension and output [14].

Diagnosis

Usually a cardiogenic obstructive shock is present, with hypotension, shortness of breath, tachycardia, a narrow pulse pressure, venous jugular distension, with central venous pressure increased, and muffled heart sounds, pericardial friction rub, and paradoxus pulsus. In pregnancy the clinical signs may be subtle.

Electrocardiography shows QRS voltage and electrical alternans. Chest X-ray shows an enlarged cardia silhouette [15, 16]. Echocardiography is the best diagnostic method for detection of pericardial effusion and tamponade. Pericardial effusion is usually visualized as an echo-free space between the visceral and parietal pericardium surrounding the heart, but hemorrhagic or purulent fluid may be more echogenic than simple serous fluid. The fluid first accumulates posterior to the heart, when the patient is examined in the supine position. A "swinging" heart may be observed when the effusion is massive, as well as a heart collapse, especially right atria at end diastole, and then right ventricle outflow tract at early diastole. Left chamber collapses are uncommon [17, 18].

Management

In the obstetric patient, the treatment should proceed as in the nonpregnant patient.

The treatment involves urgent drainage of the pericardial fluid, triggered by the integration of clinical and echocardiographic findings and by pericardiocentesis or surgical drainage in some cases. Fluid loading may improve cardiac index in half of patients, while the other half may require norepinephrine to increase blood pressure. Vasodilators and diuretics are not recommended [19–22].

The reduction in venous return induced by positive pressure mechanical ventilation and general anesthetics may decompensate cardiac tamponade. Intubation should therefore be cautious (with some authors suggesting the use of local anesthetics or ketamine) and high ventilatory pressures avoided [23].

Careful monitoring of thyroid functional tests and proper management should be performed in pregnant women with hypothyroidism to prevent cardiac complications of the disease, like pericardial effusion and tamponade [24].

The outcomes of pregnancies in women with pericardial disease are similar to those expected in the general population with pericardial disease. More difficult cases may require a multidisciplinary approach involving different subspecialties (e.g., cardiology, internal medicine, maternal-fetal medicine, and neonatology).

References

1. Adler Y, Charron P, Imazio M, et al. 2015 ESC guidelines for the diagnosis and management of pericardial diseases: the Task Force for the Diagnosis and Management of Pericardial Diseases of the European Society of Cardiology (ESC) endorsed by: the European Association for Cardio-Thoracic Surgery (EACTS). Eur Heart J. 2015;36:2921–64.
2. Risti AD, Imazio M, Adler Y, et al. Triage strategy for urgent management of cardiac tamponade: a position statement of the European Society of Cardiology Working Group on Myocardial and Pericardial Diseases. Eur Heart J. 2014;35:2279.
3. Swaminathan A, Kandaswamy K, Powari M, Mathew J. Eur Heart J. Dying from cardiac tamponade 35:2279–2284. World J Emerg Surg. 2007;2:22.
4. Imazio M, Brucato A, Rampello S, et al. Management of pericardial diseases during pregnancy. J Cardiovasc Med (Hagerstown). 2010;11:557–62.
5. Matsuki R, et al. Cardiac tamponade in pregnancy during the treatment of severe pre-eclampsia: report of a case. J Obstet Gynecol Res. 2014;40(3):826–8.
6. Haiat R, Halphen C. Silent pericardial effusion in late pregnancy: a new entity. Cardiovasc Intervent Radiol. 1984;7:267–9.
7. Enein M, Zina A, Kassem M, El-tabbakh G. Echocardiography of the pericardium in pregnancy. Obstet Gynecol. 1987;69:851–3.
8. Abduljabbar HSO, Marzouki KMH, Zawawi TH, Khan AS. Pericardial effusion in normal pregnant women. Acta Obstet Gynecol Scand. 1991;70:291–4.

9. Gabbe SG, Niebyl JR, Simpson JL. Obstetrics, normal and problem pregnancies. 1st ed. Edinburgh: Churchill Livingstene; 1986. p. 137–53.
10. Vitse M, Lesbre JP, Boulanger JG, Kalisa A, Camier B. Notre experience du depistage des epanchements pericardiques latents au troisieme trimester de la grossesse. Rev Fr Gynecol Obstet. 1984;79:765–9.
11. Yuan L, Duan Y, Cao T. Echocardiographic study of cardiac morphological and functional changes before and after parturition in pregnancy-induced hypertension. Echocardiography. 2006;23:177–82.
12. Reddy PS, Curtiss EI, Uretsky BF. Spectrum of hemodynamic changes in cardiac tamponade. Am J Cardiol. 1990;66:1487–91.
13. Sagrista-Sauleda J, Angel J, Sambola A, et al. Low-pressure cardiac tamponade: clinical and hemodynamic profile. Circulation. 2006;114:945–52.
14. Hamzaoui O, Monnet X, Teboul J-L. Pulsus paradoxus. Eur Respir J. 2013;42:1696–705.
15. Argulian E, Herzog E, Halpern DG, Messerli FH. Paradoxical hypertension with cardiac tamponade. Am J Cardiol. 2012;110:1066–9.
16. Gauchat HW, Katz LN. Observations on pulsus paradoxus (with special reference to pericardial effusions): I. Clinical. Arch Intern Med. 1924;33:350–70.
17. Grumann A, Baretto L, Dugard A, et al. Localized cardiac tamponade after open-heart surgery. Ann Thorac Cardiovasc Surg. 2012;18:524–9.
18. Gillam LD, Guyer DE, Gibson TC, et al. Hydrodynamic compression of the right atrium: a new echocardiographic sign of cardiac tamponade. Circulation. 1983;68:294–301.
19. Tsang TSM, Enriquez-Sarano M, Freeman WK, et al. Consecutive 1127 therapeutic echocardiographically guided pericardiocenteses: clinical profile, practice patterns, and outcomes spanning 21 years. Mayo Clin Proc. 2002;77:429–36.
20. Furst B, Liu C-JJ, Hansen P, Musuku SR. Concurrent pericardial and pleural effusions: a double jeopardy. J Clin Anesth. 2016;33:341–5.
21. Sagristà-Sauleda J, Angel J, Sambola A, Permanyer-Miralda G. Hemodynamic effects of volume expansion in patients with cardiac tamponade. Circulation. 2008;117:1545–9.
22. Martins JB, Manuel WJ, Marcus ML, Kerber RE. Comparative effects of catecholamines in cardiac tamponade: experimental and clinical studies. Am J Cardiol. 1980;46:59–66.
23. Ho AM-H, Graham CA, Ng CSH, et al. Timing of tracheal intubation in traumatic cardiac tamponade: a word of caution. Resuscitation. 2009;80:272–4.
24. Kudaiberdiev T, et al. Gross pericardial effusion with tamponade in 2 nd trimester of pregnancy. Cent Eur J Med. 2010;5(3):369–71.

Chapter 37
Cardiac Arrest in Pregnancy

Carlos Montufar

Introduction

Cardiac arrest is a maternal and perinatal tragedy, with a great medical and social impact. Its exact incidence is unknown, since there is a subrecord of these events, but it has been classically estimated to occur in 0.6–1 / 30,000 pregnancies [1, 2]. However, the most recent UK confidential enquiry reports an incidence of cardiac arrest in 1:20 000 pregnancies [3].

There has been an increase in pregnancies in women over 35, largely due to the rise in assisted reproduction. These pregnancies in older reproductive ages lead to patients with a higher probability of both direct obstetric complications, as well as a higher incidence of medical complications.

The pregnant patient who undergoes a cardiac arrest will have a different pathophysiological connotation, with a physiology that generates great changes in her hemodynamic and respiratory physiology, which will produce variations in her approach. In addition, the pathologies of pregnancy, such as amniotic fluid embolism and the presence of the fetus, complicate the challenge.

The survival rates of out-of-hospital cardiac arrests continue to decrease (2–5%), with improved rates reported for in-hospital cardiac arrests (15%) [4].

Most out-of-hospital cardiac arrests occur in shockable rhythms (ventricular tachycardia or ventricular fibrillation), unlike most patients who undergo cardiac arrest inside hospitals, where cardiac arrests with non-shockable rhythms are most frequent (asystole or pulseless electrical activity) [4].

C. Montufar (✉)
Obstetrics Critical Care Unit, Fellowship Program of Critical Care Obstetrics, Complejo Hospitalario, Caja de Seguro Social, Panama City, Panama

C. Montufar et al. (eds.), *Obstetric Catastrophes*,
https://doi.org/10.1007/978-3-030-70034-8_37

Physiological Considerations

The most important respiratory changes are edema and hyperemia of the vocal cords, a decrease in functional residual capacity, a decrease in compliance with the chest wall, an increase in minute ventilation, and an increase in oxygen consumption. These changes will generate the need for the use of smaller caliber endotracheal tubes, increased difficulty with bag-mask ventilation, greater rapidity in producing hypoxemia, and a marked intolerance to hypo-oxygenated states [5]. Failed intubation is eight times more frequent in pregnant than in non-obstetric patients [6].

Regarding the physiology of the cardiovascular system, the pregnant woman has an increase in cardiac output; as a result of the size of the pregnant uterus, a compression of both the aortic artery and the inferior vena cava originates, leading to an obstruction of the aortic flow and a decrease in venous return [7–9].

These changes cause a decrease in preload, a very limited cardiac output during resuscitation. In addition, it reduces the effectiveness of chest compressions and forces the uterus to move to the left to decompress the aorto-caval vascular system [10].

The gastrointestinal system of pregnant women has an increased intragastric pressure, a delay in gastric emptying, and a relaxation of the lower esophageal sphincter, which facilitates gastroesophageal reflux and bronchoaspiration [11]. Another important change is the dilutional anemia that the pregnant patient develops as a result of the increase in plasma volume, which, if not treated with an oral iron supplement during her prenatal evaluation, can aggravate hypoxemic or hemorrhagic states.

Causes

Knowing better the underlying cause of the cardiac arrest, as well as the rate of cardiac arrest, it is possible to improve the survival rates of these patients. In addition, it is necessary to know the maternal physiology, for the correct approach to this subgroup of patients.

Like all complications in the pregnant patient, the scenarios or conditions that can lead to cardiac arrest are divided into direct obstetrics, underlying medical causes, and iatrogenic (magnesium sulfate overdose).

In general, the most common causes of cardiac arrest are thromboembolism, preeclampsia/eclampsia, sepsis, trauma, massive obstetric hemorrhage (ectopic pregnancy and uterine atony), stroke, asthma, anesthetic complications, preexisting chronic cardiac or pulmonary disease, and amniotic fluid embolism [12].

The causes of cardiac arrest are different when compared to developed countries with countries with lower economic incomes. In the United States as in England, the main cause of cardiac arrest is pulmonary thromboembolism [13]. But in low-income countries, the most frequent causes are obstetric hemorrhage associated with hypovolemic shock [4] and the most severe complications of preeclampsia, especially when hemolysis, elevated liver enzyme, and low platelets (HELLP) syndrome is involved [14].

The amniotic fluid embolism or anaphylactoid syndrome of pregnancy is a rare but important cause of obstetric circulatory collapse and cardiac arrest associated with a high mortality [3]. It is responsible for about 10% of maternal deaths in the United States and 8.4% in the United Kingdom [15].

In general terms, most causes of cardiac or near cardiac arrest mediate through potentially reversible causes if they are timely recognized and properly handled. The latter include the 5 Hs and the 5 Ts: hypovolemia, hypoxia, acidosis (hydrogen ions), hypokalemia and hyperkalemia, hypothermia, hypoglycemia (Hs), and trauma, cardiac tamponade, tension pneumothorax, thrombosis, and drug toxicity (Ts) [16].

Approach

In most serious or critical clinical situations, the approach of the pregnant patient does not change with respect to the approach established in the non-obstetric population, with some exceptions.

Basic Life Support (BLS) and Advanced Cardiovascular Life Support (ACLS) guidelines for nonpregnant patients pertain in large part to maternal cardiac arrest, including basic cardiopulmonary resuscitation (CPR), pharmacology, and defibrillation. But these exceptions in the pregnant patient are important for better results.

It is decisive to understand that the chances of a successful resuscitation in cardiac arrest secondary to VF or PVT are based on effective chest compressions and early defibrillation. The management of other cardiac arrest rhythms such as PEA and asystole is based on adequate CPR and administration of vasoactive drugs (mainly epinephrine).

The study by Bobrow [17] et al. demonstrated that chest compression-only CPR was associated with a significant increase in the survival rate of bystander CPR for adults who experienced out-of-hospital cardiac arrest. For this reason, the current recommendations propose beginning resuscitation with chest compressions in a CAB (compression-airway-breathing) sequence.

This aorto-caval compression is the most influential phenomenon in CPR in the pregnant woman.

Cardiac output during cardiopulmonary resuscitation (CPR) in a nonpregnant patient is approximately 30%. The fact that approximately 17% of a pregnant patient's cardiac output is diverted to the uterus suggests that blood flow to vital organs is significantly limited during CPR in the pregnant patient [18].

During pregnancy, administration of chest compressions is more efficient with the patient's abdomen on a side slope toward the left. The cardiac output produced from chest compressions is optimized when the arrested parturient is placed on a firm surface (e.g., a backboard) in the supine position with manual left uterine displacement [19]. This maneuver is optimally performed using two hands from the left side of the patient.

Basic life support begins with an acknowledgment that the victim is either not breathing or not doing so normally. Chest compressions should be initiated with the intention of depressing the chest at least 2 in. (5 cm) at a frequency of 100–120 per minute. Interruptions during compressions should be avoided or minimized, especially during resuscitator replacement.

The resuscitator who performs chest compressions should be replaced by another, ideally, every 2 min or sooner if the resuscitator becomes fatigued.

If an advanced airway is not available, chest compressions/ventilations (30:2 ratio) should be performed with the vents through a bag-mask device.

Endotracheal intubation is the optimal method for maintaining a patent and secure airway. Early intubation is recommended if experienced providers are available.

But nevertheless, bag valve mask ventilation with supplemental oxygen (if available) is recommended before intubation attempts because of the faster trend to desaturation in pregnant women [13].

Interruptions made to attempt to intubate a patient in cardiac arrest can be considered lethal. Therefore, the intubation of a pregnant woman in cardiac arrest must be carried out by an expert. Otherwise, it is better to maintain ventilation by means of a bag-mask with an oxygen reservoir and postpone the endotracheal intubation, when the patient has a return to her spontaneous circulation (ROSC) [20].

After placement of an advanced airway, it may be reasonable for the provider to deliver 1 breath every 6 s (10 breaths/min) while continuous chest compressions are being performed.

Similarly, avoid hyperventilating the patient. Hyperventilation increases intrathoracic pressure and decreases venous return; in addition, hyperventilation may decrease cerebral blood flow [21].

The most experienced provider should perform intubation to minimize attempts. A smaller endotracheal tube (6–7 mm) should be used on first attempt, and no more than two attempts at endotracheal intubation should be made before progressing to emergent invasive airway.

Breaks greater than 10 s decrease chance of return of spontaneous circulation (ROSC) and should be avoided [22].

In case the cardiac arrest occurs with a shockable rhythm (asystole or pulseless electrical activity), the patient must be defibrillated after having made a 2-min cycle of compressions/ventilations (30/2 ratio). After applying defibrillation, cardiopulmonary resuscitation should be resumed with a new cycle of compressions/ventilations (30/2). When defibrillating a patient, it should not cause delays in chest compressions or ventilation. The 2010 AHA guidelines recommend the application of 200 J (biphasic wave devices) per electrical shock [23].

Capnography reflects the quality of chest compressions because it indirectly measures cardiac output in an intubated patient under stable ventilation conditions [20]. During resuscitation, end-tidal CO_2 levels above 10 mm Hg and/or rising end-tidal CO_2 levels suggest adequacy of chest compressions and may be predictive of ROSC [24, 25].

Failure to achieve an $ETCO_2$ of 10 mm Hg by waveform capnography after 20 min of resuscitation has been associated with an extremely poor chance of ROSC and survival. However, the studies to date are limited in that they have potential confounders and have included relatively small numbers of patients, so it is inadvisable to rely solely on $ETCO_2$ in determining when to terminate resuscitation.

Pharmacologic Therapies

The purpose of the use of vasopressors in cardiac arrest is to increase the perfusion pressure to the vital organs, heart, and brain. No clinical studies have shown that the use of epinephrine improves long-term survival. Jacobs et al. [26] found equal rate of survival (to hospital discharge) with or without epinephrine (5.1% vs. 5.0%). A Swedish study [27], in which 42% of the 10,966 patients who had suffered a cardiac arrest received epinephrine, found that use of vasopressor drugs did not improve survival. Despite this, the AHA continues to recommend adrenaline as the drug of choice in cardiopulmonary resuscitation [28].

Once the compression/ventilation cycle has been performed (30:2 ratio), if the rhythm is not defibrillable, epinephrine should be administered.

Epinephrine should be administered at standard dose of 1 mg IV/IO push every 3 to 5 min during cardiac arrest [23].

In case of shockable rhythm, a load of 200 Joules should be applied with a biphasic defibrillator and immediately resume cardiopulmonary resuscitation with compressions: ventilations (30:2). Subsequently, epinephrine should be administered at the aforementioned doses. In this way the sequence in shockable rhythms is compressions/ventilations (30:2), defibrillation, compressions/ventilations, and epinephrine, and repeat the sequence until a return of spontaneous circulation is obtained.

In cases of non-shockable rhythm, the sequence is compressions/ventilations (30:2) and epinephrine, and repeat the sequence until there is return of spontaneous circulation.

When you don't get good results with epinephrine, amiodarone should be used for ventricular fibrillation or pulseless ventricular tachycardia. The first dose should be administered IV or IO at a dose of 300 mg, and a second dose of 150 mg may be administered.

An alternative to amiodarone is lidocaine at a dose of 1–1.5 mg/kg, and a second dose of 0.5–0.75 mg/kg.

Unlike cardiac arrests that occur outside the hospital, cardiac arrests that occur in-hospital benefit from replacing intravascular volume with crystalloids, because many of its causes are hypovolemic in origin. Intravenous access is essential for rapid intravascular volume repletion, including alternatives such as intraosseous access in the proximal humerus or ultrasound-assisted peripheral or central venous access. These vascular accesses should be obtained preferably, above the diaphragm.

In reference to vasopressin, a meta-analysis concluded that there was no benefit to vasopressin over epinephrine, and its suggested use was removed from the AHA guidelines in 2015 [29].

Other Considerations

Iatrogenic overdose is possible in women who have eclampsia and receive magnesium sulfate, particularly if the woman becomes oliguric. Administration of calcium gluconate (1 ampoule or 1 g) is the treatment of choice for magnesium toxicity [30]. Empiric calcium administration may be lifesaving.

The use of sodium bicarbonate to reverse metabolic acidosis during cardiac arrest has been questioned. Rapid correction of maternal (but not fetal) acidosis could lead to reduced compensatory hyperventilation and normalization of maternal $PaCO_2$, which could result in a concomitant increase in fetal $PaCO_2$ and potential worsening of fetal acidosis [31].

Perimortem Cesarean Section (PMCS)

One of the most important interventions that add to the global resuscitation protocol, specific for pregnant patients suffering from cardiac arrest, is perimortem caesarean section. The equipment to intervene in a cardiac arrest must include a surgical tray with the implements for performing a perimortem caesarean section.

Management decisions in the setting of maternal cardiac arrest are based on the status of the parturient; thus, fetal monitoring is not necessary and in fact discouraged.

Performing the caesarean section perimortem in a scene of cardiac arrest in a pregnant woman is aimed at improving the survival of the mother and in many cases the fetal survival.

The emptying of the uterus through the PMCS achieves aorto-caval vascular decompression, improving venous return and arterial perfusion in the pregnant patient who undergoes cardiac arrest. The extraction of immature fetuses without viability achieves a maternal benefit, by decompressing the inferior vena cava and abdominal aorta. In larger fetuses, with gestational age with viability, timely extraction of the fetus can generate a maternal benefit as fetal.

The study by Katz et al. reported an increase in neurological lesion in fetuses that were born and survived after 5 min of the cardiac arrest in the mother [32].

Katz et al. in 1986 derived a 4-min rule for cardiac arrest to initiation of cesarean section at 4 min and delivery of infant at 5 min, based on the knowledge that irreversible brain damage from anoxia occurs within 4–6 min of inadequate cerebral perfusion.

Cardiac arrest should be an uncommon event in pregnant patients. Either way, the staff that is responsible for the care of pregnant patients should be prepared for this catastrophic event. Obstetric care units must have all the equipment and input necessary for the attention of a cardiac arrest. The human team must receive constant and periodic training to maintain their skills and abilities, which will result in avoiding maternal death.

References

1. Brace V, Penney G, Hall M. Quantifying severe maternal morbidity: a Scottish population study. BJOG. 2004;111(5):481–4.
2. Lewis G, Drife JO. Why mothers die 2000-2002: the sixth report of the confidential enquiries into maternal deaths in the United Kingdom. London: RCOG; 2004.
3. Lewis G. Saving mothers' lives: reviewing maternal deaths to make motherhood safer–2003-2005: the seventh report of the confidential enquiries into Maternal Deaths in the United Kingdom. CEMACH; 2007. (www.cemach.org.uk).
4. Schneider AP II, Nelson DJ, Brow DD. In-hospital cardiopulmonary resuscitation: a 30-year review. J Am Board Fam Pract. 1993;6:91–101.
5. Pollard JB. Common mechanisms and strategies for prevention and treatment of cardiac arrest during epidural anesthesia. J Clin Anesth. 2002;14(1):52–6.
6. Barnardo PD, Jenkins JG. Failed tracheal intubation in obstetrics: a 6-year review in a UK region. Anaesthesia. 2002;55:690–4.
7. Mabie WC, DiSessa TG, Crocker LG, Sibai BM, Arheart KL. A longitudinal study of cardiac output in normal human pregnancy. Am J Obstet Gynecol. 1994;170(3):849–56.
8. Spatling L, Fallenstein F, Huch A, Huch R, Rooth G. The variability of cardiopulmonary adaptation to pregnancy at rest and during exercise. Br J Obstet Gynaecol. 1992;99(suppl 8):1–40.
9. Assali NS, Rauramo L, Peltonen T. Measurement of uterine blood flow and uterine metabolism. VIII. Uterine and fetal blood flow and oxygen consumption in early human pregnancy. Am J Obstet Gynecol. 1960;79:86–98.
10. Vanden Hoek TL, Morrison LJ, Shuster M, et al. Part 12: cardiac arrest in special situations: 2010 American Heart Association guidelines for cardiopulmonary resuscitation and emergency cardiovascular care. Circulation. 2010;122(18 suppl 3):S829–61.
11. Malampalli A, Powner DJ, Gardner M. CPR and somatic support of the pregnant patient. Crit Care Clin. 2004;20:747–63.
12. Farinelli CK, Hameed AB. Cardiopulmonary resuscitation in pregnancy. Cardiol Clin. 2012;30:453–61.
13. Atta E, Gardner M. Cardiopulmonary resuscitation in pregnancy. Obstet Gynecol Clin North Am. 2007;34:585–97.
14. Jayawardena L, McNamara E. Diagnosis and management of pregnancies complicated by Haemolysis, Elevated Liver Enzymes and Low Platelets (HELLP) Syndrome in the tertiary setting. Intern Med J. 2019; https://doi.org/10.1111/imj.14337. [Epub ahead of print]
15. Tuffnell DJ. United Kingdom amniotic fluid embolism register. BJOG. 2005;112:1625–9.
16. Maternal Collapse in Pregnancy and Puerperium. RCOG Green-top Guideline No 56. January 2011. (www.cemach.org.uk).
17. Bobrow BJ, Spaite DW, Berg RA, et al. Chest compression-only CPR by Lay Rescuers and Survival from out-of-hospital cardiac arrest. JAMA. 2010;304:1447–54.
18. Ramsay G, Paglia M, Bourjeily G. When the heart stops: a review of cardiac arrest in pregnancy. J Intensive Care Med. 2013;28:204 originally published online 17 January 2012.

19. Vanden Hoek TL, Morrison LJ, Shuster M, Donnino M, Sinz E, Lavonas EJ, Jeejeebhoy FM, Gabrielli A. Part 12: cardiac arrest in special situations: 2010 American Heart Association guidelines for cardiopulmonary resuscitation and emergency cardiovascular care. Circulation. 2010;122:S829–61.
20. Montufar-Rueda C, Gei A. Cardiac arrest during pregnancy. Clin Obstet Gynecol. 2014;57(4):871–81.
21. Yannopoulos D, Nadkarni VM, McKnite SH, et al. Intrathoracic pressure regulator during continuous-chest-compression advanced cardiac resuscitation improves vital organ perfusion pressures in a porcine model of cardiac arrest. Circulation. 2005;112:803–11.
22. Cheskes S, Common MR, Byers PA, Zhan C, Morrison LJ. Compressions during defibrillator charging shortens shock pause duration and improves chest compression fraction during shockable out of hospital cardiac arrest. Resuscitation. 2014;85(8):1007–11.
23. Committee ECC. Subcommittes and Task Forces of the American Heart Association. 2010 American Heart Association guidelines for cardiopulmonary resuscitation and emergency cardiovascular care. Circulation. 2010;122:S640–861.
24. Pernat A, Weil MH, Sun S, Tang W. Stroke volumes and end-tidal carbon dioxide generated by precordial compression during ventricular fibrillation. Crit Care Med. 2003;31:1819–23 21.
25. Wayne MA, Levine RL, Miller CC. Use of end-tidal carbon dioxide to predict outcome in prehospital cardiac arrest. Ann Emerg Med. 1995;25:762–7.
26. Jacobs IG, Finn JC, Felinek GA, et al. Effect of adrenaline on survival in out-of-hospital cardiac arrest: a randomised double′-blind placebo controlled trial. Resuscitation. 2011;82:1138–43.
27. Holmberg M, Holmberg S, Herlitz J. Low chance of survival among patients requiring adrenaline (epinephrine) or intubation after out-of-hospital cardiac arrest in Sweden. Resuscitation. 2002;4:37–45.
28. Lindner KH, Ahnefeld FW, Bowdler IM. Comparison of different doses of epinephrine on myocardial perfusion and resuscitation success during cardiopulmonary resuscitation in a pig model. Am J Emerg Med. 1991;9:27–31.
29. Jeejeebhoy FM, Zelop CM, Lipman S, Carvalho B, Joglar J, Mhyre JM, et al. Cardiac arrest in pregnancy: a scientific statement from the American heart association. Circulation. 2015;132(18):1747–73.
30. Munro PT. Management of eclampsia in the accident and emergency department. J Accid Emerg Med. 2000;17:7–11.
31. Bar-Joseph G, Ambramson NS, Jansen-McWilliams L, et al. Clinical use of sodium bicarbonate during cardiopulmonary resuscitation: is it used sensibly? Resuscitation. 2002;54:47–55.
32. Katz VL, Dotters DJ, Droegmueller W. Perimortem cesarean delivery. Obstet Gynecol. 1986;68:571–6.

Chapter 38
Pregnancy-Related Infective Endocarditis

**Rania Magdi Ali, Bahaa El-Din Ewees Hassan,
and Noura M. Youssri Mahmoud**

Introduction

Infective endocarditis (IE) is an uncommon infectious disease with an annual incidence ranging from 3 to 7 per 100,000 person/years [1], whereas during pregnancy, the reported incidence is 1 in 100,000 pregnancies [2]. Globally, infective endocarditis continues to be illustrated by increased morbidity and mortality despite being relatively rare and is considered the third or fourth most common life-threatening infection syndrome, after sepsis, pneumonia, and intra-abdominal abscess [3]. Maternal and fetal mortality are significantly high [4, 5]. Most of maternal deaths are related to congestive heart failure or embolic manifestations. IE in pregnancy can present challenge in management, considering the choice of appropriate antibiotic treatment and the choice of optimal time for delivery and cardiac surgery.

Pathogenesis and Risk Factors

Over the past few decades, there were continuous changes in epidemiology, microbiology, and predisposing risk factors of IE [6]. IE is an infection of the endocardium with microorganisms that have high affinity to damaged endothelium [7]. The bacteremia can be transient; thus up to 14% of cases of IE and much more in developing countries are associated with negative blood cultures [8]. Approximately 80% of cases with IE are caused by *Staphylococcus aureus*, streptococci, and enterococci [2]. *Streptococcus viridans* is part of the normal skin, oral, respiratory, and gastrointestinal tract flora. Enterococci are part of the normal gastrointestinal and genitourinary tract flora, while *Staphylococcus aureus* is a common skin organism [9].

R. M. Ali (✉) · B. E.-D. E. Hassan · N. M. Y. Mahmoud
Anesthesia, Intensive Care and Pain Management, Faculty of Medicine, Ain Shams University, Cairo, Egypt

C. Montufar et al. (eds.), *Obstetric Catastrophes*,
https://doi.org/10.1007/978-3-030-70034-8_38

Streptococcus viridans used to be the most common causative organism of community-acquired native valve endocarditis (NVE) not associated with intravenous drug use. Nowadays, the epidemiological profile of IE has changed, and *Staphylococcus aureus* became the most common causative organism in most of the industrialized world. *Staphylococcus aureus* IE is partly due to healthcare contact as a leading risk associated with infection [3]. *Staphylococcus lugdunensis* is another rare aggressive causative organism that has high mortality. It is a coagulase-negative staphylococcus that colonizes the perineum as a skin commensal and has been isolated from amniotic fluid in several cases [10]. Fungal IE, caused by *Candida* and *Aspergillus* spp., is most frequently observed in prosthetic valve IE (PVE) and in IE affecting intravenous drug abusers and immunocompromised patients [11].

Development of IE requires a preexisting cardiac lesion or damaged endothelium. Damaged endothelium releases tissue factors that facilitate adherence of pathogens and formation of vegetations [12]. It may affect native or prosthetic valves (NVE or PVE). It can also affect large intrathoracic vessels and occasionally may extend to mural thrombi, ventricular septal defects, and patent ductus arteriosus [2]. Bicuspid aortic valve is the most common predisposing factor of native valve endocarditis. The valve-specific maternal mortality is estimated to be greater for the aortic valve followed by the mitral valve and then the tricuspid valve [13].

The major predisposing risk factor of IE includes rheumatic heart disease especially in the developing nations. Although there is a decrease in rheumatic heart disease cases worldwide, there is a concomitant increase in patients with congenital heart disease surviving to adulthood and childbearing period. Intracardiac device implants and increasing nosocomial infections are new risk factors [14, 15]. Intravenous drug abuse is a substantial risk factor of IE in the industrial nations of which only 6–40% have preexisting structural cardiac abnormality [16]. During injection microorganisms or particles from the skin or the injected drug can cause transient or permanent endothelial damage on valve leaflet, thus facilitating formation of infected vegetations [17]. Most common affected valve is the tricuspid valve, but if the particles are <10 micrometers, it may cross pulmonary capillaries and affect aortic and mitral valves [18].

Diagnosis

Diagnosis of IE in nonpregnant patient is challenging because of the highly variable clinical presentations; however, during pregnancy the challenge is even bigger as the changing cardiovascular physiology mimics the clinical picture of cardiac diseases [19]. The typical physiologic cardiac changes in pregnancy include prolonged, moderate tachycardia, high preload, and low afterload [20].

Diagnosis of IE is based on multiple findings including clinical presentations, laboratory tests, imaging techniques, and microbiological diagnosis [21].

Diagnostic Criteria

The highly variable clinical presentations of IE rendered its diagnosis a real challenge especially during pregnancy. Diagnosis of IE mainly relies on validating the presence of both infection and endocardial involvement. The Modified Duke Criteria have provided a diagnostic guide that is both sensitive to detect the disease and specific to exclude it. It classified IE into definite, possible, and rejected IE (summarized in Table 38.1) [3, 22] according to the number of major and minor criteria fulfilled (Described in Table 38.2) [21].

When the diagnosis remains only possible or even rejected according to the Modified Duke Criteria but still highly suspected clinically, echocardiography and blood culture should be repeated, and other imaging techniques should be used, either for diagnosis of cardiac involvement using cardiac computed tomography, 18F-FDG PET/CT or radiolabeled leucocyte single photon emission CT (SPECT/CT), or for imaging embolic events using cerebral magnetic resonance imaging (MRI), whole-body CT, and/or PET/CT [23].

Clinical Features

Clinical presentations vary according to the causative organism, presence or absence of preexisting cardiac lesions, prosthetic valves or intracardiac devices, as well as mode of presentation. IE may manifest as an acute rapidly progressive infection and deterioration or with a misleading subacute or chronic course with low grade fever and nonspecific symptoms [21].

Table 38.1 Definition of IE according to the Modified Duke Criteria [3, 56]

Definite IE
Pathological criteria
Microorganisms demonstrated by culture or histological examination of a vegetation, a vegetation that has embolized, or an intracardiac abscess specimen; or pathological lesions; vegetation or intracardiac abscess confirmed by histological examination showing active endocarditis
Clinical criteria
2 major criteria
1 major criterion and 3 minor criteria, or
5 minor criteria
Possible IE
1 major criterion and 1 minor criterion, or
3 minor criteria
Rejected IE
Firm alternative diagnosis explaining evidence of IE; or
Resolution of IE syndrome with antibiotic therapy for ≤4 days; or
No pathological evidence of IE at surgery or autopsy with antibiotic therapy for ≤4 days; or
Does not meet criteria for possible IE as above
IE indicates infective endocarditis

Table 38.2 Definition of terms used in the Modified Duke Criteria for the diagnosis of IE [3, 56]

Major criteria
Blood culture positive for IE
1. Typical microorganisms consistent with IE from two separate blood cultures: viridans streptococci, *Streptococcus bovis*, HACEK group, *Staphylococcus aureus*; or Community-acquired enterococci in the absence of a primary focus
2. Microorganisms consistent with IE from persistently positive blood cultures defined as follows: At least two positive cultures of blood samples drawn >12 h apart or All three or a majority of ≥4 separate cultures of blood (with first and last sample drawn at least 1 h apart)
3. Single positive blood culture for *Coxiella burnetii* or antiphase 1 IgG antibody titer ≥1:800
Evidence of endocardial involvement
Echocardiogram positive for IE defined as follows:
1. Oscillating intracardiac mass on valve or supporting structures, in the path of regurgitant jets, or on implanted material in the absence of an alternative anatomic explanation
2. Abscess
3. New partial dehiscence of prosthetic valve or new valvular regurgitation (worsening or changing or preexisting murmur not enough)
Minor criteria
Predisposition, predisposing heart condition, or IDU
Fever, temperature >38 °C
Vascular phenomena, major arterial emboli, septic pulmonary infarcts, mycotic aneurysm, intracranial hemorrhage, conjunctival hemorrhages, and Janeway lesions
Immunological phenomena: glomerulonephritis, Osler nodes, Roth spots, and rheumatoid factor
Microbiological evidence: positive blood culture but does not meet a major criterion as noted above (excludes single positive cultures for coagulase-negative staphylococci and organisms that do not cause endocarditis) or serological evidence of active infection with organism consistent with IE

HACEK indicates *Haemophilus* species, *Aggregatibacter* species, *Cardiobacterium hominis*, *Eikenella corrodens*, and *Kingella* species
IDU injection drug use
IE infective endocarditis
IgG immunoglobulin G
TEE transesophageal echocardiography
TTE transthoracic echocardiography

In the presence of cardiac lesion such as structural or congenital heart disease or prosthetic valve, IE should be considered in any patients with unexplained fever, night sweats, and systemic illness or with embolic manifestation or cardiac murmur [14]. Suspicion should increase in presence of source of bacteremia as in case of history of IV drug use or recent healthcare exposure or invasive procedure such as wound care, hemodialysis, or invasive dental care [24]. Rapid detection of endocarditis and appropriate treatment are important in reducing the risk of both maternal and fetal mortality.

Classical stigmata of endocarditis may be observed in subacute cases, including petechial hemorrhages in mucous membranes, Roth spots (retinal hemorrhages with pale centers), and splinter hemorrhages, Janway lesions (macular or nodular hemorrhagic lesions), or Osler nodules (painful raised lesions) on the extremities [25]. Glomerulonephritis is also common. Emboli to the lung, brain, and spleen occur in 30% of patients and may be the presenting symptoms [21].

In addition, IE may present right away with its complications. Heart failure is the most common complication that can be attributed to acute valve regurgitation from rupture chorda tendinea or perforation and to a lesser extent as a result of valve obstruction by vegetation [26]. Heart failure symptoms include dyspnea, orthopnea, and lower limb edema which are easily mistaken for normal manifestation of pregnancy.

Another extremely common complication is embolic manifestations that may be silent in 20–50% of cases. Left-sided IE usually sends emboli to the brain and spleen, while right-sided IE sends emboli to pulmonary vessels. The best way to handle the risk of embolization is appropriate antimicrobial therapy. However, persistent or recurrent emboli after 1 week of therapy or large mobile vegetation is a strong indication for surgery [21].

Another common complication of IE is uncontrolled infection. It may be in the form of persistent infection and fever more than 10 days despite appropriate specific antimicrobial therapy or paravalvular extension of the infection that may lead to ventricular septal defect, atrioventricular block, or acute coronary syndromes [27].

Other complications include mycotic aneurism, intracranial hemorrhages, myocarditis, and musculoskeletal arthralgia or myalgia. Besides, rheumatological symptoms are frequent and may be the first presentation delaying appropriate diagnosis [21].

Finally, acute renal dysfunction occurs in 6–30% of cases of IE. It may be due to immune complex vasculitis, renal emboli, antibiotic nephrotoxicity, or severe hypotension from heart failure or sepsis [28].

Laboratory Tests

Laboratory tests are nonspecific, and all demonstrate sepsis but are not diagnostic of IE. It may show leukocytosis or leucopenia, anemia, thrombocytopenia, elevated CRP and ESR, lactatemia, hyperbilirubinemia, elevated serum creatine level, and microscopic hematuria [29].

Imaging Techniques

The most important imaging technique in IE is echocardiography. It is essential for diagnosis, management, and prognosis of IE. Once IE is suspected, transthoracic echocardiography (TTE) should be performed. Echocardiographic findings are major criteria of diagnosis, and they include vegetation, abscesses or pseudoaneurysm, and new dehiscence of prosthetic valve [30].

If TTE is negative, transesophageal echocardiography (TEE) should be done, as visualization of vegetations with TTE may be difficult in prosthetic valves due to shadowing, small vegetation <2–3 mm, recent embolization, intracardiac devices, and mitral valve prolapse or degenerative calcified lesion. Additionally, TEE is recommended for patients rated at least possible IE by clinical criteria or complicated IE as in case of paravalvular abscess. If both TTE and TEE are negative, echocardiography should be repeated after 5–7 days if clinical suspicion of IE remains high [31]. Follow-up TTE or TEE is done to monitor complication such as appearance of new murmur and response to treatment. Finally, TTE should be repeated at the end of antimicrobial therapy to establish complete resolution [3].

There are other imaging modalities such as multi-slice computed tomography (MSCT), magnetic resonance imaging (MRI), and nuclear imaging, which can be used for diagnosis, follow-up, and decision-making [32].

MSCT may be superior over TEE in detecting perivalvular extension of vegetation and anatomy of pseudoaneurysm, abscesses, and fistula [33]. However, during pregnancy MSCT is better avoided and replaced by MRI for fear of adverse effect of radiation of fetus. Cerebral MRI should be performed to detect cerebral lesions even in the absence of neurological symptoms. Abdominal MRI can detect splenic infarctions [21].

Imaging techniques such as radiolabeled white blood cells single photon emission CT (SPECT/CT) or F-FDG PET/CT have proven to be effective in detecting peripheral silent embolic lesion. They detect leukocytes, monocytes, macrophages, and lymphocytes that accumulate at the site of infection [34, 35].

The ESC guidelines recommended to add findings of nuclear imaging as one of Duke's criteria for diagnosis of IE to increase its sensitivity by detecting silent embolic events [21]. However, their use in pregnant women is still a matter of debate and needs to weigh up the maternal benefits from early diagnosis and the risks of radiation on the fetus after considering the gestational age and dose of radiation.

Microbiological Diagnosis

A. *Blood Cultures*

Blood culture not only recognizes the causative organisms, but it also recommends the specific antimicrobial treatment by susceptibility tests. Once IE is suspected, three sets of blood culture should be withdrawn, via complete aseptic technique, from a peripheral vein to avoid contamination from a central venous line, with 30-min interval and before initiation of empirical antibiotics. Withdrawing blood cultures during peaks of fever is no longer recommended [21, 36]. After positive blood culture, identification of microorganism, and initiation of specific antimicrobial treatment, at least two sets of blood cultures should be obtained every 48–72 h to test efficacy of treatment and determine day one of therapy (the day on which blood cultures turn negative) [21, 36].

Blood culture-negative infective endocarditis (BCNIE) may be obtained in 30% of IE cases. This may result from previous antibiotic administration; in this case antibiotic should be discontinued and blood culture be repeated or infection by atypical, fastidious, or obligatory intracellular bacteria such as *Brucella* spp., *Coxiella burnetii*, *Bartonella* spp., *Tropheryma whipplei*, *Mycoplasma* spp., *Legionella* spp., or *Fungi*. These are characterized by slow growth and requires a specialized media for incubation. In this case, according to clinical presentation and local epidemiology, some serology tests of most probable organism are required [37]. If all serological and micro-assays came negative, and IE still strongly suggested clinically, non-infection IE should be considered. In this case, tests may be indicated to investigate the presence of antinuclear antibody, antiphospholipid antibody, and antipork antibodies in patients with porcine bio-prosthesis [21, 38].

B. *Histopathology of Excised Tissues*

In case of cardiac intervention, all excised infected tissues (native or prosthetic valves, vegetations) should be sent for histopathological examination for definitive identification of causative organism [21].

Prognosis in IE

Predictors of poor outcome in patients with IE are influenced by the patient characteristics, the presence or absence of cardiac and noncardiac complications, the infecting organism, and the echocardiographic findings. Patients with HF, peri-annular complications, or *S. aureus* infection are at highest risk of death and need for surgery in the active phase of the disease. A high degree of comorbidity, diabetes, septic shock, moderate-to-severe ischemic stroke, brain hemorrhage, and the need for hemodialysis are also predictors of poor outcome. Persistence of positive blood cultures 48 to 72 h after initiation of antibiotic treatment indicates a lack of infection control and is an independent risk factor for mortality [21].

Management

According to ESC and AHA 2015 recommendations, treatment of pregnancy related IE is much like that of nonpregnant patients. Once IE is diagnosed or even considered, selection of appropriate treatment strategy and decision-making should depend on multidisciplinary team approach. The multidisciplinary team should include a cardiologist, cardiothoracic surgeon, and infectious disease specialist in addition to the obstetrician [39].

Appropriate treatment strategies in pregnancy-related IE include antimicrobial therapy, optimal timing of surgical intervention if indicated, and optimal timing and mode of pregnancy termination to minimize both maternal and fetal mortality and morbidity [40].

Antimicrobial Therapy

Antimicrobial therapy is the cornerstone in the treatment of IE, with a main goal to eradicate microorganism and sterilize vegetations. Surgery, if indicated, helps achieve that goal by removing infected materials and draining abscesses. Empirical antibiotic therapy should be started immediately once IE is suspected or diagnosed by Modified Duke's Criteria and initial blood cultures are withdrawn. Prompt use of antibiotics decreases the risk of embolization. The choice of empirical antimicrobial therapy should be based on most susceptible organism according to local epidemiology and clinical presentation, whether native NVE or PVE [21].

Antibiotics that can be given during all trimesters of pregnancy are penicillin, ampicillin, amoxicillin, daptomycin, erythromycin, mezlocillin, oxacillin, and cephalosporins. There is a definite risk to the fetus in all trimesters of pregnancy with aminoglycosides and tetracyclines, and they should therefore only be used for vital indications [41].

Consequently, the proposed antibiotic regimens for initial empirical treatment before pathogen identification in case of community-acquired native valves or late prosthetic valves more than 12 months post-surgery are ampicillin with mezlocillin/oxacillin or daptomycin for penicillin-allergic patients or in case of early PVE less than 12 months post-surgery or nosocomial or non-nosocomial healthcare-associated endocarditis. Once blood culture results and antibiotic susceptibility are available, shift to specific antimicrobial therapy is mandatory [21].

Specific antimicrobial therapies in cases of BCNIE are doxycycline for *Bartonella* spp., doxycycline plus cotrimoxazole for *Brucella* spp., doxycycline plus hydroxychloroquine for *C. burnetii* and *T. whipplei*, mezlocillin/oxacillin for *Mycoplasma* spp., and mezlocillin/oxacillin or erythromycin for *Legionella* spp. [21].

Duration of antimicrobial therapy depends on causative organisms: for NPE from 2 to 6 weeks whereas for PVE more than 6 weeks. Prolonged antimicrobial therapy is crucial to avoid regrowth of tolerant and dormant organisms as they can resume growth after therapy discontinuation. These organisms can be found deeply embedded in vegetations and more commonly in biofilms [21].

Surgical Intervention

About 50–60% of pregnancy-related IE requires cardiac surgical intervention to remove any residual infected parts and to restore cardiac morphology in patients' damaged valves as in case of valve perforation or regurgitation [21].

Cardiac operation should be performed after complete eradication of microorganism embedded in the vegetation, as valve replacement in the presence of active infection leads to a high risk of reinfection. However, early cardiac surgery during the active phase and before completion of appropriate antibiotic course may be needed on emergency within less than 24 h or urgently within less than 7 days, while continuous careful clinical and echocardiographic evaluations are done to detect any deterioration or appearance of new risk factors [42, 43].

Early cardiac surgery may be indicated in many circumstances as uncontrolled fever after 1 week of culture-specific antibiotic treatment or infection with multiresistant organism, shock, severe heart failure due to acute valve regurgitation, or persistent embolic events. In addition, persistent mobile vegetation more than 10 mm and large isolated vegetations more than 15 mm on aortic or mitral valve or more than 20 mm on tricuspid valve or perivalvular abscess, fistula, aneurysm, or enlarging vegetation indicate early cardiac surgery [3, 21, 40, 44].

Another challenge in early cardiac intervention is patients with stroke or subclinical cerebral emboli as cardiac surgery is recommended to prevent further embolization. Conversely, anticoagulation during CPB may lead to hemorrhagic transformation, and intraoperative hypotension may aggravate cerebral ischemia. Urgent cardiac surgery is considered in these patients after exclusion of intracranial hemorrhage. However, in cases with major stroke or intracranial hemorrhage, cardiac intervention should be delayed at least 4 weeks [3].

Regarding the type of cardiac intervention to be performed, valve repair is not always feasible but is preferable and safer against valve replacement as it avoids the use of prosthetic material and thus reduces the risk of reinfection and reoperation. The only limiting factor of valve repair would be the near total destruction of the leaflets [45–49].

Termination of Pregnancy

Another difficulty to make correct management plan is to decide either birth induction followed by antibiotic therapy and cardiac surgery or specific antibiotic therapy followed by gestation termination with concomitant cardiac surgery.

There are no definite guidelines suggested by the ESC or AHA, so decision must be made on individual basis depending on maternal clinical condition, gestational age, and local advances in neonatal care. Theoretically, delivery is preferred before cardiothoracic surgery or massive antibiotics treatments for the sake of the fetus despite a higher risk of maternal embolism [40].

Cardiac surgery should be avoided in the first and second trimesters before 24 weeks of gestation because of the high risk of developing congenital anomalies probably from drug administration and cardiopulmonary bypass, but when emergent open-heart surgery is inevitable, early delivery by caesarean section and intervention on the patient's heart at a later stage is the most rational strategy [49].

After 24 weeks of gestation, there is lower risk of congenital malformation; however, cardiac operation is better postponed if possible after 28 weeks of gestation, as fetal mortality is still high due to fetal immaturity [50]. After 28 weeks of gestation, the fetus is considered viable as a result of new advances of neonatal care and improvement of premature infant survival rates. Thus, delivery before cardiac surgery is advisable [48]. Notably, neonatal care may be less advanced in developing countries rendering a fetus of 28 weeks of gestation less viable, so surgery should be delayed further if possible.

There is no special recommendation regarding mode of delivery whether caesarean section or natural childbirth; it should be determined via obstetrician and endocarditis team according to maternal and fetal conditions. Termination of pregnancy and cardiac surgery are better to be performed with a few days apart as it allows abdominal wound healing before heparization during surgery or in one stage where caesarean section being performed before cardiopulmonary bypass. Measures to decrease risk of postpartum bleeding should be taken such as B-lynch sutures in CS [2].

If cardiac intervention is to be performed during gestation, intraoperative monitoring of fetal heart rate, and uterine contractility, using cardiotocography is mandatory. Intraoperative fetal bradycardia as well as absence of fetal heart variability may be noticed with spontaneous recovery to normal values postoperatively [51]. Persistent postoperative fetal bradycardia denotes placental insufficiency resulting in fetal distress, and emergency delivery is indicated [52]. Administration of intravenous tocolytic such as ritodrine can be used intraoperatively to prevent preterm labor [53].

Anticoagulation, Thrombolytic, and Antiplatelet Adjunct Therapy

Anticoagulation in IE is controversial, although it may reduce the risk of embolization especially in PVE; however, it increases the risk of developing intracranial hemorrhage. In patients suffering PVE with CNS embolic manifestation, it is recommended to stop anticoagulation for at least 2 weeks in order to give chance for thrombus organization and reduce the risk for hemorrhagic transformation. After 2 weeks, reintroduction of anticoagulation may be considered using unfractionated IV heparin with a target activated thromboplastin time of 50–70 s [3].

Thrombolytic therapy is contraindicated as it increases the risk of intracranial hemorrhage, but thrombectomy can be performed in patients with ischemic stroke. Regarding antiplatelet therapy, it is not recommended to initiate it in a patient with IE. However, if patients are on long-term therapy at the time of diagnosis with IE, antiplatelet can be continued once there is no evidence or risk of bleeding. This can be seen with antiphospholipid syndrome [3].

Prophylaxis Against IE

The concept of antibiotic prophylaxis against IE was developed to avoid or at best minimize its high mortality and serious morbidity. Its main aim was to prevent attachment of bacteria to the endocardium following transient bacteremia from invasive procedures. This resulted in recommendations for antibiotic prophylaxis in all patients with rheumatic heart or congenital heart disease subject to many procedures [54].

However, the restriction of indications for antibiotic prophylaxis was initiated in 2002 because of changes in risk–benefit analyses. The main reasons for this constraint are the fact that IE is more related to cumulative low-grade bacteremia associated with routine daily activity rather than transient high-grade bacteremia following invasive procedures. Besides, the widespread use of antibiotic helped in emergence of resistant microorganisms, the risk of anaphylaxis and drug eruption from antimicrobials despite being rare significantly increased with the widespread use, and finally efficacy of antibiotic prophylaxis in preventing IE was of low evidence [21].

In 2015 both the ESC [21] and AHA guidelines [55] restricted the antibiotic prophylaxis against IE to the highest-risk patients undergoing a high-risk procedure as these patients have the worst prognosis if they develop IE. Patients with the highest risk include those with a prosthetic valve or with prosthetic material used for cardiac valve repair, patients with transcatheter-implanted prostheses and homograft, patients with previous episode of IE, and patients with untreated cyanotic congenital heart disease (CHD) and those with CHD who have postoperative palliative shunts, conduits, or other prostheses. It is recommended prophylaxis for the first 6 months after surgical repair with no residual defects until endothelialization of the prosthetic material has occurred.

Antibiotic prophylaxis is not recommended for patients at intermediate risk of IE as in case of any form of native valve disease including bicuspid aortic valve, mitral valve prolapse, and calcific aortic stenosis [21].

The high-risk procedures only include dental procedures in which there is manipulation of gingival or periapical tissues or perforation of oral mucosa. Regarding respiratory tract, gastrointestinal, or genitourinary procedures, antibiotic prophylaxis is not recommended unless there is established infection [21]. Consequently, antibiotic prophylaxis against IE is no more recommended in women with high risk of IE before caesarian or vaginal delivery unless there is established infection. However, if antibiotics are prescribed to prevent wound infection or sepsis, it is advisable that antimicrobial regimen include active agents against enterococci such as ampicillin or amoxicillin or vancomycin in women who cannot tolerate beta-lactams [21].

Pregnant women with high risk of developing of IE undergoing high-risk dental procedure should receive antibiotic prophylaxis 30 to 60 min prior the procedures up to 2 h after the procedure. Recommended regimen is 2 mg amoxicillin or ampicillin or 1 mg ceftriaxone or 600 mg clindamycin or 500 mg azithromycin in patients allergic to beta-lactams [21].

References

1. Khan O, Shafi AMA, Timmis A. International guideline changes and the incidence of infective endocarditis: a systematic review. Open Heart. 2016;3:e000498.
2. Connolly C, O'Donoghu K, Doran H, McCarthy FP. Infective endocarditis in pregnancy case report and review of the literature. Obstetr Medi. 2015;8(2):102–4.
3. Baddour LM, Wilson WR, Bayer AS, Fowler VG Jr, Tleyjeh IM, Rybak MJ, Barsic B, Lockhart PB, Gewitz MH, Levison ME, Bolger AF, Steckelberg JM, Baltimore RS, Fink AM, O'Gara

P, Taubert KA. On behalf of the American Heart Association Committee on Rheumatic Fever, Endocarditis, and Kawasaki Disease of the Council on Cardiovascular Disease in the Young, Council on Clinical Cardiology, Council on Cardiovascular Surgery and Anesthesia, and Stroke Council. Infective endocarditis in adults: diagnosis, antimicrobial therapy, and management of complications: a scientific statement for healthcare professionals from the American Heart Association. Circulation. 2015;132:1435–86.
4. Campuzano K, Roquè H, Bolnick A, Leo MV, Campbell WA. Bacterial endocarditis complicating pregnancy: case report and systemic review of the literature. Arch Gynecol Obstet. 2003;268:251–5.
5. Krcmery V, Gogová M, Ondrusová A, Buckova E, Doczeova A, Mrazova M, Hricak V, Fischer V, P & M. On behalf of the Slovak Endocarditis Study Group Etiology and Risk Factors of 339 cases of infective endocarditis: report from a 10-year National Prospective Survey in the Slovak Republic. J Chemother. 2003;15(6):579–83.
6. Kebed KY, Bishu K, Al Adham RI, Baddour LM, Connolly HM, Sohail MR, Steckelberg JM, Wilson WR, Murad MH, Anavekar NS. Pregnancy and postpartum infective endocarditis: a systematic review. Mayo Clin Proc. 2014;89(8):1143–52.
7. Shi-Min Yuan. Infective endocarditis during pregnancy. J Coll Phys Surg Pakistan. 2014;25(2):134–9.
8. Tower C, Nallapeta S, Vause S. Prophylaxis against infective endocarditis in obstetrics: new NICE guidance: a commentary. BJOG. 2008;115(13):1601–4.
9. Beynon RP, Bahl VK, Prendergast BD. Infective endocarditis. BMJ. 2006;333:334–9.
10. Marchocki Z, Collins K, Lehane E, Reilly PO, O'Donoghue K. Staphylococcus lugdunensis cultured from the amniotic fluid at Caesarean section. PLoS One. 2013;8(2):e56373.
11. Tattevin P, Revest M, Lefort A, Michelet C, Lortholary O. Fungal endocarditis: current challenges. Int J Antimicrob Agents. 2014;44:290–4.
12. Moreillon P, Que YA. Infective endocarditis. Lancet. 2004;363:139–49.
13. Abbassi-Ghanavati M, Greer LG Cunningham FG. Pregnancy and laboratory studies: a reference table for clinicians. Obstet Gynecol. 2009;114:1326–31.
14. Habib G, Hoen B, Tornos P, Thuny F, Prendergast B, Vilacosta I, Moreillon P, de Jesus Antunes M, Thilen U, Lekakis J, Lengyel M, Müller L, Naber CK, Nihoyannopoulos P, Moritz A, Zamorano JL. ESC Committee for practice guidelines. Guidelines on the prevention, diagnosis, and treatment of infective endocarditis (new version 2009): the task force on the prevention, diagnosis, and treatment of infective endocarditis of the European Society of Cardiology (ESC). Endorsed by the European Society of Clinical Microbiology and Infectious Diseases (ESCMID) and the International Society of Chemotherapy (ISC) for infection and cancer. Eur Heart J. 2009;30(19):2369–413.
15. Prendergast BD. The changing face of infective endocarditis. Heart. 2006;92:879–85.
16. Correa de Sa DD, Tleyjeh IM, Anavekar NS, Schultz JC, Thomas JM, Lahr BD, Bachuwar A, Pazdernik M, Steckelberg JM, Wilson WR, Baddour LM. Epidemiological trends of infective endocarditis: a population-based study in Olmsted County, Minnesota. Mayo Clin Proc. 2010;85(5):422–6.
17. Sande MA, Lee BL, Mills J, Chambers HF. Endocarditis in intravenous drug users. In: Kaye D, editor. Infective endocarditis. New York: Raven Press; 1992. p. 345.
18. Mathew J, Addai T, Anand A, Morrobel A, Maheshwari P, Freels S. Clinical features, site of involvement, bacteriologic findings, and outcome of infective endocarditis in intravenous drug users. Arch Intern Med. 1995;155(15):1641–8.
19. Foley M. Cardiac disease. In: Dildy G, Belfort M, Saade G, Phelan J, Hankins G, Clark S, editors. Critical care obstetrics. 4th ed. Oxford: Blackwell; 2004. p. 252–74.
20. Liu LX, Arany Z. Maternal cardiac metabolism in pregnancy. Cardiovasc Res. 2014;101(4):545–53.
21. Habib G, Lancellotti P, Antunes MJ, Bongiorni MG, Casalta JP, DelZotti F, Dulgheru R, El Khoury G, Erbaa PA, Iung B, Mirob JM, Mulder BJ, Plonska-Gosciniak E, Price S, Roos-Hesselink J, Snygg-Martin U, Thuny F, Mas PT, Vilacosta I, and Zamorano JL. 2015 ESC guidelines for the management of infective endocarditis: the Task Force for the Management of Infective Endocarditis of the European Society of Cardiology (ESC)Endorsed by: European

Association for Cardio-Thoracic Surgery (EACTS), the European Association of Nuclear Medicine (EANM) European Heart Journal 2015; 36(44): 3075–3128.
22. Li JS, Sexton DJ, Mick N, Nettles R, Fowler VG Jr, Ryan T, Bashore T, Corey GR. Proposed modifications to the Duke criteria for the diagnosis of infective endocarditis. Clin Infect Dis. 2000;30:633–8.
23. Sarrazin JF, Philippon F, Tessier M, Guimond J, Molin F, Champagne J, Nault I, Blier L, Nadeau M, Charbonneau L, Trottier M, O'Hara G. Usefulness of fluorine-18 positron emission tomography/computed tomography for identification of cardiovascular implantable electronic device infections. J Am Coll Cardiol. 2012;59:1616–25.
24. Pierce D, Calkins BC, Thornton K. Infectious endocarditis: diagnosis and treatment. Am Fam Physician. 2012;85(10):981–6.
25. Durack DT, Lukes AS, Bright DK. Duke Endocarditis Service. New criteria for diagnosis of infective endocarditis: utilization of specific echocardiographic findings. Am J Med. 1994;96(3):200–9.
26. Piper C, Hetzer R, Korfer R, Bergemann R, Horstkotte D. The importance of secondary mitral valve involvement in primary aortic valve endocarditis; the mitral kissing vegetation. Eur Heart J. 2002;23:79–86.
27. Anguera I, Miro JM, Evangelista A, Cabell CH, San Roman JA, Vilacosta I, Almirante B, Ripoll T, Farinas MC, Anguita M, Navas E, Gonzalez-Juanatey C, Garcia-Bolao I, Munoz P, de Alarcon A, Sarria C, Rufi G, Miralles F, Pare C, Fowler VG Jr, Mestres CA, de Lazzari E, Guma JR, Moreno A, Corey GR. Periannular complications in infective endocarditis involving native aortic valves. Am J Cardiol. 2006;98:1254–60.
28. Mahr A, Batteux F, Tubiana S, Goulvestre C, Wolff M, Papo T, Vrtovsnik F, Klein I, Iung B, Duval X. Brief report: prevalence of antineutrophil cytoplasmic antibodies in infective endocarditis. Arthritis Rheumatol. 2014;66:1672–7.
29. Yu CW, Juan LI, Hsu SC, Chen CK, Wu CW, Lee CC, Wu JY. Role of procalcitonin in the diagnosis of infective endocarditis: a meta-analysis. Am J Emerg Med. 2013;31:935–41.
30. Habib G, Badano L, Tribouilloy C, Vilacosta I, Zamorano JL, Galderisi M, Voigt JU, Sicari R, Cosyns B, Fox K, Aakhus S. Recommendations for the practice of echocardiography in infective endocarditis. Eur J Echocardiogr. 2010;11:202–19.
31. Eudailey K, Lewey J, Hahn RT, George I. Aggressive infective endocarditis and the importance of early repeat echocardiographic imaging. J Thorac Cardiovasc Surg. 2014;147:e26–8.
32. Bruun NE, Habib G, Thuny F, Sogaard P. Cardiac imaging in infectious endocarditis. Eur Heart J. 2014;35:624–32.
33. Feuchtner GM, Stolzmann P, Dichtl W, Schertler T, Bonatti J, Scheffel H, Mueller S, Plass A, Mueller L, Bartel T, Wolf F, Alkadhi H. Multislice computed tomography in infective endocarditis: comparison with transesophageal echocardiography and intraoperative findings. J Am Coll Cardiol. 2009;53:436–44.
34. Rouzet F, Chequer R, Benali K, Lepage L, Ghodbane W, Duval X, Iung B, Vahanian A, Le Guludec D, Hyafil F. Respective performance of 18F-FDG PET and radiolabeled leukocyte scintigraphy for the diagnosis of prosthetic valve endocarditis. J Nucl Med. 2014;55:1980–5.
35. Saby L, Laas O, Habib G, Cammilleri S, Mancini J, Tessonnier L, Casalta JP, Gouriet F, Riberi A, Avierinos JF, Collart F, Mundler O, Raoult D, Thuny F. Positron emission tomography/computed tomography for diagnosis of prosthetic valve endocarditis: increased valvular 18F-fluorodeoxyglucose uptake as a novel major criterion. J Am Coll Cardiol. 2013;61:2374–82.
36. La Scola B, Raoult D. Direct identification of bacteria in positive blood culture bottles by matrix-assisted laser desorption ionisation time-of-flight mass spectrometry. PLoS One. 2009;4:e8041.
37. Raoult D, Casalta JP, Richet H, Khan M, Bernit E, Rovery C, Branger S, Gouriet F, Imbert G, Bothello E, Collart F, Habib G. Contribution of systematic serological testing in diagnosis of infective endocarditis. J Clin Microbiol. 2005;43:5238–42.
38. Loyens M, Thuny F, Grisoli D, Fournier PE, Casalta JP, Vitte J, Habib G, Raoult D. Link between endocarditis on porcine bioprosthetic valves and allergy to pork. Int J Cardiol. 2013;167:600–2.

39. Chirillo F, Scotton P, Rocco F, Rigoli R, Borsatto F, Pedrocco A, De Leo A, Minniti G, Polesel E, Olivari Z. Impact of a multidisciplinary management strategy on the outcome of patients with native valve infective endocarditis. Am J Cardiol. 2013;112(8):1171–6.
40. Fan F, Zhou Q, Pan J, Wang D. Open-heart surgery for a pregnant woman with infective endocarditis after cesarean. J Med Cases. 2016;7(8):348–50.
41. Regitz-Zagrosek V, Blomstrom Lundqvist C, Borghi C, Cifkova R, Ferreira R, Foidart JM, Gibbs JSR, Gohlke-Baerwolf C, Gorenek B, Iung B, Kirby M, Maas AHEM, Morais J, Nihoyannopoulos P, Pieper PG, Presbitero P, Roos-Hesselink JW, Schaufelberger M, Seeland U, Torracca L. ESC guidelines on the management of cardiovascular diseases during pregnancy: the task force on the management of cardiovascular diseases during pregnancy of the European Society of Cardiology (ESC). Eur Heart J. 2011;32:3147–97.
42. Habib G, Avierinos JF, Thuny F. Aortic valve endocarditis: is there an optimal surgical timing? Curr Opin Cardiol. 2007;22:77–83.
43. Thuny F, Beurtheret S, Mancini J, Gariboldi V, Casalta JP, Riberi A, Giorgi R, Gouriet F, Tafanelli L, Avierinos JF, Renard S, Collart F, Raoult D, Habib G. The timing of surgery influences mortality and morbidity in adults with severe complicated infective endocarditis: a propensity analysis. Eur Heart J. 2011;32:2027–33.
44. Malhotra A, Prendergast BD. Evaluating treatment options for patients with infective endocarditis. When is it the right time for surgery? Futur Cardiol. 2012;8:847–61.
45. Dreyfus G, Serraf A, Jebara VA, Deloche A, Chauvaud S, Couetil JP, Carpentier A. Valve repair in acute endocarditis. Ann Thorac Surg. 1990;49:706–13.
46. Podesser BK, Rödler S, Hahn R, Eigenbauer E, Vodrazka M, Moritz A, Laufer G, Simon P, Wolner E. Mid-term follow up of mitral valve reconstruction due to active infective endocarditis. J Heart Valve Dis. 2000;9:335–40.
47. Sternik L, Zehr KJ, Orszulak TA, Mullany CJ, Daly RC, Schaff HV. The advantage of repair of mitral valve in acute endocarditis. J Heart Valve Dis. 2002;11:91–8.
48. Aoyagi S, Akasu K, Amako M, Yoshikawa K, Hori H. Infective endocarditis during pregnancy: report of a case. Ann Thorac Cardiovasc Surg. 2005;11(1):51–4.
49. Vizzardi E, De Cicco G, Zanini G, D'Aloia A, Faggiano P, Lo Russo R, Chiari E, Dei Cas L. Infectious endocarditis during pregnancy, problems in the decision-making process: a case report. Cases J. 2009;2:6537.
50. Mahli A, Izdes S, Coskun D. Cardiac operations during pregnancy: review of factors influencing fetal outcome. Ann Thorac Surg. 2000;69:1622–6.
51. Marcoux J, Rosin M, Mycyk T. CPB-assisted aortic valve replacement in a pregnant 27-year-old with endocarditis. Perfusion. 2009;24:361–4.
52. Kaoutzanis C, Evangelakis E, Kokkinos C, Kaoutzanis G. Urgent aortic valve replacement for infective endocarditis during the 23rd week of pregnancy. Gen Thorac Cardiovasc Surg. 2013;61:296–300.
53. Güler A, Sahin MA, Küçükarslan N, Kürklüoglu M, Kirilmaz A, Tatar H. A case of infective endocarditis, during pregnancy: should we keep the fetus? Anadolu Kardiyol Derg. 2010;10:291–2.
54. Duval X, Leport C. Prophylaxis of infective endocarditis: current tendencies continuing controversies. Lancet Infect Dis. 2008;8:225–32.
55. Nishimura RA, Otto CM, Bonow RO, Carabello BA, Erwin JPIII, Guyton RA, O'Gara PT, Ruiz CE, Skubas NJ, Sorajja P, Sundt TMIII, Thomas JD. 2014 AHA/ACC guideline for the management of patients with valvular heart disease: executive summary: a report of the American College of Cardiology/American Heart Association Task Force on Practice Guidelines. Circulation. 2014;129:2440–92.
56. Li JS, Sexton DJ, Mick N, Nettles R, Fowler VG Jr, Ryan T, Bashore T, Corey GR. Proposed modifications to the Duke criteria for the diagnosis of infective endocarditis. Clin Infect Dis. 2000;30:633–8.

Part IX
Neurology

Chapter 39
Seizures and Pregnancy

Javier Pérez-Fernández, Gloria Rodríguez-Vega, and Alberto Sirven

Seizures and Pregnancy

Seizure disorders affect over three million Americans, and one third of them are women of childbearing age [1]. Seizures during pregnancy can slow fetal heart rate, decrease oxygen supply to the fetus, and cause fetal injury, placental abruption, preterm labor, premature birth, and even miscarriage due to trauma, such as a fall during a seizure. On the other hand, antiepileptic drugs (AEDs) can interfere with the metabolism of oral contraceptives resulting in unplanned pregnancies and inadvertent exposure of the fetus to some of these medications. It is also recognized that antiepileptic drugs or epilepsy itself can be associated to increased risks of labor induction, C-sections, or postpartum hemorrhage [2]. Some antiepileptic drugs are teratogenic, creating a dilemma for patients and families and a great challenge for critical care personnel when confronted to the pregnant patient with seizures [3, 4].

The frequency of seizures does not usually increase during pregnancy. Half of the patients with epilepsy will have no change in seizure frequency, while others will have a worsening in their condition. Those who are sleep deprived or are not compliant with their medications are at increased risk of seizures. Conditions such preeclampsia, fetal growth restriction, or stillbirth have been associated to an increased risk of seizures [5].

J. Pérez-Fernández (✉)
Critical Care Services, Baptist Hospital of Miami, Florida International University, Herbert Wertheim College of Medicine, Miami, FL, USA

G. Rodríguez-Vega
Neurocritical Care Services, HIMA-Caguas, Caguas, Puerto Rico

A. Sirven
Women and Children Department, West Kendall Baptist Hospital, Florida International University, Herbert Wertheim College of Medicine, Miami, FL, USA
e-mail: Drsirven@wkobgyn.com

C. Montufar et al. (eds.), *Obstetric Catastrophes*,
https://doi.org/10.1007/978-3-030-70034-8_39

Table 39.1 Causes of seizures in pregnancy

Primary epilepsy	Secondary seizures
	Eclampsia Structural (AVMs, neoplasms, CVT, strokes, intracranial hemorrhages) Metabolic (hyperemesis gravidarum, acute hepatitis, fatty liver, eclampsia) Hematologic (HELLP, porphyria) Infections (meningitis, encephalitis, sepsis, malaria) Pseudo-seizures

Most seizures during pregnancy affect women with history of epilepsy. However, critical care clinicians must be ready to differentiate seizures in the setting of a prior history of epilepsy from others with a secondary etiology most commonly associated to structural changes such as intracranial hemorrhage, cerebral venous sinus thrombosis, or ischemic stroke or metabolic causes including hyperemesis gravidarum, acute hepatitis (fatty liver of pregnancy or viral hepatitis), HELLP, and eclampsia (Table 39.1) [6, 7]. Although less frequently reported, acute porphyria or infections such as malaria should also be included in the differential diagnosis.

The Effects of Pregnancy on Seizure Control

While most women with epilepsy (WWE) have their seizures well-controlled, approximately 15–30% have an increase in the frequency of their seizures [8]. Many factors have been attributed to this increased frequency: those affecting the levels of AEDs such as changes in the volume of distribution of some medications, alterations in protein binding, increased renal clearance, or impaired intestinal absorption. Other factors are associated to poor compliance with treatment usually motivated by fear of possible drug-related fetal complications [9].

Clinicians, concerned about fetal adverse drug reactions, might relinquish the use of adequate medication treatment, sometimes attempting monotherapy regimens, changing medications to less effective ones, or miscalculating pharmacokinetics of such drugs [8–10].

All these factors have created fragmentation on the care of women with epilepsy and have been the motive for recent guidelines and joint forces in an attempt to standardize the management of epilepsy during pregnancy [11].

It is important for the clinician to remember that seizures, and more specifically epilepsy, could cause maternal death as well as damage to the fetus. Maternal death is highly associated to uncontrolled tonic-clonic seizures [12, 13].

It is generally accepted that seizure control and stability are preferred over potential fetal effects of AEDs, and it is recommended that only essential changes be made when women with epilepsy become pregnant [14].

Seizures are most likely to occur in the first trimester and in the peripartum. It has been reported that almost 5% of women with epilepsy will have peripartum seizures [8].

Differential Diagnosis

Eclampsia is the most common cause of new-onset seizures during pregnancy. A woman who presents with new-onset seizures in the second half of the pregnancy should be treated with existing protocols to control eclampsia. The diagnosis may rest on a good history, by excluding history of epilepsy, and confirming risk factors for preeclampsia [15–17].

As other structural changes can be associated to seizures, the use of neuroimages might be required. Computerized tomography and magnetic resonance imaging are considered safe during pregnancy with application of radiation exposure mitigation to the fetus [18, 19].

Intracranial hemorrhages and cerebral ischemic events are increased in pregnancy, especially in the postpartum period [20]. Subarachnoid hemorrhage occurs with more frequency during pregnancy [21]. Arteriovenous malformations (AVMs) are also more prone to appear with higher risk of bleeding during the first pregnancy and subsequent ones [22].

Special considerations must be given to cerebral venous thrombosis (CVT), more frequently present in the peripartum but with increased risk throughout pregnancy [23]. The typical presentation includes headache, seizures, or focal neurologic deficits. CT scan provides a classical diagnostic sign, a delta-shaped clot near the confluence of the sagittal and transverse sinus referred as "empty delta sign." MRI can be more sensitive avoiding the use of contrast although MRA might be required for a definitive diagnosis (Fig. 39.1) [24].

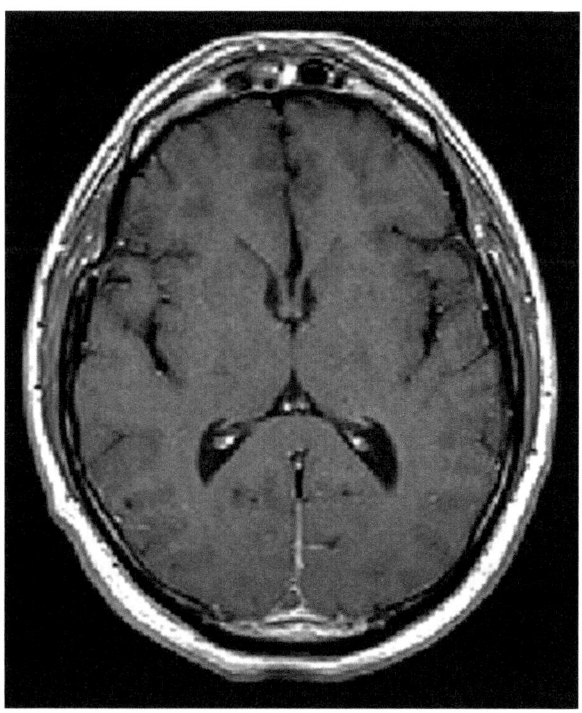

Fig. 39.1 The empty delta sign as seen on a contrast-enhanced CT. Reproduced with permission from the personal file of Dr. Kevin Abraham

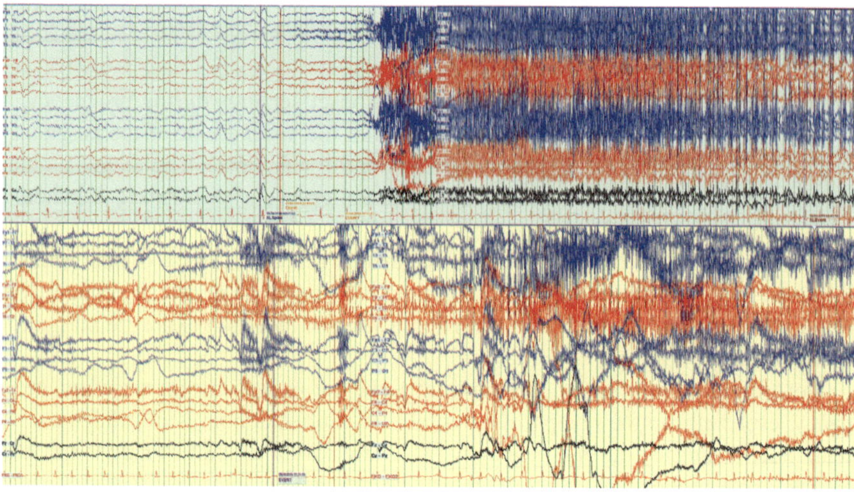

Fig. 39.2 EEG trace demonstrating tonic-clonic seizure (top) activity versus psychogenic activity (pseudo-seizures) (bottom). Reproduced with permission from the personal file of Dr. Ignacio Pita

Electrolyte abnormalities must always be ruled out in the presence of seizures. Not only can they decrease the threshold of seizures in women with epilepsy, but they can also independently cause seizures. Addisonian crisis and hypoglycemia are increased in frequency in patients with poor prenatal care. Vasovagal syndromes, cardiac arrhythmias, carotid sinus syndrome, and, in general, syncopal episodes could trigger seizures [25].

Porphyria is of special interest as it sometimes might be triggered by some AEDs [26].

Acute intermittent porphyria has been reported in cases of seizures during pregnancy [27].

Nonepileptic seizures also referred as psychogenic seizures or pseudo-seizures must be in the differential of drug-resistant attacks [28]. In these cases, EEG results are of extreme value to establish the differential diagnosis (Fig. 39.2).

Eclampsia

Eclampsia is one of the most frequent causes of seizures during pregnancy. If eclampsia occurs during the first pregnancy, it increases the odds in the subsequent pregnancies [29]. The triad of hypertension, edema, and proteinuria (preeclampsia) accompanied by seizures or coma defines eclampsia. The clinician must be aware that not all elements of the triad must be present prior to the development of eclampsia with up to one third of the patients presenting with seizures with no antecedent of proteinuria [30]. Eclampsia can occur in the antepartum, during, shortly after, or more than 48 h postpartum.

Eclampsia can sometimes be complicated by clotting disorder and bleeding diathesis associated to intracranial hypertension, a syndrome defined as HELLP. Hemolysis is seen, with elevated liver enzymes and low platelets, which carries significant morbidity and mortality [31].

Posterior reversible encephalopathy syndrome (PRES) or reversible posterior leukoencephalopathy syndrome (RPLS) is a clinical syndrome characterized by seizures, confusion, headache, and visual abnormalities. It may occur due to a number of causes including preeclampsia/eclampsia. Diagnosis must be made early, and neuroimaging findings are crucial (Fig. 39.3). Early detection followed by timely aggressive management and the elimination of the cause are crucial for satisfactory recovery and outcomes.

While therapy for eclampsia is largely aimed to control hypertension, neurology consultation should be promptly requested. Critical care departments should establish protocols for management of eclampsia and preeclampsia. The role of magnesium sulfate to treat gestational hypertension and prevent progression to eclampsia and to decrease recurrence of seizures has been historically demonstrated [32, 33]. Although magnesium sulfate is not an anticonvulsant agent, it acts as vasospastic

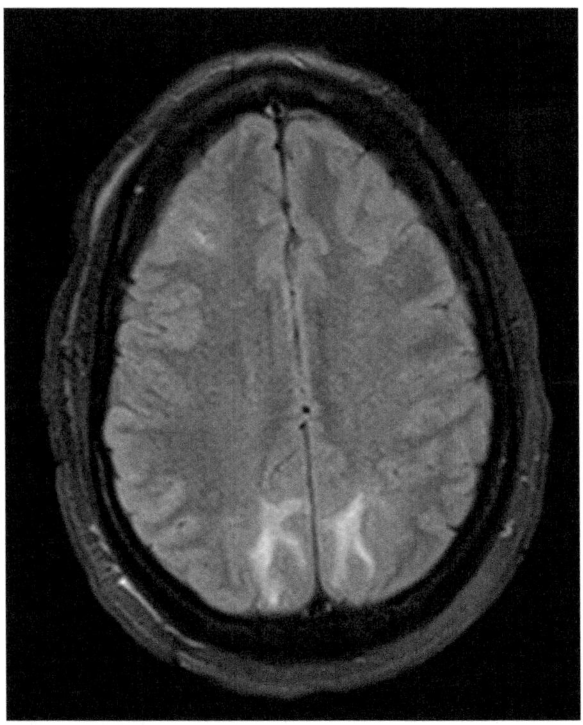

Fig. 39.3 Posterior reversible encephalopathy syndrome (PRES) visible on MRI as multiple cortico-subcortical areas of T2-weighterd hyperintense (white) signal involving the occipital lobes. Reproduced with permission from the personal file of Dr. Kevin Abraham

agent, increasing cerebral blood flow and perfusion. Its role in the increased production of prostacyclin, an endothelial vasodilator, has also been reported [34]. For eclamptic seizures refractory to magnesium sulfate, the use of other anticonvulsant medications is recommended [35].

Status Epilepticus

Status epilepticus occurs in only 1–2% of pregnancies. The risk for status epilepticus during pregnancy is similar to the nonpregnant women. The risk for maternal as well as fetal morbidity and mortality is elevated if not treated appropriately and aggressively [8]. Convulsions increase acid lactic levels causing transient increase in uterine pressure making these the primary morbid factor. Treatment must be standardized and aimed to control seizures as fast as possible. In order to facilitate fetal blood flow, a left lateral decubitus position for the mother is recommended. Clinicians must also cover all other aspects of the care of a critical care patient, including electrolyte surveillance, securing airway and oxygen administration, and a rapid evaluation of the AED levels.

Magnesium sulfate, the treatment of choice for eclampsia, should not be used for non-eclamptic seizures. Treatment should be based on AEDs. It is especially important to obtain serum levels of the patient's regular AEDs. Valproate and phenobarbital should be avoided unless the seizures are believed to be secondary to withdrawal of those medications. The role of thiamine has only been described in alcohol-related seizures or thiamine deficiency [36].

Seizures in Labor

The majority of patients should have a normal vaginal delivery despite their seizure disorder history. The incidence of seizures during labor is calculated at a rate of 1–2% of women with epilepsy. The rate increases in about 1–2% in the 24 h following the delivery [37]. Recent studies have calculated the occurrence of seizures in 3.5% of women with epilepsy in labor [38].

As seizures in labor expose the mother to hypoxia, increased lactic acidemia, and fetal hypoxia and uterine hypertonus, it becomes extremely important to control those episodes [39, 40].

Many factors have been invoked to explain the increased incidence of seizures during labor. Perhaps one of the most preventable is the missed doses of AEDs in the pre-labor period. As preventing seizures becomes a key factor in reducing morbidity for the pregnant woman, clinicians must ensure adequate administration of regular AEDs and must be prepared to respond with extreme celerity to any seizure activity. Hyperemesis might reduce intestinal absorption and availability of some AEDs, and clinicians must treat nausea and vomiting, even considering alternative routes of administration such as intravenous. Additional risk factors associated with seizures during labor include sleep deprivation, dehydration, and pain [41]. Neuraxial analgesia during the first stage of labor helps aid in sleep deprivation and pain management.

Risks of Obstetric Complications

Critical care clinicians must be aware of the small but significant increase in obstetric risks to women with epilepsy and those exposed to AEDs and promptly involve multidisciplinary care including neurology, obstetrics, and, if needed, neonatology.

Epilepsy itself can increase the risks of spontaneous miscarriages, hypertensive disorders, hemorrhage, preterm delivery, and fetal growth retardation [41]. In a recent systematic review, women exposed to AEDs demonstrated higher odds of induction of labor, increased frequency of newborn admission to neonatal intensive care unit, fetal growth retardation, or postpartum hemorrhage [42]. The same study also showed an increased number of C-sections in those patients exposed to polytherapy compared to monotherapy.

Pharmacotherapy

Pregnant women present a challenge in adjusting some medications. In general, pregnancy leads to variable pharmacokinetics of some drugs with challenging to reach therapeutic levels. Changes in absorption, metabolism, hemodilution, and excretion in pregnancy provoke that levels of medications like lamotrigine fall by up to 70% [43, 44].

Plasma binding protein levels are decreased although free (unbound) and active concentrations of medications remain stable. In this case, total serum levels might be misleading; thus the addition of extra doses of medications might not be needed and could increase potential side effects. Current practice calls for a regular serum drug monitoring with adjustments based on clinical features [41, 45]. Monitoring drug levels is likely more appropriate for phenytoin, lamotrigine, and oxcarbazepine although it must be proposed for all AEDs where pregnancy-induced metabolic changes have not been fully identified.

The role of vitamin K to prevent hemorrhagic disease in both the newborn and the mother exposed to AEDs has been advocated in the literature. This measure, although not supported with any randomized trial, has been widely accepted [46]. AEDs (carbamazepine, phenytoin, primidone, oxcarbazepine, topiramate, and eslicarbazepine) inhibit the precursors of clotting factors and increase the degradation of vitamin K. Two observational studies up to date failed to demonstrate any beneficial effect of preventive use of vitamin K, although in both studies babies born were routinely injected 1 mg of subcutaneous vitamin K at birth [47, 48].

Treatment Considerations

Seizure activity is potentially more harmful that any possible effect of AEDs. Thus, the goal for a woman admitted to critical care for any condition should be to control seizure activity and to prevent possible recurrences.

If seizures are non-epileptic in origin, inappropriate use of AEDs should be avoided. A firm diagnosis must be stablished first prior to considering delivery. Electroencephalogram (EEG) will help to differentiate psychogenic seizures from epilepsy (Fig. 39.3). Sedatives such as lorazepam or clonazepam should be used as needed.

Any seizure activity must be terminated as soon as possible to minimize hypoxia and acidosis potentially affecting the fetus. The mother must be positioned in left lateral decubitus with surveillance and patency of airway, maintaining an adequate oxygenation.

Although there is no clear evidence on the management of seizures during labor, benzodiazepines remain the drug of choice. If seizures are not controlled, phenytoin or fosphenytoin must be administered according to their regular doses [40]. Tocolytic agents should be considered if uterine hypertonus is present.

Maternal and fetal monitoring is essential. Clinicians should exercise careful attention to neonatal withdrawal syndrome if several doses of benzodiazepines are used to abort seizure activity [49].

Conclusions

The majority of seizures during pregnancy are associated with a preexisting neurological condition, or they are secondary to an increase in blood pressure as a result of eclamptic episodes. Primary care provider (obstetrician) and critical care clinician, in conjunction with a neurologist, should monitor the levels of AEDs in the preconception period. Controlling seizures should be prioritized over reducing exposure to AEDs. However, if possible, monotherapy with the least teratogenic drugs should be preferred. Medications should be administered during pregnancy and especially while in labor and adjustments must be made as needed.

Eclampsia is a very serious and dangerous condition for the pregnant patient. It can increase the mortality of both mother and fetus. It is extremely important to monitor and control patient blood pressure throughout the entire pregnancy. Current guidelines recommend delivery after 37 weeks of gestation for those patients with increased blood pressure. Magnesium sulfate has been found to be an adequate medication for the treatment of eclampsia as well as preeclamptic episodes and should be continued for at least 24 h after delivery to decrease maternal mortality. The use of AEDs in eclampsia-associated seizures rebel to the administration of magnesium sulfate is highly recommended.

Status epilepticus is the most dangerous condition due to its association and risk of placental abruption. Intravenous benzoxazepine (lorazepam) is the drug of choice in treatment. An immediate delivery, usually by C-section, is recommended once the mother is stabilized.

Although the majority of the seizures in pregnancy are associated with a preexisting condition or related to pregnancy-induced conditions, clinicians must always consider differential diagnosis such neoplasms, AVM, or CVT, especially if confronted to new-onset seizures.

References

1. Zack MM, Kobau R. National and state estimates of the numbers of adults and children with active epilepsy — United States, 2015. MMWR. 2017;66:821–5.
2. Borthen I, Eide MG, Daltveit AK, Gilhus NE. Delivery outcome of women with epilepsy- a population-based cohort study. BJOG. 2010;117(12):1537–43.
3. Laganà AS, Triolo O, D'Amico V, Cartella SM, Sofo V, Salmeri FM, et al. Management of women with epilepsy- from preconception to post-partum. Arch Gynecol Obstet. 2016;293(3):493–503.
4. Tomson T, Battino D. Teratogenic effects of antiepileptic drugs. Lancet Neurol. 2012;11:803.
5. Patel SI, Pennell PB. Management of epilepsy during pregnancy: an update. Ther Adv Neurol Disord. 2015;9(2):118–29.
6. Mikolasevic I, Filipec-Kanizaj T, Jakopcic I, et al. Liver disease during pregnancy: a challenging clinical issue. Med Sci Monit. 2018;24:4080–90.
7. Beach RL, Kaplan PW. Seizures and pregnancy: diagnosis and management. Int Rev Neurobiol. 2008;83:259–71.
8. Battino D, Tomson T, Bonizzoni E, Craig J, Lindhout D, Sabers A, et al. EURAP Study Group. Seizure control and treatment changes in pregnancy: observations from the EURAP epilepsy pregnancy registry. Epilepsia. 2013;54:1621–7.
9. Tomson T, Battino D, Bonizzoni E, Craig J, Lindhout D, Sabers A, et al. EURAP study group. Dose-dependent risk of malformations with antiepileptic drugs: an analysis of data from the EURAP epilepsy and pregnancy registry. Lancet Neurol. 2011;10:609–17.
10. Hernández-Díaz S, Smith CR, Shen A, Mittendorf R, Hauser WA, Yerby M, et al. North American AED Pregnancy Registry. Comparative safety of antiepileptic drugs during pregnancy. Neurology. 2012;78:1692–9.
11. Royal College of Obstetricians and Gynecologists. RCOG Green -Top Guideline No. 68. Epilepsy in Pregnancy. June 2016. Accessed online.
12. Shorvon S, Tomson T. Sudden unexpected death in epilepsy. Lancet. 2011;378:2028–38.
13. Christensen J, Vestergaard C, Hammer Bech B. Maternal death in women with epilepsy. Neurology. 2018;91(18):e1716.
14. Practice parameter: management issues for women with epilepsy (summary statement). Report of the Quality Standards Subcommittee of the American Academy of Neurology. Neurology. 1998;51:944.
15. Lopes-Cendes IE, Andermann E, Cendes L, Dansky L, Andermann F. Risk factors for changes in seizure frequency during pregnancy of epileptic women: a cohort study. Epilepsia. 1992;33(3):57.
16. Enye S, Ganapathy R, Braithwaite O. Proteinuria in status epilepticus or eclampsia; a diagnostic dilemma. Am J Emerg Med. 2009;27:625.e5–6.

17. Pandey R, Garg R, Darlong V, Punj J, Khanna P. Recurrent seizures in pregnancy-epilepsy or eclampsia: a diagnostic dilemma? A case report. AANA J. 2011;79:388–90.
18. Gaillard WD, Cross JH, Duncan JS, Stefan H, Theodore WH. Task Force on practice parameter imaging guidelines for the International League Against Epilepsy, Commission for Diagnostics. Epilepsy imaging study guideline criteria: commentary on diagnostic testing study guidelines and practice parameters. Epilepsia. 2011;52:1750–6.
19. ACOG Committee on Obstetric Practice. ACOG Committee Opinion. Number 299, September 2004 (replaces No. 158, September 1995). Guidelines for diagnostic imaging during pregnancy. Obstet Gynecol. 2004;104:647–51.
20. Kittner SJ Stern BJ, Feeser BR, et al. Pregnancy and the risk of stroke. N Engl J Med. 1996;335:768–74.
21. Limaye K, Patel A, Lahoti S, et al. Secular increases in spontaneous subarachnoid hemorrhage during pregnancy. Presented at: International Stroke Conference. January 24-26, 2018; Los Angeles, CA. Abstract 36.
22. Trivedi RA, Kirkpatrick PJ. (2003). Arteriovenous malformations of the cerebral circulation that rupture in pregnancy. J Obstet Gynaecol. 2003;23:484–9.
23. Gupta R, Aggarwal M, Patil S, Vyas V. Cerebral venous thrombosis associated with pregnancy: a case report. IOSR J Dental Med Sci. 2015;14(5):43–5.
24. Ferro JM, Canhao P, Stam J, et al. Prognosis of cerebral vein and dural sinus thrombosis: results of the international study on cerebral vein and dural sinus thrombosis (ISCVT). Stroke. 2004;35:664–70.
25. Seizures in pregnancy: diagnosis and management. Int Rev Neurobiol. 2008;83:259–71.
26. Hahn M, Gildemeister OS, Krauss GL, Pepe JA, Lambrecht RW, Donohue S, Bonkovsky HL. Effects of new anticonvulsant medications on porphyrin synthesis in cultured liver cells: potential implications for patients with acute porphyria. Neurology. 1997;49(1):97–106.
27. Zadra N, Grandi R, Mirabile D, et al. Treatment of seizures in acute intermittent porphyria: safety and efficacy of gabapentin. Seizure. 1998;7(5):415–6.
28. Reuber M, Baker GA, Gill R, Smith DF, Chadwick DW. Failure to recognize psychogenic nonepileptic seizures may cause death. Neurology. 2004;62:834–5.
29. Hernandez-Diaz S, Toh S, Cnattingius S. Risk of pre-eclampsia in first and subsequent pregnancies: a prospective cohort study. BMJ. 2009;b2255:338.
30. Douglas K, Redman CW. Eclampsia in the United Kingdom. BMJ. 1994;309:1395–400.
31. Sibai BM, Ramadan MK, Usta I, Salama M, Mercer BM, Friedman SA. Maternal morbidity and mortality in 442 pregnancies with hemolysis, elevated liver enzymes, and low platelets (HELLP syndrome). Am J Obstetr Gynecol. 1993;169:1000–6.
32. Lucas L, Leveno K, Cunningham G. A comparison of magnesium sulfate with phenytoin for the prevention of eclampsia. N Engl J Med. 1995;333:201–5.
33. Euser A, Cipolla MJ. Magnesium sulfate for the treatment of eclampsia. Stroke. 2009;40:1169–75.
34. Tang J, He A, Li N, et al. Magnesium sulfate-mediated vascular relaxation and calcium channel activity in placental vessels different from non-placental vessels. JAHA. 2018;e009896:7.
35. Gulmezoglu AM, Duley L. Use of anticonvulsants in eclampsia and pre-eclampsia: survey of obstetricians in the United Kingdom and Republic of Ireland. BMJ. 1998;316:975–6.
36. Botez MI, Botez T, Ross-Chouinard A, Lalonde R. Thiamine and folate treatment of chronic epileptic patients: a controlled study with the Wechsler IQ scale. Epilepsy Res. 1993;16:157–63.
37. Viale L, Allotey J, Cheong-See F, et al. Epilepsy in pregnancy and reproductive outcomes: a systematic review and meta-analysis. Lancet. 2015;386:1845.
38. MacDonald SC, Bateman BT, McElrath TF, Hernández-Díaz S. Mortality and morbidity during delivery hospitalization among pregnant women with epilepsy in the United States. JAMA Neurol. 2015;72:981.
39. Teramo K, Hiilesmaa V, Bardy A, Saarikoski S. Fetal heart rate during a maternal grand mal epileptic seizure. J Perinat Med. 1979;7:3–6.

40. Ozdemir O, Sari ME, Ertugrul FA, et al. The effects of a history of seizures during pregnancy on umbilical arterial blood gas values in pregnant women with epilepsy. J Turk Ger Gynecol Assoc. 2014;15:135–9.
41. Practice parameter: management issues for women with epilepsy (summary statement). Report of the Quality Standards Subcommittee of the American Academy of Neurology. Neurology. 1998;51:944.
42. National Institute for Health and Care Excellence. The epilepsies: the diagnosis and management of the epilepsies in adults and children in primary and secondary care. NICE clinical guideline 137. [Manchester]: NICE; 2012.
43. Adab N. Therapeutic monitoring of antiepileptic drugs during pregnancy and in the postpartum period: is it useful? CNS Drugs. 2006;20:791–800.
44. Pennell PB, Hovinga CA. Antiepileptic drug therapy in pregnancy I: gestation-induced effects on AED pharmacokinetics. Int Rev Neurobiol. 2008;83:227–40.
45. Scottish Intercollegiate Guidelines Network. Diagnosis and management of epilepsy in adults: A national clinical guideline. SIGN publication no. 143. Edinburgh: SIGN; 2015.
46. Harden CL, Pennell PB, Koppel BS, Hovinga CA, Gidal B, Meador KJ, et al. American Academy of Neurology; American Epilepsy Society. Practice parameter update: management issues for women with epilepsy—focus on pregnancy (an evidence-based review): vitamin K, folic acid, blood levels, and breastfeeding. Neurology. 2009;73:142–9.
47. Choulika S, Grabowski E, Holmes LB. Is antenatal vitamin K prophylaxis needed for pregnant women taking anticonvulsants? Am J Obstet Gynecol. 2004;190:882–3.
48. Yamasmit W, Chaithongwongwatthana S, Tolosa JE. Prenatal vitamin K1 administration in epileptic women to prevent neonatal hemorrhage: is it effective? J Reprod Med. 2006;51:463–6.
49. McElhatton PR. The effects of benzodiazepine use during pregnancy and lactation. Reprod Toxicol. 1994;8:461–75.

Chapter 40
Neurogenic Shock in Pregnant Women

Jorge Sinclair, Jorge E. Sinclair De Frías, Sabrina Da Re Gutiérrez, and Jorge Hidalgo

Introduction

Neurogenic shock is a type of shock characterized by hypotension and reflex bradycardia. Most cases occur after a severe cervical spine trauma, especially in complete injuries above T6 [36]. Spine injuries affect around 17,000 people in the United States [27], being 20–30% of these individuals fertile women [9]. Other nontraumatic causes of neurogenic shock include spinal anesthesia, Guillain-Barre syndrome, and autonomic nervous system toxins.

Diagnosis is only considered after other systemic causes of shock have been ruled out, since critically ill neurologic patients are in risk of other conditions such as sepsis, dehydration, acute cardiac failure, acute blood loss, or pulmonary embolism [22].

When this entity presents in pregnant women, gestational age of the fetus and physiological changes during pregnancy must be taken in account. These changes overlap with complications due to neurogenic shock, requiring an interdisciplinary management, including an obstetrician or subspecialist in maternal-fetal medicine.

J. Sinclair
Critical Medicine, Chief UCI Hospital Pacifica Salud/Johns Hopkins Medicine, Faculty of Medicine University of Panama, Panama City, Panama

J. E. Sinclair De Frías (✉)
Santo Tomas Hospital, Faculty of Medicine University of Panama, Panamá City, Panamá

S. Da Re Gutiérrez
Critical and Intensive Care Medicine, Maternal and Child Hospital, Caja Nacional de Salud (CNS), La Paz, Bolivia

J. Hidalgo
Division of Critical Care, Karl Heusner Memorial Hospital, Belize City, Belize

C. Montufar et al. (eds.), *Obstetric Catastrophes*,
https://doi.org/10.1007/978-3-030-70034-8_40

Hemodynamic Changes During Pregnancy

During pregnancy, multiple changes occur in the cardiovascular system. Blood volume expands, with an increase of 40–50% of the plasmatic volume and 20–30% of the red blood cells [37]. This unproportional increase of plasmatic volume and red blood cells results in physiologic anemia of pregnancy [19]. Blood pressure decreases gradually until mid-pregnancy, posteriorly returning to baseline levels by late pregnancy [29]. This decrease is mainly due to a fall in systemic vascular resistance (SVR) that occurs normally during pregnancy [3]. By week 12, heart rate increases and continues to be elevated until week 32.

Cardiac output (CO) increases from 30% to 50% due to an increase in heart rate and stroke volume. Uterine blood flow increments during pregnancy, compromising up to 20% of CO at term. This system is very sensitive to catecholamines and changes in maternal intravascular volume; thus, maternal hypovolemia can first manifest as fetal distress [37].

SVR decreases, reaching its lowest point around week 24, and progressively rises until term. Tendency to venous blood pooling during pregnancy may lead to hypotension or syncope when passing from a supine position to a standing position. Supine hypotensive syndrome presents when a pregnant woman is in a supine position as the gravid uterus compresses the aorta and inferior vena cava. It manifests as dizziness, pallor, and tachycardia.

Pathogenesis

Neurovasodilatory Shock

The hallmark of neurogenic shock is the association of hypotension and bradycardia due to a loss of autonomic tone secondary to an interruption of sympathetic pathways. Descending sympathetic fibers originate at the hypothalamus and are located in the intermediolateral and dorsolateral aspects of the lateral funiculus of the spine [26].

Disruption of descending pathways results in loss of sympathetic tone and unopposed vagal tone, leading to vascular smooth muscle relaxation below the level of spine cord injury, decreased venous return and CO, atrioventricular conduction abnormalities, and reflex bradycardia [5]. Over time, hyperactivity of peripheral adrenoreceptors develops due to low basal levels of catecholamines, accounting for the excessive vasopressor response seen in this scenario.

Patients are at increased risk of secondary spinal cord ischemia due to impairment of autoregulation mechanisms [21]. Severe hypotension results in hypoperfusion of the spinal cord, decreasing the potential of recovery of neurological functions [12, 32].

Neurocardiogenic Shock

Pathologies such as subarachnoid hemorrhage (SAH) and traumatic brain injuries might cause neurocardiogenic shock. It is most often recognized in the electrocardiogram as arrhythmias, QRS, ST segment, and T wave abnormalities [7, 20]. It is suggested that this process is neurally mediated [38], and it is not related to coronary atherosclerosis. Patients with SAH can have elevated levels of norepinephrine within the first 10 days or longer after injury [25]. High levels of catecholamines may lead to selective myocardial cell necrosis [2] resulting in reduced inotropy, increased cardiac preload due to venous constriction, and increased cardiac afterload due to peripheral arterial constriction. Subsequently, stroke volume (SV) diminishes and cannot be compensated by reflex tachycardia, leading to decreased CO and shock [22]. Neurocardiogenic shock is usually transient, resolving within several days to 2 weeks after SAH. Management focuses on preventing secondary brain damage due to hypoxia and decreased cerebral perfusion.

Neuroendocrine Shock

Neurogenic shock can also be caused by a neuroendocrine dysfunction due to insufficiency of the hypothalamic-pituitary-adrenal axis. There is an inappropriate release of cortisol during stress situations, resulting in decreased systemic vascular resistance, reduced cardiac contractility, and hypovolemia [33]. This secondary adrenal insufficiency is due to injury of the hypothalamus, pituitary gland, or connecting structures, developing within 4 days after injury [22].

Signs and Symptoms

Evaluation of circulatory system in pregnant women with neurogenic shock, especially in the context of trauma, is complicated. Hemodynamic parameters can be obscure by physiologic hemodynamic alterations of pregnancy, autonomic alterations due to neurogenic shock, and cardiovascular instability caused by acute blood loss. Decrease of blood pressure due to shock may be confused with physiological reduction of blood pressure during pregnancy. Physiologic dilutional anemia can be misperceived as a sign of blood loss.

There is no definitive test, but patients classically present with hypotension associated to bradycardia (Table 40.1). Symptoms can present anytime from the onset of the injury or illness to several weeks after the onset. Hypotension is caused by peripheral vasodilation; therefore, extremities may be warm and dry with normal capillary refill time resulting in heat loss and hypothermia, which can lead to

Table 40.1 Clinical manifestations of the different types of neurogenic shock vs hemorrhagic shock ([22])

	Vasodilatory	Neurocardiogenic	Neuroendocrine	Hemorrhagic
Skin	Dry and warm	Dry or wet, cold	Dry and warm	Wet and cold
Blood Pressure	↓	↓	↓[a]	↓
Heart Rate	↓	↑	↓ or ↑	↑
SVR	↓	↑	↓	↑
Stroke volume	↓	↓	↓	↓
Cardiac output	↓	↓	↓	↓
CVP	↓ or **N**	↑ or **N**	↓ or **N**	↓
PCWP	↓	↑	↓	↓
EDVI	–	↑	–	–
Chest X-ray	–	Apical ballooning	–	–
Echo LVEF	–	↓ with global or segmentary wall motion abnormalities different from coronary artery territory	–	–

Abbreviations: *SVR* systemic vascular resistance, *CVP* central venous pressure, *PCWP* pulmonary capillary wedge pressure, *EDVI* end-diastolic volume index, *LVEF* left ventricular ejection fraction, ***N*** normal

[a]Hypotension not responsive to vasopressors

bradycardia and fetal distress [30]. On the other hand, hypovolemic shock presents with reflex tachycardia and cool and wet extremities.

Central venous pressure (CVP) may be normal or reduced, and SVR will be usually low. SV and CO may also be decreased due to vagal tone. Bradycardia is the most frequent arrhythmia associated to neurogenic shock. It can be exacerbated by suctioning, defecation, turning, and hypoxia [16]. Other arrhythmias may be seen, including supraventricular and ventricular tachycardia. Orthostatic hypotension without reflex tachycardia is also common.

Neurocardiogenic shock presents with hypotension and tachycardia, increased systemic vascular resistance, cold and wet extremities, and prolonged capillary refill time caused by peripheral vasoconstriction observed in these cases. CVP is usually normal or high, while SV and CO are low due to myocardial dysfunction. Cardiac enzymes might be elevated, but peak levels are not as high as in myocardial infarction [22].

Neuroendocrine neurogenic shock presents with hypotension that does not respond to vasopressor infusion. The hallmark of this entity is low baseline cortisol levels. CVP, SVR, SV, and CO are low [22].

Diagnosis

In every neurointensive care patient, common systemic causes of hypotension such as sepsis, dehydration, and hemorrhage must be ruled out.

In paralyzed patients, signs of hypovolemic shock may be absent due to loss of sympathetic tone under the level of injury. Pallor of the extremities, reflex tachycardia, and signs of peritoneal irritation may also be absent.

Every patient should undergo serial electrocardiograms, serial cardiac enzymes, and chest radiographs, as pulmonary edema can present independently or concomitantly with neurocardiogenic injuries. Hemodynamic monitoring should be performed, including CVP and blood pressure through a central venous line and an arterial line, respectively.

Central venous access is required to guide fluid and vasopressor administration in pregnant women with neurogenic shock. CVC site of placement plays an important role. Subclavian vein is the preferred site, especially in patients with elevated intracranial pressure, as venous catheters within the internal jugular vein produce venous stasis increasing the risk of venous thrombosis [34]. Additionally, patients with cervical trauma usually require cervical collars; therefore, there is difficulty in jugular access.

Intracranial pressure measurement devices do not have a role in diagnosis but are important in the management of neurogenic shock. They are used to titrate the mean arterial pressure (MAP) in order to maintain cerebral perfusion.

In neurocardiogenic shock, hemodynamic monitoring must be extensive. Echocardiography is important to define the etiology of shock. The typical echocardiographic findings include atypical ballooning [42] and segmentary wall motion abnormalities that do not match the territory of any coronary artery. Despite this, acute myocardial infarction is more common and thereby should be ruled out initially.

In the setting of fever and shock, blood cultures must be obtained, and empirical antibiotics should be started until blood cultures yield results. Cerebral spinal fluid cultures are important in the setting of neurointensive care, especially in pregnant women after head trauma with skull fracture or sinus disease, or instrumentation of head or spinal canal.

Adrenal insufficiency should always be considered. Random serum cortisol levels should be measured in early stages of shock. These levels can be altered when patients receive steroids, especially in patients with neurologic injuries that frequently receive glucocorticoid therapy. The administrated dose may be sufficient to alter the results of a random serum cortisol level but not enough to treat the adrenal insufficiency appropriately. To avoid this, one could either treat empirically with higher doses of steroids at a dose that also treats adrenal insufficiency or withhold steroid administration for 12 h and then obtain serum cortisol levels and resume steroid therapy. The decision will depend on the clinical condition of the patient, since hypotension is frequently severe enough that immediate treatment is warranted. Glucocorticoid treatment is not associated to teratogenicity or increased fetal loss during pregnancy. On the other hand, there are no studies of mineralocorticoid replacement therapy during pregnancy in women with adrenal insufficiency; therefore, blood pressure and electrolytes should be monitored closely [41].

Management

Management of shock in pregnant women differs from the one in general population due to physiological changes that occur during pregnancy and that both, the mother and the fetus, are vulnerable [1].

Defining the origin of hypotension in a pregnant woman is a challenge for the clinician, especially after a severe cervical trauma. For that reason, fluid therapy may be initiated even before hypovolemia is clinically evident [8]. Due to the increase in plasmatic volume, significant blood loss may occur before changes in vital signs become evident [37].

Vena cava compression should be taken in account, since its compression can reduce up to 30% of the CO [13]. In patients without risk of spinal injury, placing the patient in left lateral decubitus avoids caval compression [11]. In pregnant women with potential spinal injury, displacement of the uterus to the left or tilting the back board at a 15° angle is preferred [37].

The main goal is to maintain perfusion of the injured spinal tissue and oxygen supplementation, lowering the risk of secondary ischemic injuries of the traumatized tissue [18]. In all cases, hemodynamic stability through fluid therapy and early vasopressor therapy is crucial. Pregnant women are at increased risk of pulmonary edema during fluid resuscitation, due to a low colloid oncotic pressure and hypoalbuminemia [15]; thus, if neurogenic shock is not recognized and is managed as other type of shock, pregnant women are at higher risk of complications secondary to aggressive fluid resuscitation. Overhydration can also lead to spinal cord edema, worsening spinal cord perfusion and prognosis [31].

In neurogenic shock, resuscitation with fluids is not enough to overcome the vasodilation and decrease in CO. In a previous study, up to 82% of the patients with incomplete cervical injury required vasopressor therapy to maintain a MAP >90 mmHg [17]. Another study correlated the severity and level of spinal injury with the need of vasopressors, where cervical and complete injuries required vasopressors more frequently than thoracic and incomplete injuries [39].

If after 1 to 2 L of IV fluids hypotension persist, vasopressor therapy is indicated. The choice of vasopressors/inotropes during pregnancy is controversial. Main concerns include its efficacy and hemodynamic effects, adverse effects on uterine blood flow, and fetal acid-base status.

Vasopressors with alpha- and beta-adrenergic effect such as dopamine and norepinephrine are preferred in nonpregnant patients, as they increase vascular tone and have a positive chronotropic effect. Epinephrine and vasopressin infusions may be used in refractory cases [35].

These drugs should be used with caution during pregnancy, that is, only when potential benefits outweigh potential risks, as most of them have shown adverse effects on the fetus in animal studies, and there are no well-controlled studies in humans (Table 40.2).

The vasopressors with most data available in obstetric patients are ephedrine and phenylephrine, which have been studied mainly in hypotension induced by spinal anesthesia during cesarean section (Table 40.3). Phenylephrine is an exclusive

Table 40.2 Vasopressor and inotropic drugs [12, 14, 23]

Drug	Mechanism of action	US FDA pregnancy category
Dopamine	Dose dependent *Low*: dopamine-1 agonist *Medium*: beta-1 agonist *High*: alpha-1 agonist	**C**
Dobutamine	Beta-1 Agonist	**B**
Norepinephrine	Alpha-1 and beta-1 agonist	**C**
Ephedrine	Alpha and beta agonist	**C**
Phenylephrine	Alpha-1 agonist	**C**
Methoxamine	Alpha-1 agonist	**C**
Mephentermine	Alpha and beta agonist	**C**
Metaraminol	Alpha and beta agonist	**C**

Abbreviations: *US FDA* United States Food and Drug Administration

Table 40.3 Phenylephrine vs ephedrine: advantages and disadvantages [12, 14, 28]

Drug	Mechanism	Primary effects	Advantages	Disadvantages
Phenylephrine	Alpha-1 agonist	Vasoconstriction	Growing supporting evidence High efficacy Easy to titrate Rapid onset and short duration of action Low incidence of nausea and vomiting No adverse effect in fetal acid-base status	Few data available in preterm, emergency, laboring patients, or in preexisting fetal compromise Reflex bradycardia and reduction in cardiac output
Ephedrine	Dose dependent *Low*: beta-1 agonist *High*: alpha-1 and beta-1 agonist	*Low dose*: increased cardiac output *High dose*: increased cardiac output and vasoconstriction	Available data with few reports of adverse clinical outcomes Economical Minimal effect on uteroplacental blood flow No reflex bradycardia	Limited efficacy (large doses required) Does not correct vasodilation Slow onset and long duration of action Difficult titration Increased heart rate and contractility may lead to palpitations and arrhythmias Fetal acidosis

alpha-adrenergic vasopressor, with no chronotropic effect and can produce reflex bradycardia; therefore, anticholinergic drugs may be required in association with phenylephrine. Drugs such as norepinephrine and epinephrine may present some benefits in comparison to ephedrine/phenylephrine due to their beta-adrenergic effects, but less data is available to support their use [14].

Management of arrhythmias includes continuous cardiac monitoring, and, when symptomatic bradycardia develops, oxygen, atropine, and inotropes could be used. If bradycardia persist, patients may require a cardiac pacemaker.

Caution must be taken in vasodilatory neurogenic shock when using vasopressor infusions. Although vagal tone predominates, patients usually have peripheral alpha adrenoceptor hypersensitivity, limiting the use of epinephrine and norepinephrine as they can lead to severe blood fluctuations.

Despite being the mainstay of treatment, vasopressors should be used with discretion as they may cause vasoconstriction of the placental vasculature leading to an increased risk of fetal hypoxia [13]. Vasopressor infusion should be titrated to maintain an adequate MAP and cerebral perfusion pressure (CPP). Blood pressure targets are not well defined. The American Association of Neurological Surgeons and the Congress of Neurological Surgeons recommend a MAP goal of 85–90 mmHg during the first 7 days [40], but certain individuals may benefit from longer management [32]. Optimal CPP is not known, but it is recommended a goal CPP of 65 mmHg or greater [22]. Some studies suggest that sustaining CPP higher than 70 mmHg is associated to better outcomes [10, 24], while others demonstrated that adverse effects are not observed unless CPP decreases lower than 50–60 mmHg [4, 6].

Blood pressure, heart rate, and urine output should be monitored continuously. Echocardiography can assess CO and filling. Inotropic support with dobutamine, milrinone, or norepinephrine may be necessary. Both dopamine and milrinone have vasodilatory effects, worsening hypotension and requiring concomitant use of alpha agonist such as phenylephrine or norepinephrine. Beta-blockers are not recommended, since tachycardia is necessary to maintain and adequate CO.

Neuroendocrine neurogenic shock caused by primary or secondary adrenal insufficiency is managed with steroid replacement therapy. Hydrocortisone can be used, 50 mg every 6 h.

References

1. Alkhatib A. The role of laboratory medicine for health during pregnancy. EJIFCC. 2018;29(4):280–4.
2. Baroldi G, Mittleman RE, Parolini M, et al. Myocardial contraction bands. Definition, quantification and significance in forensic pathology. Intern J Legal Med. 2001;115(3):142–51.
3. Borovac-Pinheiro A, Pacagnella RC, Morais SS, Cecatti JG. Standard reference values for the shock index during pregnancy. Int J Gynaecol Obstet. 2016;135(1):11–5.
4. Bullock R, Chesnut RM, Clifton G, et al. Guidelines for the management of severe head injury. Brain Trauma Foundation. Eur J Emerg Med. 1996;3(2):109–27.
5. Chong SU, Worm M, Zuberbier T. Role of adverse reactions to food in urticaria and exercise-induced anaphylaxis. Int Arch Allergy Immunol. 2002;129:19–26.
6. Czosnyka M, Guazzo E, Iyer V, et al. Testing of cerebral autoregulation in head injury by waveform analysis of blood flow velocity and cerebral perfusion pressure. Acta Neurochir. 1994;60:468–71.
7. Davies KR, Gelb AW, Manninen PH, et al. Cardiac function in aneurysmal subarachnoid haemorrhage: a study of electrocardiographic and echocardiographic abnormalities. Br J Anaesth. 1991;67(1):58–63.

8. Desjardins G. (2008). Management of the injured pregnant patient. Trauma Org. Trauma in Pregnancy.
9. DeVivo MJ. (2012) Epidemiology of traumatic spinal cord injury: trends and future implications. Spinal Cord 2012(50):365–372.
10. Eisenberg HM, Frankowski RF, Contant CF, et al. High-dose barbiturate control of elevated intracranial pressure in patients with severe head injury. J Neurosurg. 1988;69(1):15–23.
11. Goyena R. Acute spinal cord injury. J Chem Inf Model. 2019;53:1689–99.
12. Haller J, Bice M, Lawrence B. Mediating the secondary effects of spinal cord injury through optimization of key physiologic parameters. J Am Acad Orthop Surg. 2016;24:160–71.
13. Jain V, Chari R, Maslovitz S, et al. Guidelines for the management of the pregnant trauma patient. J Obstet Gynaecol Can. 2015;37(6):553–71.
14. Kinsella SM, Carvalho B, Dyer RA, et al. International consensus statement on the management of hypotension with vasopressors during caesarean section under spinal anaesthesia. Anaesthesia. 2018;73:71–92.
15. Lapinsky SE. Acute respiratory failure in pregnancy. Obstet Med. 2015;8(3):126–32.
16. Lehmann KG, Lane JG, Piepmeier JM, Batsford WP. Cardiovascular abnormalities accompanying acute spinal cord injury in humans: incidence, time course and severity. J Am Coll Cardiol. 1987;10:46–52.
17. Levi L, Wolf A, Belzberg H. Hemodynamic parameters in patients with acute cervical cord trauma: description, intervention, and prediction of outcome. Neurosurgery. 1993;33(6):1007–16.
18. Lin VW. Spinal cord medicine: principles and practice. 2nd ed. New York: Demos Medical; 2010.
19. Lund CJ, Donovan JC. Blood volume during pregnancy. Significance of plasma and red cell volumes. Am J Obstet Gynecol. 1967;98(3):394–403.
20. Macrea LM, Tramer MR, Walder B. Spontaneous subarachnoid hemorrhage and serious cardiopulmonary dysfunction–a systematic review. Resuscitation. 2005;65(2):139–48.
21. Mack EH. Neurogenic shock. Open Pediatr Med J. 2013;7:16–8.
22. Muehlschlegel S, Greer D. Neurogenic Shock. In: Grabielli A, Layon AJ, Yu M, editors. Civetta, Taylor & Kirby's critical care. 4th ed. Philadelphia: Lippincott Williams & Wilkins; 2008.
23. Nag DS, Samaddar DP, Chatterjee A, Kumar H, Dembla A. Vasopressors in obstetric anesthesia: a current perspective. World J Clin Cases. 2015;3:58–64.
24. Narayan RK, Kishore PR, Becker DP, et al. Intracranial pressure: to monitor or not to monitor? A review of our experience with severe head injury. J Neurosurg. 1982;56(5):650–9.
25. Naredi S, Lambert G, Eden E, et al. Increased sympathetic nervous ac-tivity in patients with nontraumatic subarachnoid hemorrhage. Stroke. 2000;31(4):901–6.
26. Nathan PW, Smith MC. The location of descending fibres to sympathetic preganglionic vasomotor and sudomotor neurons in man. J Neurol Neurosurg Psychiatry. 1987;50(10):1253–62.
27. National Spinal Cord Injury Statistical Center. Facts and figures at a glance. Birmingham: University of Alabama at Birmingham; 2016.
28. Ngan Kee WD, Khaw KS. Vasopressors in obstetrics: what should we be using? Curr Opin Anaesthesiol. 2006;19:238–43.
29. Norwitz ER, Robinson JN, Malone FD. Pregnancy-induced physiologic alterations. In: Dildy III GA, Belfort MA, Saade GR, Phelan JP, Hankins GDV, Clark SL, editors. Critical care obstetrics. 4th ed. Malden: Blackwell Publishing; 2004. p. 19–42.
30. Popov I, Ngambu F, Mantel G, Rout C, Moodley J. Acute spinal cord injury in pregnancy: an illustrative case and literature review. J Obstet Gynaecol (Lahore). 2003;23(6):596–8.
31. Raw DA, Beattie JK, Hunter JM. Anaesthesia for spinal surgery in adults. Br J Anaesth. 2003;91:886–904.
32. Ruiz I, Squair J, Phillips A, Lukac C, Huang D, Oxciano P, et al. Incidence and natural progression of neurogenic shock after traumatic spinal cord injury. J Neurotrauma. 2018;35(3):461–6.
33. Silverman HJ, Van Hook C, Haponik EF. Hemodynamic changes in human anaphylaxis. Am J Med. 1984;77:341–4.
34. Stephens PH, Lennox G, Hirsch N, et al. Superior sagittal sinus thrombosis after internal jugular vein cannulation. Br J Anaesth. 1991;67(4):476–9.

35. Stratman RC, Wiesner AM, Smith KM, Cook AM. Hemodynamic management after spinal cord injury. Orthopedics. 2008;31(3):252–5.
36. Taylor MP, Wrenn P, O'Donnell AD. Presentation of neurogenic shock within the emergency department. EMJ. 2016;34(3):157–62.
37. Tsuei BJ. Assessment of the pregnant trauma patient. Injury. 2006;37(5):367–73.
38. Tung P, Kopelnik A, Banki N, et al. Predictors of neurocardiogenic injury after subarachnoid hemorrhage. Stroke. 2004;35(2):548–51.
39. Vale FL, Burns J, Jackson AB, et al. Combined medical and surgical treatment after acute spinal cord injury: results of a prospective pilot study to assess the merits of aggressive medical resuscitation and blood pressure management. J Neurosurg. 1997;87(2):239–46.
40. Walters BC, Hadley MN, Hurlbert RJ, Aarabi B, Dhall SS, Gelb DE, Theodore N. Guidelines for the Management of Acute Cervical Spine and Spinal Cord Injuries. Neurosurgery. 2013;60:82–91.
41. Yuen KC, Chong LE, Koch CA. Adrenal insufficiency in pregnancy: challenging issues in diagnosis and management. Endocrine. 2013;44(2):283–92.
42. Zaroff JG, Rordorf GA, Ogilvy CS, et al. Regional patterns of left ventricular systolic dysfunction after subarachnoid hemorrhage: evidence for neutrally mediated cardiac injury. J Am Soc Echocardiogr. 2000;13(8):774–9.

Chapter 41
Prolonged Somatic Support in Brain Death During Pregnancy and Perinatal Survival: Medical, Legal, and Bioethical Aspects

Previgliano Ignacio and Poliszuk Julieta

Introduction

Brain death (BD) or death under neurological criteria is recognized as a cause of death in most of the countries and by most of religions. Since Mollaret and Goulon's [1] first description of "coma depassé" trough Harvard's criteria in 1968 [2], BD is considered as the irreversible cessation of functions of both cerebral hemispheres and the brain stem, accomplishing the whole-brain criteria of death.

In Argentina BD communication is mandatory by law, with independence of organ donation with the purpose of withdrawal of support of a death body. Exceptions for this are the candidates for organ donation and pregnant women.

BD in pregnant woman is a devastating situation that poses a bioethical dilemma to the family and the health team. Although BD in pregnant woman has a low incidence [3] (2.8% of 252 BD were pregnant women between 15 and 45 years old), it has a great entity as an ethical and medical problem according the disparity in fetal viability and outcomes and the cost-benefit relation.

The aim of this chapter is to review BD diagnosis in the pregnant women, its relation with prolonged somatic support, reviewing pathophysiology and management, as well as ethical analysis of fetus rights and organ donation.

P. Ignacio (✉)
Maimonides University, Buenos Aires, Argentina

Hospital General de Agudos J. A. Fernández, Buenos Aires, Argentina
e-mail: iprevigliano@buenosaires.gob.ar

P. Julieta
Hospital General de Agudos J. A. Fernández, Buenos Aires, Argentina

Organ Procurement and Transplantation Section – Hospital General de Agudos J. A. Fernández, Buenos Aires, Argentina

C. Montufar et al. (eds.), *Obstetric Catastrophes*,
https://doi.org/10.1007/978-3-030-70034-8_41

Brain Death Diagnosis According to Argentinean Law

Argentina has a law for Organ and Human Anatomic Material Transplantation since 1977. Protocol for BD diagnosis has been adequate according to knowledge and ancillary test technology evolution, the last one in 2019.

Law 27.447 [4] states three steps for BD diagnosis:

(a) Prerequisites
  (a) Known cause of structural brain damage, with sufficient and properly documented magnitude
  (b) Lack of effect of CNS depressant drugs and/or neuromuscular relaxants
  (c) Rectal temperature >32 °C
  (d) Systolic arterial pressure >90 mmHg or mean arterial pressure >60 mmHg
  (e) Absence of metabolic and/or endocrine disorders
(b) Neurological examination
  (a) Glasgow Coma Scale 3/15
  (b) Absence of brain stem reflexes
  (c) Positive apnea test
(c) Diagnosis ancillary test
  (a) Absence of cerebral blow flow
    (i) Arteriography of the four vessels
    (ii) Transcranial Doppler
    (iii) Radioisotopic brain angiography
  (b) Absence of neurophysiologic function
    (i) Electroencephalogram
    (ii) Evoked potentials

Regarding pregnant woman, article 40 subsection b establishes that "the removal of organs and tissues on the body of a woman of gestational age is prohibited, without previously checking the absence of the pregnancy in progress." If the absence of fetal beats is determined by daily cardiotocography or a miscarriage occurs, the procedure is according to the general donor treatment protocol.

Brain Death Pathophysiology and Management in the Pregnant Woman

Catastrophic brain injuries, either primary or secondary, generate a raise in intracranial pressure (ICP) which promotes a decrease in cerebral perfusion pressure (CPP). Sustained in time CPP evolves to cerebral circulatory arrest (CCA) that will trigger encephalic tissue necrosis, in either the brain or brain stem. Before CCA, medullar compression and ischemia triggers the Cushing reflex (hypertension, bradycardia, and respiratory changes) by means of massive acetylcholine release that generates a synergic sympathetic and parasympathetic response, the so-called adrenergic storm

[5] that allows to an stabilization phase followed by cardiovascular collapse. BD will lead to multiorgan failure and cardiac arrest. Hypothalamic and pituitary nucleus injury compromise antidiuretic hormone, adrenocorticotrophine, cortisol, and thyroid hormones release that contributes to hemodynamic instability due to hypovolemia, hypotension, impaired myocardial contractility, and arrhythmias, which contribute to ischemic multiorgan failure development.

Hemodynamic Disorders

Adrenergic response has a biphasic pattern with a peak immediately after CCA and a second peak at 60 minutes secondary to norepinephrine levels in myocardial fibers sympathetic terminals. At this time auricular and ventricular arrhythmias, electrocardiographic changes (T wave inversion, changes in ST segment, and prolonged QT segment) appears. Myocardial ischemia, neurogenic pulmonary edema, and severe ventricular function impairment are frequent consequences of coronary blood flow.

After this hemodynamic stress, the lack of medulla registration of vascular baroreceptors, medulla nucleus, and circunventricular organs injury conduce to vasomotor collapse. This is meaningful in the pregnant woman due to the lack of uterine arterial system autorregulation that can't avoid placental hypoperfusion secondary to hypotension [6]. So, medical hemodynamic control should be initiated almost immediately with crystalloid or colloids solutions in order to improve placental perfusion.

Arterial hypertension is a self-limited phenomenon and doesn't need active treatment [7, 8]. In the case of needing it, urapidil, labetalol, or sodium nitroprusside should be the drugs of choice.

The aim of the treatment is to guarantee a MAP above 65 mmHg to maintain an adequate placental perfusion. If volume expansion is not enough, vasopressor drugs as vasopressin, noradrenalin, or dopamine should be used. In refractory hypotension invasive hemodynamic monitoring should be considered.

There is no evidence of which is the best vasopressor drug, but vasopressin [9] must be avoided due to placental hypoperfusion secondary to vasoconstriction.

Respiratory Disorders

Lungs are one of the most fragile organs after BD, and lung injury is one of the first organ failures due to several mechanisms.

Physiological lung changes in pregnancy are induced by progesterone at the respiratory center and consist in larger tidal volumes and in an increment in respiratory rate [10]. As a consequence, respiratory alkalosis develops, and hypocapnea will enhance fetal CO_2 elimination. Respiratory alkalosis is compensated by renal mechanisms.

Protective lung ventilation should be instituted:

(a) TV 6–8 ml/kg.
(b) RR oriented to maintain PCO_2 between 28 and 32 mmHg.
(c) FiO_2 will be the minor possible in order to maintain SaO_2 greater than 90%.
(d) Assist control ventilation.
(e) Positive end expiratory pressure (PEEP) 5 cm of water.
(f) Plateau pressure <30 cm H_2O.
(g) Peak flow <60 l/min.

It has been demonstrated that PCO_2 <30 mmHg for more than 24 hours reduces placental blood flow. In the other hand, it must be remembered that some patients may develop pulmonary edema either neurogenic or cardiogenic.

Temperature Regulation

Hypothermia is a constant phenomenon in BD [11] due to the hypothalamic thermoregulation center. It contributes to hemodynamic instability and represents a threat to the fetus which has a limited thermoregulatory capability. Hypothermia can produce fetal death or severe fetal growth deficit.

Hemodynamic changes secondary to hypothermia are arrhythmias, conduction delay (prolonged PR and QT segments), T wave inversion, Osborn's J wave, ST segment elevation, and above 30 °C ventricular fibrillation.

Hypothermia also reduces glomerular filtration rate and generates "cold diuresis" (loss of tubular concentration gradients). Regarding other effects hepatic dysfunction, hemoglobin dissociation curve shift to the left, metabolic acidosis, and coagulopathies are the most prevalent ones.

Management includes temperature control between 36 and 37 °C diminishing exposed body surface and 38 °C heated crystalloids.

In some cases hyperthermia was observed, which can be interpreted as secondary to the reflex of poikilothermia or to infections.

Endocrine Disturbances

Panhypopituitarism frequently accompanies BD. It is caused by hypothalamic lesion (supraoptic and ventricular nuclei) and neurohypophysis and must be corrected with the replacement of all hormones during pregnancy. The first manifestation is central diabetes insipidus [12] due to the absence of ADH, clinically characterized by polyuria, arterial hypotension, and hypernatremia.

- Diabetes insipidus diagnostic criteria are the following:
- Diuresis >4 ml/kg/h or >250 ml/h
- Hypernatremia >150 mEq/l
- Plasmatic osmolarity >300 mOsm/l
- Hypotonic urine (urine gravidity <1005)
- Urine osmolarity >300 mOsm/l <300 mOsm/l

The treatment of diabetes insipidus should be focused on maintaining urine output between 75 and 100 ml/h (1 ml/Kg/h) and natremia below 150 mEq/l. Treatment is started with 1ug of intravenous desmopressin add to water replacement with half saline (500 ml of distilled water plus 10 ml 20% ClNa), according urinary loss volume. If in the next hour, urine output is greater than 200 ml/h, a second 1ug desmopressin dose should be given.

Subcutaneous or intramuscular desmopressin administration is not encouraging due to the erratic absorption of the drug in BD, since tissue perfusion varies depending on the hemodynamic state and body temperature.

As in other critical illness, there is a decrease in plasma levels of triiodothyronine (T3) and thyroxine (T4) in BD patients, up to 81% and 29%, respectively [13]. As this decrease compromise myocardial function and ensures anaerobic metabolism, T3 and T4 should be administered to the pregnant corpse according to laboratory results.

Adrenal insufficiency should be corrected. The preferred drugs are methylprednisolone or prednisone because they do not easily cross the placenta and in such manner avoids prolonged fetal exposure to steroids [14].

Hyperglycemia is a common finding in BD, and it is almost secondary to peripheral insulin resistance, steroid usage, and increased endogenous catecholamines [15]. Treatment should be aimed to maintain normal glucose values (80–110 mg%) with intravenous insulin administration.

Nutritional Support

Nutritional support is essential for fetal development. Caloric requirements calculation is obtained through the Harris Benedict equation or Basal Energy Expenditure:

$$\mathrm{BEE} = 655\,\mathrm{Kcal} + \left(9.6 \times \mathrm{Weight}\left(\mathrm{Kg}\right)\right) + \left[\left(1.8 \times \mathrm{height\ in\,cm}\right) - (4.7 \times \mathrm{age}\left(\mathrm{years}\right)\right]$$

BD pregnant woman consumes only 75% of calories compared to a healthy one. This drop in consumption is due to muscle inactivity and brain metabolism.

The recommended amount of daily protein in pregnancy is 0.8–1 g/kg/day, plus a supplement of 1.6 g/kg/d in the first trimester, 6.1 g/kg/d in the second trimester, and 10, 7 g/kg/day in the third trimester of pregnancy. The nitrogen balance should always be positive and correlate with the weight gain and growth of the fetus.

Although enteral nutrition is the route of choice, intestinal absorption capacity in BD is unknown, and in more than half of the reported cases, total parenteral nutrition was used, either as a complement to enteral feeding or as the main nutritional source. Both artificial nutrition plans have complications; bacterial and fungal infections are associated with parenteral nutrition as well visceral distention, bacterial translocation, and feedback syndrome with enteral nutrition.

Near 20–25% of non-protein calories must come from fatty acids. Folic acid, iron, and calcium should be added at the recommended doses according to the corresponding trimester of pregnancy [16].

Obstetric Considerations

Daily ultrasound monitoring is recommended to determine fetal viability. If no heartbeat is detected, proceed according to the potential organ donor protocol. In the presence of fetal heartbeat, ultrasound control should continue to rule out malformations or chromosomal alterations. In cases of inconclusive findings, the possibility of amniocentesis should be discussed with the family, because the results may influence decision-making.

In addition, laboratory analysis should be performed to determine cell count, electrolytes (Na^+, K^+, Ca^{++}), liver and kidney function, albumin, and total proteins. After 24th gestation week, treatment with corticosteroids should be started for fetal lung maturity and as prophylaxis of respiratory distress syndrome.

Prolonged immobility and lack of muscle contractions, associated with changes in hemostasis related to pregnancy, favor thromboembolic phenomena development, which would indicate heparin prophylaxis.

Premature uterine contractions should be prevented, mostly during the first gestation weeks, so treatment with tocolytics (beta-agonists, prostgalandin inhibitors, etc.) may be necessary. Somatic support should be extended until the 28th week of pregnancy. A second corticosteroids dose should be administered if hemodynamic and fetal stability permitted it. According to the literature, there is no evidence to prolong pregnancy after 32 weeks [17]. Caesarean section is the method of choice for fetal extraction.

One of the most important factors for decision-making is gestational age. The first 12 weeks of gestation is the most vulnerable period in fetal maturity. Hemodynamic instability, panhypopituitarism typical of BD, and infections secondary to prolonged support result in fetal complications, such as oligohydramnios, placental insufficiency, growth restriction, fetal distress, and the need to perform an emergency caesarean section to maximize premature neonate survival.

Bioethical Issues

The Committee on Ethics, Human Reproduction and Women's Health of the International Federation of Gynecology and Obstetrics (FIGO) considers that doctors are responsible for providing and prioritizing care in deceased women and in the second instance of viable fetus, considering that women have the right to die with dignity [18].

The objective of maintaining prolonged life support is to allow the viability of the fetus until maturity, but does not exonerate the team trying to respect the main right of women: that of autonomy.

The prolonged somatic support of the fetus exposes the deceased in a position of a "biological container" – as a means to an end – violating her right to the autonomy and integrity of her body.

But this opinion is controversial for some authors, since the woman has brain death and no longer has the moral responsibility for the life of the fetus. However, this statement is debatable, since the fact that morality and bioethics have the same etymological significance has resulted in many cases that are used interchangeably, but are not the same. Morality refers to behavior that, by agreement or consensus of society, is considered as correct or incorrect. It is about lived morals, accepted by people, without necessarily having been subjected to the mediation of systematic rational criticism.

The term ethical is reserved for the philosophical discipline that rationally studies human behavior, from the point of view of moral duties and virtues. Therefore, ethics is rational knowledge, as a critical reflection on the fact of moral life [19].

Several authors have expressed themselves against prolonged life support in pregnant women with ME or in a vegetative state and argue that this practice is experimental in nature [20, 21].

There are also controversies in different laws, the ones that protect the fetus rights and the others that establish the right to die with dignity. As a matter of example, Argentinean Constitution in the article 75, inc. 23 establish the rights for the "child to be born" giving a special and comprehensive social security regime for the protection of children in situations of helplessness, from pregnancy. These statements enters in controversy with the F.A.L. ruling of the Argentinean Supreme Court of Justice (2012) that established that those who are in the conditions described in art. 86 subsection 2 of the Criminal Code that "... cannot and should not be required to request a judicial authorization to terminate the pregnancy, since the law does not mandate it, nor can it and should not be deprived of the right that assists the interruption of same as this, far from being prohibited, is allowed and is not punishable ... " and with the Law of Dignified Death that was sanctioned in 2012 by the National Congress and allows patients and families to limit therapeutic efforts in cases of "an irreversible, incurable or terminal stage disease."

Regarding the ablation of organs for transplantation after caesarean section, data reported is limited. Some series reported the discard for not meeting the selection criteria, due to multiorgan failure during hospitalization. In others cases, there was a family refusal toward donation. Only five cases became real donors, with good outcomes 1 year after graft implantation, although the information in these data is also limited. Regarding organ transplantation, the cost-effectiveness is not entirely determined.

From another point of view, prolonged somatic support to ensure fetus life is a form of organ donation.

Costs of prolonged somatic support in BDP are another issue to be highlighted. Direct and indirect costs as well as insurance coverage and fetal outcome should be borne in mind in the decision-making process. According to the literature review, the time of the somatic support of pregnancy in BD was in the range of 2–168 days, reporting complications related to the pathophysiology of BD itself and prolonged hospitalization that increases the hospitalization costs.

Three meta-analyses [3, 22, 23] analyze the incidence and outcome of BD pregnant patients, the last one involved 43 cases, including two where the mother was in a vegetative state, for the period from 1979 to 2015. Those 43 cases of somatic support were reported from 1976 to 2015. Thirty-two viable fetuses were delivered and survived the neonatal period. Three were not delivered; one mother was removed from support due to abnormal fetal growth; one mother was removed from support by a court order, leading to fetal demise; and one family made the decision to remove the mother from support, leading to fetal demise. There is a publication bias regarding perinatal survival due to the lack of long-term follow-up of neonates, although intrauterine death, spontaneous abortion, neurological disabilities, and other complications related to prematurity were reported, such as maturational delay, language disorders, and retinopathy.

However, prior to week 24, the neonate would have a 20–30% chance for survival, with a 40% probability of severe neurological disorders. The prognosis improves for neonates delivered between weeks 24 and 28, when the survival increases to 80%, and the risk of neurological complications is 10%.

According to Erlinger [3] some estimations predict that there are annually approximately 1060 cases globally. Cartolovny and Habek [24] developed the “Guidelines for the management of the social and ethical challenges in brain death during pregnancy” which we found very useful for BD pregnant woman. They evaluated the ethical, legal, and social issues referring to the legitimacy and justification of the procedure, to the fetus, and to the mother with BDP. After that they use the Grading of Recommendations Assessment, Development and Evaluation System (GRADE) [25] in order to establish the strength of recommendation (1 (strong), 2 (weak)) and quality of evidence (A (high), B (moderate), C (low)).

A summary of these guidelines is presented in Table 41.1.

Table 41.1 Guidelines for prolonged somatic support

Grade	Guideline
A1	Adequately determine mother's brain death state, avoiding procedures that might endanger the condition of the fetus
B1	Assess the viability of the fetus (weeks of pregnancy), its actual condition, diagnosis, and prognosis, primarily focusing on the chances of survival and how the continuation of the corporeal support will contribute to it
C2	Check with the father of the child, next of kin, family, or the mother' s previously expressed wishes referring to situations regarding brain death pregnancy in living wills, advance directives, and so forth
B1	Organize a combined meeting of the interdisciplinary team comprising physicians, caregiving team, hospital ethics committee, and members of the family in order to discuss primary fetal prognosis, including all uncertainties, mother's wishes, and emotional and financial factors in addition to always keeping in mind the interests of the fetus which might prevail in some situations
A1	In the decision-making process, the primary focus should be the interests of the fetus, and precedence in this decision-making process should be given to the father of the child, regardless of whether he is the woman's legal next of kin or not
C1	Organize adequate counseling and psychological support to the father, next of kin, or members of the family from the beginning of the decision-making to the end of the corporeal life support, regardless of the positive or negative outcome of the corporeal life support
B1	Seek to establish a decision within a clinical setting, avoiding the Court if possible, and only appeal to the Court in cases when decisions cannot be made between the members of the family and father or when it is perceived that their decision is not in the interests of the fetus and is contrary to good obstetric practice
B2	Costs should not be underestimated in the clinical decision-making. However, they should not be the primary concern and focus; different options for funding sources can be considered, even in low-income countries
A1	Establish an international registry of BDP cases where the positive and negative outcomes could be collated, leading to the accumulation of the outcome data which could provide more accurate and firm conclusions regarding such cases

Conclusions

Prolonged somatic support in brain death during pregnancy and perinatal survival is a controversial issue that involves medical, bioethical, and legal aspects.

Beyond radical points of view regarding mother or fetus rights, a decision-making process that considerer fetal viability and gestational age, family (father, mother parents or next of a kin) wishes or anticipated directives, and cost of medical attention should be established in each medical facility.

Although the lack of evidence, developed guidelines appear as the best way to manage such a complex situation.

References

1. Mollaret P, GoulonM. The depassed coma (preliminary memoir). Rev Neurol (París). 1959;101:3–15.
2. Beecher HK. A definition of irreversible coma. Report of the Ad Hoc Committee of the Harvard Medical School to examine the definition of brain death. JAMA. 1968;205:337–40.
3. Erlinger LR. Guidelines for supporting a pregnant patient with brain death: a case discussion and literature review. J Nurs Educ Pract. 2017;7:86.
4. Ley 27.447 de Trasplantes de órganos, Tejidos y Células. https://www.boletinoficial.gob.ar/#DetalleNorma/188857.
5. Rosner MJ, Newsome HH, Becker DP. Mechanical brain injury:the simpatoadrenal response. J Neurosurg. 1981;61:76–86.
6. Field D, Gates E, Creasy R, Jonsen A, Laros R. Maternal brain death during pregnancy. JAMA. 1988;260:816–22.
7. Dictus C, Vienenkoetter B, Esmaeilzadeh M, Unterberg A, Ahmadi R. Critical care management of potential organ donors: our current standard. Clin Transpl. 2009;23(Suppl 21):2–9.
8. Hoemme R, Neeser G. Organ donation. Anesth. 2007;56:1291–302.
9. Hauksson A, Akerlund M, Melin P. Uterine blood flow and myometrial activity at menstruation, and the action of vasopressin and a synthetic antagonist. Br J Obstet Gynaecol. 1988;95:898–904.
10. Bhatia P, Bhatia K. Pregnancy and the lungs. Postgrad Med J. 2000;76:683–9.
11. Smith M. Physiologic changes during brain stem death: lessons for management of the organ donor. J Heart Lung Transplant. 2004;23(9 Suppl):S217–22.
12. Keller F, Dennhardt R, Voigt K. Acute endocrine failure after brain death? Transplantation. 1992;54:851–7.
13. Howlett TA, Keogh AM, Perry L, Touzel R, Rees LH. Anterior and posterior pituitary function in brain-stem-dead donors: a possible role for hormonal replacement therapy. Transplantation. 1989;47:828–34.
14. Van Runnard Heimel PJ, Franx A, Schobben AF, Huisjes AJ, Derks JB, Bruinse HW. Corticosteroids, pregnancy, and HELLP syndrome. Obstet Gynecol Surv. 2005;60:57–70.
15. Mallampalli A, Guy E. Cardiac arrest in pregnancy and somatic support after brain death. Crit Care Med. 2005;33:325–31.
16. Hamaoui E, Hamaoui M. Nutritional assessment and support during pregnancy. Gastroenterol Clin N Am. 2003;32:59–121.
17. Haas DM, Imperiale TF, Kirkpatrick PR, Klein RW, Zollinger TW, Golichowski AM. Tocolytic therapy: a meta-analysis and decision analysis. Obstet Gynecol. 2009;113:585–94.
18. Dickens B. FIGO, Committee for Ethical Aspects of Human Reproduction and Women's Health. "Brain death and pregnancy". Int J Gynaecol Obstet. 2011;115:84–5.
19. Magnante D (Editora). Bioética Clínica. Final de la vida. Legislación internacional. Primera edición. Editorial Corpus; 2020.
20. Peart NS, Campbell AV, Manara AR, et al. Maintaining pregnancy following loss of capacity. Med Law Rev. 2000;8:275–99.
21. Farragher R, Marsh B, Laffey JG. Maternal brain death-an Irish perspective. Ir J Med Sci. 2005;174(4):55–9.
22. Feldman D, Borgida A. Irreversible maternal brain injury during pregnancy: a case report and review of the literature. Obstet Gynecol Surv. 2000;55:708–14; Erlinger LR. Guidelines for supporting a pregnant patient with brain death: a case discussion and literature review. J Nurs Educ Pract. 2017;7:86.
23. Esmaeilzadeh M, Dictus C, Kayvanpour E, et al. One life ends, another begins: management of a brain-dead pregnant mother-A systematic review. BMC Med. 2010;8:74.
24. Čartolovni A, Habek D. Guidelines for the management of the social and ethical challenges in brain death during pregnancy. Int J Gynaecol Obstet. 2019;146:149–56.
25. Guyatt GH, Oxman AD, Vist GE, Kunz R, Falck-Ytter Y, Alonso-Coello P, Schünemann HJ. GRADE Working Group. GRADE: an emerging consensus on rating quality of evidence and strength of recommendations. BMJ. 2008;336:924–6.

Part X
Renal

Chapter 42
Oliguria

Leonardo Bonilla Cortés

Definition

Oliguria is defined as urinary output of less than 0.5 ml/Kg/h [1] or a urinary output of less than 400 ml in 24 hours [2]. Decreased urine output is an appropriate physiological response during prolonged fasting periods, hypovolemia, postoperative period, or consecutive to stress, pain, or response to trauma [3]. In obstetric patients, oliguria is associated with a higher mortality risk than any other renal function test alone (44.4% vs 5.3%) [4].

The 2012 Kidney Disease: Improving Global Outcomes (KDIGO) defined acute kidney injury (AKI) as one or more of three criteria. The first two were a rise in serum creatinine of at least 0.3 mg/dl over a 48-hour period and/or >1.5 times the best line value within the seven previous days. The third one was a urine volume ≤0.5 ml/kg/h in 6 hours [5].

Etiology

The vast majority of AKI cases occur postnatally; only 7% of cases occur antenatally [8]. AKI usually occurs in women with previously healthy kidneys [6], pre-existing kidney disease occurs in 4% of pregnant patients, and 10% of these will develop severe renal deterioration during pregnancy [7].

L. Bonilla Cortés (✉)
Maternal – Fetal Medicine Division, Hospital Universitario Clínica San Rafael, Bogotá, Colombia

Obstetrics Department at EPS Sanitas, Bogotá, Colombia

Department of Maternal – Fetal Medicine, Universidad El Bosque, Bogotá, Colombia

C. Montufar et al. (eds.), *Obstetric Catastrophes*,
https://doi.org/10.1007/978-3-030-70034-8_42

Table 42.1 Functional AKI causes

Hypovolemia	Hemorrhage	Placental abruption Placenta previa Postpartum hemorrhage
	Fluid loss	Hyperemesis gravidarum Sepsis Ovarian hyperstimulation syndrome Acute fatty liver of pregnancy
	Abdominal compartment syndrome	
Obstructive	Obstetric complication	Ureteral injury due to cesarean section

The etiology of AKI differs in low-/middle-income countries (LMICs) and in high-income countries (HIC) [6]. In LMICs, the main cause is preeclampsia representing 46.9% of cases, followed by sepsis and postpartum hemorrhage. In contrast, in HICs preeclampsia remains the most common cause and is followed by HELLP syndrome, hemorrhage, and acute fatty liver of pregnancy [6].

To approach the different possible etiologies, AKI has been classified as prerenal, renal, and post-renal causes. However, this classification leads to limited diagnostic and therapeutic clarity. For instance, the Acute Dialysis Quality Initiative (ADQI) proposed a different classification to differentiate between functional AKI, defined as secondary to hypovolemia and obstructive phenomena, and AKI due to renal injury [10]. Due to the clinical applicability of this classification, it will be used for the rest of this manuscript (Table 42.1).

Functional Acute Kidney Injury

Hypovolemia

Hypovolemia is the main risk factor for developing AKI. And it can be further divided into three broad categories based upon etiology: hemorrhagic, fluid loss, and abdominal compartment syndrome (ACS) [12, 13]. Oliguria is usually the earliest manifestation. Additionally, it is a diagnostic criteria according to the KDIGO guidelines [11]; usually in this situation the tubular and glomerular function are undamaged, and the glomerular filtration is affected by hypoperfusion.

Fluid Loss

Hyperemesis Gravidarum

Hyperemesis gravidarum is the main cause of AKI in the first trimester of pregnancy in LMICs but very rarely occurs in HIC. It is characterized by the presence of nausea and vomiting leading to dehydration and renal hypoperfusion. It is characterized by the loss of ≥5% of pregestational weight, ketonuria, and secondary hypokalemic metabolic alkalosis [14].

Infection

Sepsis is the result of an unmodulated reaction to an infection. The excessive inflammatory response includes extravasation of albumin and fluids, resulting in hypovolemia that, associated with the release of cytokines, causes a decrease in peripheral vascular resistance with hypotension and hypoperfusion [15]. The most prevalent causes are pyelonephritis, pneumonia, and chorioamnionitis. Most common isolated pathogens are endotoxin-producing gram-negatives, and in some cases the infection is polymicrobial.

Fatty Liver

Acute fatty liver of pregnancy is a rare complication characterized by hypertension, thrombocytopenia, with hepatocellular necrosis, elevated transaminases, and ultimately, liver dysfunction [16]. Approximately 60% of patients with acute fatty liver of pregnancy have acute renal failure due to hypoperfusion secondary hyperemesis [17], associated with disseminated intravascular coagulation (DIC) and splanchnic vasodilation. In the majority of cases after pregnancy termination, the hypovolemia component is rapidly reversible; patients who have persistent elevated creatinine levels usually have concomitant intrinsic renal injury [16].

Anaphylactoid Shock of Pregnancy

Anaphylactoid shock in pregnancy (also called amniotic fluid embolism) is a syndrome characterized by an endogenous proinflammatory reaction that triggers severe pulmonary hypertension as a result of vasospasm with secondary right ventricular failure, and sudden loss of preload. It presents with abrupt presentation of hypoxia, hypotension, seizures, and DIC during labor or birth [18].

Ovarian Hyperstimulation Syndrome

In the ovarian hyperstimulation syndrome, the most relevant phenomenon is the increase in capillary permeability. The release of vascular endothelial growth factor of follicular origin induces fluid and protein displacement from the intravascular space to the third space, leading to hypovolemia and secondary hypotension, oliguria, ascites, increased blood viscosity, hyponatremia, and hyperkalemia [19].

Hemorrhagic

During the second and third trimester of pregnancy the most important causes of hypovolemia are placenta previa, placental abruption, and postpartum hemorrhage (uterine atony, trauma, uterine rupture) [1].

Abdominal Compartment Syndrome

In the third trimester of pregnancy, intra-abdominal pressure (IAP) ranges from 10.9 ± 4.7 mm Hg to 17.8 ± 3.6 mm Hg; then at 24 hours postpartum it falls between 9.6 ± 0.89 and 10.7 mm Hg [20]. Compensated intra-abdominal hypertension is defined as IAP >14 mm Hg antenatal or IAP >12 mm Hg after birth. Certain obstetric conditions such as preeclampsia, HELLP syndrome, DIC, and massive transfusion and other non-obstetric conditions can evolve to an abdominal compartment syndrome (defined as IAP >25 mm Hg before natal or >20 mm Hg postpartum) leading to decreased cardiac output, direct compression of organs, and their vasculature [21]. Ultimately, it impairs organ perfusion and tissue viability.

Obstructive

Although stasis and compression of the urinary system is relatively frequent during pregnancy, the presentation of oliguria or AKI is rare, and it can occur in pregnancies complicated with polyhydramnios, with uterine myomatosis, or in multiple gestations [1].

Ureteral and bladder lesions are the two most prevalent types of urinary tract complications associated with caesarean section. Unlike the bladder injury that is usually diagnosed during the operative act, the ureteral injury goes unnoticed. Patients with higher risk are those with pelvic adhesions, previous caesarean section, need for obstetric hysterectomy, or patients requiring hemostatic points at the hysterotomy angles [20]. The clinical presentation is characterized by oliguria, or anuria if both ureters were ligated. In cases were the lesion is unilateral, it can go unnoticed and only diagnosed at the onset of late complications due to obstructive uropathy.

Intrinsic AKI

It is caused by a renal parenchyma lesion, usually as a result of an alteration in a primary site (tubules, interstitium, vessels, or glomerulus). The most common mechanism of intrarenal AKI is acute tubular ischemia. The oxygen partial pressure

Table 42.2 Intrinsic AKI causes

Acute tubular necrosis	Extended hypotension	Antepartum hemorrhage Postpartum hemorrhage
	Sepsis	Septic abortion Pyelonephritis Puerperal sepsis
	Preeclampsia	Glomeruloendothelioses HELLP
	Other thrombotic microangiopathy	Acute fatty liver of pregnancy Hemolytic uremic syndrome Thrombotic thrombocytopenic purpura
Pre-existing renal disease	Lupus Glomerulopathies	

in the renal medulla is between 5 and 10 mm Hg, compared to 50 mm Hg in the cortex; this low oxygen pressure and high metabolic activity make it susceptible to periods of ischemia. Parenchymal edema and necrosis of the tubular epithelium obstruct the lumen of the tube, resulting in a decrease in the glomerular filtration rate, thus, causing granular cylinders in the urinary sediment [2]. In most cases this injury is reversible if the triggering cause is reversed in a timely manner (Table 42.2).

In preeclampsia, oliguria can be presented antenatally, and it is considered by the American College of Obstetrics and Gynecology (ACOG) [22] as a sign of severity that would indicate the termination of pregnancy. During the postpartum period, the evolution to AKI is unusual unless there is significant hemodynamic instability. Most cases resolve within the first 2 weeks after delivery and rarely require dialysis. Only 2% of patients with AKI will progress to cortical necrosis (CN) [2]; in most cases it is associated with HELLP, acute fatty liver of pregnancy, hemolytic uremic syndrome, thrombotic thrombocytopenic purpura, placental abruption, or sepsis. The main presentation is anuria, hematuria, and flank pain. The percentage of affected glomeruli determines the duration of the symptoms [23].

Differential Diagnosis

AKI diagnosis has traditionally been based on an elevation of serum creatinine and/or oliguria.

Changes in urinary output occur before the biochemical changes become apparent, causes of functional AKI (hypovolemic and obstructive) are characterized by presenting oliguria, whereas the causes of AKI due to intrinsic renal injury can present a spectrum of urinary pattern that goes from anuria to polyuria [9].

When it is reported that the patient presents oliguria, the first thing is to verify that the registry of urine output is being done reliably; this implies adequate recording of the fluid balance and that in case the patient has bladder catheterization, verify that the catheter is permeable and in upright position.

Table 42.3 Intrinsic AKI distinct studies

Causes	Distinct studies
Preeclampsia/HELLP	CBC, smear, lactic dehydrogenase, transaminases, proteinuria
Thrombotic thrombocytopenic purpura/ hemolytic uremic syndrome	CBC, smear Activity level of ADAMTS 13
Acute fatty liver of pregnancy	Liver function, cholesterol, albumin, glycemia, coagulation tests
Autoimmune nephritis/vasculitis	Antinuclear antibodies, double-stranded DNA antibody, extractable antibodies, serum complement levels
Sepsis	Blood cultures, urine culture

Diagnostic algorithms are mainly used to differentiate functional AKI from AKI due to intrinsic renal injury. The clinical approach involves (Table 42.3):

1. Clinical history and physical examination
2. Urinary sediment: It is useful when taken from a fresh sample and taken with an appropriate technique; the presence of crenated red blood cells guides the diagnosis toward pathologies with glomerular involvement. The presence of bacteria or leukocyturia supports the diagnosis of sepsis [3]. Hyaline cylinders are present in hypovolemia, and granular or cellular cylinders suggest renal cause.
3. Urinary electrolytes: In situations associated with transient hypovolemia or hypoperfusion, healthy kidneys respond by increasing urinary osmolarity and reducing sodium excretion, urea, and uric acid; therefore a low sodium excretion (<1%), uric acid (<12%), and urea (34%) support the functional AKI diagnosis [3].

Management

Functional AKI

The initial therapy is aimed to restore renal perfusion and prevent further renal damage (Fig. 42.1).

Hemorrhage

In cases of hemorrhage crystalloid solutions can be used to restore intravascular volume. In the presence of severe hemorrhage, identification of the cause and proper hemostasis is paramount. The use of massive transfusions may be required to

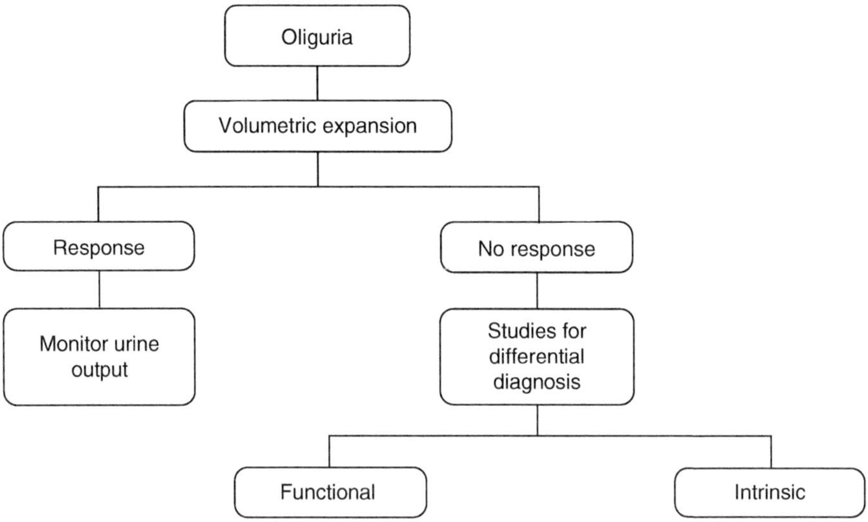

Fig. 42.1 Initial management algorithm for oliguria

maintain hemodynamic stability; early administration of fresh frozen plasma (FFP), red blood cells, and platelets in a ratio 1:1:1 prevents DIC.

Fluid Loss

In cases of fluid loss hypovolemia such as dehydration due to hyperemesis gravidarum, initial volumetric expansion with hypotonic solutions (saline solution at 0.45%) is indicated. Subsequent correction should be done according to laboratory tests results [24] (Fig. 42.1).

Management of sepsis requires an effective resuscitation with crystalloids. It is recommended to start with a volume of 30 ml/kg for the first 3 hours; some patients will require a higher volume until achieving appropriate end-organ perfusion [25]. After initial fluid resuscitation, volumetric expansion must be done according to dynamic preload measurements (SMFM).

Abdominal Compartment Syndrome

Abdominal intraluminal contents should be evacuated (place a nasogastric tube, use gastrointestinal motility promoters), evacuate lesions that occupy the intra-abdominal space, use analgesia and sedation, and proceed with decompressive laparotomy in cases where it does not resolve [13] (Fig. 42.2).

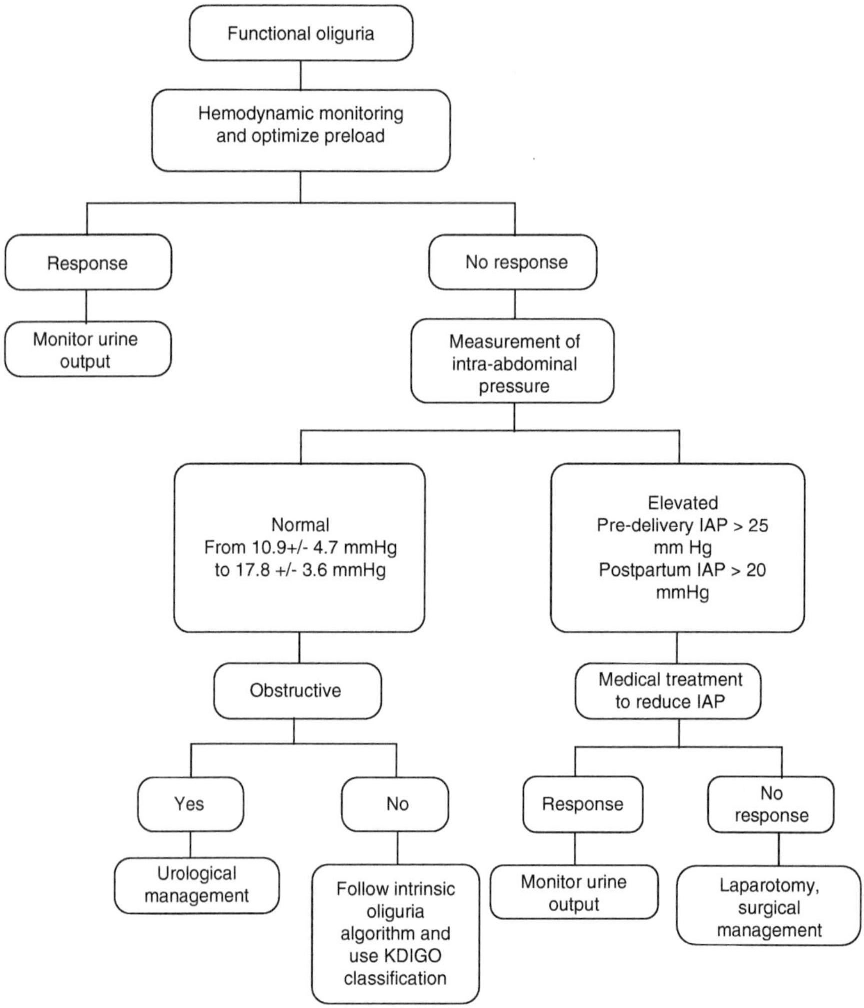

Fig. 42.2 Management algorithm of functional oliguria

Intrinsic AKI

Accurate and frequent monitoring of urine output and renal function test (serum creatinine) is recommended in patients with high risk to develop AKI. Patients' early diagnosis is necessary to establish early interventions. Close monitoring allows the clinician to stage severity and formulate treatment plans [5].

In 2012 the RIFLE (2004) and AKIN (2007) criteria were combined resulting in the KDIGO classification [3] (Table 42.4).

AKI is diagnosed with one of the following criteria:

Table 42.4 AKI KDIGO classification

Stage	Serum creatinine	Urine output
1	1.5–1.9 times baseline or ≥0.3 mg/dl (≥26.5 μmol/l) increase	<0.5 ml/kg/h for 6–12 hours
2	2.0–2.0 times baseline	<0.5 ml/kg/h for ≥12 hours
3	3.0 times baseline or increase in serum creatinine to ≥4 mg/dl or initiation of renal replacement therapy or, in patients <18 years, decrease in eGFR to <35 ml/min per 1.7 m^2	<0.3 ml/kg/h for ≥24 hours or anuria for ≥12 hours

Table 42.5 AKI differential diagnosis

	Functional AKI	Intrinsic AKI
Urinary sediment	Intact red blood cells Hyaline casts	Crenated red blood cells Granular casts
Urine osmolality (mmol/kg)	>500	>300
Sodium excretion fraction (%)	<1	>1
Uric acid excretion fraction	<7	>15
Urea excretion fraction	<35	>35

- Serum creatinine increase >0.3 mg/dl in 48 hours
- Serum creatinine increase >1.5 times baseline
- Urinary volume <0.5 ml/kg/hour for 6 hours

Severity stages are determined according to the grade of renal dysfunction (Table 42.5). The diagnosis of intrinsic AKI should be performed after ruling out functional AKI (due to hypovolemia or obstruction) [27].

In patients at risk of developing acute renal failure, it is indicated to discontinue all nephrotoxic agents, to avoid contrast imaging studies and hyperglycemia. Consider close hemodynamic monitoring as well as frequent measurement of urinary output and serum creatinine levels. Particular emphasis is placed in maintaining adequate blood volume and perfusion pressure [5].

Initially in the oliguric phase of preeclampsia or thrombotic microangiopathy, volumetric expansion must be performed (recommended that 500–1000 cc crystalloid boluses can be administered without the risk of acute pulmonary edema) [12, 26]. It is indicated to continue the fluids infusion according to hemodynamic monitoring if there is no response, and if persistent, intrinsic renal AKI (acute tubular necrosis) compromise should be suspected and rule out abdominal compartment syndrome.

The use of dopamine, fenoldopam, and N-acetylcysteine as continuous infusions failed to demonstrate benefit in preventing progression to acute renal failure [1]. The use of loop diuretics is relatively frequent in critically ill patients with AKI. Animals have demonstrated that loop diuretics reduce oxygen consumption by decreasing the sodium active transport, thus limiting potential tubular damage [28]. Even though, there is a potential benefit, other retrospective studies suggested an increase in mortality; thus its use in patients with AKI is not recommended [29].

Established Acute Renal Failure

After 7 days of unresolved AKI, it is considered that acute renal failure has been established, and the recommended management is outlined by the KDGO guidelines.

KDIGO Stage 1

Most cases of AKI that complicate pregnancy occur in the puerperium. Eventually in cases of severe preeclampsia/HELLP, termination of pregnancy must be considered [22]. Usually AKI under these circumstances has a favorable course; if patient develops acute renal failure, it is appropriate to perform studies in order to rule out other microangiopathies such as hemolytic uremic syndrome, pregnancy acute liver, or autoimmune profile in order to rule out autoimmune nephritis.

When diagnosis is not clear, non-invasive studies such as renal ultrasound or CAT scan are useful to evaluate renal structure and rule out collecting system obstruction; loss of corticomedullary differentiation and decrease in renal size are suggestive of base chronic kidney disease [3]; hypodense or hypoechoic areas could be indicative of cortical necrosis or renal abscesses in sepsis cases [4].

Renal biopsy is rarely performed in critically ill pregnant patients, mainly because of the risk of bleeding and its low utility adopting therapeutic measures [3]; thus renal biopsy would be indicated in patients who persist with anuria for a long time (30 days) [30] (Fig. 42.3).

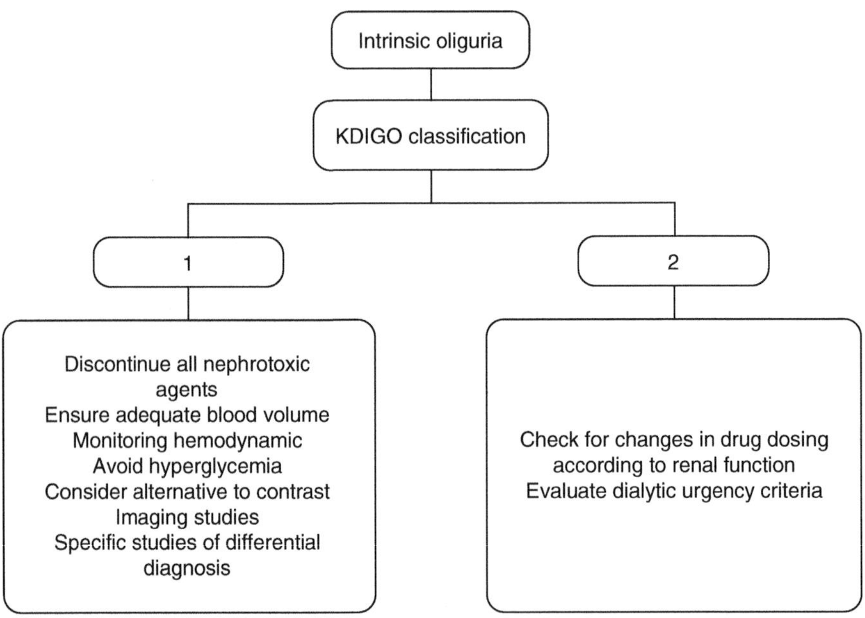

Fig. 42.3 Management algorithm of intrinsic oliguria

Table 42.6 Acute hemodialysis criteria

Acute hemodialysis criteria
Severe acidosis that does not respond to bicarbonate therapy
Severe hydroelectrolytic imbalance (hyperkalemia, hypercalcemia)
Intravascular volume overload that does not respond to diuretics
Clinical evidence of uremia (nausea, vomiting, anorexia, altered mental status in renal failure scenario, pericardial rub)
Prophylactic when BUN >50–70 or serum creatinine >4 mg/dl

KDIGO Stages 2 and 3

Check for changes in drug dosing according to renal function.

In still pregnant KDIGO2 patients with BUN>50 mg/dl, prophylactic hemodialysis can be considered due to the risk of fetal compromise. In patients with KDIGO3 meeting urgent dialysis criteria (Table 42.6), they should undergo renal replacement therapy (Fig. 42.3).

In KDIGO3 patients, subclavian catheters should be avoided.

References

1. Ari B. Renal failure in pregnancy. Crit Care Clin. 2016;32(1):78–83.
2. Mantel GD. Care of the critically ill parturient: oliguria and renal failure. Best Pract Res Clin Obstet Gynaecol. 2001;15(4):563–81.
3. Ostermann M, Joannidis M. Acute kidney injury 2016: diagnosis and diagnostic workup. Crit Care. 2016;20:299.
4. James D. Renal disorders in pregnancy. In: High risk pregancy, St. Louis, MO: Elsevier Saunders; 2017. p. 1322–7.
5. Khwaja A. KDIGO clinical practice guidelines for acute kidney injury. Nephron Clin Pract. 2012;120(4):c179–84.
6. Prakash J, Ganiger VC, Prakash S, Iqbal M, Kar DP, Singh U, et al. Acute kidney injury in pregnancy with special reference to pregnancy-specific disorders: a hospital based study (2014–2016). J Nephrol. 2018;31(1):79–85.
7. Van Hook JW. Acute kidney injury during pregnancy. Clin Obstet Gynecol. 2014;57(4):851–61.
8. Gurrieri C, Garovic VD, Gullo A, Bojanic K, Sprung J, Narr BJ, et al. Kidney injury during pregnancy: associated comorbid conditions and outcomes. Arch Gynecol Obstet. 2012;286(3):567–73.
9. Lameire N, Van Biesen W, Vanholder R, Van Biesen W. Seminar acute renal failure. Lancet. 2005;365(9457):417.
10. Endre ZH, Kellum JA, Di Somma S, Doi K, Goldstein SL, Koyner JL, et al. Differential diagnosis of AKI in clinical practice by functional and damage biomarkers: workgroup statements from the tenth acute dialysis quality initiative consensus conference. Contrib Nephrol. 2013;182:30–44.
11. Perner A, Prowle J, Joannidis M, Young P, Hjortrup PB, Pettilä V. Fluid management in acute kidney injury. Intensive Care Med. 2017;43(6):807–15.
12. Creasy RK, Resnik R, Iams JD. Creasy & Resnik's maternal-fetal medicineprinciples and practice. Saunders/Elsevier. 2009. p. 907–8.
13. Lozada MJ, Goyal V, Levin D, Walden RL, Osmundson SS, Pacheco LD, et al. Management of peripartum intra-abdominal hypertension and abdominal compartment syndrome. Acta Obstet Gynecol Scand. 2019;98(11):1386–97.

14. Prakash J, Ganiger V. Acute kidney injury in pregnancy-specific disorders. Indian J Nephrol. 2017;27(4):258.
15. Plante LA, Pacheco LD, Louis JM. SMFM Consult Series #47: sepsis during pregnancy and the puerperium. Am J Obstet Gynecol. 2019;220(4):B2–10.
16. Nelson DB, Yost NP, Cunningham FG. Acute fatty liver of pregnancy: clinical outcomes and expected duration of recovery. Am J Obstet Gynecol. 2013;209(5):456-e1.
17. Vigil-De Gracia P, Montufar-Rueda C. Acute fatty liver of pregnancy: diagnosis, treatment, and outcome based on 35 consecutive cases. J Matern Neonatal Med. 2011;24(9):1143–6.
18. Pacheco LD, Saade G, Hankins GDV, Clark SL. Amniotic fluid embolism: diagnosis and management. Am J Obstet Gynecol. 2016;215(2):B16–24.
19. Humaidan P, Nelson SM, Devroey P, Coddington CC, Schwartz LB, Gordon K, et al. Ovarian hyperstimulation syndrome: review and new classification criteria for reporting in clinical trials. Hum Reprod. 2016;31(9):1997–2004.
20. Lo TS, Wijaya T, Lo LM, Kao CC, Wu PY, Cortes EFM, et al. Clinical relevance and treatment selection of ureteral injury after cesarean section. Female Pelvic Med Reconstr Surg. 2016;22(5):303–6.
21. Tyagi A, Singh S, Kumar M, Sethi AK. Intra-abdominal pressure and intra-abdominal hypertension in critically ill obstetric patients: a prospective cohort study. Int J Obstet Anesth. 2017;32:33–40.
22. American College of Obstetricians and Gynecologists, Task Force on Hypertension in Pregnancy. Hypertension in pregnancy. Report of the American College of Obstetricians and Gynecologists' Task Force on Hypertension in Pregnancy. Obstet Gynecol. 2013;122(5):1122–31.
23. Beji S, Hajji M, Rais L, Kheder R, Jebali H, Smaoui W, et al. Acute renal cortical necrosis in pregnancy: clinical course and changing prognosis. Nephrol Ther. 2017;13(7):550–2.
24. Myburgh JA, Finfer S, Bellomo R, Billot L, Cass A, Gattas D, et al. Hydroxyethyl starch or saline for fluid resuscitation in intensive care. N Engl J Med. 2012;367(20):1901–11.
25. Rhodes A, Evans LE, Alhazzani W, Levy MM, Antonelli M, Ferrer R, et al. Surviving sepsis campaign: international guidelines for management of sepsis and septic shock: 2016. Intensive Care Med. 2017;43(3):304–77.
26. Foley M. Obstetric intensive care manual. 5th ed. New York: McGraw-Hill Education; 2018.
27. Lopes JA, Jorge S. The RIFLE and AKIN classifications for acute kidney injury: a critical and comprehensive review. Clin Kidney J. 2013;6(1):8–14.
28. Bagshaw SM, Delaney A, Jones D, Ronco C, Bellomo R. Diuretics in the management of acute kidney injury: a multinational survey. Contrib Nephrol. 2007;156:236–249.
29. Choudhury D. Acute kidney injury: current perspectives. Postgrad Med. 2010;122(6):29–40.
30. Ye W, Shu H, Wen Y, Ye W, Li H, Qin Y, et al. Renal histopathology of prolonged acute kidney injury in HELLP syndrome: a case series and literature review. Int Urol Nephrol. 2019;51(6):987–94.

Chapter 43
Acute Kidney Injury During Pregnancy

Ahmed Reda Taha

Introduction

Parturient with kidney diseases experience failure of physiological and endocrinal adaptation that takes place during a normal pregnancy. Numerous etiological disorders can lead to acute kidney injury (AKI) during pregnancy. Sepsis and pregnancy-induced hypertensive disorders being the most common causes of AKI or may be CKD. Regardless of the cause, acute kidney injury is a critical obstetric complication associated with significant maternal and fetal morbidity and mortality. Although the rates of acute kidney injury in pregnancy are declining worldwide, it remains a significant public health concern in developing countries. Pregnancy and AKI is challenging clinical scenario, where the effects on maternal and fetal outcomes need to be observed strictly. Women with acute kidney injury should be considered high-risk and managed by a multidisciplinary team involving nephrology, intensive care, and obstetrics staff.

The adaptive physiological dynamics in pregnancy and associated changes form essential inputs to provide the required care of parturient with renal impairment. It is crucial that the team who provide the care be familiar with such adaption and the mainstay management to be initiated early in the context of suspected pregnancy-related acute kidney injury (PR-AKI) utilizing evidence-based clinical practice in order to achieve the best outcomes [1].

Recently published literature demonstrates the increased awareness of kidney injury in pregnancy and the management of PR-AKI, with a focus on the correlation between sepsis, preeclampsia, pregnancy-induced hypertensive disorders, thrombotic angiopathies, and AKI [2].

A. R. Taha (✉)
Cardiac Intensive Care Institute of Critical Care – Cleveland Clinic Abu Dhabi, Abu Dhabi, UAE

C. Montufar et al. (eds.), *Obstetric Catastrophes*,
https://doi.org/10.1007/978-3-030-70034-8_43

Current consensus criteria (RIFLE, AKIN, and KDIGO) that developed to provide quantitative definition of AKI do not look useful in pregnancy, where glomerular filtration rate (GFR) increases significantly by approximately 50%, resulting in lowered serum creatinine compared with an average nonpregnant person, so parturient with normal range may represent a significant increase from their baseline, and their clinician can easily miss this [3, 4].

The true incidence is difficult to estimate due to variable clinical criteria, but it's less in developed country where adequate antenatal care was provided.

Physiologic Changes in Pregnancy

There are several hemodynamic and immunologic shifts that occur during the course of healthy pregnancy, including increased blood volume, decreased systemic vascular resistance, and increased cardiac output. There is elevation of nitric oxide, and relaxin leads to more vasodilatation and decrease of systemic blood pressure and relative resistance to vasoconstrictors, such as angiotensin II. Glomerular filtration rate (GFR) increases by ~50%, resulting in a physiologic reduction in serum creatinine (Scr) level in the setting of hyperfiltration. The normal Scr level in pregnancy is in the 0.4 to 0.6 mg/dL range. The smooth muscle relaxation due to elevated progesterone in combination with mechanical compression by the enlarging uterus can cause physiologic hydronephrosis and retention of urine in the collecting system during pregnancy [5].

Urine protein excretion increases during the course of normal pregnancy, from 60 to 90 mg/d to 180 to 250 mg/d, as measured by a 24-hour urine collection. As a consequence of this physiologic increase in proteinuria, the threshold for elevated proteinuria in pregnancy has been set at a higher level of protein excretion of 300 mg/d. This increase in proteinuria has been attributed to hyperfiltration, as described, but may also be due to changes in glomerular permeability [6]. Some studies have demonstrated an increase in tubular proteinuria, reflected as an increase in urinary retinol-binding protein, as opposed to an increase in albuminuria, which would reflect a glomerular source. The use of spot urine protein-creatinine ratio (UPCR) has gained favor in the diagnosis of preeclampsia, which is typically characterized by proteinuria (UPCR >0.3 g/g). UPCR is a faster test that has acceptable sensitivity and specificity. There may be increased UPCR in the absence of hypertension or kidney disease, a phenomenon known as isolated proteinuria, present in as many as 15% of pregnancies [6].

Changes in the function of the innate and adaptive immune systems in pregnancy may have important impacts on the behavior of autoimmune diseases, a common cause of impaired renal function in young women.

The immunology of pregnancy is complex, in that the mother must tolerate the "foreign" fetus and thus requires a degree of immunosuppression while on the other

Table 43.1 Renal changes of normal pregnancy

Parameter	Trend compared to nonpregnant state	Normal values in pregnancy
Serum creatinine	Lower	~0.5 mg/dL (<0.9 mg/dL)
Blood urea nitrogen (BUN)	Lower	~9.0 mg/dL
Serum sodium	Lower	129–135 mmol/L
Plasma uric acid	Lower	2.0–3.0 mg/dL
pCO_2	Lower	27–32 mmHg
pH	Higher	7.40–7.45
Serum bicarbonate	Lower	18–20 mEq
Creatinine clearance	Higher	~25% above baseline (>100 cc/min)
GFR	Higher 50%	150–200 ml/min
Urinary protein excretion	Variable to higher	<300 mg/24 hours
Th1:Th2 profile	In favor of Th2 profile	Th2 > Th1
Blood osmolality	Lower	270 mosm/kg
Urinary glucose excretion	Variable to higher	May be present

Data quoted from Refs. [1, 5–9]

hand needs to maintain immune function to fight off infection. So a cytokine bias trend switches from the T helper 1 (Th1) pro-inflammatory cytokine profile to the T helper 2 (Th2) anti-inflammatory cytokine profile, which is important for tolerance to fetal antigens; increased Th1 profile may correlate with increased risk for pregnancy complications, such as preterm labor, preeclampsia, and poor fetal and maternal outcomes [7] (Table 43.1).

Etiology

PR-AKI can be classified according to the mechanism of injury to prerenal, intrarenal, and post-renal causes [5, 8].

Prerenal

- Hyperemesis gravidarum
- Hemorrhage
- Heart failure
- Sepsis
- Amniotic fluid embolism

Intrarenal

- Acute tubular necrosis
- Acute cortical necrosis
- Acute fatty liver of pregnancy
- Preeclampsia/HELLP
- Thrombotic thrombocytopenic purpura/atypical hemolytic uremic syndrome
- Pyelonephritis
- Amniotic fluid embolism
- Pulmonary embolism
- Lupus nephritis
- Acute interstitial nephritis

Post-renal

- Hydronephrosis due to uterine compression
- Injury to ureters or bladder during C-section
- Ureteral obstruction from stones or tumor
- Obstruction at bladder outlet

Timing of AKI

The timing of PR-AKI is dependent mainly on the underlying etiology (Fig. 43.1). In developing countries, PR-AKI that occurs in the first trimester in most is due to septic abortions or lupus nephritis. Approximately 75% of PR-AKI cases occurring in the second and third trimesters is due to hypertensive complications such as preeclampsia/HELLP, TTP/HUS, abruption placentae, severe hemorrhage, or DIC, or AFLP. Atypical HUS, however, generally occurs late in the third trimester or postpartum. Making these diagnoses may be evident, but many overlapping features, such as preeclampsia/HELLP, lupus nephritis, TTP/HUS, and AFLP, make the interpretation more difficult [10].

Prerenal Causes

Prerenal azotemia is the result of decreased renal perfusion, due to either decreased cardiac output, true intravascular volume depletion, or impaired renal perfusion as a consequence of liver cirrhosis, nephrotic syndrome, renal artery stenosis, or the use of nonsteroidal anti-inflammatory agents. Mostly prerenal azotemia is reversible with restoration of renal perfusion [1].

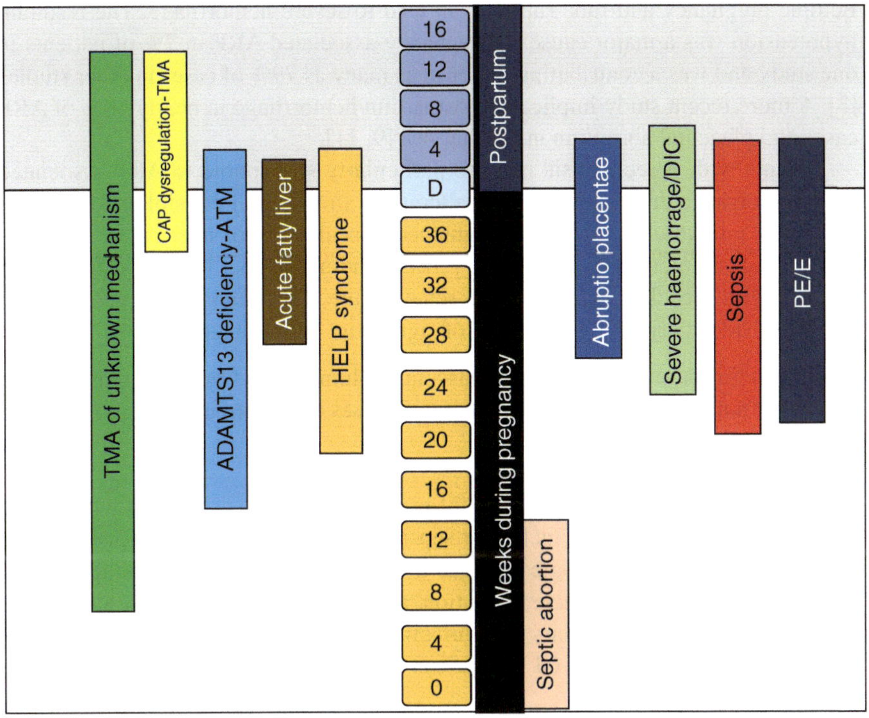

Fig. 43.1 Main causes of pregnancy-related AKI depending on their predominant timing of occurrence during pregnancy. CAP complement alternative pathway, D delivery, DIC disseminated intravascular coagulation, PE/E preeclampsia/eclampsia, TMA thrombotic microangiopathy. (Data quoted from Refs. [1, 10])

During first trimester, hyperemesis gravidarum is one of the more common causes of ARF secondary to profound volume depletion resulting from poor oral intake and vomiting. Similarly, any gastrointestinal illness with vomiting or diarrhea, excessive use of cathartics or laxatives, or bulimia may result in prerenal azotemia. Generally, these disorders are readily apparent on the basis of history and laboratory findings, including urinary electrolytes and osmolality. The urine sodium is typically low, as is the fractional excretion of sodium [(urine Na^+/serum Na^+)/(urine creatinine/serum creatinine) × 100%], reflecting a sodium-avid state, and urine osmolality is high, indicating intact urine concentrating ability. A low urine chloride may also provide a clue to surreptitious vomiting [3].

Uterine hemorrhage is an important cause of hypovolemia and subsequent prerenal azotemia late in pregnancy. Uterine blood flow increases from 50 cc/min prior to pregnancy to approximately 1000 cc/min at term. Thus, pregnancy-related bleeding can be rapid and massive, resulting in acute intravascular volume depletion and AKI. Although usually presenting as profuse vaginal bleeding, hemorrhage from placental abruption may be concealed or may occur in the postpartum period secondary to lacerations, uterine atony, inversion, or retained products of conception.

Ectopic pregnancy and tube rupture can lead to severe hemorrhage. The resultant hypotension was a major cause of pregnancy-associated ARF in 7% of patients in one study and was a contributing factor in as many as 79% of cases in other studies [3]. A more recent study implicated postpartum hemorrhage in nearly 10% of ARF cases and placental abruption in another 4% [9, 11].

Patients with preeclampsia may be particularly susceptible to ARF associated with hemorrhage due to pre-existing alterations in maternal physiology, including decreased intravascular volume, heightened vascular responsiveness to catecholamines and angiotensin II, and altered prostaglandin synthesis [12]. In a study of 31 patients with preeclampsia and acute renal failure, Sibai and colleagues reported that 90% had experienced some form of significant hemorrhage [13, 14].

Infection Sepsis can lead to intravascular volume depletion, hypotension, and organ dysfunction including AKI. Common causes of infection leading to sepsis in pregnancy are:

Pyelonephritis This occurs in 1–2% of pregnancies and is associated with maternal and fetal complications including sepsis, preterm labor, and adult respiratory distress syndrome. Physiologic changes of pregnancy including ureteral dilation, stasis related to smooth muscle relaxation, and pressure on the bladder and ureters predispose to ascending urinary tract infections. *E. coli* is the most common organism, followed by other GI organisms such as *Klebsiella*, *Proteus*, and *Enterococcus* [15].

Chorioamnionitis Intrauterine infection involving the Chorioamniotic membranes. This most commonly results from ascending infection of organisms colonizing the lower genital tract. These infections are usually polymicrobial with lower genital tract organisms, *Peptostreptococcus*, *Gardnerella*, *E. coli*, Group B streptococcus, and anaerobes.

Septic abortion This has become uncommon in the United States with the legalization of abortion, but it is a significant cause of maternal mortality and morbidity, including AKI, worldwide [9].

Hypertensive Disorders of Pregnancy

Hypertensive disorders of pregnancy are common, occurring in 6–8% of pregnancies. The differential diagnosis of hypertensive events during pregnancy includes chronic hypertension, gestational hypertension, or preeclampsia. Patients who have a known history of hypertension before pregnancy or those who are found to have BPs $\geq$ 140/90 mm Hg before 20 weeks of gestation are considered to have chronic hypertension. Women with chronic hypertension have an increased risk for superimposed preeclampsia, which can occur in up to 35% of their pregnancies. Some hypertensive patients with unknown histories of hypertension before pregnancy may present with BPs in the normal range during the first and second trimesters due to the normal physiologic decrease in BP during this time, thus masking the diagnosis of pre-existing hypertension. This may lead to the erroneous assumption that the finding of an elevated BP later during the pregnancy is related to gestational hypertension. The correct diagnosis ultimately is confirmed during the postpartum period because BP should normalize in those with true gestational hypertension. Gestational hypertension occurs during the second half of pregnancy in patients with no history of pre-existing hypertension and has an incidence of 6–7% [14].

Preeclampsia affects 3–10% of pregnancies. Diagnosis is based on new-onset hypertension and proteinuria after 20 weeks' gestation. In severe forms of the syndrome, maternal brain, lungs, kidneys, liver, and platelets as well as placental function and fetal well-being can be affected. Serial blood pressures, timed urine collection for protein excretion, creatinine, liver transaminases, and platelets are helpful in making the diagnosis and classifying severity. Systemic features include increased peripheral vascular resistance, endothelial dysfunction, vasospasm, activation of coagulation and inflammatory pathways, and platelet aggregation leading to ischemia and multi-organ dysfunction, including AKI [16]. Renal plasma flow and GFR are reduced by approximately 24% and 32%, respectively, with preeclampsia; however, the majority of women with preeclampsia do not develop AKI [17]. On the other hand, preeclampsia and other hypertensive disorders of pregnancy are the most common cause of PR-AKI, with an incidence of 1.5–2%. Often, there is a superimposed insult such as hemorrhage or DIC in a preeclamptic woman, which can lead to acute intravascular volume depletion and AKI [18].

Acute tubular necrosis is most commonly seen with preeclampsia-associated AKI. Short-term renal replacement therapy may be required. The precise cause of preeclampsia is unknown. Reduced placental perfusion leading to maternal vascular dysfunction is hypothesized. A diagnosis of preeclampsia also can be made in the absence of proteinuria in the presence of clinical features of severity [18] (Table 43.2).

Table 43.2 DD of common causes of PR-AKI during pregnancy

	Pregn. specific	GCS	Platelets	HB	INR	LDH	AKI	Proteinuria	BP	Management
Sepsis	No	↔↓	↔↓	↔↓	↑	↑	↑	↔↑	↓	TUC
Hemorrhage	No	↔↓	↑↔↓	↓↓	↔↑	↔	↑	↔	↓	TUC
DIC	No	↔↓	↔↓	↔↓	↔↑	↑	↑	↔↑	↓	TUC/Delv
PE	Yes	↓	↓↓	↔↓	↔	↑↑↑	↑↑	↑↑	↑	Delv
HELLP	Yes	↓	↓↓↓	↔↓	↔	↑↑↑	↑↑	↑↑	↑	Delv
AFLP	Yes	↔↓	↓	↔↓	↑↑↑	↑↑↑	↑	↔↑	↔↓	Delv
TTP	No	↓↓	↓↓↓	↓↓	↔	↑↑↑	↑	↑	↔↓	PP
aHUS	No	↔	↓↓	↓↓	↔	↑↑↑	↑↑↑	↑↑	↔↓	PP

Data quoted from Refs. [16–20]

BP blood pressure, *GCS* Glasgow Coma Scale, *Plt* platelets, *HB* hemoglobin, *INR* international normalized ratio, *PE* preeclampsia, *PF* plasmapheresis, *LDH* lactate dehydrogenase, *AKI* acute kidney injury, *TUC* treat underlying condition, *Dilv* delivery

Acute Fatty Liver of Pregnancy

With reported incidence of AFLP between 1 in 5000 and 1 in 10,000 deliveries, it is relatively uncommon cause of AKI in pregnancy [8]. The pathophysiological pathway is triggered by a fetal autosomal recessive defect in the beta oxidation of long-chain 3-hydroxyacyl-CoA dehydrogenase accounts for excessive fetal long-chain mitochondrial fatty acids to be transported across the placenta into the maternal circulation. Fetal long-chain fatty acids are then deposited into the maternal liver, resulting in hepatic dysfunction and, if not recognized and treated by delivery of the fetus, fulminant maternal liver failure [21].

This disease usually presents in the third trimester of pregnancy with nausea, vomiting, fever, malaise, and mental status changes [5, 22]. Laboratory evaluation reveals mild elevation of serum transaminase levels, hypocholesterolemia, thrombocytopenia, leukocytosis, and coagulation abnormalities (low Antithrombin III) as well as hypoglycemia [22, 23].

Ultrasound imaging of the liver may demonstrate increased echogenicity; however, ultrasound is not as sensitive as CT and MRI in making the diagnosis. CT of the liver in a case of AFLP may show decreased or diffuse attenuation throughout the liver. Although imaging may aid in the diagnosis of AFLP, liver biopsy is considered the gold standard. And, although biopsy will reveal microvesicular fatty infiltration, the diagnosis of AFLP is usually made based on clinical presentation and laboratory analysis [20]. A study by Knight et al., performed in the United Kingdom, evaluated 57 cases, 55 Of these women were confirmed to have AFLP based on Swansea criteria (Table 43.3) and clinical presentation, and 2 were diagnosed by clinical presentation alone [24].

Autoimmune causes could be the primary etiologies such as acute glomerulonephritis, IgA nephropathy, or secondary causes such as systemic lupus erythematosus which should be considered. Differentiating between acute glomerulonephritis and

Table 43.3 Swansea diagnostic criteria for diagnosis of AFLP [24]

Six or more of the following features in the absence of another explanation:
1. Vomiting abdominal pain
2. Polydipsia/polyuria
3. Encephalopathy
4. Elevated bilirubin
5. Hypoglycemia
6. Elevated urate
7. Leukocytosis
8. Ascites or bright liver on ultrasound
9. Elevated transaminases
10. Elevated ammonia
11. Renal impairment
12. Coagulopathy
13. Microvesicular steatosis on liver biopsy

preeclampsia can be challenging in the late second and third trimester, but is important since the treatments are different. Features that are more suggestive of glomerulonephritides include systemic symptoms (lupus symptoms, preceding infection), active urinary sediment (hematuria, red cell casts), nephrotic-range proteinuria (>2 g), positive ANA, autoantibodies, and abnormal complement levels [25].

Acute bilateral renal cortical necrosis is an ischemic destruction of the renal cortex either partial or complete due to a prolonged decrease in renal perfusion [19]. Obstetric renal cortical necrosis commonly occurs following a massive obstetric hemorrhage, which accounts for approximately 50–70% of all BRCN cases [26] with 80% of the cases due to uterine atony, the remaining etiologies attributed to DIC, placental abruption, or amniotic fluid embolism. Long-term renal function for patients with renal cortical necrosis is extremely poor, with many patients requiring dialysis and only 20–40% having partial recovery of renal function [19]. Symptoms include pain, gross hematuria, and hypotension. The diagnosis may be established by ultrasonography, contrast-enhanced CT demonstrating areas of cortical lucency, and MRI; however, renal biopsy remains the gold standard [19].

Post-renal

Urinary Obstruction

Although urinary obstruction is a relatively uncommon cause of ARF in pregnancy, it is readily reversible and, therefore, must be considered in the differential. Obstruction may occur at any level of the urinary tract due to a wide variety of causes, many of which are not unique to pregnancy. Ureteral compression by the gravid uterus, with resultant ARF and hypertension, has been reported [19], and large leiomyomata have even been reported to cause ureteral obstruction in the first trimester [19]. Another cause unique to pregnancy is an incarcerated uterus, which may cause urinary retention as the gravid uterus enlarges but becomes trapped in the pelvis secondary to significant retroflexion and then compresses the bladder [27]. Other risk factors for urinary obstruction in pregnancy include polyhydramnios, multi-fetal gestation, large uterine fibroids, pyelonephritis, renal calculi, ureteral narrowing, and low abdominal wall compliance [28].

Renal ultrasound is the first step in the evaluation of possible urinary tract obstruction, although results may be inconclusive due to the physiologic dilation of the collecting system often seen in pregnancy due to both the effects of progesterone and the mechanical pressure of the gravid uterus. Thus, anterograde or retrograde pyelography may be necessary for definitive diagnosis. Relief of the obstruction may be accomplished by ureteral stent placement, percutaneous nephrostomy, manual reduction of an incarcerated uterus, or amnioreduction in the case of polyhydramnios [20, 28]. If the fetus is significantly premature, correcting the obstruction should allow for a substantial delay in delivery as well as recovery of renal function. If the patient is near term, however, delivery may be indicated to remove both the mechanical and hormonal causes of the obstruction. It should be noted that the fetal mortality rate for reversible obstructive uropathy with associated renal failure has been reported to be as high as 33% [28].

Management of AKI (Fig. 43.2)

General measures to treat pregnancy-related AKI include quick and accurate assessment and correction of the underlying etiology and prevention of further damage and deterioration. As in the nonpregnant patient, fluid management is the most important initial therapy. Appropriate volume resuscitation, with the goal of restoring and maintaining urine output and renal perfusion to reverse preischemic changes and to limit further damage, even after tubular necrosis has occurred [5].

Van Hook et al. in their review from a renal functional perspective revealed that the use of lactated Ringer's solution and Plasmalyte is associated with less renal injury than normal saline because higher concentrations of chloride can lead to vasoconstriction and ischemia [8].

Timely initiation of renal replacement therapy (RRT) and prompt delivery of fetus are sometimes necessary dictated by the etiology. Volume repletion is crucial in prerenal states although the rate of volume replacement needs to be carefully monitored, as women with either endotoxin-mediated injury or preeclampsia can easily develop pulmonary edema. Complications of AKI can be treated as in nonpregnant patients, i.e., hyperkalemia in most circumstances can be treated with cation exchange resins, metabolic acidosis with alkali therapy, volume overload with loop diuretics, and anemia with blood transfusion. If these measures prove unsuccessful or if the renal injury progresses, initiation of renal replacement therapy will be necessary. Specific measures to treat PR-AKI depend on the underlying etiology of the injury. Steroid and immunosuppressive therapy may be warranted for biopsy-proven cases of glomerulonephritis. For the diagnoses of severe preeclampsia, AFLP, and HELLP syndrome, prompt delivery of the fetus is the only definitive therapy. Treatment of the thrombotic microangiopathy, including TTP, and atypical HUS, requires plasmapheresis and administration of eculizumab (for atypical HUS). Administration of glucocorticoids is indicated should delivery of the fetus be required prior to 34 weeks of gestation in order to reduce the risk of neonatal respiratory distress syndrome [29].

Additional important steps include the removal and avoidance of nephrotoxins, adjustment of medication dosing for renal clearance (particularly magnesium), and the prevention and treatment of infection because sepsis is the most common cause of mortality of in ARF [15].

Overt blood loss should be replaced early because hemorrhage near term may be hard to detect and early and appropriate management can prevent or limit irreversible change [5].

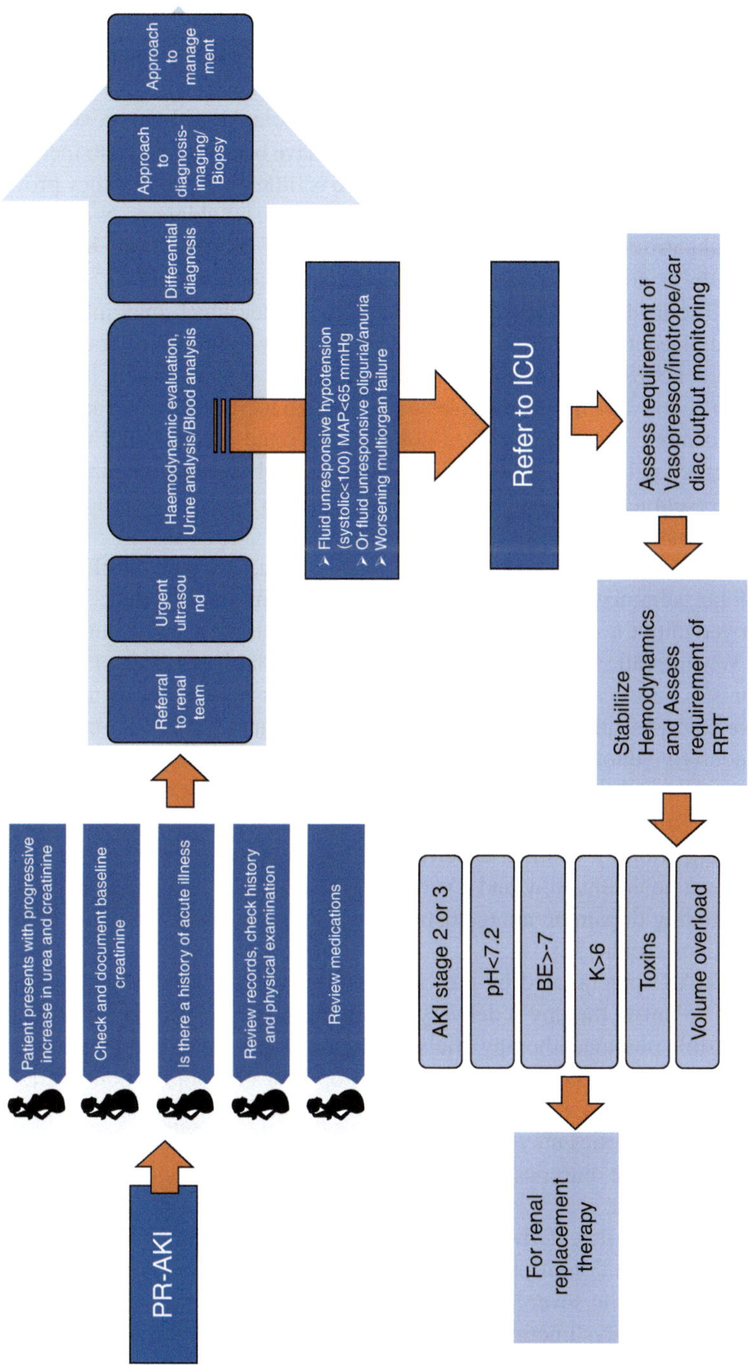

Fig. 43.2 Stepwise approaches for diagnosis and management of AKI. (Data quoted from Refs. [1, 5, 8, 15, 29])

Pharmacologic Management

Medication in general is considered second line for ARF, and it's use to maintain perfusion and urinary output has not been associated with improved outcomes. Although multiple alternatives of medications have been suggested to increase renal blood flow and maintain urinary output, there is little evidence that they provide any benefit. The use of dopamine infusion, loop diuretics, fenoldopam, N-acetylcysteine, and atrial natriuretic peptide, for the maintenance of urinary output, have been studied and have not shown any benefit in the treatment of ARF [8, 15]. Although diuretic use leads to decreased intravascular volume, which may inhibit labor and decrease placental perfusion, thiazide diuretics may be indicated for severe intractable preeclampsia or pulmonary edema. Although serum albumin levels are often found to be low and infusions have been shown to increase both serum albumin and colloid osmotic pressures, it does not stabilize renal function and was associated with higher fetal mortality [30]. The use of mannitol should be theoretically beneficial in preventing ARF in high-risk patients, but no trials have been done in pregnant women to assess the efficacy [1].

In the case of sepsis-induced acute renal failure, source control includes early antibiotic administration, and starting broad empiric coverage is commonly employed until the determination can be made for a more specific antibiotic therapy [31]. When treating septic abortion or chorioamnionitis, evacuation of the uterine contents is necessary for effective treatment because antibiotic penetration of the uterine cavity is suboptimal [15]. Managing the complications of renal failure and the underlying etiologies should be treated as appropriate.

Because renal failure occurring during pregnancy is not one specific entity, but rather a result of a variety of processes, pharmacotherapy must be tailored to the underlying etiology. Women experiencing hyperemesis gravidarum should receive thiamine supplementation, and a variety of medications can be used to control nausea, including dopamine antagonists, phenothiazines, histamine receptor blockers, and corticosteroids [32].

In PR-AKI precipitated by preeclampsia treatment is primarily supportive, and the only definitive therapy is delivery. Although corticosteroids have been suggested as a possible pharmacotherapy, trials have shown no benefit with regard to duration of hospitalization, recovery speed, or development of complications [33]. Despite the existence of peripheral edema, decreasing intravascular volume is not recommended, and diuretics may inhibit labor and decrease placental perfusion, although the use of thiazide diuretics may be indicated for severe intractable preeclampsia or pulmonary edema.

Magnesium sulfate delivered intravenously is the most important pharmacotherapy for the prevention of progression to seizures. Although tending to be rare, side effects can be quite severe, including loss of patellar reflexes, respiratory depression, and cardiac dysfunction, and extra care should be taken to monitor magnesium levels and urine output in the patient with existing renal failure because magnesium excretion may be decreased [34, 35]. Lorazepam and phenytoin may be used for refractory seizures not responsive to magnesium therapy [30].

For TTP and HUS, steroids are recommended as the initial immunosuppressive therapy in the cases of a suspected ADAMTS-13 deficiency. The use of cyclosporine, rituximab, and vincristine has been reported in more severe cases, and the use of heparin anticoagulation is potentially harmful. Fresh frozen plasma can be given for the correction of ADAMTS-13 deficiency [33].

When AFLP is the underlying etiology, therapies consist of stabilizing maternal glucose with dextrose, correction of anemia and coagulopathy with blood transfusion, fresh frozen plasma, and cryoprecipitate and treatment of hepatic encephalopathy with a low-protein diet and oral lactulose [33, 34]. As with preeclampsia, treatment is mainly supportive, and delivery is the definitive therapy. Renal failure develops in approximately 60% of cases, and, if left untreated, patients may progress to fulminant hepatic failure with jaundice, encephalopathy, DIC, gastrointestinal hemorrhage, and death [8]. Maternal and fetal mortality rates as high as 85% were seen in the past, although with earlier diagnosis and treatment, maternal mortality now ranges between 0% and 12.5%, and perinatal mortality occurs in 6.6–15% of cases [5].

The incidence of contrast-induced (CI) AKI has been progressively increasing, now accounting for approximately 10.5% of AKI in the nonpregnant population. Screening for kidney disease in patients who require iodinated contrast has been suggested as a way to prevent CI-AKI, as well as the use of the lowest possible dose of iso-osmolar or low-osmolar contrast medium. Intravenous isotonic sodium chloride (>1–1.5 ml/kg/h for 2–12 h before and 6–12 h after contrast media exposure, to achieve a UO >150 ml/h) or sodium bicarbonate solutions are to be used in patients at risk of AKI. Hydration is the only intervention associated with prevention of CI-AKI; the addition of sodium bicarbonate is not necessary. High-dose oral N-acetylcysteine (1200 mg PO q12h the day before and the day of the study) may be added despite the fact that the evidence for benefit is very limited [36].

Nonpharmacologic Management

Renal failure can progress to the point of requiring dialysis to prevent maternal morbidity and mortality and allow for progression of pregnancy to a point where delivery is feasible. It is a purely supportive measure, and there is no evidence that it shortens the course of ARF [2]. Both peritoneal dialysis and hemodialysis have been used successfully to treat renal failure occurring during pregnancy [37]. Although there are no studies to determine the optimal mode of dialysis in the pregnant patient, intermittent hemodialysis is the most commonly chosen modality, although continuous hemofiltration has come into use more recently, because it allows for control of volume and solute loads, and to prevent the hemodynamic fluctuations that occur with intermittent dialysis.

Dialysis should be undertaken early because urea, creatinine, and other metabolites that accumulate can cross the placenta, and fetal survival and gestational age are improved with a lower serum blood urea nitrogen and creatinine [38].

Indications for initiating dialysis include uremic symptoms, volume overload, and metabolic acidosis and hyperkalemia unresponsive to medical therapy, although other recommended parameters are serum creatinine of 3.5–5.0 mg/dL or GFR decreasing to less than 20 mL/min [37]. The placement of a peritoneal dialysis catheter is technically feasible in pregnancy, and the peritoneal membrane has been shown to maintain clearance and ultrafiltration capabilities. There are a number of advantages with peritoneal dialysis, including minimizing fluid and electrolyte shifts, reduction of hypotension, better management of hypertension, and the ability to administer insulin and magnesium as needed [37].

Although plasmapheresis is likely not helpful for most causes of ARF, it is used therapeutically for thrombotic microangiopathies by clearing large thrombogenic multimers or autoantibodies [8], and plasma infusion and plasma exchange are used to treat atypical HUS [33]. No trials have been done studying plasma exchange for preeclampsia/HELLP, but it seems to be an option with low risk during pregnancy and may be promising for otherwise refractory preeclampsia [30, 34]. There is no strong evidence for plasma exchange to treat AFLP, but the use of molecular adsorbent recirculating systems may present a promising mode of therapy [34].

Surgical Management

When renal failure occurs as a result of obstruction, treatment includes procedures to relieve the obstruction such as cystoscopy, stents, and percutaneous nephrostomy [8]. In the case of severe preeclampsia, uterine curettage immediately after delivery can accelerate recovery [30]. Definitive surgical therapy after the failure of all other therapies is eventual renal transplantation.

Kidney Transplant Recipients and Pregnancy

Women with ESRD could pursue pregnancy after successful kidney transplantation. Complications, such as preterm delivery and preeclampsia, are much less, and fertility is always better. Pregnancy is also a sensitizing state, which can result in the formation of anti-HLA antibodies that may make finding a future suitable donor more difficult. Recommendations from the current KDIGO (Kidney Disease: Improving Global Outcomes) guidelines state that women should wait for 1 year post-transplantation before pursuing pregnancy, provided kidney function is stable. However, a more recent study suggested that waiting 2 years may be prudent to reduce the risk of allograft failure [39].

There have been several single-center studies that have evaluated the impact of pregnancy on graft survival. However, it has been difficult to draw firm conclusions from these results given methodologic differences, including different eras, study populations, immunosuppressive agents, and control groups [39].

The combined results of 50 different studies that reported pregnancy-related outcomes in kidney transplant recipients published in metanalysis [39]. Study included more than 4700 pregnancies in 3570 kidney transplant recipients. They found that the live birth rate was similar to that for the general population (73.5% vs 66.7%). However, rates of preeclampsia (27% vs 3.8%), gestational diabetes (8% vs 3.9%), and preterm delivery (45.6% vs 12.5%) were much higher. The risk for graft loss in the cohorts was low (5.8% at 1 year and 6.9% at 5 years) [40]. Women with kidney transplants require close monitoring in pregnancy by both obstetricians and nephrologists [40]. The immunosuppressive regimen needs to be modified to medications that are safe in pregnancy, usually a combination of AZA, tacrolimus/cyclosporine, and prednisone. Tacrolimus doses often need to be increased substantially in pregnancy, though recent pharmacologic studies have shown that whole-blood measurements of tacrolimus do not accurately reflect free tacrolimus levels in the setting of pregnancy, meaning that women may experience toxicity with seemingly therapeutic levels [41].

Kidney donors may also have a need for more careful monitoring in pregnancy, given increased risk for preeclampsia that has been reported in several observational studies. A study by Garg et al. published in 2015 suggested that kidney donors had 2.4 times increased odds of having preeclampsia or gestational hypertension (11% vs 5%), but did not have increased risk for preterm delivery or low birth weight [42].

Prognosis

The prognosis for recovery of renal function determined by multiple variables, including underlying renal status, duration of renal failure, and the etiology of the ARF. For example, if the patient had normal renal function before ARF from an acute obstructive process that is relieved in a timely manner, then a full recovery should be expected. On the other hand, as previously discussed, studies have demonstrated that, of patients with compromised renal function who develop preeclampsia with ARF, up to 80% may require long-term dialysis [22].

Conclusion

Although the overall incidence of AKI in pregnancy in most of the world is declining, the absolute numbers of deaths from AKI remain unacceptably high. Diagnosis of pregnancy-related AKI is not always straight-forward and can be quite challenging in those with overlapping features such as preeclampsia/HELLP, AFLP, HUS/

TTP, atypical HUS, and lupus nephritis. Clinical judgment and experience become paramount in making an accurate diagnosis. Measuring angiogenic factors may prove to be helpful in making the diagnosis of preeclampsia. Sophisticated genetic or serologic testing may have the potential to help identify patients with AFLP and atypical HUS, but they are presently not available for everyday clinical use. Excluding the use of eculizumab for atypical HUS and plasma exchange for TTP, treatment of AKI in pregnancy is generally supportive, often coupled with expedient delivery. Research should focus on disease-specific diagnostic markers, with awareness that prompt availability of results is necessary to affect management decisions and impact outcomes. These issues are especially relevant if the incidence of AKI is increasing in the developed world, with the rise possibly related to the trend toward delaying childbirth, which may be accompanied by increases in maternal comorbidities. Furthermore, the increasing use of reproductive technologies that frequently result in multiple gestations may also increase the risk of AKI. Hence, the need for prompt and accurate diagnosis followed by appropriate treatment for pregnancy-related AKI continues to grow with the changes in the epidemiology of women of reproductive age.

Key Points

- Although the incidence of pregnancy-related acute kidney injury declined in the developed world between 1950 and 2019, rates have increased in the past decade. Furthermore, mortality and the risk of long-term renal failure remain significant in such cases.
- An approach to the management of pregnancy-related acute kidney injury must be informed by a thorough understanding of maternal renal adaptations to pregnancy, including alterations in renal hemodynamics and substrate handling.
- Management strategies should incorporate an understanding of fetal considerations, including the importance of maintaining uteroplacental blood flow and interventions that may ameliorate fetal compromise.
- In addition to causes of acute renal failure that may occur coincident with pregnancy, several disease processes unique to pregnancy should be considered in the pregnant patient. The most common of these is preeclampsia.
- The determination of the specific cause of pregnancy-related acute renal failure can allow for the differentiation of conditions that require delivery for treatment from those that would not be altered by delivery. This distinction allows for minimization of iatrogenic prematurity and its associated complications. In making this distinction, prudent use of renal biopsy may be indicated.
- When indicated, renal replacement therapy can be administered to pregnant women, and care should be taken to minimize hemodynamic and solute fluctuations. Intermittent or continuous therapy may be helpful in these patients.
- A multidisciplinary team approach is imperative for optimal management of the pregnant woman with acute renal failure.

References

1. Mantel GD. Care of the critically ill parturient: oliguria and renal failure. Best Pract Res Clin Obstet Gynaecol. 2001;15:563–81.
2. Bellomo R, Ronco C, Kellum JA, et al. Acute renal failure – definition, outcome measures, animal models, fluid therapy and information technology needs: the Second International Consensus Conference of the Acute Dialysis Quality Initiative (ADQI) Group. Crit Care. 2004;8:R204–12.
3. Hussein W, Lafayette RA. Renal function in normal and disordered pregnancy. Curr Opin Nephrol Hypertens. 2014;23:46–53.
4. Abosaif NY, Tolba YA, Heap M, Russell J, El Nahas AM. The outcome of acute renal failure in the intensive care unit according to RIFLE: model application, sensitivity, and predictability. Am J Kidney Dis. 2005;46:1038–48.
5. Balofsky A, Fedarau M. Renal failure in pregnancy. Crit Care Clin. 2016;32(1):73–83.
6. Kattah A, Milic N, White W, Garovic V. Spot urine protein measurements in normotensive pregnancies, pregnancies with isolated proteinuria and preeclampsia. Am J Physiol Regul Integr Comp Physiol. 2017;313(4):R418–24.
7. Aluvihare VR, Kallikourdis M, Betz AG. Regulatory T cells mediate maternal tolerance to the fetus. Nat Immunol. 2004;5(3):266–71.
8. Van Hook JW. Acute kidney injury during pregnancy. Clin Obstet Gynecol. 2014;57:851–61.
9. Odutayo A, Hladunewich M. Obstetric nephrology: renal hemodynamic and metabolic physiology in normal pregnancy. Clin J Am Soc Nephrol. 2012;7(12):2073–80.
10. Fakhouri F, Vercel C, Frémeaux-Bacchi V. Obstetric nephrology: AKI and thrombotic microangiopathies in pregnancy. Clin J Am Soc Nephrol. 2012;7:2100–6.
11. Munnur U, Bandi V, Guntupalli KK. Management principles of the critically ill obstetric patient. Clin Chest Med. 2011;32:53–60.
12. Piccoli GB, Gaglioti P, Attini R, et al. Pre-eclampsia or chronic kidney disease? The flow hypothesis. Nephrol Dial Transplant. 2013;28:1199–206.
13. Sibai BM, Villar MA, Mabie BC. Acute renal failure in hypertensive disorders of pregnancy. Pregnancy outcome and remote prognosis in thirty-one consecutive cases. Am J Obstet Gynecol. 1990;162(3):777–83.
14. Henderson JT, Thompson JH, Burda BU, Cantor A. Preeclampsia screening: evidence report and systematic review for the US Preventive Services Task Force. JAMA. 2017;317(16):1668–83.
15. Gammill HS, Jeyabalan A. Acute renal failure in pregnancy. Crit Care Med. 2005;33:S372–84.
16. Sibai BM, Ramadan MK, Usta I, Salama M, Mercer BM, Friedman SA. Maternal morbidity and mortality in 442 pregnancies with hemolysis, elevated liver enzymes, and low platelets (HELLP syndrome). Am J Obstet Gynecol. 1993;169(4):1000–6.
17. Conrad K, Lindheimer M. Renal and cardiovascular alterations. In: Lindheimer M, editor. Chesley's hypertensive disorders in pregnancy. Stamford: Appleton & Lange; 1999. p. 263–326.
18. Brown M, Child RP, O'Connor M, et al. Pregnancy-induced hypertension and renal failure: clinical importance of diuretics, plasma volume, and vasospasm. Aust N Z J Obstet Gynaecol. 1989;29:230–2.
19. Myers DL, Scotti RJ. Acute urinary retention and the incarcerated, retroverted, gravid uterus: a case report. J Reprod Med. 1995;40(6):487–90.
20. Jena M, Mitch WE. Rapidly reversible acute renal failure from ureteral obstruction in pregnancy. Am J Kidney Dis. 1996;28(3):457–60.
21. Wei Q, Zhang L, Liu X. Clinical diagnosis and treatment of acute fatty liver of pregnancy: a literature review and 11 new cases. J Obstet Gynaecol Res. 2010;36:751–6.
22. Prakash J. The kidney in pregnancy: a journey of three decades. Indian J Nephrol. 2012;22(3):159–67. https://doi.org/10.4103/0971-4065.98750.
23. Sibai BM. Imitators of severe pre-eclampsia/eclampsia. Manag High-Risk Pregnancy. 2004;31(4):835–52.

24. Knight M, Nelson-Piercy C, Kurinczuk JJ, et al. A prospective national study of acute fatty liver of pregnancy in the UK. Gut. 2008;57(7):951–6.
25. Colombo DF. Renal disease in pregnancy. In: Obstetrics: Normal and problem pregnancies. Philadelphia: Elsevier/Saunders; 2012. p. 850–61.
26. Nwoko R, Plecas D, Garovic VD. Acute kidney injury in the pregnant patient. Clin Nephrol. 2012;78(12):478–86.
27. Nelson MS. Acute urinary retention secondary to an increased gravid uterus. Am J Emerg Med. 1986;4(3):231–2.
28. Gary CF. Renal and urinary tract disorders. In: Williams obstetrics. 24th ed. New York: McGraw-Hill Education; 2014. p. 1051–68.
29. ACOG Committee Opinion No. 475: antenatal corticosteroid therapy for fetal maturation. Obstet Gynecol. 2011;117(2 Pt 1):422–4.
30. Müller-Deile J, Schiffer M. Preeclampsia from a renal point of view: insides into disease models, biomarkers and therapy. World J Nephrol. 2014;3:169–81.
31. Galvagno SM, Camann W. Sepsis and acute renal failure in pregnancy. Anesth Analg. 2009;108:572–5.
32. Wegrzyniak LJ, Repke JT, Ural SH. Treatment of hyperemesis gravidarum. Rev Obstet Gynecol. 2012;5:78–84.
33. Machado S, Figueiredo N, Borges A, et al. Acute kidney injury in pregnancy: a clinical challenge. J Nephrol. 2012;25:19–30.
34. Ganesan C, Maynard SE. Acute kidney injury in pregnancy: the thrombotic microangiopathies. J Nephrol. 2011;24:554–63.
35. Smith JM, Lowe RF, Fullerton J, et al. An integrative review of the side effects related to the use of magnesium sulfate for pre-eclampsia and eclampsia management. BMC Pregnancy Childbirth. 2013;13:34.
36. KDIGO clinical practice guideline for acute kidney injury. Kidney Int. 2012;2(Suppl.):1–138.
37. Krane N. Peritoneal dialysis and hemodialysis in pregnancy. Hemodial Int. 2001;5:97–101.
38. Hladunewich MA, Hou S, Odutayo A, et al. Intensive hemodialysis associates with improved pregnancy outcomes: a Canadian and United States cohort comparison. J Am Soc Nephrol. 2014;25:1103–9.
39. Deshpande NA, James NT, Kucirka LM, et al. Pregnancy outcomes in kidney transplant recipients: a systematic review and meta-analysis. Am J Transplant. 2011;11(11):2388–404.
40. Kidney Disease: Improving Global Outcomes Transplant Work Group. KDIGO clinical practice guideline for the care of kidney transplant recipients. Am J Transplant. 2009;9(suppl 3):S1–55.
41. Zheng S, Easterling TR, Umans JG, et al. Pharmacokinetics of tacrolimus during pregnancy. Ther Drug Monit. 2012;34(6):660–70.
42. Garg AX, Nevis IF, McArthur E, et al. Gestational hypertension and preeclampsia in living kidney donors. N Engl J Med. 2015;372:124–33.

Part XI
Hematology

Chapter 44
Hematological Emergencies

Janice Zimmerman

Introduction

Hematological emergencies may be a primary disorder in pregnancy (i.e., thrombotic thrombocytopenic purpura) or complicate other serious conditions (i.e., thrombocytopenia in severe preeclampsia or HELLP). Although most hematological disorders in pregnancy are acquired, congenital disorders such as sickle cell anemia also lead to potential complications. Little or no data exists on the incidence of hematological emergencies in pregnancy.

Hematological Adaptations During Pregnancy

The evaluation of hematological complications during pregnancy must take into account physiological changes that occur during this period. Beginning at 8–10 weeks of gestation, the number of red blood cells increases and will be 20–30% higher by the end of pregnancy compared to nonpregnant women. This increment results from increased production of erythropoietin that supports the requirement for increased oxygen delivery during pregnancy. The plasma volume increases 10–15% by 6–12 weeks gestation and continues until weeks 30–34, reaching 30–50% more compared to nonpregnant women. This increase in plasma volume facilitates the delivery of nutrients and waste removal from the fetus and protects the mother from excessive blood loss during delivery. These changes explain the dilutional decrease in hemoglobin concentration and the physiological anemia of pregnancy.

J. Zimmerman (✉)
Baylor College of Medicine, Houston, TX, USA

C. Montufar et al. (eds.), *Obstetric Catastrophes*,
https://doi.org/10.1007/978-3-030-70034-8_44

The number of white blood cells starts to increase after the second month of pregnancy up to the third trimester, when the count can reach 10 to 15,000/mm^3. The white blood cell count usually returns to normal by 1 week postpartum. The presence of Dohle bodies (oval, basophilic inclusions in the periphery of granulocytes) can be normal during pregnancy.

The platelet count can be mildly reduced during pregnancy (gestational thrombocytopenia/incidental thrombocytopenia) but should remain within the normal range. Counts less than 100,000/mm^3 must be properly investigated.

During pregnancy there is a reduction in fibrinolysis, explained by an increase in thrombin cleavage products and a decrease in the concentrations of protein S and antithrombin. Clotting factor concentrations also increase, which helps in prevention of excessive bleeding during placental separation. However, these changes in the coagulation cascade increase the risk of thrombosis in the mother. Despite increases in clotting factors, coagulation test results (PT and aPTT) remain within the normal range.

Evaluation of Hematological Disorders

The complete blood count and coagulation studies are the most commonly used diagnostic tests for hematological disorders in pregnancy. Visual inspection of the peripheral blood smear should also be performed when evaluating potential hemolytic disorders, thrombocytopenia, thrombotic microangiopathies, and hemoglobinopathies. Hemoglobin electrophoresis may be ordered if an undiagnosed hemoglobinopathy is suspected. Coagulation abnormalities may require further evaluation with specific factor levels or mixing studies to distinguish factor deficiency from an inhibitor. If available, an ADAMTS 13 level is helpful in confirming the diagnosis of thrombotic thrombocytopenic purpura (TTP).

Severe Anemia in Pregnancy

Physiologic anemia is the most common hematological finding of pregnancy but is not severe. Iron deficiency anemia may cause severe anemia in pregnancy, but it usually does not present as an obstetric emergency. Aplastic anemia is one hematological emergency that may occur in pregnancy.

Aplastic anemia associated with pregnancy or induced by pregnancy is uncommon, but it is a serious condition that usually presents as a progressive pancytopenia. The etiology is related to an immunological disorder with an overproduction of bone marrow inhibiting cytokines induced by abnormal T cell response in an individual that is genetically predisposed. Common complications in these patients include postpartum bleeding, premature rupture of membranes, endometritis, growth restrictions, and placental abruption. Severe thrombocytopenia (platelet count less than 20,000/mm^3) is associated with more complications [1, 2]. The most frequent causes of maternal mortality are bleeding and sepsis.

Patients may present with symptoms of fatigue or dyspnea but also more serious manifestations such as bleeding or infection. Bone marrow biopsy is required for diagnosis and reveals hypoplasia of all cell lines. Management while pregnant includes transfusions to maintain platelet count greater than 20,000/mm^3 and adequate hemoglobin concentrations [3]. Higher platelet counts may be needed at the time of delivery especially with operative deliveries. Prophylactic antibiotics are indicated for neutropenia to prevent infection. Growth factors such as granulocyte/monocyte colony-stimulating factor can be administered, and cyclosporine has also been used in pregnancy [3]. Hematopoietic stem cell transplant is not an option during pregnancy. Spontaneous remission may occur after delivery in 50–70% of women, but standard therapies are indicated for those that do not recover [4].

Sickle Cell Anemia

Sickle cell disease (SCD) during pregnancy increases the risk of obstetric and non-obstetric complications including infections, thrombotic events, acute chest syndrome, pulmonary hypertension, postpartum hemorrhage, preeclampsia, stillbirths, spontaneous abortions, preterm labor, and infants with low birth weight. Maternal and perinatal mortality are also increased. Worsening anemia in SCD may be precipitated by malaria infection, preeclampsia, postpartum hemorrhage, aplastic crisis, and vaso-occlusive pain crisis [4]. A multidisciplinary approach to care involving hematologists, obstetricians, and primary care physicians is needed to optimize outcomes. The optimal approach to treating anemia in pregnant patients with SCD is unclear. Options are limited to treating the precipitant of worsening anemia and support with blood transfusion. A Cochrane review found insufficient evidence to recommend prophylactic transfusion over standard care [5]. A meta-analysis of 11 cohort studies suggested prophylactic transfusion was associated with decreased maternal and perinatal mortality, vaso-occlusive pain crises, and pulmonary complications, but the studies had a high risk of bias [6]. Additional data on prophylactic transfusion will be available from a trial in progress (https://clinicaltrials.gov/ct2/show/NCT03975894) [7]. Currently, routine prophylactic transfusion is not recommended [8]. Serious complications of SCD in pregnancy such as severe anemia (hemoglobin < 6 g/dL), stroke, organ failure, or acute chest syndrome are likely to require simple transfusion to increase the hemoglobin or exchange transfusion to lower hemoglobin S levels. Once transfusion is initiated for a serious complication, it may be appropriate to continue a transfusion program for the duration of the pregnancy. Unfortunately, blood transfusion in the pregnant patient with SCD is associated with higher risk of alloimmunization, delayed hemolytic transfusion reactions, and hemolytic disease in the infant. Compatible blood for transfusion may also be difficult to obtain due to alloimmunization from prior transfusions.

Immune Thrombocytopenia (ITP)

There are many causes of thrombocytopenia in pregnancy (Table 44.1) [9], and some of these conditions have been discussed in other chapters. Immune thrombocytopenia more commonly develops in the first trimester but can occur at any gestational age [10]. The peripheral blood smear shows thrombocytopenia without small or giant platelets. The presence of antiplatelet antibodies is neither sensitive nor specific for the diagnosis.

Although the lowest platelet count in ITP in pregnancy is usually above 50,000/mm^3, some women develop severe thrombocytopenia and bleeding [10]. Treatment of ITP during the first and second trimester is similar to nonpregnant women. The use of oral corticosteroids (10–30 mg prednisone daily) and intravenous immunoglobulin (1 g/kg) should be considered for platelet counts below 20,000/mm^3, active bleeding, or when an invasive procedure is required.

Therapy during the third trimester should be based on the risk of maternal bleeding during delivery. The mode of delivery is determined by the risk of obstetrical complications rather than the presence of ITP. If a cesarean section or spinal anesthesia is planned, a short course of corticosteroids or immunoglobulin and platelet transfusions can be initiated with the goal to increase the platelet count above 75,000 to 80,000/mm^3. A platelet count of 50,000/mm^3 or greater is recommended for a vaginal delivery [10]. In the event of refractory thrombocytopenia, splenectomy can be considered during the second trimester or at the time of cesarean section. Cytotoxic agents are generally not recommended due to their teratogenic effects.

Thrombotic Microangiopathies

Thrombotic microangiopathies are characterized by hemolytic anemia, thrombocytopenia, and microvascular thrombosis leading to organ dysfunction. Although systemic lupus and antiphospholipid syndrome are thrombotic microangiopathies that

Table 44.1 Causes of thrombocytopenia in pregnancy

Gestational thrombocytopenia
Preeclampsia/eclampsia
HELLP
Immune thrombocytopenia
Acute fatty liver
Thrombotic thrombocytopenic purpura
Hemolytic uremic syndrome
Disseminated intravascular coagulation
Hemorrhage
Sepsis
Drug-induced thrombocytopenia

can occur in pregnancy, this chapter will limit discussion to thrombotic thrombocytopenic purpura (TTP) and hemolytic uremic syndrome (HUS). Preeclampsia and HELLP have been discussed in Chap. 10.

Thrombotic Thrombocytopenic Purpura (TTP)

TTP is caused by a severe congenital (Upshaw-Schulman syndrome) or acquired deficiency in ADAMTS13, a metalloprotease that cleaves ultra-large von Willebrand factor multimers. These large multimers increase platelet adhesiveness and aggregation and impair fibrinolytic activity that predisposes to thrombotic occlusion of the microvasculature. The acquired deficiency of ADAMTS13 is most commonly due to an autoantibody. Pregnancy may be the initiating event in approximately 7% of TTP cases (congenital and acquired). More than 80% of TTP cases occur after 30 weeks gestation or during the postpartum period [10, 11].

Clinically TTP consists of the following classic conditions: microangiopathic hemolytic anemia, thrombocytopenia, fluctuating central nervous system abnormalities, fever, and renal dysfunction. Only microangiopathic hemolysis and thrombocytopenia are required for diagnosis, and other elements of the pentad may not be present. TTP may be difficult to distinguish from severe preeclampsia or HELLP syndrome. Manifestations that are more suggestive of TTP are listed in Table 44.2.

Examination of the peripheral blood smear should be performed to assess for typical findings of thrombocytopenia, polychromasia of reticulocytes, and fragmented red blood cells. Other laboratory manifestations include elevated lactate dehydrogenase (LDH) and bilirubin. Renal findings may be subtle, such as proteinuria, or more overt with elevated BUN and creatinine. Measurement of ADAMTS13 activity is helpful in the diagnosis of congenital and acquired TTP. Activity levels are usually less than 10% [10]. However, testing may not be readily available, and treatment may need to be initiated based on clinical suspicion. A low ADAMTS13 antigen level or the absence of antibody to ADAMTS13 suggests congenital deficiency.

The treatment of choice in pregnant patients with acquired TTP is urgent plasma exchange therapy to remove the antibody and infusion of fresh frozen plasma to

Table 44.2 Manifestations suggesting a diagnosis of TTP rather than preeclampsia or HELLP

Absence of hypertension
Lower platelet count (<50,000/mm^3, especially if <10,000/mm^3)
Mental status changes more common
Liver function abnormalities less common
More severe hemolysis
Normal coagulation parameters (PT/PTT)
Presence of fever
Failure to resolve or worsening after delivery

replace ADAMTS13. Corticosteroids are also initiated for immunosuppression in acquired TTP. Fresh frozen plasma alone may be effective in congenital TTP and can be infused in acquired TTP when there are delays in initiation of plasma exchange. Once platelet counts have normalized, the frequency of plasma exchange will depend on the subsequent platelet counts. More intense plasma exchange may be required prior to delivery if time allows. Platelet transfusions are usually avoided unless severe bleeding develops. Caplacizumab, an antibody fragment that inhibits interaction of von Willebrand factor with platelets, is approved for use in TTP along with plasma exchange, but there is no data on safety and efficacy in pregnancy [12]. Maternal mortality is usually not compromised significantly by TTP, but fetal morbidity and mortality are increased [13]. Fetal loss more commonly occurs in the second trimester [11].

Hemolytic Uremic Syndrome (HUS)

Hemolytic uremic syndrome is a thrombotic microangiopathy with prominent renal involvement, and two types have been characterized. Typical HUS is mediated by exposure to Shiga toxin and is more common in children. Bloody diarrhea is a characteristic manifestation but may not be present in all cases. Atypical HUS (aHUS) is associated with mutations in genes regulating the alternative complement pathway and more likely to be associated with pregnancy. Almost 80% of aHUS in pregnancy occurs postpartum [13, 14].

Diagnosis of aHUS is based on clinical manifestations consistent with the syndrome, laboratory findings of hemolytic microangiopathy and thrombocytopenia, and exclusion of other causes. Low complement levels are not specific for aHUS, and activity levels of ADAMTS13 are near normal in aHUS. Findings of genetic mutations associated with aHUS support the diagnosis, but testing may not be available or results are delayed for weeks.

Treatment for HUS is often initiated with plasma exchange, but benefit has not been established, and improvement in renal function is frequently poor [13]. Hemodialysis is usually required, and progression to end-stage renal disease is high. Eculizumab (a monoclonal antibody inhibitor of complement C5) is indicated for aHUS and has been used effectively in a limited number of reports of pregnancy-associated aHUS [15].

Coagulopathies

Bleeding disorders during pregnancy can be the result of inherited or acquired coagulopathy. Acquired bleeding disorders during pregnancy are usually secondary to disseminated intravascular coagulation (DIC).

Disseminated Intravascular Coagulation

Disseminated intravascular coagulation in pregnancy occurs secondary to precipitating events such as massive postpartum hemorrhage, sepsis, amniotic fluid embolism, placental abruption, and acute fatty liver of pregnancy. Systemic activation of clotting is thought to lead to microvascular thrombi and organ dysfunction, while depletion of platelets and coagulation factors contributes to bleeding. Although DIC is a common indicator of severe maternal morbidity, it is rarely a sole cause of maternal mortality [16].

Obstetrical emergencies due to bleeding from DIC usually do not pose a diagnostic dilemma. Prolongation of the PT, aPTT along with thrombocytopenia are expected findings. Due to physiological increases in fibrinogen and D-dimer in pregnancy, normal values may be consistent with DIC. Trends in results for fibrinogen and D-dimer may be more helpful than single test results [17]. DIC scores have not been specifically applied in pregnancy [16].

Effective treatment of severe DIC requires control of the precipitating condition and support with blood products. Transfusion of red blood cells, fresh frozen plasma, platelets, cryoprecipitate, or fibrinogen concentrates provides hematological support based on coagulation studies and status of the patient (See Chap. 46).

Acquired Hemophilia

Acquired hemophilia in pregnancy is rare and usually due to an antibody inhibitor against factor VIII. Acquired hemophilia typically develops in the postpartum period and may be associated with clinically significant bleeding. Patients may present with unexpected vaginal bleeding weeks after delivery or hematomas and ecchymoses months after delivery. Laboratory results show a prolonged aPTT that does not correct with normal plasma in mixing studies. Treatment for significant bleeding includes the use of activated prothrombin complex concentrates (aPCC) or rFVIIa to bypass the inhibitor. Although corticosteroids, intravenous immunoglobulin, and rituximab have been used in acquired hemophilia, experience is limited.

Summary

Acquired and congenital hematological emergencies can occur as primary disorders or complicate other conditions in pregnancy. Abnormal bleeding and bruising should be investigated with standard tests taking into account the physiological changes associated with pregnancy. Treatment depends on the specific diagnosis, gestational age, status of the mother and fetus, and availability of resources.

References

1. Shin JE, Lee Y, Kim SJ, Shin JC. Association of severe thrombocytopenia and poor prognosis in pregnancies with aplastic anemia. PLoS One. 2014;9(7):e103066.
2. Chen K-J, Chang Y-L, Chang H, Su S-Y, Peng H-H, et al. Long-term outcome of pregnancy complicating with severe aplastic anemia under supportive care. Taiwan J Obstet Gynecol. 2017;56:632–5.
3. Killick SB, Brown N, Cavenagh J, Dokal I, Foukaneli T, et al. Guidelines for the diagnosis and management of adult aplastic anemia. Br J Haematol. 2016;172:187–207.
4. Lee AI, Okam MM. Anemia in pregnancy. Hematol Oncol Clin N Am. 2011;25:241–59.
5. Okusanya BO, Oladapo OT. Prophylactic versus selective blood transfusion for sickle cell disease in pregnancy. Cochrane Database Syst Rev. 2016;(12):CD010378.
6. Malinowski AK, Shehata N, D'Souza R, Kuo KH, Ward R, et al. Prophylactic transfusion for pregnant women with sickle cell disease: a systematic review and meta-analysis. Blood. 2015;126:2424–35.
7. Oakley LL, Awogbade M, Brien S, Briley A, Chorozoglou M, et al. Serial prophylactic exchange blood transfusion in pregnant women with sickle cell disease (TAPS-2): study protocol for a randomized controlled feasibility trial. Trials. 2020;21:347.
8. Chou ST, Alsawas M, Fasano RM, Field JJ, Hendrickson JE, et al. American Society of Hematology 2020 guidelines for sickle cell disease: transfusion support. Blood Adv. 2020;4:327–55.
9. Bergmann F, Rath W. The differential diagnosis of thrombocytopenia in pregnancy. Dtsch Arztebl Int. 2015;112:795–802.
10. Piatek CI, El-Hemaidi I, Feinstein DI, Liebman HA, Akhtari M. Management of immune-mediated cytopenias in pregnancy. Autoimmun Rev. 2015;14:806–11.
11. Scully M, Thomas M, Underwood M, Watson H, Langley K, et al. Thrombotic thrombocytopenic purpura and pregnancy: presentation, management and subsequent pregnancy outcomes. Blood. 2014;124:211–9.
12. Scully M, Cataland SR, Peyvandi F, Coppo P, Knobl P, et al. Caplacizumab treatment for acquired thrombotic thrombocytopenic purpura. N Engl J Med. 2019;380:335–46.
13. Neave L, Scully M. Microangiopathic hemolytic anemia in pregnancy. Transfus Med Rev. 2018;32:230–6.
14. Fakhouri F, Roumenina L, Provot F, et al. Pregnancy-associated hemolytic uremic syndrome revisited in the era of complement gene mutations. J Am Soc Nephrol. 2010;21:859–67.
15. Gately R, San A, Kurtkoti J, Parnham A. Life-threatening pregnancy-associated atypical haemolytic uraemic syndrome and its response to eculizamab. Nephrology. 2017;22(Suppl 1):32–5.
16. Cunningham FG, Nelson DB. Disseminated intravascular coagulation syndromes in obstetrics. Obstet Gynecol. 2015;126:999–1011.
17. Thachil J, Toh C-H. Disseminated intravascular coagulation in obstetric disorders and its acute haematolgical management. Blood Rev. 2009;23:167–76.

Chapter 45
Immune Thrombocytopenia and Microangiopathies in Pregnancy

Alcibiades E. Villarreal and Lineth López

Immune Thrombocytopenic Purpura

Introduction

Immune thrombocytopenic purpura (ITP) is an acquired disease that raises diagnostic and therapeutic doubts in the clinician for being a diagnosis of exclusion, fear of bleeding, and not being able to correct the event with simple transfusion measures. Although it was previously defined as a purpura, waiting for a hemorrhagic clinical presentation, today its name has changed to "immune thrombocytopenia," not only because of its immune pathological origin but because paradoxically it is not usual for it to bleed at the time of its debut, unless other clinical factors are added. However, in the medical nomenclature, the term ITP continues to be used.

In the pregnant patient, other clinical challenges are added for the control or prevention of bleeding, such as the time of delivery, the administration of epidural anesthesia, and fetal and newborn safety according to the trimester of onset.

A. E. Villarreal
Centro de Neurociencias y Unidad de Investigacion Clínica, Instituto de Investigaciones Científicas y Servicios de Alta Tecnología (INDICASAT AIP), Panama City, Republic of Panama
e-mail: avillarreal@indicasat.org.pa; http://www.indicasat.org.pa/; http://www.indicasat-times.org.pa/

L. López (✉)
Department of Hematology, Complejo Hospitalario Dr. Arnulfo Arias Madrid de la Caja de Seguro Social, Panama City, Republic of Panama
e-mail: linlopez@css.gob.pa

C. Montufar et al. (eds.), *Obstetric Catastrophes*,
https://doi.org/10.1007/978-3-030-70034-8_45

Epidemiology

Usually 7–10% of pregnant women will have thrombocytopenia [1]. ITP is the second most frequent cause of thrombocytopenia in pregnant women after gestational thrombocytopenia, representing 1–4% of the causes of thrombocytopenia [2]. ITP in pregnant women has one case incidence per 10,000 to 100,000 women [3], but in the general adult population, the incidence of ITP is 2.64 in 100,000 people [4], and the average age of presentation is 56 years. It usually occurs more frequently in the first trimester of pregnancy, most often in women with a history of ITP, and has a very low maternal morbidity and mortality; sometimes when the ITP is mild, it can be indistinct from one another. Controversial cases are in third trimester due to the choice of the delivery route, use of epidural anesthesia, and the safety of the newborn among others. The percentage of neonatal condition with the passage of antibodies is estimated at around 22%, with 6% of intracranial hemorrhages in newborn, but fortunately less than 1% mortality [3].

Physiopathology

ITP is a non-specific disease of pregnancy; its pathophysiological basis is due to an autoimmune disease. The disease is increasingly understood, which is why its name has changed over time from idiopathic to immune thrombocytopenia [5].

The protagonists in this case "platelets" are enucleated fragments, with 7 fl. diameter, which come from megakaryocytes in the bone marrow and are produced by polyploidization; once they reach peripheral blood, they have a half-life of 7–10 days [6]. There are many transmembrane receptors that are potential target for antibodies such as CD41, CD61 (integrin αIIbβ3), CD42 (glycoprotein Ib) and glycoprotein V, which allow them to adhere by Gap (glycoproteins) to von Willebrand multimers, aggregation between them and actively participate in the establishment of coagulation as seen in the new cell model, hence its susceptibility to autoimmune phenomena despite being one of the smallest of the hematological parameters [7].

Its immune base manifests itself in the same way as in non-pregnant patients with IgG antibodies against glycoproteins, mainly GpIIb-IIIa and GpIb-IX, and increased clearance by tissue macrophages; these antibodies bind both platelets and megakaryocytes [8]. It is also known that c-mpl receptor antibodies are produced with intracellular and extracellular domains, which are found in both megakaryocytes and circulating platelets [9]. Normally thrombopoietin (TPO) acts as an agonist cytokine in the c-mpl favoring megakaryopoiesis; this concept has been key in the use of new therapies for the ITP treatment, with TPO agonists; however, they have not proved safety in pregnant women yet. Also, these labeled platelets are cleared by the reticuloendothelial system mainly of the spleen, hence splenectomy as a therapeutic option [10]. See Fig. 45.1.

Primary ITP is diagnosed if other underlying diseases or conditions have been excluded and is equivalent to 70–80% of cases [11]. Depending on its evolution

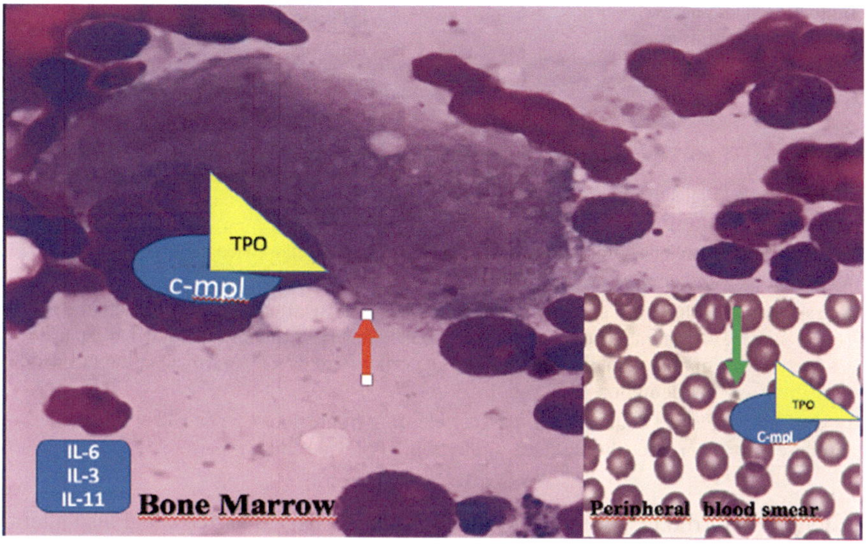

Fig. 45.1 This figure represents the presence of c-mpl receptors both in the bone marrow megakaryocyte and in the platelets observed in peripheral blood, and their interaction with TPO. In red arrow a megakaryocyte is observed and in green arrow a platelet in peripheral blood. Blood taken from patient from the Centro Hemato Oncológico of Panama. (Figure taken by Dr. Lineth López)

Table 45.1 Causes of ITP, according to the International Working Group [12]

Primary	Isolated thrombocytopenia Platelets <100 × 10^9/L No secondary cause of ITP
Secondary	All autoimmune, infectious, or drug forms

time it can be acute or chronic; in adults, a large percentage of acute ITP will evolve to chronic patients despite treatment, and of these a large part despite not obtaining a complete remission will remain under observation. Here we summarize the ITP causes (see Table 45.1), ITP phases (see Table 45.2), and ITP response criteria (see Table 45.3), according to the International Working Group.

Clinical Presentation

The presentation is mostly asymptomatic; usually low platelet count is detected in routine blood laboratory during obstetric follow-up, which is why it is no longer so frequent to talk about purpura [13]. Thrombocytopenia increases the risk of bleeding, but it is not until values reach <30 × 10^9/L, a spontaneous hemorrhagic event can occur. The bleeding risk is increased with antiplatelet agents (non-steroidal anti-inflammatory drugs, acetylsalicylic acid, or others), coagulopathies with underlying

Table 45.2 ITP phases according to the International Working Group [12]

Acute	Presentation in less than 3 months
Persistent	Duration between 3 and 12 months
Chronic	Duration greater than 12 months

Table 45.3 ITP response criteria according to the International Working Group [12]

Complete remission	Platelets count >100 × 10^9/L and absence of bleeding
Partial remission	Platelets count ≥30 × 10^9/L, increase by more than twice the baseline and absence of bleeding
Refractary	Failure to achieve response or loss of response after splenectomy, with the need of continuous treatment to reduce bleeding risk. Having responded to the use of immunoglobulin or high doses of corticosteroids temporarily also can fall within this definition
Loss of response	Platelet count <100 × 10^9/L or bleeding (if previous CR) or <30 × 10^9/L or less than twice the baseline, or bleeding (if previous PR)

lesion, as in cirrhotic patients who suffer from esophageal varices, and also alteration of secondary hemostasis [13].

Platelets are part of primary hemostasis, and the hemorrhagic manifestations are mucocutaneous, as gingivorrhagia, petechiaes, epistaxis, and there could be transvaginal or gastrointestinal bleeding [14].

The diagnosis is made with exclusion of other thrombocytopenia causes. The first assessment is always clinical where there are no other symptoms or signs that force to rule out another etiology, can't be weight loss, fever, joint manifestations, adenopathies, and/or visceromegalies, and has to exclude the use of medications that cause thrombocytopenia; if there is any alteration, it should only be hemorrhagic [13].

In laboratory test, the most important is the evaluation of the blood count and the analysis of the peripheral blood spread; exclusively it has a decrease in the platelet series, with normal or high average platelet volume; if there are other alterations, another clinical entity should be suspected.

Based on the clinic, perform kidney and liver tests; viral or infectious as human immunodeficiency virus (HIV), hepatitis B virus (HBV), hepatitis C virus (HCV), dengue, and *Helicobacter pylori*, either with stool antigen or urea breath test (if there is a possibility of treatment); screening of autoimmune diseases according to other clinical manifestations (ANA, C3, C4, direct Coombs) and for antiphospholipid syndrome (AFS) lupus anticoagulant, anticardiolipins, and B2 glycoproteins; thyroid function for some cases associated with hypothyroidism, DIC coagulation tests (disseminated intravascular coagulopathy), prothrombin time (PT), activated partial thromboplastin time (PTT), and fibrinogen [1, 15].

There is no indication for bone marrow studies in patients under 60 years old, and it is not recommended to perform routine antiplatelet antibodies for diagnosis or to predict the risk of neonatal thrombocytopenia [1].

Differential Diagnosis

Within the causes of thrombocytopenia, there are differences between specific and non-specific conditions in pregnancy; this is important in the diagnosis and treatment of each entity. ITP is not specific; in fact the most frequent cause is gestational thrombocytopenia in 70–80% of cases, unlike ITP in 1–4% [1, 16]. The timing of the presentation can also be correlated, for example, gestational thrombocytopenia usually occurs in the second and third trimesters and ITP in the first, although it may appear at any stage of pregnancy [17]. See Table 45.4.

Treatment

The mainstay of treatment is based on avoiding bleeding, and this is achieved with a multidisciplinary management: the obstetrician, anesthesiologist, hematologist, and neonatologist. And although only one third of the patients will require treatment, we must consider the platelet value, if there are previous stigmas of bleeding, if there is any associated coagulopathy, and mode of delivery as well as use of epidural and neonate safety.

The first line will always be corticosteroids, especially prednisone at 0.5–2 mg/kg/day in the general population, but in pregnant women a dose of 10–20 mg/day is

Table 45.4 Differential diagnosis of thrombocytopenia [1, 18]

Specific causes of pregnancy	Non-specific causes
Gestational thrombocytopenia (70–80%)	Isolated thrombocytopenia
Hypertensive disorders	Pseudotrombocytopenia by antibodies to EDTA[a]
Preeclampsia (15–20%)	ITP (1–4%)
HELLP (<1%)[d]	Drugs[b] (<1%)
Fatty liver (<1%)	von Willebrand IIB (<1%)
	Congenital (<1%)
	Secondary-viral-infectious ITP (<1%)[c] [19]
	Thrombocytopenia associated with systemic diseases
	DIC
	Thrombotic thrombocytopenic purpura (TTP), hemolytic uremic syndrome (HUS) (<1%)
	Autoimmune (e.g., lupus, AFS) (2–5%) [20]
	Myeloptisis
	Liver disease
	HIT (heparin-induced thrombocytopenia)
	Vitamin B12 deficiency, folic acid (<1%)

[a]Ethylenediaminetetraacetic acid (EDTA)
[b]Quinine, antibiotics, glycoprotein IIb/IIIa inhibitors, antiplatelet, antireumatic, antiepileptic, cardiac, biological agents
[c]HIV, CMV, HBV, HCV, tuberculosis, *H. pylori*, chicken pox, Epstein-Barr virus, parvovirus B19, bunyavirus
[d]HELLP (hemolysis, elevated liver enzyme levels, and low platelet levels)

Table 45.5 ITP treatment [21]

First line	Second line
Corticosteroid	Splenectomy
Prednisone 0.5–2 mg/kg/day per 3 weeks[a]	Azatioprina1–2 mg/kg/day
Metilprednisolona 1 g/dia per 3 days	Ciclosporina
Immunoglobulin anti IgG 1 g/kg/day, until 2 days	
Inmunoglobulin anti-D 50–75 ug/kg unic dose	

[a]Prednisone after administered for 3 weeks, the dose should be progressively decayed to avoid adrenal insufficiency

recommended, due to its adverse effects and potential complications. Among the adverse effects of steroids in the first trimester, there is an increased risk of cleft palate, and in the rest of pregnancy weight gain, hyperglycemia, osteoporosis, psychosis, and hypertension exacerbation among others. Also, in the first line in cases of acute bleeding or imminent procedure (cesarean section or epidural), the use of immunoglobulins is proposed [21]. See Table 45.5.

The second therapeutic line that is proposed is splenectomy; this is preferably performed in the second trimester, before week 20. Although there are advances with thrombopoietin agonists such as eltrombopag and romiplostin, studies show class C safety for now, like rituximab. For now, the use of immunodulators such as azathioprine has been proven safe. See Table 45.5.

A platelet value >50 × 10^9/L is recommended for a cesarean section and >75–80 × 10^9/L for a regional epidural block [22, 23]; this is controversial because of the balance between the prothrombotic effect of pregnancy vs the hemorrhagic ITP; a thromboelastogram could be used to guide this decision. Women with platelet count >20–30 × 10^9/L and without bleeding do not require treatment until approximately 36 weeks; once near the date of delivery, it is recommended to use prednisone or prednisolone 10 mg/day [1].

If there is bleeding and/or surgical or epidural intervention is required, immunoglobulin is recommended at a dose of 1 g/kg every day for a maximum of 2 days, and its response is seen in 1–2 days, or anti-D 50–75 ug/kg in RH-positive patients; for this the response is seen at 4–5 days [22, 23]. The use of platelet transfusion is reserved for acute situations with life-threatening bleeding, in case there is no response to steroids and the effect of immunoglobulin use or concomitant use is not yet seen [23]. If the patient has a basic disease that increases the risk of thrombosis such as FAS with platelet values >50 × 10^9/L, aspirin or prophylaxis low molecular weight heparin may be used [22].

The delivery mode is based on the obstetric indication; studies indicate that there is no impact on morbidity and mortality in deciding vaginal or cesarean delivery. Hemorrhagic events in neonates, if any, occur within 24–48 hours delivery, and occur in less than 1% [22, 23].

There is no clear predictor to know if the neonate will have ITP, and there is no impact on the use of peripartum steroids, so this is not an indication to start them in the mother [23]. It is not recommended to perform platelet counts to neonates during childbirth, nor tests of the umbilical cord by drainage (they are only admitted by direct venipuncture to the cord) and of course the use of forceps or maneuvers, or administration of intramuscular vitamin K (at less until platelet value is obtained) in infants or mothers diagnosed with ITP [23].

Monitoring

Blood test samples are required every 2 weeks at least, and if platelet values >50 × 10^9/L. If platelets descend to <30 × 10^9/L, monitoring should be weekly until the time of delivery or until a hemorrhagic phenomenon occurs. The neonate should be monitored daily until day 5 postpartum; a rise in values around day 7 is observed in those with thrombocytopenia [22, 23]. The use of transcranial ultrasound in infants with ITP is also recommended [23].

Thrombotic Microagiopathies: Thrombotic Thrombocytopenic Purpura (TTP) and Hemolytic Uremic Syndrome (HUS)

Introduction

Thrombotic thrombocytopenic purpura (TTP) and hemolytic uremic syndrome (HUS) are thrombotic microangiopathies, both acute, rare life-threatening conditions, and the biggest challenge is timely and rapid diagnosis. There are microangiopathies related to pregnancy, like preeclampsia and HELLP, often difficult to differentiate from each other. They cause microvascular and macrovascular occlusion causing thrombosis and hence its clinical manifestations. TTP is characterized by hemolytic anemia, thrombocytopenia, acute renal failure, neurological disorders, and fever [24] and shares with the HUS the first three characteristics; however, the treatment differs in each one. In pregnant women both incur the danger of death to both the mother and the product, so the success of treatment is its early diagnosis [25].

Thrombotic Thrombocytopenic Purpura (TTP)

Epidemiology

TTP can be congenital or acquired; 75% of cases in total occur in women and is more frequent in black youth [26]. The annual incidence for acquired is 3.1 per million persons, and the congenital is less than 1 per million persons in the United

States [27]. A prevalence was observed to be 13 per million persons in the national registry of France between 1999 and 2013 [28]. TTP can be precipitated by pregnancy in 10–30% of cases, and of these cases 24–60% could be congenital [23].

Physiopathology

One step of normal hemostasis, after an endothelial lesion, is the exposure of the high molecular weight von Willebrand glycoprotein, which is secreted in the endothelial cells, creating an elongated base for platelet adhesion and aggregation with subsequent thrombus generation [29]. In this glycoprotein, there are ADAMTS13 binding domains (a disintegrin and metalloproteinase with athrombospondin type 1 motif, member 13), which cleave the von Willebrand protein to regulate its activity and regulate sustained thrombus generation. In TTP, also called Moschcowitz syndrome, there is quantitative or qualitative deficiency of ADAMTS13 creating giant von Willebrand multimers that initiate the thrombus production cascade [30]. This can occur congenitally (Upshaw-Schulman syndrome) due to the absence or mutation of ADAMTS13 that produces protein activity less than 5% or acquired by the production of antibody, usually IgG against ADAMTS13, triggered by infections, autoimmune diseases, transplantation, pregnancy, or cancer among others and other times idiopathic [31].

The generation of these thrombi in the microvasculature generates ischemic events in the kidney, brain, and heart, excessive consumption of platelets, and hemolytic anemia due to fragmentation of red blood cells; generally, these events occur when the values of ADAMTS13 fall below 10% [32].

In pregnancy it can develop in the second or third trimester although there is more possibility of complication between week 20 and 29 due to severe intrauterine growth restriction, so they have a better prognosis if it occurs before week 20 or after 30.

Diagnosis

The real challenge is to differentiate this entity from other pregnancy conditions that have some similarities, for example, in hypertensive disorders of pregnancy, HELLP (hemolysis, elevated liver enzymes, low platelets) share inclusive pathophysiological bases such as increase in von Willebrand multimers and complement activation, but with normal or slightly decreased ADAMST13 activity [33, 34].

The clinical manifestations are variable; all alterations may be present (in 5% of patients, the following: fever, neurological manifestations, renal alteration, thrombocytopenia, and hemolytic anemia) as one or two, always accompanied in laboratories of a hemolytic anemia microangiopathic and thrombocytopenia 100% of the time [35]. See Figure 45.2 of a characteristic TTP peripheral blood smear patient.

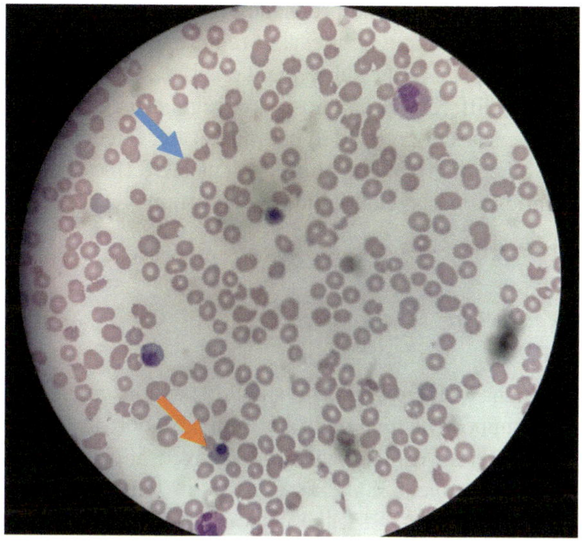

Fig. 45.2 Peripheral blood smear where schistocytes (blue arrow) and nucleated red blood cells or normoblasts (red arrow) are identified. Blood taken from patient from the Centro Hemato Oncológico of Panama. (Figure taken by Dr. Lineth López)

Anemic syndrome of rapid onset (weakness, fatigue, fatigue, paleness) and hemorrhagic manifestations (petechiae, purpura, bruises, intestinal bleeding, hematuria among others) are usual when platelets $<10 \times 10^9$/L; neurological abnormalities (dizziness, delirium, seizures, headache, changes in vision) and manifestations of cerebrovascular events; cardiac disorders such as heart failure, arrhythmias, dyspnea, and also renal manifestations such as uremic syndrome (it is not usual to require dialysis unlike atypical HUS that usually is an alternative diagnosis); and finally and less frequent fever (22%) [35].

To establish the diagnosis, the initial assessment should always include a peripheral blood smear, to observe the schistocytes and nucleated red blood cells, and a direct negative Coombs. Other laboratories to corroborate hemolysis are lactate dehydrogenase (LDH), elevated reticulocytes, elevated indirect bilirubin, decreased haptoglobin, negative CID profile, and elevated creatinine. In the case of pregnant women, this condition per se is the most obvious trigger, but to complement the diagnosis, tests will be requested to rule out viral infections such as HIV, HBV, and HCV among others, ANA, and complement values to rule out autoimmune alterations, if the clinic is suggestive [36].

As a confirmatory test, ADAMTS13 must be requested before treatment initiation and can be used for monitoring and response: (1) the percentage of activity that will be less than 10%; (2) assess antibody titers; (3) antigenic titers; and (4) mutational genetic screening of this protein.

This panel of tests will also guide us to rule out whether it is of acquired or congenital etiology [36].

Pregnancy is the main trigger in women with congenital etiology who have double heterozygous or homozygous mutations, and generally the diagnosis is made during the first pregnancy; it is important to clarify this aspect since 100% will relapse during second pregnancy [25]. In the acquired causes, pregnancy is a mild trigger, and although the risk of relapse is not so high, if there is an increased risk of preeclampsia, in the subsequent ones.

The differential diagnosis in pregnant is CID, HELLP, and preeclampsia; and other causes not related to pregnancy are: infections, tumors, autoimmune diseases, and other microangiopathies such as HUS (the last one, very important if the main manifestation is renal failure with normal ADAMTS13 levels) [37].

Treatment

Pregnant women with TTP should start plasma exchange therapy (PEX) urgently, give supportive treatment and induce labor; at the same time steroids should be administered; if this measure is delayed, it could result in the death of the mother and the product [38]. PEX consists in removing the antibodies and replacing the depleted ADAMTS13; the response to PEX is the same as the general population and reduces mortality by 80% and should not be delayed until confirmatory tests such as ADAMTS13 are obtained [38]. Replace 1.5 times the volume daily at least 2 days until platelets reach values greater than >150 × 10^9/L. If replacement is not available right away, infuse fresh frozen plasma 25–30 cc/kg in the meantime; studies show that survival rates in replacement use vs. plasma infusion are 96% vs. 84%, with platelets increased at 9 days from 78% vs. 49%, respectively, so a measure does not replace the other [39].

Red blood cells can be transfused, if there is severe anemia; however, platelet transfusions should be avoided because it is more substratum to the disease unless there is bleeding that compromises life. Thromboprophylaxis with low heparin can be used if platelets are greater than 50 × 10^9/L [39].

Concomitantly start steroids either prednisone 1 mg/Kg/day or methylprednisolone 1 g/day for 3 days. Another measure used is the application of rituximab, an anti-CD20 monoclonal (CD cluster differentiation) at a dose of 375 mg/m^2 iv every week for 4 weeks, taking into account that 60% is eliminated after plasmapheresis [40]. It should be infused after replacement and not before, used in cases where there is refractoriness or severe neurological or cardiac alterations, always rule out the following diseases before use rituximab: HIV and hepatitis B virus; its average response time is 10 days, but it can take up to 3 weeks or more. Its use has been shown to decrease relapse rates 10% vs. 57% in combination with steroids and replacement in both cases [41]. There is no indication of the use of aspirin.

Follow-up in subsequent pregnancies is appropriate due to its high recurrence 15–20% [23] in those acquired and up to 100% in congenital ones [25]. In congenital TTP, it is recommended to use rituximab if ADAMTS 13 levels are below 20% before delivery and start plasmapheresis if they fall below 10%; also, infuse 10 ml/Kg plasma from week 8 to 10 every 2 weeks, and the frequency can be increased if platelets descend to less than 150 × 10^9.

Other immunosuppressant may be added to treatment such as cyclosporine, vincristine, and cyclophosphamide. Other options for emerging therapeutics are the use

Table 45.6 Criteria for response to TTP [42]

Clinical response	Platelets >150 × 10^9/L and LDH less than 1.5 times after plasmapheresis
Clinia remission	Clinical response greater than 30 days
Exacerbation	Decrease in platelet value, within 30 days of the last plasmapheresis, if there was a clinical response
Relapse	Decrease of platelet values after 30 days of the last plasmapheresis, if there was a clinical response
Refractoriness	Persistent thrombocytopenia (<10 × 10^9/L after 5 plasmapheresis and steroids

of recombinant ADAMST13 [42], yet in clinical studies phase another and recently approved by FDA (February 2019) is an anti-von Willebrand monoclonal, caplacizumab, that prevents platelet interaction by Ib-IX-V glycoprotein, demonstrating decrease of platelet recovery time and relapse rates, but it is too early to assess safety in pregnancy.

About fetal well-being, fetal monitoring and arterial Doppler of the placental flow and intrauterine growth rates should be performed, with greater relevance in patients who debut with the condition in the first trimester and remain stable with plasma exchanges [43]. If TTP is acquired, it is recommended to perform levels of ADAMTS13 to predict adjuvant therapy, and if it is congenital ADAMTS13 should be supplemented throughout pregnancy and postpartum; theoretically infusions of fresh frozen plasma are sufficient, but plasma exchanges may be required to maintain adequate levels [43]. Finally, counseling should be given for subsequent pregnancies due to high risk of relapse and in those that require contraceptives to assess thromboembolic risk [43]. See Table 45.6 to detail the criteria for response to TTP.

Hemolytic Uremic Syndrome (HUS)

Hemolytic uremic syndrome is a type of microangiopathy that manifests with a clinical triad of hemolytic anemia, thrombocytopenia, and acute renal failure and differs considerably from TTP in its pathogenesis [44]. It is usually preceded by a gastrointestinal infection caused by Shiga toxin-producing *Escherichia coli* (STEC), O157: H7 or Shigella, although it can be caused by other bacteria such as *Streptococcus pneumoniae* [45]. In 5–10% an infection is not found as a trigger, and they are called atypical HUS, just by dysregulation of the complement system [45].

Epidemiology

In the HUS, the most affected population is children, and its annual incidence in the general population is 1–2 cases per 100,000 people [27]. A greater relationship has been observed between atypical HUS and pregnancies, almost 1 in 25,000; its postpartum presentation (80%) is more frequent at the third or fourth week; the rest usually occurs in the first trimester. It has a 30% risk of recurrence in future pregnancies [46].

Physiopathology

It is an entity not directly related to pregnancy, unlike preeclampsia and HELLP, which have differential diagnoses related to pregnancy. The pathophysiology can be divided into two causes: infectious and through complement activation. Patients with atypical HUS are confused with a picture of TTP but with the particularity that the renal failure stands out and does not meet the total requirements for a TTP [25]. It is caused by mutations in complement regulatory proteins, some hypofunctional such as CFH, CFI, MCP (CD46), and THBD (thrombomodulin gene) the latter in 5% and others hyperfunctional such as CFB or C3 [25].

The importance of differentiating these microangiopathies is to choose the correct treatment; usually the HUS is treated with support measures, while TTP and atypical HUS are treated with plasma exchange; although the definitive treatment of the atypical HUS are complement inhibitors such as eculizumab, this is a direct monoclonal antibody of C5 which, upon binding, inhibits it [27].

Diagnosis

Clinically, the patient comments on a previous gastrointestinal picture one or two prior weeks, with varied manifestations such as mild abdominal pain, diarrhea which is often bloody, cramping, and nausea: subsequently anemic syndrome of rapid establishment and neurological alterations from irritability until seizures [47].

The alterations in the laboratories are generally presented in a particular order with thrombocytopenia and subsequent renal failure, and microangiopathic hemolytic anemia [47].

In the atypical form, it can be normal or low levels of complement C3, normal levels of C4, and increase of C3b, C3c, and C3d, but for its definitive diagnosis, it will be necessary to demonstrate the mutational alterations [48]. The key to obtain a correct diagnosis is to exclude other causes of microangiopathies, so that timely treatment can be directed. See Table 45.7 for differential diagnosis of microangiopathies in pregnancy.

Treatment

In the typical HUS support measures may include delivery of the fetus (some cases), fluid management, and temporary renal replacement therapy (dialysis), but 25% of cases show permanent renal failure condition [49].

Table 45.7 Differential diagnosis of microangiopathies in pregnancy [2]

	Microangiopathies	Related	To pregnancy	Microangiopathies	NOT related	To pregnancy
	Preclampsia	HELLP	AFLP	TTP	HUS atypical	HUS
Initial presentation	Incidence 5–8% Second and third trimester	Incidence 1% Second and third trimester (70%) Post delivery (30%)	Incidence <0.1% Third trimester	Incidence <0.1% Second and third trimester	Incidence <0.1% First trimester and post delivery	Incidence <0.1% Anytime
Clinic	Headache and visual disturbances Hypertension Proteinuria	Preeclampsia, symptoms	Nausea, vomiting, abdominal pain, jaundice	Neurological symptoms, fever, acute anemic syndrome	Fever, acute anemic syndrome, and renal failure	Enterohemorrhagic infection with previous diarrhea and subsequent anemic syndrome and renal failure
Labs	Low PLT Proteinuria Elevated LFTs 2x	Low PLT Proteinuria Elevated LFTs MAHA Elevated LDH	Low PLT Marked elevated LFTs Elevated LDH CID Low Glc	Low PLT MAHA Elevated LDH ARF Low ADAMST 13	Low PLT MAHA, Elevated LDH Intense ARF Proteinuria	Low PLT MAHA Elevated LDH +Shigatoxin
Treatment	Pregnancy interruption	Pregnancy interruption	Pregnancy interruption	Plasma turnover	Plasma turnover Eculizumab	Support

MAHA microangiopathic hemolytic anemia, *PLT* platelet, *ARF* acute renal failure, *LFTs* liver function tests, *LDH* lactate dehydrogenase, *DIC* disseminated intravascular coagulation, *Glc* glucose

In the atypical HUS plasma turnover is a measure used but the response rates are low; its indication is important because of the difficult differentiation between TTP and atypical HUS. The main treatment is eculizumab which is safe during pregnancy and breastfeeding. The fetus delivery and support measures are recommended; also consider eculizumab treatment.

In cases of severe neurological abnormalities, immunoglobulin could be used, but risk-benefit assessment should be made due to risk of fatal renal failure [50].

References

1. Gernsheimer T, James AH, Stasi R. How I treat thrombocytopenia in pregnancy. Blood. 2013;121(1):38–47. https://doi.org/10.1182/blood-2012-08-448944. Epub 2012/11/13. PubMed PMID: 23149846
2. Rajasekhar A, Gernsheimer T, Roberto S, James AH. 2013 Clinical practice guide on thrombocytopenia in pregnancy. In: Hematology So, editor. American Society of Hematology; 2013.
3. Alonso MAnS, García VV. Directrices de diagnóstico, tratamiento y seguimiento de la PTI: Documento de Consenso. In: López A, editor. 2011.
4. Frederiksen H, Schmidt K. The incidence of idiopathic thrombocytopenic purpura in adults increases with age. Blood. 1999;94(3):909–13. Epub 1999/07/27. PubMed PMID: 10419881
5. Neunert C, Lim W, Crowther M, Cohen A, Solberg L Jr, Crowther MA, et al. The American Society of Hematology 2011 evidence-based practice guideline for immune thrombocytopenia. Blood. 2011;117(16):4190–207. https://doi.org/10.1182/blood-2010-08-302984. Epub 2011/02/18. PubMed PMID: 21325604
6. Vainchenker W, Raslova H. Megakaryocyte polyploidization: role in platelet production. Platelets. 2019:1–10. https://doi.org/10.1080/09537104.2019.1667497. Epub 2019/09/24. PubMed PMID: 31544577
7. Kaushansky K. Historical review: megakaryopoiesis and thrombopoiesis. Blood. 2008;111(3):981–6. https://doi.org/10.1182/blood-2007-05-088500. Epub 2008/01/29. PubMed PMID: 18223171; PubMed Central PMCID: PMCPMC2214745
8. Hirokawa M, Fujishima N, Togashi M, Saga A, Omokawa A, Saga T, et al. High-throughput sequencing of IgG B-cell receptors reveals frequent usage of the rearranged IGHV4-28/IGHJ4 gene in primary immune thrombocytopenia. Sci Rep. 2019;9(1):8645. https://doi.org/10.1038/s41598-019-45264-2. Epub 2019/06/16. PubMed PMID: 31201346; PubMed Central PMCID: PMCPMC6570656
9. Zufferey A, Kapur R, Semple JW. Pathogenesis and therapeutic mechanisms in Immune Thrombocytopenia (ITP). J Clin Med. 2017;6(2) https://doi.org/10.3390/jcm6020016. Epub 2017/02/18. PubMed PMID: 28208757; PubMed Central PMCID: PMCPMC5332920
10. Rosa Maria RN, Laura RL, Angeles PB, Laura LB. Use of Romiplostim during pregnancy as a rescue therapy in primary immune thrombocytopenia: literature review and case description. Platelets. 2019:1–4. https://doi.org/10.1080/09537104.2019.1615613. Epub 2019/05/23. PubMed PMID: 31116059
11. Gil WR. Diagnosis and treatment of immune thrombocytopenic purpura. Rev Med Hered. 2015;26:246–55.
12. Rodeghiero F, Stasi R, Gernsheimer T, Michel M, Provan D, Arnold DM, et al. Standardization of terminology, definitions and outcome criteria in immune thrombocytopenic purpura of adults and children: report from an international working group. Blood. 2009;113(11):2386–93. https://doi.org/10.1182/blood-2008-07-162503. Epub 2008/11/14. PubMed PMID: 19005182
13. Kistangari G, McCrae KR. Immune thrombocytopenia. Hematol Oncol Clin North Am. 2013;27(3):495–520. https://doi.org/10.1016/j.hoc.2013.03.001. Epub 2013/05/30. PubMed PMID: 23714309; PubMed Central PMCID: PMCPMC3672858

14. Páramo Fernández JA, Alfonso Piérola A, Varea Díaz S. Alteraciones de la hemostasia primaria. Púrpuras y alteraciones de las plaquetas. Medicine – Programa de Formación Médica Continuada Acreditado. 2012;11(22):337–1344. https://doi.org/10.1016/s0304-5412(12)70460-2.
15. Jang JH, Kim JY, Mun YC, Bang SM, Lim YJ, Shin DY, et al. Management of immune thrombocytopenia: Korean experts recommendation in 2017. Blood Res. 2017;52(4):254–63. https://doi.org/10.5045/br.2017.52.4.254. Epub 2018/01/16. PubMed PMID: 29333401; PubMed Central PMCID: PMCPMC5762735
16. Gill KK, Kelton JG. Management of idiopathic thrombocytopenic purpura in pregnancy. Semin Hematol. 2000;37(3):275–89. Epub 2000/08/15. PubMed PMID: 10942222
17. Khellaf M, Loustau V, Bierling P, Michel M, Godeau B. Thrombocytopenia and pregnancy. Rev Med Interne. 2012;33(8):446–52. https://doi.org/10.1016/j.revmed.2012.05.011. Epub 2012/06/30. PubMed PMID: 22742709
18. Payne YC, González DC. Thrombocytopenia in pregnancy: gestational, immune and congenital Revista Cubana de Hematol. Inmunol y Hemoter. 2014;30(3):196–207.
19. Yu XJ, Liang MF, Zhang SY, Liu Y, Li JD, Sun YL, et al. Fever with thrombocytopenia associated with a novel bunyavirus in China. N Engl J Med. 2011;364(16):1523–32. https://doi.org/10.1056/NEJMoa1010095. Epub 2011/03/18. PubMed PMID: 21410387; PubMed Central PMCID: PMCPMC3113718
20. Cines DB, Bussel JB, Liebman HA, Luning Prak ET. The ITP syndrome: pathogenic and clinical diversity. Blood. 2009;113(26):6511–21. https://doi.org/10.1182/blood-2009-01-129155. Epub 2009/04/28. PubMed PMID: 19395674; PubMed Central PMCID: PMCPMC2710913
21. Goldman BG, Hehir MP, Yambasu S, O'Donnell EM. The presentation and management of platelet disorders in pregnancy. Eur J Haematol. 2018;100(6):560–6. https://doi.org/10.1111/ejh.13049. Epub 2018/02/22. PubMed PMID: 29464836
22. Provan D, Stasi R, Newland AC, Blanchette VS, Bolton-Maggs P, Bussel JB, et al. International consensus report on the investigation and management of primary immune thrombocytopenia. Blood. 2010;115(2):168–86. https://doi.org/10.1182/blood-2009-06-225565. Epub 2009/10/23. PubMed PMID: 19846889
23. Hematology ASo, editor. Self-assessment program seventh edition. American Society of Hematology; 2019.
24. Amorosi EL, Ultmann JE. Thrombotic thrombocytopenic purpura: report of 16 cases and review of the literature. Medicine. 1966;45(2):139–60.
25. von Auer C, von Krogh AS, Kremer Hovinga JA, Lammle B. Current insights into thrombotic microangiopathies: Thrombotic thrombocytopenic purpura and pregnancy. Thromb Res. 2015;135(Suppl 1):S30–3. https://doi.org/10.1016/S0049-3848(15)50437-4. Epub 2015/04/24. PubMed PMID: 25903530
26. Scully M, Yarranton H, Liesner R, Cavenagh J, Hunt B, Benjamin S, et al. Regional UK TTP registry: correlation with laboratory ADAMTS 13 analysis and clinical features. Br J Haematol. 2008;142(5):819–26. https://doi.org/10.1111/j.1365-2141.2008.07276.x. Epub 2008/07/22. PubMed PMID: 18637802
27. Scully M, Hunt BJ, Benjamin S, Liesner R, Rose P, Peyvandi F, et al. Guidelines on the diagnosis and management of thrombotic thrombocytopenic purpura and other thrombotic microangiopathies. Br J Haematol. 2012;158(3):323–35. https://doi.org/10.1111/j.1365-2141.2012.09167.x. Epub 2012/05/26. PubMed PMID: 22624596
28. Mariotte E, Azoulay E, Galicier L, Rondeau E, Zouiti F, Boisseau P, et al. Epidemiology and pathophysiology of adulthood-onset thrombotic microangiopathy with severe ADAMTS13 deficiency (thrombotic thrombocytopenic purpura): a cross-sectional analysis of the French national registry for thrombotic microangiopathy. Lancet Haematol. 2016;3(5):e237–45. https://doi.org/10.1016/S2352-3026(16)30018-7. Epub 2016/05/03. PubMed PMID: 27132698
29. Marchi R, Rojas H. Effect of von Willebrand factor on clot structure and lysis. Blood Coagul Fibrinolysis. 2015;26(5):533–6. https://doi.org/10.1097/MBC.0000000000000284. Epub 2015/03/27. PubMed PMID: 25811448

30. Beranger N, Benghezal S, Savigny S, Capdenat S, Joly BS, Coppo P, et al. Loss of von Willebrand factor high-molecular-weight multimers at acute phase is associated with detectable anti-ADAMTS13 IgG and neurological symptoms in acquired thrombotic thrombocytopenic purpura. Thromb Res. 2019;181:29–35. https://doi.org/10.1016/j.thromres.2019.07.012. Epub 2019/07/23. PubMed PMID: 31330376
31. Moatti-Cohen M, Garrec C, Wolf M, Boisseau P, Galicier L, Azoulay E, et al. Unexpected frequency of Upshaw-Schulman syndrome in pregnancy-onset thrombotic thrombocytopenic purpura. Blood. 2012;119(24):5888–97. https://doi.org/10.1182/blood-2012-02-408914. Epub 2012/05/02. PubMed PMID: 22547583
32. van Dorland HA, Mansouri Taleghani M, Sakai K, Friedman KD, George JN, Hrachovinova I, et al. The International Hereditary Thrombotic Thrombocytopenic Purpura Registry: Key findings at enrolment until 2017. Haematologica. 2019; https://doi.org/10.3324/haematol.2019.216796. Epub 2019/02/23. PubMed PMID: 30792199
33. La Rubia JD, Pérez F, Navarro A. Síndrome HELLP. Med Clin. 2001;117(2):64–8.
34. Lattuada A, Rossi E, Calzarossa C, Candolfi R, Mannucci PM. Mild to moderate reduction of a von Willebrand factor cleaving protease (ADAMTS-13) in pregnant women with HELLP microangiopathic syndrome. Haematologica. 2003;88(9):1029–34. Epub 2003/09/13. PubMed PMID: 12969811
35. Page EE, Kremer Hovinga JA, Terrell DR, Vesely SK, George JN. Thrombotic thrombocytopenic purpura: diagnostic criteria, clinical features, and long-term outcomes from 1995 through 2015. Blood Adv. 2017;1(10):590–600. https://doi.org/10.1182/bloodadvances.2017005124. Epub 2018/01/04. PubMed PMID: 29296701; PubMed Central PMCID: PMCPMC5728353 interests
36. Chiasakul T, Cuker A. Clinical and laboratory diagnosis of TTP: an integrated approach. Hematology Am Soc Hematol Educ Program. 2018;2018(1):530–8. https://doi.org/10.1182/asheducation-2018.1.530. Epub 2018/12/07. PubMed PMID: 30504354; PubMed Central PMCID: PMCPMC6246034 Bayer, Bioverativ, Novo Nordisk, Pfizer, Shire, Spark, and Syntimmune and has consulted for Genzyme, Kedrion, and Synergy. T.C. declares no competing financial interests
37. Bommer M, Wolfle-Guter M, Bohl S, Kuchenbauer F. The differential diagnosis and treatment of thrombotic microangiopathies. Dtsch Arztebl Int. 2018;115(19):327–34. https://doi.org/10.3238/arztebl.2018.0327. Epub 2018/06/08. PubMed PMID: 29875054; PubMed Central PMCID: PMCPMC5997890
38. Scully M, Goodship T. How I treat thrombotic thrombocytopenic purpura and atypical haemolytic uraemic syndrome. Br J Haematol. 2014;164(6):759–66. https://doi.org/10.1111/bjh.12718. Epub 2014/01/07. PubMed PMID: 24387053; PubMed Central PMCID: PMCPMC4163720
39. Rock GA, Shumak KH, Buskard NA, Blanchette VS, Kelton JG, Nair RC, et al. Comparison of plasma exchange with plasma infusion in the treatment of thrombotic thrombocytopenic purpura. Canadian Apheresis Study Group. N Engl J Med. 1991;325(6):393–7. https://doi.org/10.1056/NEJM199108083250604. Epub 1991/08/08. PubMed PMID: 2062330
40. Schwartz J, Padmanabhan A, Aqui N, Balogun RA, Connelly-Smith L, Delaney M, et al. Guidelines on the Use of Therapeutic Apheresis in Clinical Practice-Evidence-Based Approach from the Writing Committee of the American Society for Apheresis: The Seventh Special Issue. J Clin Apher. 2016;31(3):149–62. https://doi.org/10.1002/jca.21470. Epub 2016/06/21. PubMed PMID: 27322218
41. Scully M, McDonald V, Cavenagh J, Hunt BJ, Longair I, Cohen H, et al. A phase 2 study of the safety and efficacy of rituximab with plasma exchange in acute acquired thrombotic thrombocytopenic purpura. Blood. 2011;118(7):1746–53. https://doi.org/10.1182/blood-2011-03-341131. Epub 2011/06/04. PubMed PMID: 21636861
42. Scully M, Knobl P, Kentouche K, Rice L, Windyga J, Schneppenheim R, et al. Recombinant ADAMTS-13: first-in-human pharmacokinetics and safety in congenital thrombotic thrombocytopenic purpura. Blood. 2017;130(19):2055–63. https://doi.org/10.1182/

blood-2017-06-788026. Epub 2017/09/16. PubMed PMID: 28912376; PubMed Central PMCID: PMCPMC5680611
43. Scully M, Thomas M, Underwood M, Watson H, Langley K, Camilleri RS, et al. Thrombotic thrombocytopenic purpura and pregnancy: presentation, management, and subsequent pregnancy outcomes. Blood. 2014;124(2):211–9. https://doi.org/10.1182/blood-2014-02-553131. Epub 2014/05/27. PubMed PMID: 24859360
44. Jokiranta TS. HUS and atypical HUS. Blood. 2017;129(21):2847–56. https://doi.org/10.1182/blood-2016-11-709865. Epub 2017/04/19. PubMed PMID: 28416508; PubMed Central PMCID: PMCPMC5445567
45. Loirat C, Fremeaux-Bacchi V. Atypical hemolytic uremic syndrome. Orphanet J Rare Dis. 2011;6:–60. https://doi.org/10.1186/1750-1172-6-60. Epub 2011/09/10. PubMed PMID: 21902819; PubMed Central PMCID: PMCPMC3198674
46. S M. Thrombocytopenia in pregnancy. In: Clínica Universitaria Reina Fabiola CC, editor. XIII Congreso del Grupo CAHT; Septiembre 20182018. p. 117–24.
47. Karpman D, Loos S, Tati R, Arvidsson I. Haemolytic uraemic syndrome. J Intern Med. 2017;281(2):123–48. https://doi.org/10.1111/joim.12546. Epub 2016/10/11. PubMed PMID: 27723152
48. Rodriguez de Cordoba S, Hidalgo MS, Pinto S, Tortajada A. Genetics of atypical hemolytic uremic syndrome (aHUS). Semin Thromb Hemost. 2014;40(4):422–30. https://doi.org/10.1055/s-0034-1375296. Epub 2014/05/07. PubMed PMID: 24799305
49. Michael M, Elliott EJ, Craig JC, Ridley G, Hodson EM. Interventions for hemolytic uremic syndrome and thrombotic thrombocytopenic purpura: a systematic review of randomized controlled trials. Am J Kidney Dis. 2009;53(2):259–72. https://doi.org/10.1053/j.ajkd.2008.07.038. Epub 2008/10/28. PubMed PMID: 18950913
50. Sarno L, Tufano A, Maruotti GM, Martinelli P, Balletta MM, Russo D. Eculizumab in pregnancy: a narrative overview. J Nephrol. 2019;32(1):17–25. https://doi.org/10.1007/s40620-018-0517-z. Epub 2018/08/31. PubMed PMID: 30159857

Chapter 46
Bleeding During Pregnancy

Malini Chauhan, Kendra Gray, and Michael Foley

Introduction, Evaluation, and Differential Diagnosis

Bleeding in pregnancy at any gestational age is anxiety provoking for patients and an indication for evaluation [1]. Bleeding throughout the course of a woman's pregnancy can vary from spotting to obstetrical hemorrhage. A careful evaluation must be performed in all scenarios to determine the source bleeding. Attention to rule out non-obstetric causes of bleeding such as those from the lower genital tract, bladder, or bowel for help guide meaningful treatment and avoid potentially unnecessary intervention.

Initial evaluation includes taking a thorough obstetrical and medical history. Physical examination included evaluation of external genitalia followed by a speculum examination evaluating for discrete cervical or vaginal lesions. It is prudent to also examine the urethral meatus and the anus to rule out urinary or rectal sources of bleeding. Ultrasound evaluation of patients with first trimester bleeding is the mainstay of the examination as the most common etiologies of first trimester bleeding include spontaneous abortion, ectopic pregnancy, and gestational trophoblastic disease. The most concerning conditions in and in the third trimester of pregnancy include evaluation for placental abruption, placenta previa, and placenta accreta. In most scenarios vaginal bleeding is maternal and not fetal; however that is not the case with a bleeding vasa previa which can cause fetal demise within a few short moments. Postpartum hemorrhage remains one of the most common obstetrical emergencies providers face and remains one of the leading causes maternal mortality throughout the world.

M. Chauhan (✉)
The University of Arizona College of Medicine – Tucson, Tucson, AZ, USA
e-mail: mchauhan@email.arizona.edu

K. Gray · M. Foley
The University of Arizona College of Medicine – Phoenix, Phoenix, AZ, USA
e-mail: mike.foley@bannerhealth.com

C. Montufar et al. (eds.), *Obstetric Catastrophes*,
https://doi.org/10.1007/978-3-030-70034-8_46

First Trimester

In the first trimester approximately 15–25% of pregnant women will experience some form of vaginal bleeding. Spotting or light bleeding during the first 1–2 weeks of pregnancy may be physiologic, due to the implantation of the fertilized egg to the uterine lining. Other non-pathological causes of bleeding in the first trimester include starting or bleeding post coitus, after a routine Papanicolaou smear or after a public exam due to the increasing blood supply developing in the cervix and uterus. Non-pathologic causes of first trimester bleeding are diagnoses of exclusion, and do not necessitate treatment [2]. In the remainder of this section, we will focus on pathologic causes of first trimester bleeding.

Ectopic Pregnancy

Ectopic pregnancy accounts for approximately 2% of all reported pregnancies although this may be underdiagnosed. Pregnant women who presented to the emergency room, in the first trimester with vaginal bleeding, abdominal pain or both were noted to have a prevalence of ectopic pregnancy as high as 18%. Despite advances in ultrasound imaging and increasing knowledge in management, ruptured ectopic pregnancy continues to be a significant cause of pregnancy-related mortality and morbidity with ruptured ectopic pregnancy accounting for 2.7% of all pregnancy-related deaths with the ultimate cause of mortality being hemorrhage. The most common location for ectopic implantation is in the fallopian tube (Table 46.1). Women who receive a diagnosis of an ectopic pregnancy may have known risk factors, including prior ectopic pregnancy, history of sexually transmitted infection, use of assistive reproductive technology, or other tubal disease. While it is rare for women with intrauterine devices to become pregnant, overall under 1%, up to 52% of pregnancies that occur with an IUD are ectopic [3].

Diagnosis of and ectopic pregnancy is usually made in the setting of a positive pregnancy test and either empty uterine cavity on transvaginal ultrasound or visualization of a gestational sack with the yolk sac, for embryo, or both in the adnexa. An intrauterine gestational sac with a yolk sac should be visible between 5 and 6 weeks gestational age regardless of whether a singleton or multiple gestation pregnancy exists. Depending on the patient's hemodynamic stability, the provider may choose

Table 46.1 Common implantation sites for ectopic pregnancies and their frequencies

Location of the topic implantation	Frequency of occurrence
Fallopian tube	90%
Abdomen	1%
Cervix	1%
Ovary	1–3%
Cesarean scar	1–3%

to obtain serial quantitative hCG measurements and evaluate whether serum increases mimic a normal pregnancy. Alternatively, a "discriminatory zone" may be utilized, which describes a threshold value for hCG, above which an intrauterine pregnancy should be visualized by transvaginal ultrasound examination. The utilization of discriminatory zones has been called into question, and the threshold value varies between institutions. If a discriminatory zone is utilized, a serum hCG level is used, and a cutoff level of 3500mIU/ml would be considered appropriate to avoid interruption of a desired intrauterine pregnancy.

Depending on the clinical scenario, ectopic pregnancies may be managed medically or surgically. Candidates for medical management include women with a confirmed or high clinical suspicion of ectopic pregnancy who are hemodynamically stable, do not have a desired intrauterine gestation, have no ruptured mass, and do not have contraindications with methotrexate administration and are willing and able to perform follow-up surveillance. Methotrexate therapy is more likely to be successful in the absence of embryonic cardiac activity, an initial hCG concentration less than 5000, and a pregnancy size less than 4 cm on transvaginal ultrasound.

Candidates for medical management include women with a confirmed or high clinical suspicion of ectopic pregnancy who are hemodynamically stable, have no ruptured mass, and do not have contraindications with methotrexate administration and are willing and able to perform follow-up surveillance.

Surgical management is indicated if the patient becomes hemodynamically unstable, has symptoms of a ruptured ectopic mass such as pubic pain, or has signs of intraperitoneal bleeding. Generally, salpingectomy is the preferred approach as fertility rates do not differ from salpingostomy and severe tubal damage and bleeding may preclude salpingectomy.

Hydatidiform Mole

A hydatidiform mole is the result of abnormal fertilization and can be subclassified as either a complete mole or a partial mole. Complete moles arise from a haploid sperm cell fertilizing an ovum without a nucleus, and then duplicating its genetic material. Thus, complete moles are diploid, do not possess embryonic tissue, and can be histologically characterized by generalized edematous and hyperplastic chorionic villi. Partial moles result from a normal ovum being fertilized by two sperm cells, resulting in triploidy and the presence of embryonic tissues. Pathological evaluation of partial moles reveals focal edema and hyperplasia of chorionic villi [4]. These differences between complete and partial moles are summarized in Table 46.2.

Table 46.2 Key characteristics of molar pregnancies [4]

Characteristic	Complete mole	Partial mole
Karyotype	Diploid (46 XX, 46 XY)	Triploid
Fetal or embryonic tissue	Absent	Present
Hydropic swelling of villi	Diffuse	Focal
Trophoblastic hyperplasia	Diffuse	Focal

Hydatidiform moles are relatively rare but can evolve into a gestational trophoblastic neoplasia (choriocarcinomas, invasive moles, epithelioid trophoblastic tumors, or placental site trophoblastic tumors). Conversion to gestational trophoblastic neoplasia is more likely with complete rather than partial moles. Risk factors for a molar pregnancy include prior molar pregnancy and extremes of maternal age.

In addition to vaginal bleeding, molar pregnancies are clinically associated with sensations of pelvic pressure or pain, fundal height greater than expected for gestational age, hyperemesis gravidarum, and higher hCG levels than expected for an intrauterine pregnancy. Ultrasound examination for complete moles classically will show a "snow storm" pattern and no fetal tissue. Ovarian cysts may also be present. In contrast, partial moles may present as a fetus with congenital anomalies, growth restriction, low amniotic fluid, and placental abnormalities such as focal cysts [5]. Imaging and hCG measurements may not be definitive, so for partial moles it is imperative to rule out a viable gestation. Treatment and definitive diagnosis for both types of molar pregnancies rely on uterine evacuation with suction curettage and subsequent pathologic examination. Hysterectomy may be considered for older patients who have completed child-bearing, as progression to gestational trophoblastic neoplasia is more likely in this group. Presence of a neoplastic process necessitates consultation with an oncologist and possible chemotherapy [6].

Abortion

Most spontaneous losses of pregnancy occur during the first trimester and may be clinically silent. Previous studies have estimated that about 30% of pregnancies will terminate spontaneously, and this outcome is less likely as gestational age advances [7]. Fetal death is associated with bleeding into the decidua basalis, tissue necrosis, and finally expulsion of fetal parts [8]. There are various fetal and maternal etiologies and risk factors for spontaneous abortion, though they may not be immediately apparent. The fetus may be anembryonic, as with a complete molar pregnancy, or with a "blighted ovum." The latter usually refers to the presence of an empty gestational sac where development of a fetus has failed. About half of embryonic abortions will be due to chromosomal anomalies, such as autosomal trisomies (usually 13, 18, and 21), monosomy X (also known as Turner's syndrome), and triploidies (partial molar pregnancy). Euploid embryonic abortions occur at later gestational ages and more common with advancing maternal age. Sadly, an exact etiology may not always be found [9, 10].

Maternal factors associated with spontaneous pregnancy loss include prior miscarriage, structural uterine abnormalities, infection, autoimmune diseases, neoplastic disease, uncontrolled endocrine disease, malnutrition, obesity, and substance abuse. Infection with tuberculosis or any organism in the mnemonic "TORCH," which stands for toxoplasmosis, "other" (syphilis, varicella, parvovirus B19), rubella, cytomegalovirus, and herpes simplex virus, may be associated with abortion. Pregnant patients from South America, certain countries in Africa, and southeast Asia or with recent travel there are at risk for infection with *Zika virus* [11]. Autoimmune diseases such as systemic lupus erythematosus and celiac disease can increase risk as well. Common endocrine abnormalities encountered include uncontrolled diabetes and thyroid disorders, as well as polycystic ovarian syndrome.

Spontaneous abortion may present clinically as threatened, inevitable, incomplete, complete, and missed. Establishing presence or absence of uterine contents and a fetal heartbeat, as well as performing a sterile vaginal exam to see if the cervical os is open or closed and if products of conception can be detected, is important in classification and management. A missed abortion is one in which uterine contents of conception are not expelled, and there may not be any vaginal bleeding, but the patient may notice cessation of symptoms of pregnancy such as nausea. Sonographic presence of a fetal heartbeat is not detectable in a missed abortion. All other classifications of abortion will be accompanied by some form of vaginal bleeding and abdominal cramping. It should be noted that threatened abortion and vaginal bleeding in the first trimester, particularly later on in gestational age, carry poor prognosis for both the mother and the fetus [12]. Treatment with progestins for purposes of preventing an abortion after a threatened abortion is controversial, with studies conflicting [13]. A summary of findings and management for different types of abortion is presented in Table 46.3.

Table 46.3 Characterization and management of abortion

Type of Abortion	Uterine Contents	Cervical os	Management
Threatened	Yes	Closed	Progestins (controversial) Follow-up monitoring to confirm IUP as appropriate
Inevitable	Yes/no	Open, products of conception may be visualized	Evacuation of uterine contents
Incomplete	No	Open, products of conception often in cervical canal	Evacuation of uterine contents
Complete	No	Closed	Confirm complete evacuation of uterine contents, assess bleeding, send products of conception to pathology for confirmation
Missed	Yes	Closed	Evacuation of uterine contents

Inevitable, incomplete, and missed abortions may be managed expectantly, medically, or surgically. Patients that are at or under 12 weeks and 6 days of pregnancy and clinically present as hemodynamically stable, have no signs of infection, and do not possess a history of bleeding disorders are candidates for medical management [14]. This usually involves treatment with an anti-progestin (mifepristone) followed by a prostaglandin (misoprostol) that causes expulsion. Methotrexate, a folate antagonist, may also be used in combination with misoprostol. Advantages of medical treatment include avoidance of anesthesia and an invasive procedure, but the patient will undergo experience much heavier bleeding compared to surgical management and would require access to good follow-up.

Surgical management usually involves dilation and curettage. This is a more invasive procedure and carries risk for uterine perforation and introduction of infection but is associated with much less bleeding than medical management and does not require a stringent follow-up. This method may be the only option for patients that are clinically unstable and/or too far along in gestational age.

Hemorrhage is a complication of induced and spontaneous abortions. The patient should first be evaluated for retention of products of conception, and if present, uterine contents should be promptly evacuated. If an empty uterine cavity is confirmed and the patient continues to bleed, evaluation for uterine atony, perforation (particularly for surgical abortion), and lacerations should proceed.

Other than bleeding, another important complication to consider during spontaneous pregnancy loss is septic abortion. It is more commonly associated with induced abortions rather than spontaneous ones but can be life-threatening and requires prompt recognition. Management includes stabilization with fluids as necessary, obtaining blood and endometrial cultures, broad-spectrum antibiotic therapy, and surgical evacuation of any remaining uterine contents. Various antibiotic regimens are used for empiric treatment, including intravenous gentamicin and clindamycin, though regimens recommended based on high-quality randomized control trials are still needed [15].

Placenta Previa

Placenta previa occurs when the placenta implants partially or completely over the cervical os, classically associated with painless vaginal bleeding in a gravid patient. Previas can be classified as:

- Low-lying placenta: Margin of the placenta is 2 cm or less from the internal cervical os which may be recognized on transvaginal ultrasound but not present with vaginal bleeding.
- Complete previa: whereby the placenta completely overlies the internal os.
- Marginal and partial previas are antiquated terms and should not be used.

The most important risk factor for previa is history of cesarean section. It is also associated with other uterine surgeries, smoking, and multiparity. Like with placenta accreta (discussed later), incidence of previa has increased as more patients receive cesarean sections. It is estimated to affect 0.4% of deliveries. Diagnosis is achieved with transvaginal ultrasound examination. Often a sterile vaginal exam will be performed as well, but digital cervical exam is contraindicated. Transvaginal ultrasound examination is safe because the probe is positioned on top of the anterior cervix rather than over the os. If diagnosed, the patient should also undergo investigation for a placenta accreta. Most previas are now diagnosed antenatally with ultrasound, but a patient without prenatal care may present with fetal malpresentation and/or unstable lie in addition to vaginal bleeding.

Management for placenta previa found during second trimester ultrasound in an asymptomatic patient involves observation, as many will resolve on their own as the uterus expands and the placenta is pulled toward the fundus. At 36–38 weeks' gestation, patients should be delivered via cesarean section. In the acute setting of bleeding placenta previa, the patient's hemodynamic stability should be assessed and treated appropriately. If the patient is in active labor, non-reassuring fetal heart tones are observed, and/or maternal hemodynamic stability cannot be achieved, emergency cesarean section should proceed [16].

In the Peripartum/Postpartum Period

Bleeding following delivery is normal, with the average blood loss following a vaginal delivery being less than 500 mL and less than 1000 mL after cesarean section. Various physiologic changes occur during pregnancy that allow the pregnant patient to adapt better to blood loss. These changes include increased erythrocyte mass (though hematocrit is usually low normal because of dilutional effect from increased plasma volume), increased cardiac output, and increased concentration of clotting factors. Additionally, in the immediate postpartum period, myometrium contractions help reduce bleeding. Postpartum hemorrhage after a vaginal delivery was previously described as estimated blood loss of more than 500 mL, but is now has the same criteria as postpartum hemorrhage after a cesarean section: estimate blood loss of 1000 mL or more, or any blood loss leading to symptoms of hypovolemia. Postpartum hemorrhage may also be classified as primary or secondary, occurring within the first 24 hours and first 6 weeks after delivery, respectively [17, 18]. This section will focus on primary postpartum hemorrhage. Possible etiologies include uterine atony, lacerations, uterine rupture, uterine inversion, placenta accreta, placenta previa, coagulopathy, abruptio placentae, and amniotic fluid embolism, which are discussed in detail below.

Uterine Atony

Uterine atony, the failure of the myometrium fibers to adequately contract uterine blood vessels, is the most common cause of postpartum hemorrhage, accounting for 75% of cases [19]. Risk factors include multiple gestation, polyhydramnios, fetal macrosomia, grand multiparity, retained products of conception, and chorioamnionitis. Medications that interfere with uterine contractility include calcium channel blockers, magnesium, halogenated anesthetics, and nitroglycerin [17]. Signs of atony include a soft, boggy uterus on exam after delivery. Management includes fundal massage, oxytocin administration, uterotonic agents, uterine tamponade balloon, and surgical treatment. Common uterotonic agents other than oxytocin include methylergonovine, carboprost, misoprostol, and dinoprostone. Note that methylergonovine should not be administered to patients with hypertensive disorders, and carboprost should not be given if the patient has a history of asthma. Surgical treatment includes introduction of B-lynch sutures for uterine compression and, depending on the severity of bleeding and the patient's desires for future childbearing, hysterectomy.

Lacerations

Lacerations, or tears, are a common sequelae of vaginal deliveries and are the second most common cause of postpartum hemorrhage [17]. If bleeding persists after a delivery and uterine tone is firm, inspection for lacerations should proceed. Lacerations will commonly occur in the periurethral area and along the rectovaginal midline. If forceps are utilized, there may be tears along the vaginal wall. Lacerations are more prone to happen with operative vaginal deliveries, episiotomy, fetal macrosomia or malpresentation, and shoulder dystocia. Perineal lacerations are categorized as first degree, second degree, third degree, and fourth degree, which involve superficial skin/vaginal mucosa, perineal musculature, sphincter muscles, and from the vaginal mucosa to rectal mucosa, respectively. First degree lacerations do not require repair; all others will.

Uterine Rupture

Uterine rupture is a relatively rare event, occurring in less than 1% of deliveries [20]. It may be classified as primary, occurring spontaneously in a patient without risk factors, or secondary. The major risk factor for secondary uterine rupture is trial of labor after a prior cesarean section or uterine surgery [21]. Dehiscence will typically occur in the lower uterine segment. Signs and symptoms include loss of fetal station, loss of uterine tone, palpation of fetal parts in the abdomen, pain out of proportion, heavy bleeding, non-reassuring fetal heart tracings, and maternal hemodynamic instability. Treatment includes immediate hemodynamic stabilization with administration of blood products followed by surgical management with cesarean section followed by either uterine repair or hysterectomy.

Uterine Inversion

Like uterine rupture, uterine inversion is a rare but catastrophic event, occurring in approximately every 1 out of 1100–2500 deliveries [17]. It is most commonly caused by excessive traction on the umbilical cord while attempting to deliver the placenta and may be associated with fundal placental implantation or accreta (discussed in detail below). It may be characterized by bleeding, abdominal pain, absence of the fundus on abdominal palpation, and protrusion of a red mass appreciated in the uterine cavity or through the cervix, depending on the severity of inversion. Treatment involves managing hemodynamic instability, replacing the inverted uterus, and use of uterotonic agents. Note that if uterotonic agents are used prior to manual replacement, they should be discontinued until the inversion is corrected, and then resumed to help the uterus contract properly. Terbutaline and sevoflurane relax uterine muscles and may be used while trying to manually correct inversion. If manual correction fails, surgery should be considered.

Placenta Accreta

Placenta accreta is due to invasive placentation due to defective decidua basalis. Invasion through the decidua basalis is a placenta accreta. Invasion into and beyond the myometrium is known as incretas and percretas, respectively. "Accreta" may be used to refer to invasive placentation in general. The combination of placenta previa (discussed below) and history of multiple cesarean sections increase risk for abnormal placentation because of disruption of the decidua basalis [22]. One study comparing patients without and with placenta previa found that incidence of accreta increased from 0.03% to 3% in patients with one cesarean section, 0.2% to 11% of patients with two, and 0.1% to 40% in patients with three. Thus, presence of a previa should prompt investigation for an accreta. Structural uterine anomalies, myomectomy, or other uterine surgery are also risk factors. Prevalence of placenta accreta has increased with the number of cesarean sections, which is estimated to occur in 30% of births in the United States. During the 1950s, placenta accreta affected 1 in every 30,000 deliveries; between 2008 and 2011, number of cases increased to 1 in every 713 deliveries [23].

In a patient where prenatal history is unknown, a placenta accreta may present with life-threatening hemorrhage on attempting to deliver the placenta. Excessive traction on the adherent placenta may lead to uterine inversion. Antenatally, ultrasound imaging during the second and third trimesters may identify a placenta accreta. Findings include blurring of the hypoechoic distinction between the placenta and myometrium, thinning of the myometrium, multiple irregular placental lacunae ("moth-eaten" or "Swiss-cheese" appearance), turbulent blood flow on color Doppler, and if percreta is present bladder abnormalities may be noted as well. Sonographic findings may be supplemented with MRI, particularly when ultrasound exam is equivocal, placenta is posterior, or to better define depth of invasion.

Treatment for accreta disorders is usually cesarean section followed by cesarean hysterectomy between 34 and 36 weeks gestation to minimize risk of spontaneous labor and hemorrhage. Ideally, a multidisciplinary team consisting of at least maternal fetal medicine specialists, gynecologic oncologists, interventional radiology, and neonatologists will be present. Surgery should be coordinated with the blood bank, and the institution should have a massive transfusion protocol in place. Expectant management or more conservative measures that preserve fertility, such as partial placental removal and balloon tamponade, are still topics of research [24].

Abruptio Placentae

Abruptio placentae (also referred to as "placental abruption") is premature separation of the placenta from the decidua basalis, usually from rupture of maternal vessels leading to blood accumulation and separation between the placental and uterine planes. It complicates 0.6–1.2% of pregnancies. Any sort of vasculopathy can increase risk for abruption, including chronic hypertension, preeclampsia, diabetes, tobacco use, or cocaine use. Other risk factors include prior abruption, advanced maternal age, multiple gestations, multiparity, abdominal trauma, short umbilical cord, and prior history of stillbirth. It is associated with a number of adverse neonatal outcomes, including intrauterine growth restriction and prematurity.

Clinical signs of abruption include vaginal bleeding with painful abdominal cramping or contractions. Bleeding may be concealed, so any patient presenting in preterm labor or preterm rupture of membranes should have abruption ruled out. Monitoring may show tachysystole and non-reassuring fetal heart tones. Greater than 50% separation between the placenta and decidual layer leads to significant maternal and fetal hemodynamic instability from resulting disseminated intravascular coagulopathy (DIC) and shock. Low fibrinogen levels may be a sign of abruption with concomitant DIC. Patients may also present less dramatically with "chronic abruption," characterized by smaller amounts of bleeding periodically throughout the latter two trimesters and associated with maternal hypertensive disorders. Diagnosis is aided with sonography, which may show retroplacental clots or fluid tracking along the placenta.

Management depends on maternal and fetal stability and gestational age. Term gestations at 37 or more weeks with abruption should be delivered either vaginally or via cesarean, whichever is safer. Gestations between 34 and 36 6/7 weeks should generally be delivered. Gestations under 34 weeks, if maternal and fetal status are reassuring, should be managed expectantly until late preterm or term. For chronic abruptions in stable mothers and fetuses, patients may be monitored in an inpatient setting until bleeding ceases for several days in the event of rapid deterioration. If intrauterine fetal demise occurs, vaginal or cesarean delivery may be undertaken depending on maternal status [25].

Vasa Previa

Vasa previa occurs when fetal blood vessels overlie the internal cervical os, causing potential for fetal hemorrhage and rapid exsanguination when membranes rupture. There are two types:

- Type I: fetal vessels overlying the internal cervical os are in association with a velamentous insertion (vessels from the umbilical cord diverge before entering the placenta and are covered only by fetal membranes).
- Type II: occurs with the presence of a succenturiate or multi-lobed placenta.

Vasa previa complicates approximately 1 in every 2500 deliveries. Associated risk factors include placenta previa/low-lying placenta, in vitro fertilization, and multiple gestations.

On digital cervical exam, pulsating vessels may be palpated. Often diagnosis may be made antenatally with ultrasound using color Doppler. An arterial vessel overlying the os with pulsating rate matching the fetal heart rate should be documented. Management is centered around timing cesarean delivery adequately to avoid rupture of membranes while trying to minimize adverse effects associated with prematurity, though there is no consensus on exactly when this should be done. Caution during surgery should be taken to avoid lacerating vulnerable fetal vessels, and if one is cut, it should be immediately clamped [26].

Amniotic Fluid Embolism

Amniotic fluid embolism is an extremely rare but often fatal event that typically occurs during the peripartum or immediate postpartum period attributed to the entry of amniotic contents into maternal circulation. An estimated 70% of cases will occur during labor. Amniotic contents induce release of pulmonary vasoconstrictors like endothelin, activate factor VII, and platelets and trigger inflammatory cascades. This ultimately leads to maternal cardiopulmonary distress as well as disseminated intravascular coagulation (DIC). Epidemiological data is difficult to obtain due to lack of international consensus on diagnostic criteria. Anything that may promote exchange of amniotic fluids between fetal and maternal compartments can be a risk factor, such as operative deliveries, placental abnormalities, and uterine rupture.

Change in mental status, anxiety, and agitation may precede clinical features related to the pathophysiology described above, including respiratory distress with hypoxia, cardiac arrest, electrocardiogram abnormalities, category III fetal heart tracings, and vaginal hemorrhaging as well as hematuria on catheterization and bleeding from venipuncture sites. Management consists of cardiopulmonary stabilization, treating shock with fluids and vasopressors if present, and managing DIC with blood products if necessary. Some patients may exhibit signs of anaphylactic shock, such as respiratory compromise with urticarial rash and should be treated accordingly with airway stabilization and epinephrine administration. If the fetus is of viable gestational age and has not been delivered, cesarean section should commence following maternal stabilization [27].

Coagulopathy

Any hematologic abnormality can contribute to abnormal bleeding during pregnancy and should be sought when obtaining history from the patient. Examples include von Willebrand disease, hemophilias A and B, and thrombocytopenia. The patient may not be formally diagnosed but may have a history of abnormal uterine bleeding. Patients with procoagulation disorders like Factor V Leiden may be on heparin therapy, which may also contribute to bleeding.

A pregnant patient may also be at risk of developing a disruption of hemostasis known as disseminated intravascular coagulation (DIC), especially with massive hemorrhage. DIC associated with multiple obstetric complications including postpartum hemorrhage, preeclampsia with severe features, placental abruption, sepsis, septic abortion, retained dead fetus, amniotic fluid embolism, acute fatty liver of pregnancy, and HELLP (hemolysis, elevated liver enzymes, low platelets) syndrome. A detailed explanation of the pathophysiology of DIC is complex and beyond the scope of this text. Looking at the process broadly, DIC occurs with excessive release of activated tissue factor (found in many places including amniotic fluid, decidual cells, and damaged blood vessel endothelium) that ultimately leads to cleaving fibrinogen into fibrin and recruitment of platelets. Clots are formed faster than they can be broken down, resulting in a consumptive coagulopathy and depletion of clotting factors. Clinically, the patient presents with profuse vaginal bleeding with a firm uterus, bleeding from venipuncture sites, incisions, and mucous membranes, and shock that may be out of proportion to estimated blood loss. DIC is usually a clinical diagnosis; there are no definitive laboratory tests. Decreased fibrinogen levels is the earliest laboratory sign of DIC, preceding clinical bleeding, and should be checked in patients that have any of the above-listed associated obstetric complications. Other laboratory findings in DIC are prolonged PT/INR, prolonged aPTT, decreased hemoglobin/hematocrit, increased LDH, and increased bilirubin. It should be noted that many of these values are affected by pregnancy, and adjusted normal values for obstetric patients and trending values may be more useful.

Treatment for DIC is centered around managing the inciting condition and supportive therapy as necessary. Blood products such as fresh frozen plasma, cryoprecipitate, platelets, and PRBCs should be administered depending on the clinical scenario. Strategies for blood product therapy are listed in the table below. DIC patients will often develop vitamin K and folate deficiencies and should receive supplementation and following the event should have their fluid status closely monitored [17]. Common causes and treatments of pregnancy-related DIC are listed in Table 46.4.

Hemodynamic Monitoring

There are many normal hemodynamic changes that occur during pregnancy, differentiating obstetric from nonobstetric patients. Such changes in baseline should be taken into account when interpreting data. As early as 7–8 weeks' gestation, there is an increase in preload and total blood volume causing increases in stroke volume (SV) and cardiac output (CO). Multiple gestations are associated with larger increases in these parameters compared to singletons. Overall blood pressures do not increase in normal pregnancy because of progesterone-mediated decreases in systemic vascular resistance (SVR). Echocardiographic studies have demonstrated left ventricular hypertrophy and deviation of the heart as a whole to the patient's left due to the gravid uterus pushing up against the diaphragm. Increases in annular diameters for valves have also been noted, which can cause benign flow murmurs.

During labor, cardiac output increases even more with "auto-transfusion" of 300–500 mL of blood with every contraction. Immediately after placental delivery, and the uteroplacental shunt is closed, about 500 mL of blood is redirected to maternal circulation. This, combined with reduced aortocaval compression by the shrinking uterus, causes dramatic increases in cardiac output. The increase peaks and lasts about 10 minutes after delivery and gradually decreases over the next 3 months postpartum. Table 46.5 summarizes normal hemodynamic changes throughout pregnancy.

Table 46.4 Etiology and management for DIC in pregnancy

Inciting event of DIC in pregnancy	Treatment
Massive hemorrhage	Treat cause (uterotonics, repair lacerations, etc.)
Placental abruption	Delivery: vaginal preferred if fetus and mother stable
Preeclampsia/HELLP	Delivery
Amniotic fluid embolus	Cardiovascular support Steroids
Sepsis	Broad-spectrum antibiotics Source control
Adult respiratory distress syndrome	Ventilatory support Cardiovascular support
Retained fetal demise	Delivery Consideration of antibiotics

Table 46.5 Normal hemodynamic changes in pregnant and nonpregnant state

Parameter	Nonpregnant	Pregnant	Postpartum
Heart rate (bpm)	60–100	80 ± 10	70 ± 10
Mean arterial pressure (mmHg)	90–110	90 ± 6	80 ± 7
Cardiac output (L/min)	4.3–6.0	6 ± 1	4 ± 1
Systemic vascular resistance (dyn/s/cm^{-5})	900–1400	1200 ± 250	1500 ± 500
Pulmonary vascular resistance (dyn/s/cm^{-5})	<350	80 ± 20	120 ± 50

Hemodynamic Effects Positioning for Procedures and Neuraxial Anesthesia

A 20-week-sized uterus (fundal height at the umbilicus) can compress the inferior vena cava, leading to decreased SV and CO and ultimately decreasing blood pressure. As the pregnancy progresses and the uterus grows, this effect becomes more pronounced and is responsible for supine hypotension. Reductions in CO can be up to 30% when the patient is supine compared to lateral recumbent position. For this reason, left lateral decubitus positioning is recommended during cesarean section and other surgeries.

As mentioned earlier, CO increases during the intrapartum period. This is partially due to pain, which is blunted when regional anesthesia is utilized. Regional anesthesia will also decrease SVR and can lead to prominent hypotension. Clinically the patient may complain of dizziness, nausea, begin to vomit, have pallor, and cyanotic lips. Maternal hypotension must be addressed quickly, as hypotension for longer than 4 minutes can lead to significant fetal compromise. Strategies for managing hypotension from neuraxial anesthesia include left uterine displacement, intravenous hydration with normal saline solution, leg wrapping, and phenylephrine administration [17].

Monitoring Hemodynamics in the Pregnant Patient

Invasive monitoring with the Swan-Ganz catheter for central venous pressure (CVP) has been controversial in nonobstetric patients due to associated risk and uncertain benefit, and there is a paucity of data to support its use in critically ill pregnant patients. Thus, CVP monitoring is not commonly utilized. Mean arterial pressure (MAP) is more commonly utilized in critically ill patients, particularly in sepsis. Guidelines from the Surviving Sepsis Campaign recommend maintaining MAP pressures at 65 mmHg or higher. Because of the uteroplacental shunt, MAP goals of 70 mmHg or higher are recommended for obstetric patients with sepsis. Placement of an arterial line may be desirable when accurate MAP measurements are needed and peripheral tissues are not receiving adequate perfusion.

Noninvasive monitoring modalities commonly used in pregnant patients with cardiac morbidities other than external blood pressure monitoring include telemetry and echocardiography. Women with cardiac abnormalities such as diastolic dysfunction, congenital heart disease, and valve disorders should be monitored postpartum with telemetry and arterial-line. Because lab values such as hemoglobin and hematocrit may take time to respond during hemorrhage or resuscitation, echocardiography may be useful in monitoring a patient's volume status and their response to treatment [17, 28].

Shock

Shock can result from different types of pathological insults but is always characterized by inadequate tissue perfusion. Neural tissue is especially vulnerable to poor perfusion, with irreversible damage occurring with just minutes of ischemia. Early on, patients may appear confused or agitated and later present as obtunded or with loss of consciousness. Oxygen depletion in the heart can lead to the development of fatal arrhythmias, but skeletal muscle is relatively resistant to hypoxia. Hypoperfusion of the kidneys leads to oliguria, and anuria is a poor prognostic indicator and sign of severe hemorrhage.

Different types of shock include hypovolemic, cardiogenic, obstructive, and distributive. Hypovolemic or hemorrhagic shock is most likely to be encountered in otherwise healthy obstetric patients, cardiogenic shock should be considered in patients with known cardiac abnormalities, and distributive shock may be seen with sepsis. Obstructive shock occurs in the setting of cardiac tamponade, constrictive pericarditis, or tension pneumothorax.

Hypovolemic/Hemorrhagic Shock

Hypovolemic shock can occur in volume-overloaded states with significant third-spacing of fluids, as is the case in congestive heart failure or with severe preeclampsia, and in this clinical scenario volume resuscitation should be considered carefully. In this section, we will primarily consider hypovolemic shock in the context of hemorrhage. Massive hemorrhage is defined as the loss of a patient's total estimated blood volume over the span of 24 hours. The American College of Surgeons classifies hemorrhagic shock into four categories summarized in the table below.

Table 1. Classification of Hemorrhagic Shock

	Class I	Class II	Class III	Class IV
Blood loss, mL	<1000	1000–1500	1500–2000	>2000
Blood loss, %	<15%	15%–30%	30%–40%	>40%
Blood pressure	Normal	Orthostatic	Marked fall	Profound fall
Pulse, beats/min	<100	>100	>120	>140
Respiratory rate, breaths/min	14–20	20–30	30–40	>35
Urine output, mL/h	>30	20–30	5.0–20	Anuria
Capillary refill	Normal	May be delayed	Usually delayed	Always delayed
Mental status	Normal	Agitated	Confused	Lethargic

Adapted from Advanced Trauma Life Support.[2-4]

In class I hemorrhagic shock, which may be expected after a typical vaginal delivery, estimated blood loss is under one liter, and many vital signs remain within or close to within normal ranges. Blood pressure and urinary output are generally unaffected. In obstetrics, class II hemorrhagic shock and beyond describe postpartum hemorrhage. One to 1.5 liters of blood is lost in class II hemorrhage, or approximately 15–30% of the patient's blood volume, and they begin to exhibit symptoms such as orthostatic hypotension, tachycardia, tachypnea, decreased urinary output, and agitation. It is not until 1.5–2.0 liters of blood is lost that compensatory mechanisms fail, and the patient is confused, has marked hypotension, tachycardia >120 bpm, markedly decreased urinary output from baseline, and delayed capillary refill. Finally, when over 2.0 liters of blood is lost (at least 40% of total blood volume), the patient enters class IV hemorrhagic shock and will exhibit profound hypotension, be lethargic, and have anuria.

Additionally, at class III or IV of hemorrhagic shock, patients can enter the "lethal triad" of metabolic acidosis, coagulopathy, and hypothermia. Hypoperfusion of tissues leads to reliance on anaerobic metabolism, which produce lactate, leading to metabolic acidosis. At lower pH values, activity of pro-coagulation factors such as factor VII and prothrombin decrease, while fibrinogen breakdown increases. Lactic acidosis is often worsened iatrogenically by hyperchloremic acidemia induced from overly aggressive resuscitation with crystalloids. Concentrations of varoius coagulation factors decrease due to the dilutional effect from resuscitation strategies that center on crystalloids, lactated Ringer's solution, and/or PRBCs. Hypoperfusion will also lead to hypothermia, which is defined as core body temperature of 35 ° C or less, further decreasing activity of the coagulation cascade.

Hemodynamic Support

Hemodynamic support may be necessary for bleeding during pregnancy. Every attempt should be made to correct the pathology responsible for the bleeding (i.e., uterine inversion, uterine rupture, etc.) in concordance with steps to achieve hemodynamic stability. Hypovolemic shock can result from hemorrhage or significant third-spacing, as is the case with severe preeclampsia (due to high hydrostatic pressure and leaky capillaries).

Cardiac output = Heart Rate × Stroke volume

Increases in the heart rate are accomplished at the expense of diastolic filling time.

Cardiac output is determined by several factors including preload, afterload, heart rate, and contractility. In the setting of hemorrhage preload is decreased warranting resuscitation with a combination of crystalloid, colloid, and blood products depending on the clinical scenario. Remembering that cardiac output is a function of heart rate x stroke volume, it is notable that increases in the heart rate are accomplished at the expense of diastolic filling time. Heart rate that exceeds the difference of 220 and the patient's age in years reduces cardiac output and myocardial perfusion. The MAP goal for obstetric patients is 70 mmHg or higher [17].

Transfusion Therapy

Blood volume in the average adult represents approximately 7% of body weight, or 70 mL of blood per kilogram. Blood is a living tissue comprised of cellular and plasma compartments. Red blood cells (RBCs) contain the oxygen-carrying molecule hemoglobin. Oxygen's affinity to hemoglobin allows the transport of oxygen from the alveoli of the lungs to vital organs and peripheral tissues. Normal female adult hemoglobin levels are 12 to 15 g/dL in women; however due to the relative dilution due to pregnancy changes, a low threshold of 10.5 g/dL is considered normal.

Massive hemorrhage is a rare occurrence in the practice of obstetrics and gynecology. Early recognition of the clinical signs and symptoms of hemorrhagic shock can facilitate a rapid response to the decompensating patient. Needle size depends on the size and integrity of a patient's vein; however an 18-gauge needle is standard for transfusion and two large bore lines are advised. A needle or catheter as small as 23-gauge can be used for transfusion if necessary; however the smaller the gauge, the slower is the flow rate and the higher is the risk of clotting.

Every 500 cc of blood loss = decrease in hemoglobin by 1 point

Example: A 26-year-old G1 has just delivered vaginally. Her admission hemoglobin was 9.5. Her current estimated blood loss is 2 liters.

What would her expected current hemoglobin be?

(Answer: 7.5)

The goal of red blood cell transfusion is to improve oxygen delivery to the body's tissues and organs. Generally, the threshold for transfusion is a hemoglobin of <7 g/L; however in cases of acute or ongoing hemorrhage lab values will not equilibrate accurately and should be used with caution and delaying resuscitation or

Table 46.6 Blood component therapy

Components	Contents	Indications	Volume (mL)	Shelf life	Expected effect
PRBC	Red cells, some plasma, few WBCs	Correct anemia	300	42 days	Increase Hct 3% and Hgb 1 g per unit
Leukocyte poor blood	Red cells, some plasma, few WBCs	Correct anemia, reduce febrile reactions	250	21–24 days	Increase Hct 3% and Hgb 1 g per unit
Platelets	Platelets, some plasma, some RBC, few WBCs	Bleeding due to thrombocytopenia	50	Up to 5 days	Increases total platelet count 7500/mm^3/U
Fresh frozen plasma	Fibrinogen, plasma, clotting factors V, XI, XII	Treatment of coagulation disorders	250	2 hours thawed 12 months frozen	Increases total fibrinogen 10–15 mg/dL/U
Cryoprecipitate	Fibrinogen, plasma, clotting factors V, VIIII, XIII, von Willebrand factor	Hemophilia A, von Willebrand disease, fibrinogen deficiency	40	4–6 hours thawed	Increases total fibrinogen 10–15 mg/dL/U

transfusion based on lab values alone is inappropriate. Blood component therapy is listed in Table 46.6.

As hemorrhage remains one of the major causes of potentially preventable maternal deaths, many obstetrical units have adopted protocol-based management of these patients using massive transfusion protocols (MTPs). Protocol-based management of patients using massive transfusion protocol have shown improved outcomes. The majority of MTPs set a ratio of blood components used for transfusion approximating 1:1:1 for RBC:FFP:platelets. Once MTP is ordered for a patient, the blood bank ensures rapid delivery of all blood components to facilitate resuscitation. These protocols reduce dependency on laboratory testing during the acute resuscitation phase decreasing the need for communication between the blood bank, laboratory, and physician so that each team member can work more expeditiously. The limitations of MTP are that in the event of a non-massive blood loss situation, wastage of blood products may occur [28, 29].

References

1. Breeze C. Early pregnancy bleeding. Aust Fam Physician. 2016;45(5):283–6. Review
2. Frequently asked questions. Pregnancy FAQ038. Bleeding during pregnancy. In: American College of Obstetricians and Gynecologists. https://www.acog.org/Patients/FAQs/Bleeding-During-Pregnancy. Accessed 30 Jun 2019.

3. Long-acting reversible contraception: implants and intrauterine devices. Practice Bulletin No. 186. American College of Obstetricians and Gynecologists. Obstet Gynecol. 2017;130:e251–69.
4. Berkowitz RS, Goldstein DP. Molar pregnancy. N Engl J Med. 2009;360:1639–45.
5. Lazarus E, Hulka C, Siewert B, Levine D. Sonographic appearance of early complete molar pregnancies. J Ultrasound Med. 1999;18:589–94.
6. Elias KM, Shoni M, Bernstein M, Goldstein DP, Berkowitz RS. Complete hydatidiform mole in women aged 40 to 49 years. J Reprod Med. 2012;57(5–6):254–8. PubMed PMID: 22696822
7. Wilcox AJ, Weinberg CR, O'Connor JF, Baird DD, Schlatterer JP, Canfield RE, Armstrong EG, Nisula BC. Incidence of early loss of pregnancy. N Engl J Med. 1988;319(4):189–94. https://doi.org/10.1056/NEJM198807283190401. PubMed PMID: 3393170
8. Cunningham FG. Williams obstetrics. New York: McGraw-Hill Education; 2018.
9. Kajii T, Ferrier A, Niikawa N, Takahara H, Ohama K, Avirachan S. Anatomic and chromosomal anomalies in 639 spontaneous abortuses. Hum Genet. 1980;55:87–98.
10. Stein Z, Kline J, Susser E, et al. Maternal age and spontaneous abortion. In: Porter IH, Hook EB, editors. Human embryonic and fetal death. New York: Academic Press; 1980. p. 107.
11. (2019) Maps of areas with risk of Zika. In: Center for Disease Control. https://wwwnc.cdc.gov/travel/files/zika-areas-of-risk.pdf. Accessed 27 Mar 2019.
12. Saraswat L, Bhattacharya S, Maheshwari A, Bhattacharya S. Maternal and perinatal outcome in women with threatened miscarriage in the first trimester: a systematic review. BJOG Int J Obstet Gynaecol. 2009;117:245–57.
13. Early pregnancy loss. ACOG Practice Bulletin No. 200. American College of Obstetricians and Gynecologists. Obstet Gynecol. 2018;132:e197–207.
14. Neilson JP, Gyte GM, Hickey M, Vazquez JC, Dou L. Medical treatments for incomplete miscarriage. Cochrane Database Syst Rev. 2013; https://doi.org/10.1002/14651858.cd007223.pub3.
15. Udoh A, Effa EE, Oduwole O, Okusanya BO, Okafo O, Iya J. Antibiotics for treating septic abortion. Cochrane Database Syst Rev. 2015; https://doi.org/10.1002/14651858.cd011528.
16. Oyelese Y, Canterino JC. Placenta Previa and Placenta Accreta. In: Sheiner E, editor. Bleeding during pregnancy. New York: Springer; 2011.
17. Foley MR, Strong TH, Garite TJ. Obstetric intensive care manual. New York: McGraw-Hill Education; 2018.
18. Postpartum hemorrhage. Practice Bulletin No. 183. American College of Obstetricians and Gynecologists. Obstet Gynecol. 2017;130:e168–86.
19. Marshall A, Durani U, Bartley A, Hagen C, Ashrani A, Rose C, Go R, Pruthi R. The impact of postpartum hemorrhage on hospital length of stay and inpatient mortality. Obstet Anesth Dig. 2018;38:66–7.
20. Guise JM, Eden K, Emeis C, Denman MA, Marshall N, Fu RR, Janik R, Nygren P, Walker M, McDonagh M. Vaginal birth after cesarean: new insights. Evid Rep Technol Assess (Full Rep). 2010;(191)1–397. Review. PubMed PMID: 20629481; PubMed Central PMCID: PMC4781304.
21. Vaginal birth after cesarean delivery. ACOG Practice Bulletin No. 205. American College of Obstetricians and Gynecologists. Obstet Gynecol 2019;133:e110–27.
22. Placenta Accreta: Spectrum of US and MR Imaging Findings. In: RadioGraphics. https://pubs.rsna.org/doi/full/10.1148/rg.287085060. Accessed 30 Jun 2019.
23. Silver RM, Landon MB, Rouse DJ, Leveno KJ, Spong CY, Thom EA, Moawad AH, Caritis SN, Harper M, Wapner RJ, Sorokin Y, Miodovnik M, Carpenter M, Peaceman AM, O'Sullivan MJ, Sibai B, Langer O, Thorp JM, Ramin SM, Mercer BM. Maternal morbidity associated with multiple repeat cesarean deliveries. Obstet Gynecol. 2006;107(6):1226–32. https://doi.org/10.1097/01.AOG.0000219750.79480.84. PubMed PMID: 16738145
24. Placenta accreta spectrum. Obstetric Care Consensus No. 7. American College of Obstetricians and Gynecologists. Obstet Gynecol. 2018;132:e259–75.

25. Ananth CV, Kinzler WL. Placental Abruption. In: Sheiner E, editor. Bleeding during pregnancy. New York: Springer; 2011.
26. Alouini S, Megier P, Fauconnier A, Huchon C, Fievet A, Ramos A, Megier C, Valéry A. Diagnosis and management of placenta previa and low placental implantation. J Matern Fetal Neonatal Med. 2019:1–6.
27. #37: Diagnosis and management of vasa previa Sinkey, Rachel G. et al. Am J Obstetr Gynecol. 2015;213(5):615–9
28. Backer DD, Dorman T. Surviving sepsis guidelines. JAMA. 2017;317:807.
29. Shaylor R, Weiniger CF, Austin N, Tzabazis A, Shander A, Goodnough LT, Butwick AJ. National and international guidelines for patient blood management in obstetrics. Surv Anesthesiol. 2017;61:72.

Part XII
Cancer

Chapter 47
Cancer in Obstetrics

Ramoncito Yacab and Jorge Hidalgo

Introduction

Cancer in pregnancy is the second leading cause of death during the reproductive years. It is an uncommon event that is estimated to occur in 1 per 1000 pregnancies annually and accounts for 0.1% of all malignant tumors [1]. In Europe, there are an estimated 3000 to 5000 cases per annum, and similar figures have been reported for the USA [2].

In a recent European cohort ($n = 1170$), the most common malignancies during pregnancy were breast cancer (39%), cervical cancer (13%), lymphomas (10%), and ovarian cancer (7%). Approximately one-fourth of all cases are documented during the first trimester, and up to a fourth of cases present with metastatic disease [3]. Still, most of the data might be underrepresented due to difficulties in data reporting, especially in developing countries.

During the past two decades, treatment and obstetrical outcomes have changed based on the availability of chemotherapeutic drugs, the regimen used, and the antenatal services. For every 5 years, the likelihood of receiving treatment during pregnancy increased by 10% and was associated with more live births and fewer iatrogenic preterm deliveries. Furthermore, antenatal exposure to chemotherapy drugs does not increase the frequency of congenital malformation (4%) compared to the general population nor has it been associated with neurological or psychological abnormalities [3, 4]. Oncologic management is possible during pregnancy without significantly negatively impacting maternal and fetal outcomes.

R. Yacab (✉)
Head of the Oncology Department at Karl Heusner Memorial Hospital, Belize City, Belize

J. Hidalgo
Division of Critical Care, Karl Heusner Memorial Hospital, Belize City, Belize

C. Montufar et al. (eds.), *Obstetric Catastrophes*,
https://doi.org/10.1007/978-3-030-70034-8_47

Clinical Presentation

Pregnancy is associated with physiological changes that may give rise to a myriad of clinical signs and self-limiting symptoms. Unfortunately, symptoms associated with malignancy may be vague and unspecific, often attributed to the process of pregnancy by both patients and physicians. These symptoms may include nausea, appetite changes, abdominal discomfort, anemia, increased volume of breast tissue, and fatigue [5]. A delay in diagnosis will negatively impact both mother and fetal outcomes, often associated with a grim prognosis.

Diagnostic and Staging Studies

Once there is a clinical suspicion of cancer, there are still various challenges that may limit a timely diagnosis. This includes selecting the most appropriate test without causing potential harm to the fetus. Magnetic resonance imaging (MRI) and ultrasound are imaging modalities regarded as safe during pregnancy since there is no exposure to ionizing radiation nor is there any scientific evidence of fetal complications associated with both radiological modalities [4–6]. These tests should be used prudently and only when its use will provide a benefit to the patient.

Common studies generally used during the diagnostic and staging workup include chest X-rays and computed tomography. These are generally avoided during pregnancy due to the deleterious effect of ionizing radiation on the fetus. The severity of these complications is dependent on the gestational age at exposure and the dose of radiation. Radiation exposure above 50 mGy during the gestational period has been associated with congenital abnormalities and growth restriction and severe intellectual disability when exposure occurs during the fetal period [4, 5]. The use of these studies should not be withheld when clinically indicated, but a thorough discussion on the potential risks and benefits should be made.

Tissue sampling modalities for histological confirmation will depend on both clinical suspicion and stage. Upper gastrointestinal endoscopy and colonoscopy have adequate sensitivity for the detection of gastrointestinal tumors and are considered safe during pregnancy [6]. Fine needle aspiration and core needle biopsies are generally considered safe and feasible.

Cancer Treatment in Pregnancy

Surgery

Surgery is the cornerstone of cancer treatment in solid tumors. In the oncologic patient, it may have a dual role, since it can be both diagnostic and therapeutic. Pregnancy is not a contraindication to surgery. While operations are not associated with a congenital malformation, it has been linked along with exposure to anesthesia with an increase in miscarriages during the first trimester (1–2%). Surgery is often deferred to the second trimester, when the risk to the fetus is lowest, although there is an increased risk of lower birth weight and premature delivery (two times the relative risk) [5, 7]. The complications that may derive from the procedure are higher when it involves the abdominal or the pelvic cavity. Oncological surgery should not be delayed when clinically indicated.

Chemotherapy

Chemotherapy drugs are a fundamental part of cancer care. Its use in the pregnant patient is faced with therapeutic and ethical issues. It is essential to understand the optimum time and use of cytotoxic drugs to adequately balance the well-being of the fetus.

The teratogenicity of chemotherapy drugs will depend on the time of exposure, the dose, and the pharmacokinetic properties of the drug. Chemotherapy during the first trimester increases the risk of spontaneous abortion, fetal death, and congenital malformation. During the first 2 weeks postconception, the undifferentiated embryo can either be lost or unaffected, a phenomenon known as "all or none" [8]. Any exposure during the rest of the first trimester negatively affects organogenesis, in particular, the heart, neural tube, and limbs. After organogenesis, the risk of malformation reduces significantly (1.3%); however, it is associated with intrauterine growth retardation and prematurity [8, 9]. Long-term follow-up of people exposed to chemotherapy in utero has not been associated with neurological, physiological, or physical anomalies nor is there an increase in the incidence of secondary tumors [4, 10]. Table 47.1 shows the potential risk to the fetus associated with exposure to chemotherapy agents. Based on the current evidence, chemotherapy can be used during the second and third trimester of pregnancy.

Considering that chemotherapy may decrease maternal blood production and lead to thrombocytopenia and neutropenia, the adequate timing for delivery should be planned within 3 weeks after chemotherapy. Chemotherapy should not be administered after 37 weeks of gestation due to the risk of the onset of spontaneous labor [8, 9].

Radiotherapy

Radiation therapy (RT) is an integral part within the multidisciplinary management of cancer. Technological and technical advancements during the past decade have led to the introduction of modern radiation technology, including 3D conformal RT, intensity-modulated RT (IMRT), and volumetric modulated RT (VMRT). While these technologies have improved both effectiveness and tolerability, the treatment

Table 47.1 Risks associated with chemotherapy exposure during pregnancy

Drug Family	Potential risk to a fetus
Plant alkaloids	Preterm delivery, intrauterine growth restriction
Anthracycline antibiotics	Mid trimester miscarriage, neonatal neutropenia, intrauterine growth restriction, transient myelosuppression
Alkylating agents	Ophthalmic abnormalities, cleft palate, esophageal atresia, abnormal inferior vena cava, renal agenesia
Antimetabolites	Spontaneous abortion, microcephaly, syndactyly, deficient growth and development
Platinum	Sensorineural hearing loss

Table 47.2 Adverse effects of radiation in relation to gestational stages

Stage	Period	Adverse Event
Implantation	First 2 weeks	All or nothing
Early organogenesis	Week 2 to 12	Teratogenesis, growth retardation
Late organogenesis/early fetal period	Week 12 to 20	Mental and growth retardation, microcephaly, eye, palate, and genital deformity
Late fetal stage	Week 20 up to birth	Sterility, secondary malignancies

of the pregnant patient still poses a challenge. Its selective use during pregnancy aims at improving outcomes for the mother while reducing potential harm to the fetus.

Potential harmful effects to the fetus will depend on the dose of irradiation, the embryonal age (weeks or days from fertilization), and the primary tumor. During the organogenesis phase, comprised between the second and seventh week, there is an increase in the risk of gross malformation and small head size (SHS) without retardation with doses higher to 0.5 Gy. Exposure during the rest of the first trimester has been associated with similar effects; however, there is a higher risk of mental retardation, considering that it is during this phase that brain development occurs [11]. The effects of irradiation during the second trimester have been associated with growth retardation, mental retardation, sterility, and secondary malignancies. Although exposure during the third trimester has been associated with lower rates of harmful effects, these have been reported for exposures lesser than 0.5 Gy. Table 47.2 shows the adverse effects associated with radiation.

The usual dose for radiation therapy is typically between 40 and 70 Gy. Considering the potential harms that derive from these high doses during gestation, radiation therapy is not routinely recommended during pregnancy and should be postponed until after childbirth when possible. The radiation dose to the fetus depends on the total dose required, the distance from the target lesion and the fetus, and the scattered radiation from the collimator and within the patient. The use of shielding serves as protection. Radiation dose can be kept between 40 and 200 mGy when adequately used along with a distance greater than 30 cm from the edge of the field to the fetus [11, 12]. Radiotherapy has been used in selected cases of breast cancer and lymphomas; however, patient selection must be performed on a case-by-case evaluation weighing the risk for the fetus and the benefits on the oncological outcome [12, 13].

Conclusion

The management of cancer during pregnancy is a challenge and should be optimally managed at a high-risk obstetrical unit. The prognosis of cancer is not biologically affected by a pregnancy nor is its biological behavior different from a nonpregnant patient. The physiological changes unique to pregnancy have not only been associated with a delay in diagnosis and staging, but it also accounts for the need to develop a personalized approach from standard protocols taking into account both the benefits and risks of any therapeutic procedure. A multidisciplinary team is required to evaluate each individual case to determine strategies based on gestational age and fetal viability to ensure the least potential harm on both fetal and maternal health. Surgery should not be delayed when indicated and can be performed safely during pregnancy. Systemic therapy should be delayed to the second and third trimester since the risk of anomalies, growth restriction, and prematurity are lower during these phases. The patient should receive in-depth information on these potential risks associated with treatment. Finally, radiotherapy is not recommended during pregnancy and must be delayed until after the birth when possible. Its use during pregnancy has been limited to selected cases, mostly involving oncologic emergencies or situations where waiting for resolution of the pregnancy might compromise treatment efficacy.

Bibliography

1. Van Calsteren K, Heyns L, De Smet F, Van Eycken L, et al. Cancer during pregnancy: an analysis of 215 patients emphasizing the obstetrical and the neonatal outcomes. J Clin Oncol. 2010;28(4):683–9.
2. Pentheroudakis G, Pavlidis N. Cancer, and pregnancy: Poena Magna, not anymore. Europ J Cancer. 2006;42(2):126–40.
3. De Haan J, Verheecke M, van Calsteren K, et al. Oncological management and obstetric and neonatal outcomes for women diagnosed with cancer during pregnancy: a 20-year international cohort study of 1170 patients. Lancet Oncol. 2018;19(3):337–46.
4. Hepner A, Negrini D, Hase EA, et al. Cancer during pregnancy: the oncologist overview. World J Oncol. 2019;10(1):28–34.
5. Botha MH, Rajaram S, Karunaratne K. Cancer in pregnancy. Int J Gynecol Obstet. 2018;143:137–42.
6. Peccatori FA, Azim HA, Orecchia R, Hoekstra HJ, Pavlidis N, Kesic V. Cancer, pregnancy, and fertility: ESMO Clinical Practice Guidelines for diagnosis, treatment, and follow-up. Ann Oncol. 2013;24(suppl 6):vi160–70.

7. Basta P, Bak A, Roszkowski K. Cancer treatment in pregnant women. Współczesna Onkologia. 2015;5:354–60.
8. Esposito S, Tenconi R, Preti V, Groppali E, Principi N. Chemotherapy against cancer during pregnancy. Medicine. 2016;95(38):e4899.
9. Cardonick E, Iacobucci A. Use of chemotherapy during human pregnancy. Lancet Oncol. 2004;5(5):283–91.
10. Brewer M, Kueck A, Runowics CD. Chemotherapy in pregnancy. Clin Obstet Gynecol. 2011;54(4):602–18.
11. Martin D. Review of radiation therapy in the pregnant Cancer patient. Clin Obstet Gynecol. 2011;54(4):591–601.
12. Mazzola R, Corradini S, Eidemueller M, Figlia V, Fiorentino A, et al. Modern radiotherapy in cancer treatment during pregnancy. Crit Rev Oncol Hematol. 2019;136:13–9.
13. Gök M, Bozkurt M, Guneyli S, Kara Bozkurt D, Korkmaz M, Peker N. Prenatal radiation exposure. Proc Obstetr Gynecol. 2015;5(1):2.

Chapter 48
Superior Vena Cava Syndrome in Pregnant Woman

Jorge Sinclair Ávila, Sabrina Da Re Gutiérrez, Jorge E. Sinclair De Frías, Fabricio Vera, and Maria V. Rodriguez

Introduction

SVC syndrome is a constellation of signs and symptoms caused by the obstruction of the SVC due to either external compression or internal obstruction. It was first described by William Hunter in 1757 as a complication of a saccular aortic aneurysm [23]. The etiology has evolved over centuries. Before antibiotics, infectious diseases were the main cause of SVC syndrome, specifically syphilitic infections and tuberculosis [62]. In the early twentieth century, cases were equally distributed between aortic aneurysms and malignancies [17, 24]. Since the advent of antibiotics, the role of infections declined, while malignancies became the most common etiology, causing up to 80–99% of the cases in the late 1900s [52].

Recently, there has been an increasing incidence of SVC syndrome associated to benign causes, mainly due to intravascular devices such as catheters and pacemakers [12, 61] since they predispose to thrombosis due to damage of the intima of the vessels. Clinical signs and symptoms include edema of the arms, head, and neck, distention of subcutaneous vessels, and plethora.

J. S. Ávila (✉)
Critical Medicine, UCI Hospital Pacifica Salud/Johns Hopkins Medicine, Faculty of Medicine University of Panama, Panama City, Panama

S. Da Re Gutiérrez
Critical and Intensive Care Medicine, Maternal and Child Hospital, Caja Nacional de Salud (CNS), La Paz, Bolivia

J. E. Sinclair De Frías
Santo Tomas Hospital, Faculty of Medicine University of Panama, Panamá City, Panamá

F. Vera
General de Manta Hospital, Manta, Ecuador

M. V. Rodriguez
General Verdi Cevallos Hospital, Portoviejo, Ecuador

C. Montufar et al. (eds.), *Obstetric Catastrophes*,
https://doi.org/10.1007/978-3-030-70034-8_48

In the late 1900s, chemotherapy and radiotherapy were considered the main therapy for this entity. Since the introduction of SVC stenting in 1986, the role of endovascular therapy (ET) has increased exponentially [11].

Anatomy

The superior vena cava is a thin-walled, low-pressure vein formed by the union of left and right innominate veins, measuring from 6 to 8 cm. It drains blood from the head, neck, upper extremities, and upper thorax, representing one third of the venous return to the heart. It is located in the right mediastinum where it can be compressed by surrounding structures including the trachea, right bronchus, aorta, pulmonary artery, and perihilar and paratracheal lymph nodes [77].

Etiology

Etiologies during pregnancy are similar to that in general population. It is divided into two main groups: malignant and benign SVC syndrome. Malignant SVC syndrome is often due to an extrinsic compression of the SVC by a tumor, while most cases of benign SVC syndrome are caused by thrombus formation within the SVC.

- *Malignant*: Around 90% of all SVC syndrome are caused by malignancy, especially lung cancer and non-Hodgkin lymphoma [12, 61]. Other malignancies are also associated, but in a lesser extent, including breast cancer, esophageal cancer, germ cell tumors, thymoma, thyroid carcinoma, and metastatic disease [43, 61].
- *Benign*: The remaining cases are accounted by benign causes such as intravascular devices, cardiac causes, mediastinal fibrosis, benign mediastinal tumors, vascular disease, and infections [12, 43, 61, 71].

Coexistence of two or more underlying etiologies is not rare, especially in oncologic patients who usually have indwelling catheters used to receive chemotherapy or antibiotics.

Epidemiology

Most cases occur in men between 50 and 70 years old, thus explaining the rarity of this entity during pregnancy. In addition, most contemporary cases are due to an underlying malignancy. The occurrence of malignancy during pregnancy is unusual, complicating approximately 1 per 1000 pregnant women [45]. Most common malignancies during pregnancy are breast cancer, melanoma, cervical carcinoma, an, Hodgkin lymphomas [45, 46].

Frequency of SVC syndrome varies depending on the underlying malignancy. Around 2–4% of lung cancer and non-Hodgkin lymphoma patients develop SVC syndrome during the course of the disease [71]. The incidence is higher (10%) in small cell lung cancer (SCLC) due to its predilection for mediastinal involvement and rapid growth [55, 71] but is rare in Hodgkin lymphoma despite the presence of mediastinal lymphadenopathy [49].

Both lung cancer and non-Hodkin lymphoma are rare during pregnancy. Lung cancer usually presents later in life with only 2% of cases affecting people under the age of 45 [39], while the incidence of non-Hodgkin lymphoma is reportedly 5.39 per 100,000 births [18].

In recent decades, the use of indwelling central venous catheters and cardiac pacemakers has increased, resulting in higher incidence of SVC thrombosis associated to intravascular devices [53]. Annually, more than 5 million central venous catheters and 170,000 pacemakers are implanted in the United States [34, 50, 54].

Although most cases are due to malignancy, pregnancy can be complicated by benign SVC obstruction [4]. In general population, nonmalignant causes are responsible of a significant percentage of cases. Reports have shown that up to 40% are due to benign etiologies [52, 56] and up to 75% of the patients with benign SVC syndrome have an indwelling venous device [28]. SVC syndrome is observed in 1–14% of patients with central venous catheter and in 0.2–3.3% of patients with implanted pacemakers [9, 21, 52].

Pathogenesis

Most contemporary cases of SVC syndrome can be attributed to one or more of the following pathologic mechanisms: compromised vessel anatomy, compromised vessel wall integrity, and compromised venous flow [12].

1. *Compromise of vessel anatomy*: occurs when there is an extrinsic compression of the vessel caused by a mediastinal mass. Often due to malignancies and less commonly caused by nonmalignant masses.
2. *Compromise of the vessel wall integrity*: usually caused by an intravascular device. The tip or edge of the indwelling catheter or lead irritates the venous endothelium, leading to reactive inflammation, fibrosis, and stenosis (8: [21, 31]). Another cause of SVC fibrosis is mediastinitis. Fibrosing mediastinitis can be idiopathic or a result of chest radiation, Bechet's disease, or infections such as tuberculosis, syphilis, and histoplasmosis [25, 37, 52].
3. *Compromised venous flow*: results from occlusive or near-occlusive venous thrombus. Usually happens in the setting of a hypercoagulable state, potentiated by the presence of intravascular devices.

These mechanisms may coexist and promote obstruction of the SVC, for example, a pregnant woman with an underlying malignancy and an indwelling central line. Recognizing the overlap of these mechanisms can help identify patients at risk as well as initiate prompt management if needed.

Pathophysiology

Compression and/or obstruction of the SVC increases resistance of venous blood flow leading to blood accumulation proximal to the obstruction with consequent elevation of hydrostatic pressure. This results in venous hypertension and interstitial edema, producing classic signs and symptoms found in SVC syndrome [8]. High venous pressure in collateral vessels leads to the development of a collateral blood flow network over time [35]. Collateral vessels often take weeks to dilate sufficiently to accommodate blood that normally passes through the SVC [71]. Commonly found collateral vessels include azygos, intercostal, mediastinal, paravertebral, hemiazygos, thoracoepigastric, internal mammary, thoracoacromioclavicular, and anterior chest wall veins [19].

Collateral network diverts blood flow reducing SVC venous pressure, explaining why, in rapidly developing SVC obstructions and in obstructions below the insertion of azygos vein, signs and symptoms tend to be worse [58, 59]. Moreover, this collateral network consists of small-caliber vessels that can also be compromised by the same tumor causing SVC syndrome.

Signs and Symptoms

Evaluation includes clinical history and physical examination with attention to the duration of symptoms, history of previous invasive procedures, and history of malignancies. Signs and symptoms often have a gradual onset and may be masked by physiological changes of pregnancy. In addition, concerns about exposure of fetus to complementary examination might make physicians less prone to proceed with the investigation of those symptoms [14].

Most patients complain of facial, neck, or arm swelling, dyspnea, orthopnea, cough, and dilated veins [52]. Other symptoms include chest pain, dysphagia, hoarseness, headache, confusion, dizziness, night sweats, hypoxia, hypernatremia, and syncope [59]. Stridor, confusion, and obtundation may indicate laryngeal edema or cerebral edema, which are rare but life-threatening conditions that require immediate intervention [65, 76].

The severity of symptoms will depend on the rapidity and location of the obstruction. A rapidly developing obstruction and/or obstruction below the insertion of the azygos vein tends to have more severe symptoms due to lack of collateral veins [58, 59, 71]. In the other hand, when the obstruction occurs relatively slow and/or above the azygos insertion, patients may present asymptomatic or with mild symptoms.

Physical examination findings include facial and neck edema, distended neck, and chest veins. Extremity edema, plethora, alteration in mental status, and papilledema can also be present. Facial swelling and plethora are exacerbated when the patient is supine.

Diagnosis

Diagnosis is made by history and physical examination and is confirmed by imaging studies. SVC syndrome must be considered in any patient with previous history of cancer, particularly lung cancer and non-Hodgkin lymphoma, or with previous intravascular procedures [71, 77]. Imaging plays a main role in confirming the diagnosis and identifying the underlying cause. Noninvasive modalities, such as computed tomography (CT) and magnetic resonance imaging (MRI), are usually preferred.

In pregnant patients, the physician is challenged with the choice of diagnostic image modality while limiting danger to the fetus as much as possible and still enabling management of the disease similar to that in nonpregnant patients [67, 75]. Therefore, gestational age, the suspected underlying etiology, and the mother's wishes should be taken in account when deciding which diagnostic test and therapy will be used. Another factor to consider is the target field, as the fetal radiation dose increases when the fetus is in the field of view [13] (Table 48.1).

When ionizing radiation is used for imaging, the cumulative uterine dose should be kept as low as reasonably achievable (ALARA) [67]. Ionizing radiation can cause several adverse effects on the fetus, from spontaneous abortion to teratogenesis and carcinogenesis. The higher the radiation dose, the higher the severity of impairment of the fetus, especially if exposures exceed the threshold dose of 100 mGy.

Radiation exposure over 50–100 mGy during the first 2 weeks after conception follows the *all or nothing effect*, resulting in either spontaneous abortion or a completely unaffected embryo [38, 67]. The fetus is most susceptible to teratogenic effects when exposed to radiation over 50–100 mGy during weeks 3–15, when organogenesis and rapid neural development take place [20, 38, 67]. After 16 weeks of gestation, the threshold for teratogenic effects is around 500–700 mGy [20]. After 26 weeks of gestation, teratogenic effects are extremely unlikely at dose levels reached in diagnostic radiology [75]. Exposure lower than 50 mGy has not been associated with an increase in fetal anomalies or pregnancy loss [1].

Carcinogenesis is a stochastic effect of radiation that can occur at any dose during pregnancy, but risk increases at higher doses [41, 60]. Risk is assumed to be higher when exposure occurs early in the gestation. Despite this, incidence rate of carcinogenesis is still considered low for childhood cancer [75].

Iodinated contrast is recommended if the expected information could affect treatment and if it is unjustifiable to delay the study after delivery [2]. If intravenous iodinated, water-soluble contrast agents are use during pregnancy, newborns should be routinely evaluated for hypothyroidism during the first week of life [2, 32].

Chest Radiography

Fetal radiation exposure with this modality is generally negligible and can be used safely during pregnancy [67]. Around 84% of the patients will have an abnormal

Table 48.1 Fetal radiation doses associated with common radiologic examinations [69]

Type of examination	Fetal dose[a] (mGy)
Very low-dose examinations (<0.1 mGy)	
Us	0
MRI	0
Cervical spine radiography (anteroposterior and lateral views)	<0.001
Radiography of any extremity	<0.001
Mammography (two views)	0.001–0.01
Chest radiography (two views)	0.0005–0.01
Low- to moderate-dose examinations (0.1–10 mGy)	
Radiography	
Abdominal radiography	0.1–3.0
Lumbar spine radiography	1.0–10
Intravenous pyelography	5–10
Double-contrast barium enema	1.0–20
Computed tomography	
Head or neck CT	1.0–10
Chest CT or CT pulmonary angiography	0.01–0.66
Limited CT pelvimetry (single axial section through femoral heads)	<1
Nuclear medicine	
Low-dose perfusion scintigraphy	0.1–0.5
Technetium-99 m bone scintigraphy	4–5
Pulmonary digital subtraction angiography	0.5
Higher-dose examinations (10–50 mGy)	
Abdominal CT	1.3–3.5
Pelvic CT	10–50
^{18}F PET/CT whole-body scintigraphy	10–50

Note - Annual average background radiation = 1.1–2.5 mGy
Abbreviations: US ultrasonography, *MRI* magnetic resonance imaging, *CT* computed tomography, *PET* positron emission tomography, *18F-FDG* 2-[fluorine-18]fluoro-2-deoxy-d-glucose
[a]*Fetal exposure varies with gestational age, maternal body habitus, and exact acquisition parameters*

chest radiograph, being mediastinal widening (64%) and pleural effusion (26%) the most common findings [44]. However, these findings are not diagnostic, and further imaging studies must be performed.

Chest CT Scan

CT scan can be used during pregnancy as long as it does not directly involve the fetus.

Chest CT with intravenous (IV) contrast is the most useful imaging study [57]. It is preferred over other imaging modalities, such as MRI, because of its availability, cost, and short acquisition time. In addition, CT scan provides the diagnosis of SVC syndrome, defines the level and extent of the blockage, allows evaluation of collateral pathways, gives information about the underlying cause, and can determine whether there is external compression, thrombus, or both. If caused by a malignancy, CT scan also provides diagnostic and staging information about the underlying malignancy. CT may also reveal the presence of collateral vessels, which has a sensitivity and specificity for SVC syndrome of 96% and 92%, respectively [29].

Venography

It is considered the gold standard for diagnosing thrombotic obstructions within the SVC and demonstrating the extent of the thrombus [48, 70] but is not useful for determining causes of SVC syndrome other than thrombus. Nowadays, it is primarily used if an interventional stent is planned.

Ultrasonography

Ultrasound is a safe imaging modality during pregnancy but should only be performed when indicated [3]. It can determine the presence and extent of thrombus and site of obstruction. But due to the interposition of the underlying ribs, ultrasound cannot be used to directly imaged SVC.

Magnetic Resonance Imaging (MRI)

Aside from CT scan, it can be used for initial evaluation of SVC syndrome and may be useful in patients allergic to IV contrast or with renal failure [68]. MRI should be preferred over ionizing radiation, whenever possible [67]. It can be used regardless of the gestational age [1]. It has a sensitivity and specificity of 100%; however, it is less available than other imaging studies, is more expensive, and has longer acquisition time.

In suspected malignant SVC syndrome, a complete diagnostic workup for the suspected cancer may be appropriate. Accurate imaging and histologic diagnosis should be obtained, since treatment approaches depend on histology and staging of the malignancy. If possible, treatment approach should be directed toward definitive treatment rather than palliation of symptoms.

In the absence of respiratory compromise or neurologic deterioration, initiation of therapy before obtaining a diagnosis is not recommended [71]. Interventions such as radiation, chemotherapy, and steroids may obscure a histologic diagnosis [36]. Therefore, an accurate diagnosis and biopsy should precede therapeutic interventions in most cases [76].

A thorough physical examination must be performed in search of easily accessible sites for tissue biopsy before proceeding to more invasive procedures, as they carry a greater risk of complications, predominantly bleeding and infections [71]. Minimally invasive procedures such as sputum cytology, pleural fluid cytology, and superficial lymph node biopsy can diagnose up to two-thirds of malignancies [63]. The remaining one-third may require more invasive techniques such as bronchoscopy, mediastinoscopy, and thoracoscopy. Bone marrow biopsy may provide diagnosis and stage of certain malignancies, for example, lymphomas. Benefits of biopsy for diagnostic purposes during pregnancy often overcome the risks and should not be withheld [7]. If a mediastinal infection or large vessel vasculitis is suspected, cultures and serum inflammatory markers are indicated [12].

Treatment

Management of SVC syndrome during pregnancy is determined by the gestational age, clinical condition of the patient, and the underlying etiology. These factors must be considered especially when therapeutic modalities that may affect the course of the gestation are used.

Treatment goals are symptomatic, by relieving the obstruction and, if possible, treatment of the underlying cause. In the past, it was considered a medical emergency, and almost every patient received emergent radiation or chemotherapy. Nowadays, it is not considered a major life threat in most cases, unless there is evidence of respiratory and/or neurologic compromise, which can be associated with possible fatal outcomes.

Life-threatening SVC syndrome may require prompt intervention. Treatment of the underlying cause may be indicated. Empiric therapy with stenting, radiation, and/or chemotherapy may be required, even in the absence of a histologic diagnosis. If stenting is feasible, RT is not recommended as first-line treatment, as stenting provides faster symptom relief [42].

Patients with signs and symptoms suggestive of severe airway compromise or CT findings of laryngeal edema or tracheal obstruction may require prompt interventions to protect the airway, such as endotracheal intubation.

Management of cerebral edema in the setting of SVC syndrome does not differ from the management in general population. It includes head elevation and use of osmotic diuretics, such as mannitol. Cerebral images should be obtained in order to rule out other intracranial causes of cerebral edema.

In oncologic patients, it is important to consider other cancer-related symptoms that may be more life-threatening than SVC syndrome and may need to be addressed urgently. These conditions include extrinsic compression of the major airway by the tumor, hemoptysis, or thrombosis [71].

No standardized grading system exists for evaluation of SVC syndrome. Yale University proposed a classification system for grading the severity of malignant SVC obstruction from asymptomatic (grade 0) to fatal (grade 5) [76] (Table 48.2).

The system has not been validated but provides a framework on how to approach these patients and assist in determining the urgency of intervention.

The Kishi score is another grading system developed to assist in making the decision to initiate stent therapy [30] (Table 48.3). It takes into account clinical signs including neurologic signs, laryngeal signs, facial signs, and vein dilation. A Kishi score of 4 or higher indicates a need for percutaneous stenting.

Once life-threatening conditions have been ruled out, management of SVC syndrome will vary depending on the etiology. When caused by an infectious disease, antibiotics are considered first-line treatment. Thrombolysis and

Table 48.2 Yale University proposed grading system and management for malignant superior vena cava syndrome

Grade	Category	Definition[a]	Management
0	Asymptomatic	Radiographic superior vena cava obstruction in the absence of symptoms	Perform diagnostic and staging procedures to define the tumor type and stage Develop a stage and tumor specific treatment plan
1	Mild	Edema in the head or neck (vascular distention), cyanosis, plethora	
2	Moderate	Edema in the head or neck with functional impairment (mild dysphagia, cough, mild or moderate impairment of head, jaw or eyelid movements, visual disturbances caused by ocular edema)	
3	Severe	Mild or moderate cerebral edema (headache, dizziness) or mild/moderate laryngeal edema or diminished cardiac reserve (syncope after bending)	
4	Life-threatening	Significant cerebral edema (confusion, obtundation) or significant laryngeal edema (stridor) or significant hemodynamic compromise (syncope without precipitating factors, hypotension, renal insufficiency)	Immediate intervention Urgent relief of the SVC obstruction
5	Fatal	Death	

Adapted from Yu et al. [76]

[a]*Each sign or symptom must be thought due to superior vena cava obstruction and the effects of cerebral or laryngeal edema or effects on cardiac function. Symptoms caused by other factors (e.g., vocal cord paralysis, compromise of the tracheobronchial tree, or heart as a result of mass effect) should not be considered as they are due to mass effect on other organs and not superior vena cava obstruction*

Table 48.3 Kishi score [30]

Clinical signs	Weighting
Neurological signs	
Awareness disorders, coma	4
Visual disorders, headache, vertigo, memory disorders	3
Mental disorders	2
Malaise	1
Thoracic/pharyngeal-laryngeal signs	
Orthopnea, laryngeal edema	3
Stridor, dysphagia, dyspnea	2
Coughing, pleurisy	1
Facial signs	
Lip edema, nasal obstruction, epistaxis	2
Facial edema	1
Vessel dilation (neck, face, arms)	1

Table 48.4 Advantages and disadvantages of radiation therapy, stent insertion, and chemotherapy [71]

	Advantages	Disadvantages
Radiation	Noninvasive intervention Treats underlying malignancy	Symptom relief in 7–15 days May compromise a tissue diagnosis if not yet obtained May initially worsen symptoms due to inflammation
Stent insertion	Rapid relief of symptoms usually within 24–72 h Does not compromise a tissue diagnosis Allows option for further treatment with chemotherapy, radiation, or combined-modality therapy	Invasive intervention Bleeding complications Increased risk of thrombosis due to foreign object Does not treat the underlying malignancy
Chemotherapy	Noninvasive intervention Treats underlying malignancy Does not require specialized equipment Ability to be administered in the ICU	Symptom relief in 7–15 days May compromise a tissue diagnosis if not yet obtained Patient may be too sick to tolerate chemotherapy Hematologic and other toxicity

The interventions are supported by level of evidence B; there is no level A evidence specific to the management of SVCS
Abbreviation: ICU intensive care unit

anticoagulation therapy is the mainstay in thrombus-driven SVC syndrome, being more effective if started within 5 days of thrombus development [12, 59]. Balloon angioplasty is preferred for stenosis, usually followed by stenting. Management of SVC syndrome associated to malignancy will depend on the histology of the cancer, the extent of the disease, the severity of symptoms, and the prognosis of the patient [76].

Treatment options include supportive measures, radiotherapy (RT), chemotherapy, ET, and surgical interventions. Favoring one treatment modality over the other will depend mostly on availability and clinical reasons (Table 48.4).

Supportive Measures

Although they have no effect on the underlying etiology, supportive care and medical management can be performed with minimal risk and may provide symptoms relief in the short term. These measures include oxygen support and attempts to reduce hydrostatic pressure, such as head elevation, limitation of fluid intake, and use of diuretics [71].

Steroids can be temporarily used to alleviate symptoms, especially in a patient in whom airway edema is believed to contribute to symptoms [27], but there is no data supporting the effectiveness and dose of steroids in this setting. Steroids can obscure histologic diagnosis [55], and long-term use can produce facial swelling and fluid retention that can contribute to symptoms of SVC syndrome [71]. Steroids may be also used as prophylaxis against radiation-induced edema [61], but they must not be considered a first-line treatment for SVC syndrome. Steroids and diuretics have almost no role in treatment of benign SVC syndrome [73].

Although thrombosis can contribute to SVC syndrome symptoms and may represent a major life threat, there is no evidence that support routine anticoagulation, unless the patient has a demonstrable thrombus on imaging [71]. When SVC syndrome is due to thrombus formation, catheter-based thrombolysis followed by anticoagulation is often used [72]; however, short- and long-term benefits of anticoagulation are still unproven [42, 70].

Radiotherapy

RT dose of radiation is usually in the range of 40–70 Gy, which is much higher than the dose utilized for diagnostic procedures [22]. For this reason, RT is not recommended during pregnancy and should be postponed until after childbirth whenever possible [46]. However, some areas such as the head, neck, and thorax could be irradiated with minimal radiation to the fetus; therefore, RT to those areas could be considered in selected patients.

RT is effective in the treatment of SVC syndrome due to malignancy, especially in radiosensitive tumors, such as lymphomas and SCLC. However, in most cases it should be delayed until a histologic diagnosis is obtained [6]. The rapidity of response ranges from 7 to 15 days but may be as early as 72 h after initiating RT [71] (Table 48.4). Clinical and objective response rates tend to be discordant, usually observing a higher clinical response rate [5]. This discrepancy might be explained by the decrease of tumor bulk after RT, which results in an increased capacity for collateral circulation rather than a complete relief of SVC obstruction [74].

Radiation treatment varies based on histology and the intent of treatment [71]. Radiosensitive tumors may require lower radiation levels and a shorter course of treatment in comparison to radioresistant tumors. When definitive treatment is intended, it may be administered for at least 3 weeks with smaller fractions of radiation. In the other hand, when palliative treatment is intended, the course of RT may be shorter (1 to 2 weeks) but with larger fractions of radiation with the goal of achieving a faster response. Currently, there is no evidence comparing which RT fractionations scheme is more effective; thus, decisions regarding doses and frequency of radiation may be based on clinical expertise [59].

Relative contraindications for RT include previous treatment with radiation in the same region, certain connective tissue diseases, and known radioresistant tumors [71]. Assessment of the patient is needed during RT to monitor for side effects and to identify patients that may need alternative interventions. Failure of treatment may be due to persisting tumor mass or SVC thrombosis.

Chemotherapy

Chemotherapy is reserved for SVC syndromes caused by malignancies. It is a non-invasive therapy that does not require specialized equipment and can treat the underlying malignancy but can compromise histopathology diagnosis and might not be tolerated in critical patients.

Chemotherapeutic agents can cross the placenta, and security data is limited due to the rarity of association between cancer and pregnancy [33]. They also differ in their teratogenicity, where drugs as methotrexate, cyclophosphamide, and cytarabine are associated to higher teratogenic potential [40].

Administration of chemotherapy during pregnancy can induce harmful effects on the fetus and newborn, such as malformations, mutations, carcinogenesis, and retarded development. While in the mother, it can induce spontaneous abortion and infertility. As with ionizing radiation, weeks of gestation, the clinical condition of the patient, and the underlying malignancy should be considered before initiating chemotherapy. During the first 2 weeks of gestation, it follows the *all or nothing effect*. During weeks 2 to 15, organogenesis and neural development take place; therefore, exposure during this period is more likely to cause malformations [22]. Exposure during the second and third trimester of pregnancy could result in intrauterine growth restriction, low birth weight, and preterm labor [33]. Data has shown a high incidence of major malformations in exposition during the first trimester, while during the second and third trimester the incidence was similar to that in the general population [40]. Knowing this, chemotherapy should be avoided during the first trimester, unless there exists an urgent need to start treatment. Although it is considered relatively safe during the second and third trimester, obstetrical and neonatal complications may occur more frequently in patients receiving chemotherapy during this period [33, 40].

Chemotherapy is often used as initial therapy in chemosensitive tumors such as lymphomas, SCLC, and germ cell tumors [61]. The response rate of SVC syndrome treated with chemotherapy is similar to response rates of RT, with a range of 7–15 days [55] (Table 48.4). A meta-analysis demonstrated that chemotherapy alone, radiotherapy alone, and chemoradiotherapy provided similar rates of symptoms relief in SCLC patients [55]. Therefore, RT can be used in chemosensitive tumors as well but yields poorer long-term results and hence is reserved mainly for patients who are not candidate for chemotherapy.

Once symptomatic benefit is obtained, the patient may be candidate for curative treatment, which could include the addition of RT or other treatment modalities to systemic chemotherapy, as this can decrease local recurrence rates and improve survival [71].

Endovascular Therapy

ET can include stenting, percutaneous transluminal angioplasty, and intravascular thrombolysis [51]. SVC angioplasty and stenting can be performed in any setting, as long as the patient can tolerate supine or semi-supine position.

ET benefits include a rapid relief of symptoms, it does not compromise histopathology diagnosis, and it allows future treatment with RT or chemotherapy, but it does not treat the underlying malignancy and is an invasive procedure with risk of short- and long-term complications [15] (Table 48.4). It has shown higher and faster symptom relief rates and lower recurrence rates compared to chemotherapy and RT [55].

There is increasing evidence that endovascular therapy may be the best treatment for SVC syndrome of benign origin [10, 53]. It is less invasive and has lower morbidity compared to surgical reconstruction with equal efficacy and patency in the short and midterm. However, stenting is associated with a higher need for secondary interventions over the mid- and long term [53].

In SVC syndrome associated to malignancy, stents can be used to relieve symptoms, while the histologic diagnosis is being perused in patients who have been previously treated with RT or in those with known chemotherapy- and radiation-resistant tumors. Stents do not treat the underlying malignancy; thereby in most cases, stent placement is followed by other interventions. Modern treatment usually involves prompt stent placement followed by tissue biopsy and subsequent RT and/or chemotherapy.

Endovascular stenting can provide a rapid and effective relief of symptoms, with up to 97–99% of patients experiencing rapid symptom relief [59]. Relief can be immediate, but in most cases, it is reported within 24–72 h after the procedure [71].

Complications of stent placement are infrequent with an overall major complication rate of 4% and mortality rate of 2% [72]. Most common complications are restenosis and intra-stent thrombosis. Therefore, in most patients, anticoagulation may be continued after endovascular interventions, and antiplatelet therapy may be started for indefinite time [56, 64]. Other minor complications include groin hematoma and local infections at the puncture site. Unusual major complications include stent migration, bleeding, cardiac injury, pulmonary embolism, and pericardial tamponade [51].

Surgery

In the past, surgery was considered the only invasive procedure for SVC syndrome treatment and the mainstay of treatment when caused by benign etiologies [53].

Surgical procedures and the use of anesthetic drugs are considered safe during pregnancy [47, 66]. Although complications are rare, it carries some risks such as miscarriage, low birth weight, and prematurity.

Patients with benign SVC syndrome are younger, with longer life expectancy, thus needing a durable reconstruction. Open surgery repair of these patients has been performed with low morbidity and mortality and excellent long-term results [16, 26]. Despite shift toward primary endovascular therapy in patients with benign SVC syndrome, surgery remains a viable option in selected patients, especially in patients with failed endovascular therapy or whose occlusions cannot be recanalized [12, 53].

In oncologic patients, surgery is almost never an option, as SVC syndrome is usually caused by an unresectable tumor within the mediastinum, but it may have a role after induction treatment in selected patients.

Outcome and Prognosis

The presence of SVC syndrome does not directly affect overall survival. Overall survival is determined by the underlying cause, even during pregnancy. However, median life expectancy of patients with SVC syndrome due to malignancy ranges from 1.5 to 9.5 months. Nonetheless, this range can vary widely depending on the tumor type and stage [55, 76].

SVC syndrome relapse rates are relatively low after treatment with chemotherapy, RT, or stent placement [55]. If stent fails, recanalization is possible, resulting in long-term success rates greater than 90% [59].

In conclusion, diagnosis and treatment of SVC syndrome can be performed with minimal risk for the fetus if risks and benefits of diagnostic and therapeutic procedures are taken in account and if the clinical condition of the mother allows it.

Bibliography

1. ACOG Committee on Obstetric Practice. ACOG Committee Opinion. Number 723, October 2017 (replaces No. 656, February 2016). Guidelines for diagnostic imaging during pregnancy and lactation. Obstet Gynecol. 2017;130:210–6.
2. ACR Committee on Drugs and Contrast Media. ACR Manual on Contrast Media: Version 10.3; 2019.
3. AIUM–ACR–ACOG–SMFM–SRU Practice Parameter for the Performance of Standard Diagnostic Obstetric Ultrasound Examinations. J Ultrasound Med. 2018;9999:1–12.
4. Aghaji MAC, Nnabuko REE. Life threatening superior vena caval obstruction complicating pregnancy. J Obstet Gynecol. 1988;9:113–5.
5. Ahmann FR. A reassessment of the clinical implications of the superior vena cava syndrome. J Clin Oncol. 1984;2(8):961–9.
6. Ampil F, Caldito G, Previgliano C. Palliative radiotherapy for superior vena caval obstruction by lung cancer: a major issue about tim- ing and a minor issue about efficacy. Ann Thorac Med. 2012;7:170–1.
7. Andersson TM, Johansson AL, Fredriksson I, Lambe M. Cancer during pregnancy and the postpartum period: a population-based study. Cancer. 2015;121(12):2072–7.
8. Armstrong BA, Perez CA, Simpson JR, et al. Role of irradiation in the management of superior vena cava syndrome. Int J Radiat Oncol Biol Phys. 1987;4:531–9.
9. Barakat K, Robinson NM, Spurrell RA. Transvenous pacing lead-induced thrombosis: a series of cases with a review of the literature. Cardiology. 2000;93:142–8.
10. Breault S, Doenz F, Jouannic AM, et al. Percutaneous endovascular management of chronic superior vena cava syndrome of benign causes: long term follow-up. Eur Radiol. 2017;1:97–104.
11. Charnsangavej C, Carrasco CH, Wallace S, et al. Stenosis of the vena cava: preliminary assessment of treatment with expandable metallic stents. Radiology. 1986;161:295–8.

12. Cheng S. Superior vena cava syndrome: a contemporary review of a historic disease. Cardiol Rev. 2009;17:16–23.
13. Coakley FV, Cody DD, Mahesh M. The pregnant patient: alternatives to CT and dose-saving modifications to CT technique. Image Wisely Web site. 2010. http://www.imagewisely.org/imaging-modalities/computed-tomography/medical-physicists/articles/the-pregnant-patient. Accessed November 11, 2019.
14. de Haan J, Vandecaveye V, Han SN, Van de Vijver KK, Amant F. Difficulties with diagnosis of malignancies in pregnancy. Best Pract Res Clin Obstet Gynaecol. 2016;33:19–32.
15. del Rio Sola ML, Fuente Garrido R, Gutiérrez Alonso V, Vaquero Puerta C. Endovascular treatment of superior vena cava syndrome caused by malignant disease. J Vasc Surg. 2014;59(6):1705–6.
16. Doty JR, Flores JH, Doty DB. Superior vena cava obstruction: bypass using spiral vein graft. Ann Thorac Surg. 1999;67:1111–6.
17. Ehrlich W, Ballon HC, Graham EA. Superior vena caval obstruction with a consideration of the possible relief of symptoms by mediastinal decompression. J Thorac Surg. 1934;3:352.
18. El-Messidi A, Patenaude V, Abenhaim HA. Incidence and out-comes of women with non-Hodgkin's lymphoma in pregnancy: a population-based study on 7.9 million births. J Obstet Gynaecol Res. 2015;41:582–9.
19. Eren S, Karaman A, Okur A. The superior vena cava syndrome caused by malignant disease: imaging with multi-detector row CT. Eur J Radiol. 2006;59:93–103.
20. Gomes M, Matias A, Macedo F. Risks to the fetus from diagnostic imaging during pregnancy: review and proposal of a clinical protocol. Pediatr Radiol. 2015;45:1916–29.
21. Goudevenos JA, et al. Pacemaker-induced superior vena cava syndrome: report of four cases and review of the literature. Pacing Clin Electrophysiol. 1989;12:890–1895.
22. Hepner A, Negrini D, Hase EA, Exman P, Testa L, Trinconi AF, Filassi JR, Francisco RPV, Zugaib M, O'Connor TL, et al. Cancer during pregnancy: the oncologist overview. World J Oncol. 2019;10(1):28–34.
23. Hunter W. The history of an aneurysm of the aorta, with some remarks on aneurysms in general. London: Med Obs Inq; 1757. p. 323–57.
24. Hussey HH, Katz S, Yater WM. The superior vena caval syndrome; report of thirty-five cases. Am Heart J. 1946;1:1–26.
25. Kale A, Akyildiz L, Akdeniz N, Kale E. Pregnancy complicated by superior vena cava thrombosis and pulmonary embolism in a patient with Behcet disease and the use of heparin for treatment. Saudi Med J. 2006;27:95–7.
26. Kalra M, Gloviczki P, Andrews JC, Cherry KJ Jr, Bower TC, Panneton JM, et al. Open surgical and endovascular treatment of superior vena cava syndrome caused by nonmalignant disease. J Vasc Surg. 2003;38:215–23.
27. Kaplan AP, Greaves MW. Angioedema. J Am Acad Dermatol. 2005;53(3):373–88.
28. Kee ST, Kinoshita L, Razavi MK, et al. Superior vena cava syndrome: treatment with catheter-directed thrombolysis and endovascular stent placement. Radiology. 1998;206:187–93.
29. Kim HJ, Kim HS, Chung SH. CT diagnosis of superior vena cava syndrome: importance of collateral vessels. AJR Am J Roentgenol. 1993;161(3):539–42.
30. Kishi K, Sonomura T, Mitsuzane K, et al. Self-expandable metallic stent therapy for superior vena cava syndrome: clinical observations. Radiology. 1993;189:531–5.
31. Kitamura J, Murakami Y, Shimada T, et al. Morphological observation by intravascular ultrasound in superior vena cava syndrome after pacemaker implantation. Catheter Cardiovasc Diagn. 1996;37:83–5.
32. Kochi MH, Kaloudis EV, Ahmed W, et al. Effect of in utero exposure of iodinated intravenous contrast on neonatal thyroid function. J Comput Assist Tomogr. 2012;36:165–9.
33. Koren G, Carey N, Gagnon R, Maxwell C, Nulman I, Senikas V. Cancer chemotherapy and pregnancy. J Obstet Gynaecol Can. 2013;35(3):263–78.
34. Korkeila P, Nyman K, Ylitalo A, Koistinen J, Karjalainen P, Lund J, et al. Venous obstruction after pacemaker implantation. Pacing Clin Electrophysiol. 2007;30:199–206.

35. Lacout A, Marcy PY, Thariat J, Lacombe P, El Hajjam M. Radioanatomy of the superior vena cava syndrome and therapeutic orientations. Diagn Interv Imaging. 2012;93:569–77.
36. Loeffler JS, Leopold KA, Recht A, et al. Emergency prebiopsy radiation for mediastinal masses: impact on subsequent pathologic diagnosis and outcome. J Clin Oncol. 1986;4(5):716–21.
37. Mackie GC, Thomas A, Greenspan B, et al. Focal hepatic activity during ventilation-perfusion scintigraphy due to systemic-portal shunt due to superior vena cava obstruction from histoplasmosis induced fibrosing mediastinitis. Clin Nucl Med. 2007;32:707–10.
38. McCollough CH, Schueler BA, Atwell TD, et al. Radiation exposure and pregnancy: when should we be concerned? Radiographics. 2007;27:909–17.
39. Mitrou S, Petrakis D, Fotopulos G, Zarkavelis G, Pavlidis N. Lung cancer during pregnancy: a narrative review. J Adv Res. 2016;7:571–4.
40. National Toxicology P. NTP Monograph: Developmental Effects and Pregnancy Outcomes Associated With Cancer Chemotherapy Use During Pregnancy. NTP Monogr ;i-214; 2013.
41. Nguyen CP, Goodman LH. Fetal risk in diagnostic radiology. Semin Ultrasound CTMR. 2012;33:4–10.
42. Nicholson AA, Ettles DF, Arnold A, Greenstone M, Dyet JF. Treatment of malignant superior vena cava obstruction: metal stents or radiation therapy. J Vasc Interv Radiol. 1997;8:781–8.
43. Nieto AF, Doty DB. Superior vena cava obstruction: clinical syndrome, etiology and treatment. Curr Probl Cancer. 1986;10(9):441–84.
44. Parish JM, Marschke RF Jr, Dines DE, et al. Etiologic considerations in superior vena cava syndrome. Mayo Clin Proc. 1981;56(7):407–13.
45. Pavlidis AN. Coexistence of pregnancy and malignancies. Oncologist. 2002;7:279–87.
46. Peccatori FA, Azim HA Jr, Orecchia R, Hoekstra HJ, Pavlidis N, Kesic V, Pentheroudakis G, et al. Cancer, pregnancy and fertility: ESMO Clinical Practice Guidelines for diagnosis, treatment and follow-up. Ann Oncol. 2013;24(Suppl 6):vi160–70.
47. Petraglia F, Luisi S, Benedetto C, Zonca M, Florio P, Casarosa E, Volpe A, et al. Changes of dimeric inhibin B levels in maternal serum throughout healthy gestation and in women with gestational diseases. J Clin Endocrinol Metab. 1997;82(9):2991–5.
48. Podoloff DA, Kim EE. Evaluation of sensitivity and specificity of upper extremity radionuclide venography in cancer patients with indwelling central venous catheters. Clin Nucl Med. 1992;17(6):457–62.
49. Presswala RG, Hiranandani NL. Pleural effusion and superior vena cava canal syndrome in Hodgkin's disease. J Indian Med Assoc. 1965;45(9):502–3.
50. Raad I. Intravascular-catheter-related infections. Lancet. 1998;351:893–8.
51. Rachapalli V, Boucher LM. Superior vena cava syndrome: role of the interventionalist. Can Assoc Radiol J. 2014;65(2):168–76.
52. Rice TW, Rodriguez RM, Light RW. The superior vena cava syndrome: clinical characteristics and evolving etiology. Medicine (Baltimore). 2006;85(1):37–42.
53. Rizvi AZ, Kalra M, Bjarnason H, Bower TC, Schleck C, Gloviczki P. Benign superior vena cava syndrome: stenting is now the first line of treatment. J Vasc Surg. 2008;47:372–80.
54. Rosamond W, Flegal K, Friday G, Furie K, Go A, Greenlund K, et al. Heart disease and stroke statistics—2007 update: a report from the American Heart Association Statistics Committee and Stroke Statistics Subcommittee. Circulation. 2007;115:e69–171.
55. Rowell NP, Gleeson FV. Steroids, radiotherapy, chemotherapy and stents for superior vena caval obstruction in carcinoma of the bronchus: a systematic review. Clin Oncol (R Coll Radiol). 2002;14(5):338–51.
56. Schifferdecker B, Shaw JA, Piemonte TC, et al. Nonmalignant superior vena cava syndrome: pathophysiology and management. Catheter Cardiovasc Interv. 2005;65:416–23.
57. Schwartz EE, Goodman LR, Haskin ME. Role of CTscanning in the superior vena cava syndrome. Am J Clin Oncol. 1986;9(1):71–8.
58. Stanford W, Jolles H, Ell S, Chiu LC. Superior vena cava obstruction: a venographic classification. AJR Am J Roentgenol. 1987;148:259–62.
59. Straka C, Ying J, Kong F-M, Willey CD, Kaminski J, Kim DWN. Review of evolving etiologies,implications and treatment strategies for the superior vena cava syndrome. Springerplus. 2016;5:229.

60. Streffer C, Shore R, Konermann G, Meadows A, Uma Devi P, Preston Withers J, Holm LE. ICRP publication 90 – biological effects after prenatal irradiation (embryo and fetus). Ann ICRP (International Commission on Radiological Protection). 2003;33:205–6.
61. Ostler PJ, Clark DP, Watkinson AF, et al. Superior vena cava obstruction: a modern management strategy. Clin Oncol (R Coll Radiol). 1997;9:83–9.
62. Schechter MM. The superior vena cava syndrome. Am J Med Sci. 1954;227:46–56.
63. Schraufnagel DE, Hill R, Leech JA, Pare JA. Superior vena caval obstruction. Is it a medical emergency? Am J Med. 1981;70:1169–74.
64. Sheikh MA, Fernandez BB Jr, Gray BH, et al. Endovascular stenting of nonmalignant superior vena cava syndrome. Catheter Cardiovasc Interv. 2005;65:405–11.
65. Talapatra K, Panda S, Goyle S, et al. Superior vena cava syndrome: a radiation oncologist's perspective. J Cancer Res Ther. 2016;12:515–9.
66. Talwar P, Kondareddy T, Shree P. LDH as prognostic marker in hypertensive pregnancy. Int J Reprod Contracept Obstet Gynecol. 2017;6(6):2444–6.
67. Tirada N, Dreizin D, Khati NJ, et al. Imaging pregnant and lactating patients. Radiographics. 2015;35:1751–65.
68. Thornton MJ, Ryan R, Varghese JC, et al. A three-dimensional gadolinium enhanced MR venography technique for imaging central veins. Am J Roentgenol. 1999;173:999–1003.
69. Tremblay E, Thérasse E, Thomassin-Naggara I, Trop I. Quality initiatives: guidelines for use of medical imaging during pregnancy and lactation. Radiographics. 2012;32:897–911.
70. Uberoi R. Quality assurance guidelines for superior vena cava stenting in malignant disease. Cardiovasc Intervent Radiol. 2006;29:319–22.
71. Wan JF, Bezjak A. Superior vena cava syndrome. Emerg Med Clin North Am. 2009;27:243–55.
72. Warner P, Uberoi R. Superior vena cava stenting in the 21st century. Postgrad Med J. 2013;89:224–30.
73. Watkinson AF, Yeow TN, Fraser C. Endovascular stenting to treat obstruction of the superior vena cava. BMJ. 2008;336:1434–7.
74. Wilson LD, Detterbeck FC, Yahalom J. Superior Vena Cava Syndrome with malignant causes. N Engl J Med. 2007;356:1862–69.
75. Woitek R, Prayer D, Hojreh A, Helbich T. Radiological staging in pregnant patients with cancer. ESMO Open. 2016;1:e000017.
76. Yu JB, Wilson LD, Detterbeck FC. Superior vena cava syndrome–a proposed classification system and algorithm for management. J Thorac Oncol. 2008;3(8):811–4.
77. Zimmerman S, Davis M. Rapid fire: superior vena cava syndrome. Emerg Med Clin North Am. 2018;36:577–84.

Index

C. Montufar et al. (eds.), *Obstetric Catastrophes*,
https://doi.org/10.1007/978-3-030-70034-8

D

GPSR Compliance

The European Union's (EU) General Product Safety Regulation (GPSR) is a set of rules that requires consumer products to be safe and our obligations to ensure this.

If you have any concerns about our products, you can contact us on ProductSafety@springernature.com

In case Publisher is established outside the EU, the EU authorized representative is:

Springer Nature Customer Service Center GmbH
Europaplatz 3
69115 Heidelberg, Germany

Batch number: 10732064

Printed by Printforce, the Netherlands